Glial ⇔ Neuronal Signaling

Glial ⇔ Neuronal Signaling

Edited by

Glenn I. Hatton and Vladimir Parpura

Department of Cell Biology and Neuroscience
University of California
Riverside, CA 92521 USA

KLUWER ACADEMIC PUBLISHERS
Boston / Dordrecht / London

Distributors for North, Central and South America:
Kluwer Academic Publishers
101 Philip Drive
Assinippi Park
Norwell, Massachusetts 02061 USA
Telephone (781) 871-6600
Fax (781) 681-9045
E-Mail: kluwer@wkap.com

Distributors for all other countries:
Kluwer Academic Publishers Group
Post Office Box 322
3300 AH Dordrecht, THE NETHERLANDS
Telephone 31 786 576 000
Fax 31 786 576 254
E-Mail: services@wkap.nl

 Electronic Services <http://www.wkap.nl>

Library of Congress Cataloging-in-Publication Data

A C.I.P. Catalogue record for this book is available
from the Library of Congress.

Glia Neuronal Signaling edited by Glenn I. Hatton and Vladimir Parpura
ISBN 1-4020-7936-2
e-ISBN 1-4020-7937-0

Permission for books published in Europe: permissions@wkap.nl
Permissions for books published in the United States of America: permissions@wkap.com

Printed on acid-free paper.

Printed in the United States of America.

The Publisher offers discounts on this book for course use and bulk purchases.
For further information, send email to <joseph.burns@wkap.com> .

To Our Wives

Contents

* contains electronic files of all figures, including color, tables and movies

List of contributors

Gregory Arcuino
Center for Aging and Developmental
Biology, University of Rochester
School of Medicine
Rochester, NY 14642 USA

Dwight E. Bergles
Department of Neuroscience, Johns
Hopkins University School of
Medicine, 725 N. Wolfe St., WBSB
813, Baltimore, MD 21205 USA

Angus M Brown
MRC Applied Neuroscience Group
Biomedical Sciences, University of
Nottingham Queens Medical Center
Nottingham, UK

Marisa Cotrina
Center for Aging and Developmental
Biology, University of Rochester
School of Medicine
Rochester, NY 14642 USA

Amin Derouiche
Anatomical Institute,
Cologne University, Germany

Joachim W. Deitmer
Abteilung für Allgemeine Zoologie
FB Biologie, Universität
Kaiserslautern, P.B. 3049, D-67653
Kaiserslautern, Germany

Daniel S. Evanko
Department of Neuroscience
University of Pennsylvania
School of Medicine
Philadelphia, PA 19104 USA

Angela Giangrande
Institut de Génétique et Biologie
Moléculaire et Cellulaire
IGBMC/CNRS/ULP/INSERM - BP
10142, 67404 Illkirch
c.u. de Strasbourg, France

Christian Giaume
INSERM U114, Collège de France
11 Place Marcelin Berthelot
75005 Paris, France

Jens Grosche
Paul Flechsig Institute for Brain
Research, Leipzig University
Leipzig, Germany

Menachem Hanani
Laboratory of Experimental Surgery
Hadassah University Hospital
Jerusalem, Israel

Glenn I. Hatton
Department of Cell Biology and
Neuroscience, University of
California, Riverside, CA 92521 USA

Philip G. Haydon
Department of Neuroscience
University of Pennsylvania
School of Medicine
Philadelphia, PA 19104 USA

Helmut Kettenmann
Max-Delbrück Center for Molecular
Medicine, Cellular Neurosciences
Robert-Rössle-Str. 10
13092 Berlin, Germany

Harold K. Kimelberg
Neural and Vascular Biology Theme
Ordway Research Institute
150 New Scotland Ave.
Albany, NY 12208 USA

Annette Koulakoff
INSERM U114, Collège de France
11 Place Marcelin Berthelot
75005 Paris, France

William Même
INSERM U114, Collège de France
11 Place Marcelin Berthelot
75005 Paris, France

Frederic Mercier
Laboratory of Matrix Pathobiology
Biomedical Research Center T408
University of Hawaii, 1993 East-
West Rd, Honolulu, HI 96822 USA

Maiken Nedergaard
Center for Aging and Developmental
Biology, University of Rochester
School of Medicine
Rochester, NY 14642 USA

Kimberly A. Parkerson
Department of Neurobiology and
Civitan International Research Center
University of Alabama
Birmingham, AL 35294 USA

Vladimir Parpura
Department of Cell Biology and
Neuroscience, and Center for
Nanoscale Science and Engineering
University of California
Riverside, CA 92521, USA

Frank W. Pfrieger
Max-Planck/CNRS Group, UPR 2356
Centre de Neurochimie 5, rue Blaise
Pascal, F-67084 Strasbourg, France

Bruce R Ransom
University of Washington School of
Medicine, 1959 NE Pacific Street
Seattle, WA 98195 USA

Andreas Reichenbach
Paul Flechsig Institute for Brain
Research, Leipzig University
Leipzig, Germany

Jeffrey D. Rothstein
Department of Neurology
Johns Hopkins University School of
Medicine, 725 N. Wolfe St., WBSB
813, Baltimore, MD 21205 USA

Carola G. Schipke
Max-Delbrück Center for Molecular
Medicine, Cellular Neurosciences
Robert-Rössle-Str. 10
13092 Berlin, Germany

Gerald Seifert
Experimental Neurobiology,
Neurosurgery, University of Bonn
Sigmund-Freud-Str. 25
53105 Bonn, Germany

Michal Slezak
Max-Planck/CNRS Group, UPR 2356
Centre de Neurochimie 5, rue Blaise
Pascal, F-67084 Strasbourg, France

Harald Sontheimer
Department of Neurobiology and
Civitan International Research Center
University of Alabama
Birmingham, AL 35294 USA

Laurent Soustelle
Institut de Génétique et Biologie
Moléculaire et Cellulaire
IGBMC/CNRS/ULP/INSERM - BP
10142 , 67404 Illkirch
c.u. de Strasbourg, France

Christian Steinhäuser
Experimental Neurobiology,
Neurosurgery, University of Bonn
Sigmund-Freud-Str. 25
53105 Bonn, Germany

Jai-Yoon Sul
Department of Neuroscience
University of Pennsylvania
School of Medicine
Philadelphia, PA 19104 USA

Selva Baltan Tekkök
University of Washington School of
Medicine, 1959 NE Pacific Street
Seattle, WA 98195 USA

Min Zhou
Neural and Vascular Biology Theme
Ordway Research Institute
150 New Scotland Ave.
Albany, NY 12208 USA

Qi Zhang
Department of Neuroscience
University of Pennsylvania
School of Medicine
Philadelphia, PA 19104 USA

Preface

When we think about the brain we usually think about neurons. Although there are 100 billion neurons in mammalian brain, these cells do not constitute a majority. Quite the contrary, glial cells and other non-neuronal cells are 10-50 times more numerous than neurons. Glial cells were long considered to serve merely as the supporting cast and scenery against which the starring neuronal roles would be played out. Relatively recent evidence, however, indicates that glial cells are intimately involved in many of the brain's functions, including its computational power. Besides neglecting more than 90% of brain cells, an additional "sin" that neurobiologists frequently commit is to selectively consider isolated cell types and their (homotypic) functions, to the exclusion of seriously analyzing (heterotypic) interactions between cell types. For example, we pay much attention to neurons and synaptic transmission, but relatively much less attention has been paid to the modulation of that synaptic transmission, an activity rather extensively engaged in by glial cells. One can hardly overstate the importance of this modulation since it provides the exquisite balance, subtlety and smoothness of operation for which nervous systems are held in awe. The intent of this book is to rectify, in some degree, this oversimplified "neuroncentric" view. Rather than merely developing a "gliacentric" directory listing of glial functions *per se*, we are exploring the glial⇔neuronal bi-directional signaling that adds an additional layer of complexity in the brain. We begin with a brief bit of historical background that makes clear the paths that were taken to bring us from the discovery of glia as cells to where we are today. After delineating many of the genes that are involved in bidirectional glial⇔neuronal signaling during and after development, we proceed to structural relationships between glia and neurons. We believe that in order to understand signaling between glial and neuronal cells, one has first to consider their intimate structural associations, and to appreciate the development and plasticity of these associations that has significant functional implications. The next chapters of the book are devoted to the emerging detailed story of glial⇔neuronal signaling. Those chapters discuss glial components (neurotransmitter receptors) necessary to receive signals from neurons, followed by their possible "integration" capabilities. Discussions proceed of ion channels on glia, their transporters for neurotransmitter, pH and potassium ion regulation, metabolic coupling to neurons, and glial excitability based on internal calcium ion changes. Glial signaling "output" using gap junctions and the release of transmitters are also outlined, together with a functional consequence of glial⇔neuron signaling: the formation and maintenance of synapses, as well as the modulation of synaptic transmission.

This book is meant to integrate the emerging body of information that has been accumulating, revealing the interactive nature of the brain's two major neural cell types, neurons and glia, in brain function. Additionally, this book may fill a need for a monograph/textbook that would be used in advanced courses or graduate seminars aimed at exploring glia⇔neuronal interactions.

Glenn Hatton and Vlad Parpura
Riverside, California

Chapter 1

The glial-neuronal interactions and signaling: an introduction

Selva Baltan Tekkök and Bruce R. Ransom*

Department of Neurology
University of Washington School of Medicine
Seattle, Washington, 1959 NE Pacific Street, WA 98195 USA

*Corresponding author: bransom@u.washington.edu

Contents

1.1. Introduction

It is a plausible hypothesis that glial cells participate in every brain transaction, normal and pathological. Even if we restrict ourselves, as we do for this discussion, to a single type of glial cell, astrocytes, the hypothesis remains reasonable based on current information. In fact, the real question is why this proposition would strike anyone working on the nervous system in 2004 as 'extreme'. The reasons have been discussed recently and include pervasive neuron-centric attitudes and the slower pace of glial research compared to neuronal research (Ransom et al., 2003). While glia-philes may be indignant that the truths which we hold self-evident are not universally appreciated, there is a greater concern. Continued skepticism, or ignorance, about the importance of astrocytes in brain functions among our 'unconverted' colleagues will slow scientific progress. This timely volume stakes out the new boundaries of our knowledge regarding astrocyte-neuron interactions. It highlights the emerging reality that neuroscientists, whatever their areas of interest might be, must consider how glial cells fit into the picture. Ignoring this principle puts one at risk of getting the 'story' wrong or, at least, at risk for telling it incompletely.

To set the stage for what follows, this chapter considers astrocyte-neuron interactions generally. There are anatomic and physiological features that facilitate and set limits on how these cell types interact. These are worth stating explicitly in advance of the details. It should be emphasized, of course, that these features not only inform our understanding of established astrocyte-neuron interactions, but they beg the question of what else might be possible. A brief historical review of glial-neuronal interactions is also provided; be forewarned that this is both selective and somewhat personal.

Terminology, like anatomy, may determine destiny. Such has been the case in our field. The very term 'neuroscience' inadvertently, and subliminally, focuses attention on neurons at the expense of glia. Sensitized in this way to the words we use in science, it is appropriate to consider what terms we should employ in referring to brain events in which neurons and glial cells work together. It is probable that multiple terms will be needed and we must define them clearly and use them consistently. Terms are preferred that accurately describe events and that refrain from implying more about the phenomena than is established. We suggest a classification scheme for astrocyte-neuron interactions. It is neither complete, nor will it stand the test of time. It is simply too early in our current knowledge of these phenomena to expect that we can provide a lasting framework for discussing them. But we need a place to start. The classification offered should spur critical thinking about these events and stimulate further exploration.

1.2. Anatomic and physiologic infrastructure for glial-neuronal interactions: form follows function

It is obvious that the anatomic relationship between neurons and astrocytes dictates opportunities for these cells to interact and sets limits on how they might do so. Because neurons and glial cells make no functional synaptic or gap junctional contacts with one another [some rare situations notwithstanding (e.g., Mudrick-Donnon et al., 1993; Alvarez-Maubecin et al., 2000), interactions between the two cell types must occur via the narrow separating extracellular space (ECS) (Nicholson, 1995). The features of this space are interesting and important to bear in mind as we consider the movement of ions and other molecules that mediate the dialogue between neurons and glia.

Astrocytes are often stellate cells with multiple fine processes. Dye injection studies have demonstrated that astrocytes in white matter (called fibrous astrocytes) have fifty to sixty long-branching processes that radiate from the cell body (Butt and Ransom, 1993). Astrocytes in gray matter, called protoplasmic astrocytes, have incredibly profuse vellate processes that give to these cells an appearance that have been referred to as spongiform (Bushong et al., 2002). Processes of neighboring astrocytes make contact and their somas distribute themselves in a non-random, orderly fashion that has been called contact spacing (Chan-Ling and Stone, 1991). In the hippocampus, and probably in other areas of gray matter, each protoplasmic astrocyte seems to occupy a separate anatomic domain, and processes of adjacent astrocytes do not project into neighboring domains (Bushong et al., 2002).

Astrocytes are uniformly distributed throughout the central nervous system (CNS) and virtually every neuron shares common ECS with astrocyte neighbors (Peters et al., 1991). The ubiquitous proximity of astrocytes and neurons is a necessary precondition for cooperativity. Some astrocyte processes seem to enwrap synapses. One study estimated that peri-synaptic processes constituted 70-80% of astrocytic plasma membrane (Wolff, 1970). This anatomic characteristic anticipates the remarkable richness of astrocyte-neuron interactions that take place in the vicinity of synapses (see below). The full extent of anatomic specialization that might lend itself to functional interactions between neurons and glial cells is probably not yet fully appreciated. Recent findings reinforce this suspicion. Bergmann glial cells are a special form of astrocyte in the cerebellum. Portions of Bergmann glial processes form electrically isolated compartments, or microdomains, capable of interacting with adjacent neurons in a manner that is isolated from other parts of the glial cell. In response to glutamate release from immediately adjacent synapses, these microdomains exhibit isolated increases in intracellular calcium ion concentration ($[Ca^{2+}]_i$) (Chapter 12). Astrocytic microdomains might exist elsewhere in the brain but this has not been examined. Another example of an anatomic feature that probably mediates important cell-cell interactions is astrocyte endfeet on nutritive capillaries (Nedergaard et al., 2003; also see Chapter 11).

Many astrocyte processes terminate in specialized endfeet that cover the entire surface of intraparenchymal capillaries. Astrocytic endfeet express glucose transporters (Vannucci et al., 1997), water channels called aquaporins (e.g. aquaporin-4) (Nielsen et al., 1997) and a high density of potassium channels (Newman, 1986). These endfoot specializations make it highly probable that astrocytes play important roles in glucose uptake (Chapter 11) and in water and ion balance in the brain (Nedergaard et al., 2003). Astrocyte endfeet may also be mechanistically involved in the vascular dilatation associated with neural activity (Zonta et al., 2003). These astrocyte mediated homeostatic functions are crucial for the stability of neuron function. Broadly defined, these functions constitute a form of glial-neuronal interaction. Astrocytes, and especially their endfeet, may also have a role in maintaining the integrity of the blood-brain-barrier (Abbott, 2002). Astrocytes release a number of chemical agents that can increase blood-brain-barrier permeability. That they may do this in response to 'signals' generated by neurons is intriguing and entirely feasible, although unproven (Abbott, 2002).

Astrocytes strongly express gap junction proteins called connexins. The majority of astrocytes, but perhaps not all (Sontheimer et al., 1990), are strongly coupled to one another by gap junction channels that mediate the passage of current and molecules having a molecular weight less than 1000. This anatomic feature stabilizes and equalizes membrane potential among groups of astrocytes and ensures common levels of ions (Rose and Ransom, 1997) and presumably other molecules as well. In the context of glial-neuronal interactions, this feature suggests that groups of astrocytes act in a cooperative fashion in their dealings with other cells. While there may be exceptions to this principle, for example the microdomains discussed above, it is a design feature to be kept in mind.

The CNS is composed of a great diversity of neurons. Neurons from different brain regions differ in morphology, ion channels, receptors, etc. The extent of meaningful astrocyte diversity remains a mystery. Examples of regional astrocyte differences in ion channel and transmitter receptor expression are known (Prochiantz and Mallat, 1988; Steinhauser et al., 1992; Lee et al., 1994; but see Bordey and Sontheimer, 2000), increasing the likelihood of functionally unique sub-populations of these cells. This issue is raised because it has implications for studying how neurons and glial cells interact. Obviously, the challenge of understanding these interactions will be compounded if astrocyte characteristics differ greatly from one brain region to the next (Ransom, 1991).

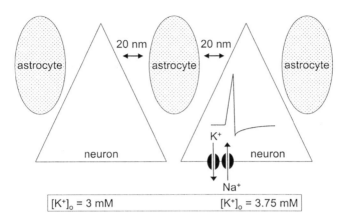

Figure 1.1. Schematic diagram illustrating the relationship of astrocytes, neurons, and brain extracellular space (ECS) Brain ECS is a narrow space with an average width of about 20 nm. This arrangement creates a highly restricted compartment for brain extracellular fluid. For example, a single action potential can instantaneously increase extracellular potassium concentration ($[K^+]_o$) from 3 mM to about 3.75 mM, a 25% increase. Spatial relationships are not to scale; ECS is measured in nanometers, while cells are measured in micrometers.

The average width of the space between brain cells is about 20 nm, which is about three orders of magnitude smaller than the diameter of either a neuron or glial cell body (Figure 1.1). However, because the surface membranes of neurons and glial cells are highly folded, brain ECS in toto has a sizable volume fraction, about 20%, of the total brain volume. This figure varies somewhat in different areas of the CNS (Perez-Pinzon et al., 1995). The physics of diffusion in this complex compartment has been intensively studied (Nicholson et al., 2000). The distance between brain cells is small enough that molecules released from one cell can diffuse to immediately adjacent cells with negligible time delay. On the other hand, molecules released into this space can diffuse laterally for hundreds of micrometers, a trip that can take many seconds. These two different latencies bracket the time domain of communications between these cell types. A particle that diffuses through brain extracellular fluid (ECF) from one side of a cell to the other must take a circuitous route that is described by a parameter called tortuosity (Nicholson, 1995). Under normal circumstances, this tortuosity reduces the rate of diffusion by approximately 60% when compared with movement of molecules in free solution.

As a consequence of its small size the composition of brain ECF fluctuates with neural activity. Even the small amount of K^+ efflux necessary for repolarization following a single action potential instantaneously increases extracellular $[K^+]$ ($[K^+]_o$) by about 0.75 mM (Ransom and Sontheimer, 1992); this is a 25% increase from the usual value of about 3 mM (Figure 1.1). Very effective mechanisms of K^+ sequestration and redistribution have evolved to prevent accumulation of $[K^+]_o$ from disrupting normal neural function (Ransom and Sontheimer, 1992; Newman, 1995).

The point is that small additions of ions or molecules to extracellular fluid can quickly reach functionally significant concentrations.

It is important to realize that brain ECS and astrocyte-neuron anatomy are not static. Intense neural activity can rapidly decrease ECS volume by as much as 15% (e.g., Ransom et al., 1985). This is probably a consequence of water movement into astrocytes along with K^+ (Ransom et al., 1985; MacVicar et al., 2002). During ischemia or inflammation, brain ECS may shrink by 50% or more (Ransom et al., 1992; Sykova et al., 1994). Reductions in brain ECS volume, called α, further slow diffusion and, more importantly, they magnify the magnitudes of fluctuations in extracellular ion concentrations caused by neural activity. In the hypothalamus, glial processes retract in relation to hormonal cycles affecting the physical relationship between glial and neuronal membranes (Chapter 4). These life-cycle changes in the hypothalamus reversibly alter neuronal signal processing (Chapter 4). The space between brain cells contains an extracellular matrix consisting of proteoglycans and glycosaminoglycans (Nicholson et al., 2000). The role of this material and its impact on the diffusion of solutes is not fully understood. Extracellular matrix appears to have little effect on the movement of ions or small molecules but may impede diffusion of macromolecules (Nicholson et al., 2000). While simple diffusion is an important contributor to solute motion in brain ECF, movement of some molecules will be affected by interaction with membrane bound transporters, receptors or ion channels. An obvious case in point is the disposition of the ubiquitous excitatory neurotransmitter, glutamate. This molecule is potentially toxic if its concentration in ECS is not rigidly controlled. Consequently, glutamate transporters are densely expressed in astrocytes and powerfully affect glutamate dynamics (Danbolt, 2001; also see Chapter 9).

1.3. History of glial-neuronal interaction

The history of glial-neuronal interactions has its roots in work and ideas that date back to the discovery of these cells. It is worthwhile revisiting some of the important events and contributions that influenced this field. History illuminates the importance of happenstance in the evolution of scientific thought and often provides explanations for the particular route progress has taken. We are not professional historians, of course, and what follows is an unabashedly personal and selective commentary.

1.3.1. Eary period (1856 to ~1910)

"Hitherto, gentlemen, in considering the nervous system, I have only spoken of the really nervous parts of it. But if we would study the nervous system in its real relations in the body, it is extremely important to have a knowledge of that substance also which lies between the proper nervous parts, holds them together and gives the whole its form in a greater or less degree" [Virchow, 1858 (Virchow, 1858)].

Rudolph Virchow coined the term *neuroglia* in 1856 and expanded on the topic two years later (see above and Kettenmann and Ransom, 2004 for details). The limitations of mid-nineteenth century microscopes and histological technique, and the vagueness of Virchow's illustrations, have left us in a quandary about whether or not he actually saw the cells that we call neuroglia today. Certainly he invented the concept of neuroglia, which is to say a non-neuronal CNS interstitial tissue. Virchow felt that neuroglia constituted a 'cement-like' substance which held neurons together and gave brain tissue its form. This sentiment is the parent of the long-held notion that neuroglial cells are purely passive elements whose primary purpose in the CNS is to provide structural integrity. Virchow also believed, however, that neuroglial tissue was important in brain pathology. He stated that "*experience shows us that this very interstitial tissue of the brain and spinal marrow is one of the most frequent seats of morbid change, as for example, of fatty degeneration* (Virchow, 1858)." If we presume that pathologic changes in neuroglia would have consequences for neighboring neurons, this might be construed as the earliest description of a glial-neuronal interaction.

Cajal's monumental treatise, *Histology of the Nervous System* (Cajal, 1995), contains an impressive chapter on neuroglia. Oligodendrocytes and microglial cells had not yet been discovered so this chapter focuses exclusively on astrocytes. When Cajal finished this portion of his book in 1897, the term astrocyte was not yet widely accepted, having been introduced only two years earlier by Lenhossek (Kettenmann and Ransom, 2004). Cajal critically summarized the hypotheses about astrocyte functions.

Cajal was skeptical of "Weigert's filling theory". This theory, whose origins lie in Virchow's original writings about neuroglia, presumed that glia served an entirely passive role, filling in spaces not occupied by neuron cell bodies or processes. Weigert further believed that glia proliferated to fill in the gaps created when neurons fell subject to pathologic processes and disappeared. In discussing Weigert's "faulty reasoning", Cajal states: "*He* (i.e. Weigert) *never dreamed that instead of resulting from empty spaces left by neurons, glial accumulations could well have been the cause of what appeared to be spaces*".

The "insolation theory" developed by Cajal's brother, Pedro, was strongly supported. This theory stated that astrocytes acted as physical insulation against the passage of neuronal impulses. Cajal argues that this insulating function is of special importance to dendrites and to axons lacking myelin. As an extension of this idea, he briefly entertained the idea that astrocytes might hold the key to understanding sleep (Cajal, Vol II): "*We thought for a while that these cells tend to extend their processes into synapses, reducing their activity. In contrast, when astrocytic processes retract, neurons would contact one another and thus become active once again.*" This idea superficially anticipated the discovery that hypothalamic glia exhibit great morphological plasticity that has functional consequences (Chapter 4).

Golgi's nutritional theory derived from the observation that astrocytes seemed to be preferentially located between capillaries and neuron cell bodies. It was believed that "nutritional fluids" were carried by glia to the neuronal cell bodies. While this theory, in modified form (Chapter 11), has been vindicated, Cajal found fault with it for several reasons. For example, as originally proposed, Golgi included the idea that dendrites made direct contact with capillaries and participated with glia in transporting nutrients to neuron somata; Cajal pointed out that dendrites never contact capillaries.

Two other theorists from the golden age of neurohistology should be mentioned. Lugaro, in 1907, proposed that glia might chemically inactivate metabolic by-products of neurons (even mentioning that this might take place at "nervous articulations", i.e. synapses), serve as guides for developing axons by providing chemotactic cues, and prevent toxic substances in blood from entering the brain (Lugaro, 1907). Lugaro's ideas are shockingly prescient. Unfortunately, his name is all but forgotten in this story. Finally, Nageotte described secretory granules in glia and suggested that these cells might release substances into blood in a manner akin to an endocrine gland (Nageotte, 1910). While this exact theory has not been validated (nor has it been entirely excluded, one might add), it is, nevertheless, the first mention of glial cells as the source of biologically significant secretion. Nageotte would not have been surprised by the eventual discovery that these cells release neurotransmitters such as glutamate (Chapters 14-16).

1.3.2. The pre-modern period (1910 to ~1980)

"What is the function of glial cells in neural centers? The answer is still not known, and the problem is even more serious because it may remain unsolved for many years to come until physiologists find direct methods to attack it." [Cajal, 1909 (Cajal, 1995)].

Surprisingly little new information about the function of astrocytes emerged during the first half of the twentieth century. Penfield (Penfield, 1932) and Glees (Glees, 1955) provided comprehensive reviews of this topic. The lack of physiological methods to effectively study glia remained the dilemma (see quote above). In regard to astrocyte function, Penfield mentions structural support and the suggestion of "nutritive and insulating capacity", already old concepts and still not proven. He also discusses the proposal that "astrocytes constitute a gland of internal secretion", an idea based primarily on the presence in astrocytes of possible secretory granules (i.e., 'gliosomes') and endfeet on capillaries (see above). In his review, Glees concludes that, *"Apart from a protective, insulating and supporting function, could neuroglia have a metabolic activity exceeding its own requirements, which would influence directly neuronal metabolism or synaptic activity? Until this dynamic concept has been proved, neuroglia will remain largely a domain of morphology and the artistic delight of neurohistologists...".*

In the early 1960s, Hyden and colleagues conducted a series of experiments to determine if biochemical changes took place in neurons and glial cells during activity, including special training protocols (Hyden and Lange, 1965). Single neurons and small clumps of glial cells were analyzed with regard to protein content, RNA content, and RNA base ratios, among other biochemical parameters (Kuffler and Nicholls, 1966). Superficially, these innovative experiments seemed to indicate that neurons and glial cells showed subtle biochemical changes in parts of the brain that should have been activated by the training procedures. Hyden and colleagues argued that neurons and glia *"form a functional unit with two parts which are eventually coupled and influence each other functionally"* (Hyden and Lange, 1965). Unfortunately, critical analysis reveals a host of experimental flaws that render this body of data almost useless (Kuffler and Nicholls, 1966).

In an elegant series of experiments in the mid-1960s, Kuffler and colleagues used direct physiological techniques to study identified glial cells in two simple preparations, the central nervous system of the leech and the optic nerves of amphibia (Kuffler and Potter, 1964; Nicholls and Kuffler, 1964). This work produced the first credible evidence of 'signaling' between neurons and glial cells. Using intracellular recording techniques, glial cells were shown to have high negative membrane potentials, selective permeability to K^+, and to be electrically connected to one another by gap junctions. Neural activity, such as a train of action potentials in optic nerve axons, caused slow depolarizing potentials in glia that were proportional to the duration and intensity of the eliciting neural activity (Orkand et al., 1966). These depolarizations were mediated by accumulation of K^+ in brain ECS. In their brilliant review on the physiology of glial cells, Kuffler and Nicholls (Kuffler and Nicholls, 1966) speculate that extracellular K^+ accumulation might constitute a special form of signaling between neurons and glia. It was apparent to them that accumulation of K^+ in brain ECS constituted an ionic signal that was directly proportional to the integral of nearby neural activity. The signal was received by adjacent glial cells that responded by graded depolarization (Orkand et al., 1966; Ransom and Goldring, 1973; Lothman and Somjen, 1975). The signal was specific for glial cells because small increases in $[K^+]_o$ had little effect on neuronal membrane potential (Kuffler and Nicholls, 1966). At the time, however, it was not clear if this 'information' had any functional consequences. Nearly forty years later, we know that the K^+ 'signal' causes astrocytes to increase K^+ uptake (Rose and Ransom, 1996), export protons leading to an extracellular acid shift (Ransom, 2000), and breakdown glycogen (Hof et al., 1988; Brown et al., 2003). The functional significance of these demonstrated effects has not been fully explored, but enhanced K^+ removal and glycogen breakdown appear highly adaptive in the face of increased neural activity (Chapter 11). The function of a K^+-induced glial-mediated extracellular acid shift is more theoretical at this time but it would tend to act as a negative feedback loop reducing neural excitability (Ransom, 2000).

The next steps in the history of glial-neuronal interactions, in what might be called the contemporary or modern period, will become obvious by reading the chapters that follow.

1.4. Astrocyte-neuron interactions

It is a valuable exercise, albeit possibly premature, to organize astrocyte-neuron interactions into a classification scheme (Table 1.1). This scheme should have the characteristic of being able to accommodate all known forms of astrocyte-neuron interaction, as well as plausible interactions that have not advanced beyond the state of hypothesis. A perfect classification would employ straightforward definitions and unequivocally define a single niche for each specific form of interaction. We make no such claims for the classification scheme offered here. Preferably, this effort will be seen as a workable draft. We did not attempt to list all presently known forms of astrocyte-neuron interaction in Table 1.1. Rather, we have chosen a few examples of specific interactions that seem to fit well in each of the subcategories, and which illustrate key features that define the subcategory.

The term volume transmission (VT) has been used to define intercellular communication "not based on any specialized structural arrangement" (Agnati et al., 1986; Agnati and Fuxe, 2000). This term is used as a contrast to wiring transmission (WT), implying intercellular communication "based on a few specialized structural arrangements" such as a chemical synapse or gap junction. There is certainly value in drawing this distinction. It is probable that the vast majority of astrocyte-neuron interactions would fall into the category of VT based on the definition provided here, rare instances of synaptic-like communication between glial cells and neurons notwithstanding (Mudrick-Donnon et al., 1993; Bergles et al., 2000). This dichotomy alone, however, fails to discriminate the several unique forms of glial-neuronal interaction that are now understood.

Table 1.1. Classification of astrocyte-neuron interactions

Interaction Categories	Physiological Events	
	Neurons	Astrocytes
A. Homeostatic or Supportive		
1. K$^+$ sequestration or redistribution	K$^+$ release	K$^+$ uptake or redistribution
2. Neurotransmitter uptake	Glutamate release	Glutamate uptake
3. Water homeostasis	H$_2$O from glucose oxidation	H$_2$O removal (aquaporins)
B. Metabolic		
1. Glutamate-glutamine cycle	Glutamine uptake	Glutamine synthesis
2. Ammonium fixation	Ammonium release	Ammonium fixation
3. Glycogen & neuron energy metabolism	Lactate uptake for energy metabolism	Glycogen breakdown to lactate
4. Detoxification of brain free radicals	Free radical generation & release	Free radical scavenging
C. Signaling		
1. Astrocyte Ca^{2+} waves	Activate glutamate receptors (modulation of EPSPs and IPSPs)	Glutamate release
2. Blood flow control	Glutamate release	Glutamate-mediated cyclooxygenase product release (vasodilation)
D. Trophic		
1. Trophic factor secretion (bFGF, GDNF, etc)	Trophic effects	Release of factors
2. Regulation of synaptogenesis	Synapse formation	Release of factors
3. Axonal guidance	Directed growth	Expression of aversive or attractive molecules
E. Pathologic		
1. Stroke	Excitotoxicity	Glutamate uptake failure & glutamate release
2. Glioma	Excitotoxicity	Glutamate uptake failure

1.4.1. Homeostatic or supportive astrocyte-neuron interactions

The widespread and uniform distribution of astrocytes throughout the brain coupled with their inevitable intimacy with neuron neighbors makes them ideally suited for homeostatic or supportive type relationships. In fact, one might speculate that the regularity and uniformity of astrocyte distribution was an obstacle to thinking about these cells as anything other than homeostatic or supportive cells.

For an interaction to fall into the category of being homeostatic or supportive, the core mission of the interaction must be to eliminate or minimize recurring extracellular perturbations. For example, active neurons release K^+ in conjunction with action potentials or synaptic potentials. Astrocytes are designed to keep $[K^+]_o$ around 3 mM (Ransom and Sontheimer, 1992). This is accomplished by transient uptake and sequestration of K^+ mediated by transport mechanisms (Rose and Ransom, 1996) and/or by the redistribution of focal increases in $[K^+]_o$ by a process known as 'K^+ spatial buffering' (Kuffler and Nicholls, 1966; Newman, 1995) (Figure 1.2). In a similar fashion, astrocytes quickly remove glutamate in their vicinity, a function primarily carried out at glutamatergic synapses throughout the brain (Anderson and Swanson, 2000; Danbolt, 2001). A plausible but unstudied example of a homeostatic astrocyte-neuron interaction relates to removal of the water generated by oxidative metabolism of glucose. Neurons derive more of their ATP from oxidative metabolism than do astrocytes and therefore impose a greater water burden (Walz and Mukerji, 1988; Ransom and Fern, 1996). Astrocytes, by virtue of their capillary endfeet and expression of aquaporins, probably play a role in bringing metabolically derived water to the brain-blood interface (Nedergaard et al., 2003). The K^+ and glutamate released by neurons do not function as 'signals' in the context of the homeostatic interactions described here. That is to say that neither K^+ or glutamate conveys specific 'information' to the nearby astrocyte acting to remove them. This is a subtle point but the ability to distinguish between a 'homeostatic' and a 'signaling' interaction hinges on just this attribute. For as we shall see, glutamate and K^+ can convey information to astrocytes, qualifying these molecules in certain contexts as signals (see below).

Homeostatic interaction: reversible K^+ sequestration

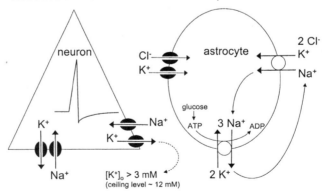

Figure 1.2. Schematic diagram of K^+ sequestration mechanisms. Active neurons extrude K^+ which is actively sequestered by astrocytes in three ways. The sodium pump and an anion transporter both take up K^+; the sodium pump requires ATP, while the anion transporter is indirectly powered by the energy stored in the transmembrane Na^+ gradient. The presence of channels for Cl^- and K^+, allow Donnan forces to produce a KCl influx. These mechanisms along with K^+ spatial buffering (not pictured), prevent $[K^+]_o$ from exceeding ~12 mM, the so-called ceiling level. Increases in astrocyte intracellular $[K^+]$ ($[K^+]_i$) are seen during neural

activity as $[K^+]_o$ increases. As $[K^+]_o$ increases dissipate with cessation of neural activity, astrocytes return the sequestered $[K^+]_i$ to the ECS.

1.4.2. Metabolic astrocyte-neuron interactions

In some respects, metabolic and homeostatic interactions are similar. Neither class of interaction involves "signaling" (as described above) and both of them serve to maintain certain baseline conditions conducive to 'normal' brain function. What distinguishes a glial-neuronal event as a metabolic interaction in this classification scheme is that one or more of its essential steps depends on the differential expression of enzymes in neurons and astrocytes. These enzymes mediate a specific, important and coordinated exchange of metabolites between the two cell types.
The glutamate-glutamine cycle is the premier example of a metabolic interaction (Westergaard et al., 1995) (Figure 1.3). Note that the glutamate uptake portion of the cycle has been split off and classified as a homeostatic function (it is not directly dependent on an enzyme-mediated event). Glutamate's conversion to glutamine by the ATP-dependent enzyme glutamine synthetase, which is located exclusively in astrocytes, is the starting point for the interaction. Glutamine is transported out of astrocytes and taken up by adjacent glutamatergic presynaptic terminals where it is converted by glutaminase to glutamate. The enzyme glutamine synthetase also mediates ammonium fixation (Figure 1.3), another metabolic interaction between neurons and astrocytes. Ammonium, of course, is neurotoxic at high concentrations (Norenberg et al., 1997). Removing ammonium by the creation of glutamine is a strategy that limits the accumulation of a potentially toxic compound by creating a relatively inert precursor metabolite.

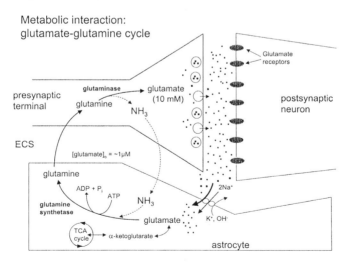

Figure 1.3. Scheme showing how astrocytes are involved in the metabolism of glutamate (i.e., the glutamate-glutamine cycle). Astrocytes, but not neurons, contain the enzyme glutamine synthetase which converts glutamate to glutamine in an ATP-requiring reaction. Glutamine is transported out of astrocytes and into nearby presynaptic terminals where it is converted to glutamate for synaptic release. Finally, the released glutamate is taken up by astrocytes via

high affinity glutamate transporters expressed predominately on astrocytes.   This diagram
also shows how astrocytes consume metabolically produced NH_3.

Glycogen is contained solely in astrocytes and can be broken down
enzymatically to lactate for distribution to adjacent neural elements during periods of
reduced glucose availability (Pellerin et al., 1998; Brown et al., 2003; also see
Chapter 11 for detailed discussion).   In some systems where glial glycogen acts as a
fuel reserve for neurons, there appears to be a 'signal' released by the neurons that
triggers glycogen breakdown (Tsacopoulos et al., 1997).   If this proves to be the case
in mammalian brain, it could justify reclassifying this event as a signaling interaction.
The detoxification of brain free radicals is listed as a metabolic astrocyte-neuron
interaction.   This interaction is substantially more complex, and less well understood,
than the examples previously mentioned.   Astrocytes contain more glutathione and
have higher levels of the enzymes involved in glutathione metabolism than do
neurons (Chen and Swanson, 2003).   Astrocytes have the capacity to protect neurons
from reactive oxygen species (Tanaka et al., 1999), and astrocytes depleted of
glutathione fail to do so (Chen et al., 2001).   Astrocytes also appear to provide
neurons with the powerful antioxidant ascorbate (Chen and Swanson, 2003).   This
example merely emphasizes the complex manner in which a metabolic interaction
might proceed.
    It is worth mentioning that alterations in the efficacy of homeostatic or
metabolic interactions could modulate neural behavior.   For example, interfering
with the normal production of glutamine deprives glutamatergic synapses of the
precursor for glutamate synthesis (Keyser and Pellmar, 1994).   Not surprisingly,
glutamate mediated synaptic transmission is diminished.   Chronic interference with
any homeostatic or metabolic interaction might have important pathophysiological
consequences.   Genetic downregulation of the main astrocyte transport proteins, i.e.,
GLAST or GLT-1, causes elevated extracellular levels of glutamate and
neurotoxicity (Rothstein et al., 1996; also see Chapter 9).

1.4.3. Signaling astrocyte-neuron interactions

The assertion that chemical signals mediate communication between astrocytes
and neurons was untenable until quite recently.   The discovery and subsequent
cataloging, of neurotransmitter receptors on astrocytes was the first step in
legitimizing this concept (Kettenmann and Ransom, 1995, 2004).   The second step
was the observation that astrocytes release glutamate and ATP when chemically (for
review see Haydon, 2001), electrically or mechanically stimulated (Newman and
Zahs, 1997).   There is now undeniable evidence that neurotransmitters released by
astrocytes can alter neural excitability (for reviews see Haydon, 2001; Newman,
2003; also see Chapters 14-16).   In other words, glia can send as well as receive
messages.   As these facts were emerging, an unusual regenerative event came to light
in cultured astrocyte monolayers (Cornell-Bell et al., 1990).   Astrocyte monolayers
focally stimulated with glutamate, exhibited slow traveling waves of increased
$[Ca^{2+}]_i$.   The mechanism(s) underlying these Ca^{2+} waves has proved unexpectedly
complex (Nedergaard et al., 2003; Newman, 2003); details are discussed elsewhere
in this volume (Chapters 13-16).   It is enough to say that both gap junctions and
ATP-dependent extracellular signaling are involved (Figure 1.4).   Gliologists are

excited about these waves because they are associated with astrocytes releasing glutamate, and possibly other neurotransmitters. The release is dependent on elevation of $[Ca^{2+}]_i$ and several competing theories exist about the release mechanism, including that it is vesicular in nature (Chapters 15 and 16). Neurons often change their behavior when astrocyte Ca^{2+} waves pass nearby and this phenomenon has become considerably more interesting with the discovery that it is seen in intact brain tissue, namely the retina (Newman, 2001). Currently, Ca^{2+}-dependent release of neurotransmitter(s) from astrocytes serves as the most dramatic example of astrocyte-neuron signaling. There is still no unequivocal evidence, however, that this type of signaling mechanism plays a role in normal brain function.

Another example of a signaling interaction derives from recent work suggesting that astrocytes may mediate neural activity-induced increased blood flow (Zonta et al., 2003). There is reason to believe, however, that other unique astrocyte-neuron interactions will be recognized as the complex relationships between astrocyte endfeet, endothelial cells and neurons are better understood (Nedergaard et al., 2003).

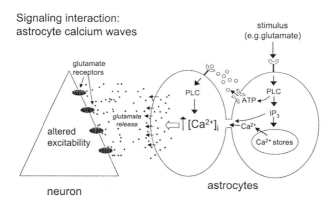

Figure 1.4. Illustration depicting how astrocyte intercellular Ca^{2+} waves propagate and how elevation in $[Ca^{2+}]_i$ leads to glutamate release that alters neuronal excitability. Astrocytes can be provoked to exhibit intercellular Ca^{2+} waves in many ways, such as the application of glutamate. Effective stimuli activate phospholipase C (PLC)- and inositol (1,4,5)-trisphosphate (IP$_3$)- dependent pathways which causes Ca^{2+} release from internal Ca^{2+} stores. IP$_3$ and Ca^{2+} could diffuse to adjacent cells through gap junctions. Astrocytes also release ATP upon activation. ATP activates purinergic P2Y receptors on nearby astrocytes and this is the predominant mode by which Ca^{2+} waves spread. Increase in astrocyte $[Ca^{2+}]_i$ causes glutamate release which modulates the excitability of neighboring neurons.

1.4.4. Trophic astrocyte-neuron interactions

Trophic astrocyte-neuron interactions are the most complex and least explored among all the subclasses of interactions considered here. They represent a subtype of signaling interaction, but we felt justified in splitting them off as a unique category based on the unique nature of the signaling molecules and the fact that these interactions take place very slowly. In contrast to the effects mediated by 'signaling' interactions, those mediated by 'trophic' interactions include neurogenesis, morphological changes such as spine formation, and axon guidance (Figure 1.5). Such events proceed on a time scale of hours to days, in contrast to the milliseconds to seconds time scale of signaling events. Another distinctive feature of trophic interactions is that they are often reciprocal. In the course of achieving a particular biological outcome, such as the growth of an axon to its target, neurons and glial cells may engage in a nearly continuous, reciprocal dialogue mediated by trophic molecules (Sepp and Auld, 2003). Finally, it is important to emphasize how early we are in the process of understanding these trophic interactions. Even so, based on information currently available, it is probable that this category of interaction will ultimately prove to be the most diverse and the most universal type of communication between astrocytes and neurons.

Trophic interactions

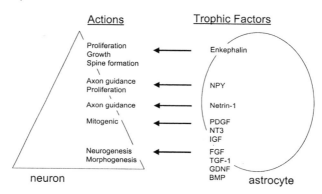

Figure 1.5. Diagram illustrating the numerous astrocyte-neuron interactions that might be mediated by trophic factors. Soluble trophic factors and neuropeptides may be released by astrocytes and activate specific neuronal receptors leading to a wide range of effects. The factors that dictate release and cellular responses are not well understood. NPY, neuropeptide Y; PDGF, platelet derived growth factor; NT3, neurotrophin 3; IGF, insulin-like growth factor; FGF, fibroblast growth factor; GDNF, glial cell-line derived neurotrophic factor; BMP, bone morphogenetic protein family.

Until very recently, the formation of synapses was viewed as a process that went on completely independent of glial cells. Convincing studies over the last few years, however, indicate that astrocytes increase the formation and enhance the function of CNS synapses (Pfrieger and Barres, 1997; Slezak and Pfrieger, 2003; also see Chapter 17). Surprisingly, cholesterol was identified as the soluble synaptogenic factor released by astrocytes (Mauch et al., 2001). It now seems probable that other factors are involved as well (Slezak and Pfrieger, 2003), including TNF-α (Beattie et al., 2002). These trophic interactions have obvious implications for development, but they may also play a crucial role in maintaining synapses throughout life and supporting the synaptic plasticity necessary for memory and learning (Slezak and Pfrieger, 2003).

1.4.5. Pathological astrocyte-neuron interactions

A final subcategory that recognizes pathological astrocyte-neuron interactions is amply justified by our growing appreciation that astrocytes play key roles in the pathophysiology of neurological diseases. The importance of astrocytes in brain pathologies should be no surprise. Astrocytes and neurons are inextricably cooperative during normal brain function (Ransom et al., 2003) and it follows logically that neurological diseases would tend to disrupt or pervert astrocyte-neuron relationships even if the primary problem were neuron-specific. We focused on those pathologic interactions between astrocytes and neurons that shed light on how a disease progresses and/or produces symptoms.

The ionic and molecular events underlying ischemic brain injury are now understood in satisfying detail (Lipton, 1999). Accumulation of excess extracellular glutamate is a crucial event that sets in motion a biochemical death spiral in neurons and, to a lesser extent, in glia as well. Astrocytes are responsible for removing glutamate from synaptic clefts and, more generally, for maintaining extracellular levels of glutamate near 1 to 2 μM (Anderson and Swanson, 2000) (Figure 1.3). Ischemia disrupts ion gradients resulting in massive increases in $[K^+]_o$ and $[Na^+]_i$. These changes are associated with membrane depolarization and uncontrolled release of glutamate from neurons (Lipton, 1999). Unfortunately, glutamate uptake by astrocytes, which is powered by the transmembrane Na^+ gradient, is also disabled by these events and extracellular glutamate rises to toxic levels. Because glutamate transporters operate in either direction, strictly dependent on transmembrane ion gradients, the collapse in ion gradients associated with ischemia will eventually cause astrocytes to release glutamate into the ECS via reverse transport. In fact, there is now consensus that most of the glutamate that accumulates in the ECS during ischemia is a consequence of reverse transport (Danbolt, 2001). These events are discussed in greater detail in recent review articles (Chen and Swanson, 2003; Ransom and Chan-Ling, 2004).

Glial tumors are notoriously resistant to treatment and produce progressive neurological deterioration and death. Beyond the obvious pathological consequences of an expansive intracranial growth, glioma cells are altered in ways that make them directly toxic to neurons (Sontheimer, 2003). Glioma cells have dramatically reduced ability to take up glutamate because of deranged glutamate transporter expression and enhanced cystine-glutamate exchange (Sontheimer, 2003; Ye et al., 1999). This results in higher levels of extracellular glutamate that are toxic to nearby neurons. This pathologic interaction between neoplastic astrocytes and neurons is a likely explanation for some of the neurological dysfunction and neuronal death seen in patients with infiltrating gliomas.

As a final challenge, let us consider some types of glial-neuronal interactions that fall slightly askew of the categories in our Table 1.1. The slow, hormonally-driven morphological changes in hypothalamic astrocytes that induce, or at least coincide with, altered synaptic function is a case in point. In an effort to avoid excessive sub-categorization, this could be considered a special type of signaling interaction. The interaction itself might be called 'spatially-mediated synaptic modulation'. To further conform to our classification, we can identify the astrocyte 'event' during the interaction as process withdrawal and the neuronal event as altered synaptic transmission. Another type of slow glial-neuronal interaction that is likely to become common place is 'signal-induced gene modulation' (Chapter 2). The proposed scheme (i.e., Table 1.1) can accommodate this as yet another subtype of signaling interaction. Splitters might wish to recognize this very contemporary type of interaction with its own category, especially as the number of discrete examples in this class increases. Finally, the category of pathologic interaction will come under pressure as more instances are uncovered of breakdowns in the normally synergistic relationships between neurons and astrocytes. For now, one category suffices but the range of pathophysiology that seems possible will likely invite sub-classification to assist in logically ordering the list.

1.5. The future

The brain is an amazing machine. The sophistication of its ability to sense and react to our environment is astounding. But those functions pale in comparison to its fantastic capacity for information storage and reasoning. Our lack of understanding about these defining features of the human brain is humbling. There is a vague sense that we are slowly making progress in solving these profound mysteries. For now, however, they remain in a class by themselves within the universe of unanswered scientific riddles. It is the philosophical premise of this book that brain functions, from the simple to the sublime, are a product of neurons and glial cells working together.

The brain's design incorporates equal volumes of glia and neurons, and phylogeny instructs that glial density increases with brain complexity. We may conclude, with no more information than this, that evolution endorsed the partnership between glia and neurons. Cajal rejected, and so may we, that glia serve only a structural role. Nevertheless, there has been a reluctance, or perhaps the inability, to rigorously test for glial participation in a whole range of vital brain transactions that support neural integration (an accepted, but poorly defined, term for the synthesis of information in support of everything the brain does). Fortunately, this is changing. The book in your hands is a timely summary of recent evidence supporting a wide range of glial-neuronal interactions. Looking forward from this vantage point, we are optimistic that work on this cellular partnership has reached a point of critical momentum and that we are on the right path to the future.

1.6. References

Abbott NJ (2002) Astrocyte-endothelial interactions and blood-brain barrier permeability. J Anat 200:629-638.

Agnati LF, Fuxe K (2000) Volume transmission as a key feature of information handling in the central nervous system possible new interpretative value of the Turing's B-type machine. In: Progress in Brain Research: Volume Transmission Revisited (Agnati LF, Fuxe K, Nicholson C, Sykova E, eds), pp 3-19. Amsterdam: Elsevier Science BV.

Agnati LF, Fuxe K, Zoli M, Ozini I, Toffano G, Ferraguti F (1986) A correlation analysis of the regional distribution of central enkephalin and beta-endorphin immunoreactive terminals and of opiate receptors in adult and old male rats. Evidence for the existence of two main types of communication in the central nervous system: the volume transmission and the wiring transmission. Acta Physiol Scand 128:201-207.

Alvarez-Maubecin V, Garcia-Hernandez F, Williams JT, Van Bockstaele EJ (2000) Functional coupling between neurons and glia. J Neurosci 20:4091-4098.

Anderson CM, Swanson RA (2000) Astrocyte glutamate transport: review of properties, regulation, and physiological functions [In Process Citation]. Glia 32:1-14.

Beattie EC, Stellwagen D, Morishita W, Bresnahan JC, Ha BK, Von Zastrow M, Beattie MS, Malenka RC (2002) Control of synaptic strength by glial TNFalpha. Science 295:2282-2285.

Bergles DE, Roberts JD, Somogyi P, Jahr CE (2000) Glutamatergic synapses on oligodendrocyte precursor cells in the hippocampus. Nature 405:187-191.

Bordey A, Sontheimer H (2000) Ion channel expression by astrocytes in situ: comparison of different CNS regions. Glia 30:27-38.

Brown AM, Tekkok SB, Ransom BR (2003) Glycogen regulation and functional role in mouse white matter. J Physiol 549:501-512.

Bushong EA, Martone ME, Jones YZ, Ellisman MH (2002) Protoplasmic astrocytes in CA1 stratum radiatum occupy separate anatomical domains. J Neurosci 22:183-192.

Butt AM, Ransom BR (1993) Morphology of astrocytes and oligodendrocytes during development in the intact rat optic nerve. J Comp Neurol 338:141-158.

Cajal R (1995) Histology of the Nervous System. New York: Oxford University Press.

Chan-Ling T, Stone J (1991) Factors determining the morphology and distribution of astrocytes in the cat retina: a 'contact-spacing' model of astrocyte interaction. J Comp Neurol 303:387-399.

Chen Y, Swanson RA (2003) Astrocytes and brain injury. J Cereb Blood Flow Metab 23:137-149.

Chen Y, Vartiainen NE, Ying W, Chan PH, Koistinaho J, Swanson RA (2001) Astrocytes protect neurons from nitric oxide toxicity by a glutathione-dependent mechanism. J Neurochem 77:1601-1610.

Cornell-Bell AH, Finkbeiner SM, Cooper MS, Smith SJ (1990) Glutamate induces calcium waves in cultured astrocytes: long-range glial signaling. Science 247:470-473.

Danbolt NC (2001) Glutamate uptake. Prog Neurobiol 65:1-105.

Glees P (1955) Neuroglia: Morphology and Function. Springfield, Illinois: Blackwell Scientific Publications.

Haydon PG (2001) GLIA: listening and talking to the synapse. Nat Rev Neurosci 2:185-193.

Hof PR, Pascale E, Magistretti PJ (1988) K+ at concentrations reached in the extracellular space during neuronal activity promotes a Ca2+-dependent glycogen hydrolysis in mouse cerebral cortex. J Neurosci 8:1922-1928.

Hyden H, Lange PW (1965) A differentiation in RNA response in neurons early and late during learning. Proc Natl Acad Sci U S A 53:946-952.

Kettenmann H, Ransom BR (1995) Neuroglia. New York: Oxford University Press.

Kettenmann H, Ransom BR (2004) Neuroglia, The concept of neuroglia: A historical perspective. New York: Oxford University Press.

Keyser DO, Pellmar TC (1994) Synaptic transmission in the hippocampus: critical role for glial cells. Glia 10:237-243.

Kuffler SW, Potter DD (1964) Glia in the Leech Central Nervous System: Physiological Properties and Neuron-Glia Relationship. J Neurophysiol 27:290-320.

Kuffler SW, Nicholls JG (1966) The physiology of neuroglial cells. Ergeb Physiol 57:1-90.

Lee SH, Kim WT, Cornell-Bell AH, Sontheimer H (1994) Astrocytes exhibit regional specificity in gap-junction coupling. Glia 11:315-325.

Lipton P (1999) Ischemic cell death in brain neurons. Physiol Rev 79:1431-1568.

Lothman EW, Somjen GG (1975) Extracellular potassium activity, intracellular and extracellular potential responses in the spinal cord. J Physiol (Lond) 252:115-136.

Lugaro E (1907) Sulle funzioni della nevroglia. Riv Pat Nerv Ment 12:225-233.

MacVicar BA, Feighan D, Brown A, Ransom B (2002) Intrinsic optical signals in the rat optic nerve: role for K(+) uptake via NKCC1 and swelling of astrocytes. Glia 37:114-123.

Mauch DH, Nagler K, Schumacher S, Goritz C, Muller EC, Otto A, Pfrieger FW (2001) CNS synaptogenesis promoted by glia-derived cholesterol. Science 294:1354-1357.

18 Glial ⇔ Neuronal Signaling

Mudrick-Donnon LA, Williams PJ, Pittman QJ, MacVicar BA (1993) Postsynaptic potentials mediated by GABA and dopamine evoked in stellate glial cells of the pituitary pars intermedia. J Neurosci 13:4660-4668.

Nageotte J (1910) Phenomenes de secretion dans le protoplasma des cellules nevrogliques de la substance grise. C R Soc Biol (Paris) 68:1068-1069.

Nedergaard M, Ransom BR, Goldman S (2003) New roles for astrocytes: Redefining the functional architecture of the brain (review). TINS 26:523-530.

Newman EA (1986) High potassium conductance in astrocyte endfeet. Science 233:453-454.

Newman EA (1995) Glial cell regulation of extracellular potassium. In: Neuroglia (Kettenmann H, Ransom BR, eds), pp 717-731. New York: Oxford University Press.

Newman EA (2001) Calcium signaling in retinal glial cells and its effect on neuronal activity. Prog Brain Res 132:241-254.

Newman EA (2003) New roles for astrocytes: regulation of synaptic transmission. Trends Neurosci 26:536-542.

Newman EA, Zahs KR (1997) Calcium waves in retinal glial cells. Science 275:844-847.

Nicholls JG, Kuffler SW (1964) Extracellular Space as a Pathway for Exchange between Blood and Neurons in the Central Nervous System of the Leech: Ionic Composition of Glial Cells and Neurons. J Neurophysiol 27:645-671.

Nicholson C (1995) Extracellular space as the pathway for neuron-glial cell interaction. In: Neuroglia (Kettenmann H, Ransom BR, eds), pp 387-397. New York: Oxford University Press.

Nicholson C, Chen KC, Hrabetova S, Tao L (2000) Diffusion of molecules in brain extracellular space: theory and experiment. In: Progress in Brain Research: Volume Transmission Revisited (Agnati LF, Fuxe K, Nicholson C, Sykova E, eds), pp 129-154. Amsterdam: Elsevier Science BV.

Nielsen S, Nagelhus EA, Amiry-Moghaddam M, Bourque C, Agre P, Ottersen OP (1997) Specialized membrane domains for water transport in glial cells: high-resolution immunogold cytochemistry of aquaporin-4 in rat brain. J Neurosci 17:171-180.

Norenberg MD, Huo Z, Neary JT, Roig-Cantesano A (1997) The glial glutamate transporter in hyperammonemia and hepatic encephalopathy: relation to energy metabolism and glutamatergic neurotransmission. Glia 21:124-133.

Orkand RK, Nicholls JG, Kuffler SW (1966) Effect of nerve impulses on the membrane potential of glial cells in the central nervous system of amphibia. J Neurophysiol 29:788-806.

Pellerin L, Pellegri G, Bittar PG, Bouras C, Martin J-L, Stella N, Magistretti PJ (1998) Evidence supporting the existence of an activity-dependent astrocyte-neuron lactate shuttle. DN 20:291-299.

Penfield W (1932) Cytology & Cellular Pathology of the Nervous System. New York: Paul Hoeber, Inc.

Perez-Pinzon MA, Tao L, Nicholson C (1995) Extracellular potassium, volume fraction, and tortuosity in rat hippocampal CA1, CA3, and cortical slices during ischemia. J Neurophysiol 74:565-573.

Peters A, Palay SL, Webster Hd (1991) The Fine Structure of the Nervous System: Neurons and Their Supporting Cells, 3 Edition. New York: Oxford University Press, Inc.

Pfrieger FW, Barres BA (1997) Synaptic efficacy enhanced by glial cells in vitro. Science 277:1684-1687.

Prochiantz A, Mallat M (1988) Astrocyte diversity. Ann N Y Acad Sci 540:52-63.

Ransom B, Behar T, Nedergaard M (2003) New roles for astrocytes (stars at last). Trends Neurosci 26:520-522.

Ransom BR (1991) Vertebrate glial classification, lineage, and heterogeneity. Ann N Y Acad Sci 633:19-26.

Ransom BR (2000) Glial modulation of neural excitability mediated by extracellular pH: a hypothesis revisited. In: Progress in Brain Research: Volume Transmission Revisited

(Agnati LF, Fuxe K, Nicholson C, Sykova E, eds), pp 217-228. Amsterdam: Elsevier Sciences BV.

Ransom BR, Goldring S (1973) Ionic determinants of membrane potential of cells presumed to be glia in cerebral cortex of cat. J Neurophysiol 36:855-868.

Ransom BR, Sontheimer H (1992) The neurophysiology of glial cells. J Clin Neurophysiol 9:224-251.

Ransom BR, Fern R (1996) Anoxic-Ischemic glial cell injury: Mechanisms and Consequences. In: Tissue oxygen deprivation (Haddad G, Lister G, eds), pp 617-652. New York: Marcel Dekker, Inc.

Ransom BR, Chan-Ling T (2004) Astrocytes. In: Youmans Neurological Surgery 5th Edition (Winn HR, ed), pp 97-115. Philadelphia, PA: Elsevier, Inc.

Ransom BR, Yamate CL, Connors BW (1985) Activity-dependent shrinkage of extracellular space in rat optic nerve: a developmental study. J Neurosci 5:532-535.

Ransom BR, Walz W, Davis PK, Carlini WG (1992) Anoxia-induced changes in extracellular K+ and pH in mammalian central white matter. J Cereb Blood Flow Metab 12:593-602.

Rose CR, Ransom BR (1996) Intracellular sodium homeostasis in rat hippocampal astrocytes. J Physiol (Lond) 491:291-305.

Rose CR, Ransom BR (1997) Gap junctions equalize intracellular Na+ concentration in astrocytes. Glia 20:299-307.

Rothstein JD, Dykes-Hoberg M, Pardo CA, Bristol LA, Jin L, Kuncl RW, Kanai Y, Hediger MA, Wang Y, Schielke JP, Welty DF (1996) Knockout of glutamate transporters reveals a major role for astroglial transport in excitotoxicity and clearance of glutamate. Neuron 16:675-686.

Sepp KJ, Auld VJ (2003) Reciprocal interactions between neurons and glia are required for Drosophila peripheral nervous system development. J Neurosci 23:8221-8230.

Slezak M, Pfrieger FW (2003) New roles for astrocytes: regulation of CNS synaptogenesis. Trends Neurosci 26:531-535.

Sontheimer H (2003) Malignant gliomas: perverting glutamate and ion homeostasis for selective advantage. Trends Neurosci 26:543-549.

Sontheimer H, Minturn JE, Black JA, Waxman SG, Ransom BR (1990) Specificity of cell-cell coupling in rat optic nerve astrocytes in vitro. Proc Natl Acad Sci U S A 87:9833-9837.

Steinhauser C, Berger T, Frotscher M, Kettenmann H (1992) Heterogeneity in the Membrane Current Pattern of Identified Glial Cells in the Hippocampal Slice. Eur J Neurosci 4:472-484.

Sykova E, Svoboda J, Polak J, Chvatal A (1994) Extracellular volume fraction and diffusion characteristics during progressive ischemia and terminal anoxia in the spinal cord of the rat. J Cereb Blood Flow Metab 14:301-311.

Tanaka J, Toku K, Zhang B, Ishihara K, Sakanaka M, Maeda N (1999) Astrocytes prevent neuronal death induced by reactive oxygen and nitrogen species. Glia 28:85-96.

Tsacopoulos M, Poitry-Yamate CL, Poitry S (1997) Ammonium and Glutamate Released by Neurons Are Signals Regulating the Nutritive Function of a Glial Cell. J Neurosci 17:2383-2390.

Vannucci SJ, Maher F, Simpson IA (1997) Glucose transporter proteins in brain: delivery of glucose to neurons and glia. Glia 21:2-21.

Virchow R (1858) Cellular Pathology. Birmingham, AL: Division of Gryphon Editions, Ltd.

Walz W, Mukerji S (1988) Lactate release from cultured astrocytes and neurons: a comparison. Glia 1:366-370.

Westergaard N, Sonnewald U, Schousboe A (1995) Metabolic trafficking between neurons and astrocytes: the glutamate/glutamine cycle revisited. Dev Neurosci 17:203-211.

Wolff JR (1970) Quantitative aspects of macroglia. In: Proceedings of the Sixth international congress of neuropathology, pp 327-352. Paris: Masson.

Ye ZC, Rothstein JD, Sontheimer H (1999) Compromised glutamate transport in human glioma cells: reduction-mislocalization of sodium-dependent glutamate transporters and enhanced activity of cystine-glutamate exchange. J Neurosci 19:10767-10777.

Zonta M, Angulo MC, Gobbo S, Rosengarten B, Hossmann KA, Pozzan T, Carmignoto G (2003) Neuron-to-astrocyte signaling is central to the dynamic control of brain microcirculation. Nat Neurosci 6:43-50.

1. 7. Abbreviations

BMP	Bone morphogenetic protein family
CNS	Central nervous system
ECF	Extracellular fluid
ECS	Extracellular space
FGF	Fibroblast growth factor
IGF	Insulin-like growth factor
GDNF	Glial cell-line derived neurotrophic factor
IP_3	Inositol (1,4,5)-trisphosphate
NPY	Neuropeptide Y
NT3	Neurotrophin 3
PDGF	Platelet derived growth factor
PLC	Phospholipase C
VT	Volume transmission
WT	Wiring transmission
$[X^+]_o$	Extracellular concentration of a cation
$[X^+]_i$	Intracellular concentration of a cation

Chapter 2

Gene function in glial-neuronal interactions

Laurent Soustelle and Angela Giangrande*

Institut de Génétique et Biologie Moléculaire et Cellulaire
IGBMC/CNRS/ULP/INSERM - BP 10142
67404 Illkirch, c.u. de Strasbourg, France

*Corresponding author: angela@titus.u-strasbg.fr

Contents

2.1. Introduction

Neurons and glial cells constitute the major components of the nervous system. Although they display distinct roles, their continuous interactions are the gage for appropriate development and function of such a complex tissue. For this reason, the more we will understand the molecular and cellular bases of neuron-glia interactions, the more we will be able to unravel the complex processes underlying the differentiation, the function and the survival of these two cell types.

In this review, we will focus on the neuron-glia interactions that occur during cell differentiation, migration, axonal navigation, as a model to understand the developmental mechanisms of neuro and gliogenesis. We will also present examples of neuron-glia interactions occurring during axon regeneration and cell survival, as a model to understand the mechanisms controlling nervous system homeostasis during ontogenesis. During the recent past, it has become more and more evident that the basic mechanisms underlying neuron-glia interactions are conserved throughout evolution and much has been integrating the information obtained in different model systems. Throughout the review, we will present examples from invertebrate and vertebrate models and compare the results whenever possible.

2.2. Neuron-glia interactions during differentiation

Gliogenesis and neurogenesis depend on the activity of different types of genes coding for secreted morphogenesis, transcription factors and transmembrane molecules. The genetic and the molecular interactions between the different pathways have been the focus of many *in vivo* and *in vitro* studies in vertebrates and invertebrates. This has made it possible to integrate the processes that control positional information and those that control cell fate choices in the nervous system. Enormous progress has also been achieved upon the identification of multipotent progenitors also called stem cells that display unexpected plastic behaviours. The important point is now to understand how is the production of glia and neurons from such precursors controlled in space and time.

2.2.1. Role of the Notch signalling pathway during gliogenesis

During development, neurons and glial cells are produced by the same population of multipotent stem cells (Rao, 1999). In most cases, neurons emerge before glia, in response to instructive signals coming from local environment. Different scenarios might be envisaged to explain the temporal switch between neurogenesis and gliogenesis. One hypothesis proposes that neurogenic, instructive, signals decay with time allowing cells to take the default, glial, fate. Alternatively, gliogenic signals might be temporally regulated and only be expressed once neurons have differentiated.

It has been shown that neural development requires a process of lateral inhibition that allows some cells to single out from the neurogenic region and to inhibit neighbouring cells from differentiating (Beatus and Lendahl, 1998). According to the first hypothesis, the cell that singles out differentiates into a neuron, due to an instructive signal, such as bone morphogenetic proteins, and *sonic hedgehog* (BMPs, *shh*) (Mehler et al., 1997; Patten and Placzek, 2000). The interplay of neurogenic signal and lateral inhibition controls the amount of neurons and undifferentiated stem cells. At late development stages, the neurogenic signal declines and neurons migrate away. This combination of events allows a second differentiative wave producing glia. In this context, neurons are actively induced to differentiate and control the differentiative state of stem cells sending back an inhibitory signal (Henrique et al., 1997).

The most likely pathway participating to the temporal switch involves the Notch receptor, which also controls lateral inhibition. The Notch family of proteins includes four known vertebrate orthologs and several ligands encoded by the *Delta* and *Jagged* gene families (for reviews see Weinmaster, 1997; Nye, 1999). During vertebrate neurogenesis, the Notch receptor is expressed ubiquitously whilst its ligand Delta/Jagged shows a punctuated expression profile, consistent with a role in lateral inhibition (Lewis, 1996; Lindsell et al., 1996). Moreover, targeted deletion of Notch in mice leads to massive and precocious overproduction of neurons (de la Pompa et al., 1997), suggesting that the resistance to the neurogenic signal depends on the activation of Notch by Delta/Jagged. These data supported a model in which Notch signalling protects stem cells from all differentiative signals (Henrique et al., 1997). According to this view, if Notch were removed at late stages, glial cells would be produced simply because the neurogenic signal would be gone. In other words, Notch represses cell differentiation in general, rather than play an instructive role in fate choice.

Recent data, however, suggest that Notch also plays an active, gliogenic, role. Using an *in vivo* gain of function approach, Fishell and collaborators have shown a gliogenic role for Notch in the early mouse central nervous system (CNS) (Gaiano et al., 2000). If the intracellular domain of Notch1 (Notch1 IC), which has been shown to work as a constitutively active Notch molecule, is introduced into cells of the developing mouse forebrain before the onset of neurogenesis, the Notch1 IC expressing cells develop into radial glial cells. Moreover, using clonal culture analysis, Anderson and collaborators have shown that Notch1 IC or soluble Notch ligand is able to not only increase but also accelerate the production of Schwann cells from peripheral nervous system (PNS) stem cells (Morrison et al., 2000). These data show that Notch does not maintain stem cells in an uncommitted state, but rather acts positively to direct neural crest stem cells towards a glial fate.

Notch also instructs gliogenesis in stem cells from the adult brain. Honjo and collaborators (Tanigaki et al., 2001) used retroviral vectors expressing Notch1 IC or Notch3 IC to stably transfect hippocampal precursor cells. They found that expression of Notch IC resulted in elevated number of cells exhibiting an astrocytic morphology and expressing the astrocyte marker GFAP (glial fibrillary acidic protein). The increase in GFAP-expressing cells was accompanied by a decrease in the number of cells expressing neuronal or oligodendrocyte markers, but not in an increase in the number of dying cells. This suggests that Notch plays an instructive role rather than preferentially allowing a glial progenitor population to survive. Finally, both Notch1 and *Hes1*, a downstream gene of the Notch signalling pathway (for a review see Kageyama et al., 1997), are expressed in retinal progenitor cells, downregulated in differentiated neurons and expressed in Müller glia, suggesting a role of these genes during retina glial differentiation (Bao and Cepko, 1997; Furukawa et al., 2000). The group of Cepko has shown that retroviral transduction of Notch1 IC or Hes1 in progenitor cells induces differentiation into Müller glial cells in the mouse retina (Furukawa et al., 2000). Because lineage analyses have shown that neurons and glia are derived from a common progenitor cell (Turner and Cepko, 1987), it is tempting to speculate that the persistent expression of these genes promotes the choice towards a glial fate at the expense of the neuronal one (for a review see Vetter and Moore, 2001). Similar results were obtained with *Hes5*, another downstream gene of the Notch signalling pathway. Indeed, a decrease in the number of Müller glial cells was reported in mice lacking *Hes5* without affecting cell survival (Hojo et al., 2000). Moreover, retroviral overpexression of Hes5 leads to an increase in the number of glial cells at the expense of neurons. These results indicate that *Hes* genes modulate glial fate specification in mouse retina.

How might Notch promote gliogenesis? The different results obtained *in vivo* and *in vitro* suggest that Notch signalling has different readouts depending on the cues available in the environment: at early stages, it prevents neuronal differentiation, at late stages, it promotes gliogenesis. Although it is known that a gene can have different roles at different stages, our understanding of Notch function relies on different approaches and models. An important step forward will be certainly achieved with the production of Notch conditional knock-out mice. Indeed, mice deficient for Notch signalling die before gliogenesis begins, which prevents their use to analyze the gliogenic role of Notch *in vivo*.

One possible explanation for the different results implies the interaction of Notch signalling with two classes of genes, one promoting neuronal differentiation, and including the proneural genes, the other including yeast unknown gliogenic factors. Within this context, Notch contributes to maintain the pool of multipotent precursors during early development. It does so by inducing the expression of *Hes* genes of the bHLH family, which have an inhibitory effect on proneural gene expression (Kageyama and Ohtsuka, 1999). At late stages, when the neurogenic signal declines, Notch actively promotes gliogenesis, in agreement with the observation that, in the absence of Mash 1, Notch and Hes signalling is still able to induce gliogenesis. This is also confirmed by the phenotype of *Hes* loss of function mutations: mice deficient for *Hes5* (Hojo et al., 2000) and mice in which *Hes1* (Furukawa et al., 2000) is inhibited show a decrease in Müller glial cells production. The identification of the gliogenic factor(s) will be crucial to understand the role(s) of Notch in nervous system development.

These results demonstrate that Notch1 activation leads to the acquisition of a glial phenotype during vertebrate development. In *Drosophila*, Notch controls gliogenesis in a lineage specific manner (Jacobs et al., 1989; Udolph et al., 2001; Van De Bor and Giangrande, 2001; Umesono et al., 2002). During embryonic development, Notch activates gliogenesis in several CNS and PNS lineages (Udolph et al., 2001; Umesono et al., 2002) but it represses it in the adult PNS (Van De Bor and Giangrande, 2001). In each case, Notch regulates (positively or negatively) the expression of Glide/Gcm (Glia cell deficient/Glia cell missing)-Glide2, two transcription factors that are specifically necessary to induce glial differentiation (Hosoya et al., 1995; Jones et al., 1995; Vincent et al., 1996; Kammerer and Giangrande, 2001). Indeed, these genes code for the whole glial promoting activity in fly and are sufficient to induce gliogenesis (see below).

2.2.2. The *Olig* genes and the temporal switch between neurons and glia

Several laboratories have recently identified a novel family of genes encoding basic helix-loop-helix (bHLH) transcription factors, the *Olig* genes (Lu et al., 2000; Takebayashi et al., 2000; Zhou et al., 2000). There are three family members (*Olig-1, Olig-2* and *Olig-3*) but only *Olig-1* and *Olig-2* are expressed in neural tissues. Although *Olig-2* orthologs have been found in chick and zebrafish (Mizuguchi et al., 2001; Novitch et al., 2001; Park et al., 2002), *Olig-1* has been identified only in mammals.

Olig-1 and *Olig-2* expression analysis suggested a role in the generation of both motor neurons and oligodendrocytes (OLs). In developing mouse embryos, *olig* gene expression overlaps but precedes the expression of any other oligodendroglial specific gene making it the earliest marker for this lineage. Olig proteins are also expressed in motor neuron precursors but are downregulated in differentiated motor neurons (Novitch et al., 2001). Ectopic expression of *Olig-2* in the chick spinal cord leads to increased number of motor neurons showing that *Olig* genes can promote motor neuron development (Novitch et al., 2001). Moreover, ectopic coexpression of *Neurogenin2*, another bHLH protein, and *Olig2*, results in the production of motor neurons in the dorsal part of neural tube (Mizuguchi et al., 2001). Finally, *Olig-2* null mice show a loss of motor neurons in the spinal cord (Lu et al., 2002). *Olig-1* expression is controversial, as one study reports it to be strictly co-expressed with *Olig-2* (Lu et al., 2000), whereas others finds its expression to be temporally delayed relative to *Olig-2* and undergoing significant variations in strength during development (Zhou et al., 2000).

Recent genetic studies provide compelling evidence that Olig proteins are essential for development of all OLs in the CNS. *Olig-1* null mice are viable, but show a delay in OLs maturation (Lu et al., 2002). *Olig-2* null mice entirely lack oligodendrocyte precursor (OLP) cells in the spinal cord but not in the brain where there is only a small alteration in the number of precursors (Lu et al., 2002). In *Olig-1/Olig-2* double mutant mice, no OLPs are seen in the CNS (Zhou and Anderson, 2002). Loss of function studies in zebrafish indicates that *Olig2* has a conserved role in formation of both OLs and motor neurons (Park et al., 2002).

How can we explain the time-dependent change in the activities of Olig proteins during the switch from motor neuron to OLP cells production? It is possible that the set of cofactors interacting with Olig proteins change during development (Mizuguchi et al., 2001; Novitch et al., 2001) (Fig. 2.1).

In this view, the presence of early cofactors drives the production of motor neurons whereas the presence of a different set of Olig interacting proteins at late stages gives rise to OLPs cells (Marquardt and Pfaff, 2001). *Nkx2.2* is probably one of these late cofactors. Another possibility is that inhibitory factors are involved in regulating the timing of initial OLPs cell specification. For example, it has been proposed that *Neurogenin2* plays a positive role in motor neuron and a negative role in glia differentiation, respectively. According to this hypothesis, *Neurogenin 2* is necessary to promote motor neuron differentiation, its downregulation being a pre-requisite for OL to differentiate (Zhou et al., 2001; Zhou and Anderson, 2002). While these data highlight the importance of spatio-temporal cues in glial differentiation, the relationship between the Notch pathway and the Olig genes remains unclear.

2.2.3. Role of *glide/gcm* in fate choice between neurons and glia in *Drosophila*

Nervous system and genome simplicity make *Drosophila* an ideal model system to look at neuron-glia interactions at early stages of differentiation. Not only all neural stem cells have been identified using specific cell markers, but lineage trees and genes acting on neuronal and glial differentiation have been extensively characterized.

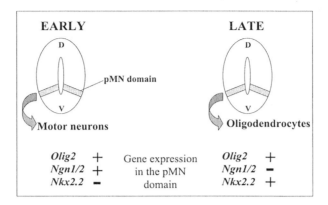

Figure 2.1. The Neuron-Oligodendrocyte fate switch in spinal cord. During spinal cord development, the same ventral region gives rise to motor neurons and to oligodendrocytes. This region is called motor neuron progenitor domain (pMN). At early developmental stages, *Olig2* and *Ngn1/2* are expressed in the pMN domain and participate to motor neuron generation. Later, *Ngn1/2* are downregulated in this area. At the same time, Nkx2.2, a homeodomain transcription factor, starts being expressed in the *Olig2* expression domain. This triggers the production of oligodendrocytes progenitors into the pMN domain. D, Dorsal; V, ventral.

The embryonic nervous system includes a brain and a metameric structure, the ventral cord, which corresponds to the vertebrate spinal cord. Within the ventral cord, *Drosophila* glial cells can be subdivided into two classes (midline and lateral glia) that display distinct origins, developmental pathways and functions. Lateral glia represent the most important class in cell number (60 per neuromere) and originate in the ventral neurogenic ectoderm. Midline glial cells (3-4 cells per neuromere) are mesectoderm-derived cells (Jacobs, 2000). In this paragraph, we will focus on lateral glia, which are subdivided into different subtypes depending on the position, on the type of precursor and on the lineage tree. In agreement with the diversity of neuronal precursors, several genes of the proneural class have been identified, each promoting the differentiation of different neuronal cell types. In contrast, mutations in a single locus eliminate all lateral glia in embryonic and adult PNS and CNS, irrespective of the precursor type (Hosoya et al., 1995; Jones et al., 1995; Vincent et al., 1996; Van De Bor et al., 2000; Kammerer and Giangrande, 2001). This locus contains the *glide/gcm* (*glial cell deficient/glial cell missing*) and *glide2* genes, which we will refer to as *glide* and *glide2*.

Glide and Glide 2 transcription factors contain a similar DNA-binding motif that recognizes an octamer sequence also called Glide-Binding Site (GBS). Several copies of this site are present in potential target genes that encode transcriptional activators of glial fate (reversed polarity and pointed) (Akiyama et al., 1996; Giesen et al., 1997) and transcriptional repressors of neuronal fate (tramtrack p69) (Giesen et al., 1997). They are also present in the glide /glide2 locus and mediate cross- and auto-regulation of the two genes (Akiyama et al., 1996; Schreiber et al., 1997; Miller et al., 1998; Kammerer and Giangrande, 2001).

In glide null mutant embryos, most presumptive glial cells are transformed into neurons showing that *glide* acts as a binary switch to promote gliogenesis in the developing nervous system (Hosoya et al., 1995; Jones et al., 1995; Vincent et al., 1996) (Fig. 2.2). The few remaining glial cells in *glide* mutant embryos express *glide2* and are lost in double *glide-glide2* mutants, suggesting that both genes contribute to the glial fate, even though *glide* plays the major role (Kammerer and Giangrande, 2001; Alfonso and Jones, 2002). Moreover, *glide* or *glide2* overexpression is sufficient to induce ectopic gliogenesis at the expense of the endogenous fates (Fig. 2.2), even in non-neural tissues (Hosoya et al., 1995; Jones et al., 1995; Vincent et al., 1996; Akiyama-Oda et al., 1998; Bernardoni et al., 1998). These results show that the *glide* locus is necessary and sufficient to promote the glial fate during development.

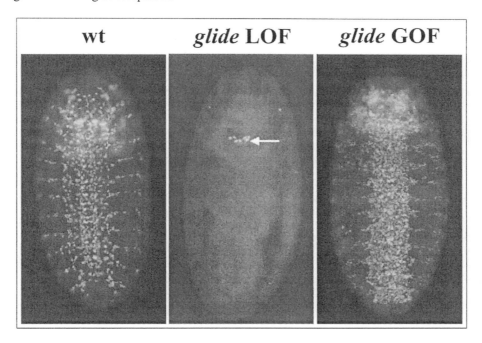

Figure 2.2. Glide is necessary and sufficient to promote gliogenesis. In wild-type fly embryos, glial cell nuclei are visualized by an anti-Repo immunolabeling (wt). Repo is the marker for *Drosophila* glial cells. In the absence of Glide (*glide* loss-of-function or LOF), only few glial cells are present (see arrow in *glide* LOF). If Glide expression is induced throughout the nervous system (*glide* gain-of-function or GOF), glial cells differentiate at ectopic positions, indicating that Glide is sufficient to promote the glial fate (*glide* GOF).

Whereas *glide* has been consistently considered as an instructive cue autonomously required in glial lineages, a specific dominant allele has revealed an unexpected potential (Van De Bor et al., 2002). The *glide^{Pyx}* mutation, as well as specific heat-shock regimens on hs-*glide* flies, induce ectopic neurogenesis in the adult PNS. Such PNS hyperplasia is caused by precocious Glide expression, which ectopically activates the expression of basic helix-loop-helix (bHLH) proneural genes. Thus, temporal misexpression transforms a glial-promoting factor into a neural-promoting factor. These new data clearly highlight the importance of temporal regulation, as seen in the case of Olig proteins.

   glide orthologs have been identified in mammals: *gcma* and *gcmb* (Akiyama et al., 1996; Altshuller et al., 1996; Kammerer et al., 1999; Kanemura et al., 1999). Mutating *gcmb* results in defects in parathyroid development (Gunther et al., 2000); *gcma* knock-out mice display implantation defects (Anson-Cartwright et al., 2000; Schreiber et al., 2000). Interestingly, *gcma* but not *gcmb* rescues the fly *glide* phenotype (Kim et al., 1998; Reifegerste et al., 1999). Moreover, introduction of the fly gene into a medulloblastoma line induces the glial fate (Buzanska et al., 2001). Although it is possible that the two genes have gained novel functions during evolution, conditional and/or double knock-outs will be necessary to determine whether vertebrate orthologs have a role in glial differentiation. These studies will also reveal whether such orthologs play a role at specific times and/or in specific subsets of glia, since gain of function experiments suggest that *gcm* genes do not induce the Müller glia fate in the retina (Hojo et al., 2000).

2.3. Cell migration

   Cell migration is a hallmark of nervous system development. Indeed, neurons and glial cells of central and peripheral nervous system move extensively to reach their final destination. The interaction between the two cell types plays a pivotal role in such process.

2.3.1. Neuronal migration along radial glia

   Neuronal positioning is critical for the formation of cytoarchitecturally distinct brain regions such as cerebral cortex, hippocampus and cerebellum. During the development of laminated brain structures, a series of coordinated migrations takes neurons from their site of origin to their final destinations, where they adopt definitive morphological phenotypes by elaborating dendritic and axonal processes (Ramon y Cajal, 1911). Embryonic neuronal precursors in the ventricular zone move to other layers within the same brain region by radial migration or to other brain regions by tangential migration (Hatten, 1999). Radial migration is defined as neuronal movement perpendicular to the surface of the brain, whereas tangential migration describes neurons moving parallel to the surface of the brain. Radial migration, but not tangential migration, requires glial fibers. Around 80-90% of the billions of neuronal precursors in mammalian cortex migrate along glial fibers.

   Radial glial cells are a morphological, biochemically, and functionally distinct cell class characterized by an elongated fiber of an even caliber that early in development spans the entire cerebral wall from the ventricular to the pial surface. Radial glia are present only during neuronal development. Subsequently, they have been proposed to transform into astrocytes in the cerebral cortex and Bergmann glia in the cerebellum, however, more recent data indicate that such cells constitute the stem cell population (Hatten, 1999; Parnavelas and Nadarajah, 2001). Since 1970, it has been known that migrating post-mitotic neurons are in close apposition with radial glial cells (Rakic, 1972). Several lines of evidence from both *in vitro* and *in vivo* analyses indicate that contact interaction between radial fibers and migrating neurons plays a crucial role in the selection of the migratory pathway as well as in generating signals for displacement and migration arrest (Hatten, 1999).

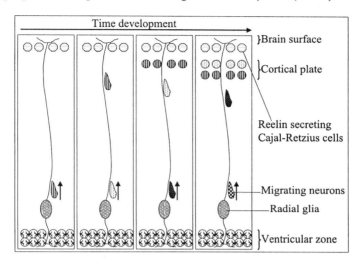

Figure 2.3. Neuronal migration along radial glia fibers. In early corticogenesis, cells proliferating in the ventricular zone undergo their last mitotic division and start to migrate to the brain periphery where the Cajal-Retzius cells are present and secrete Reelin. When neurons meet Reelin, they detach from radial glial fibers. Subsequently, the cortical plate forms by the arrival of newly generated neurons. Pattern coding is used to indicate subtypes of neurons migrating at different stages. In the cortical plate, cells are arranged in an inside-out pattern, where late-produced neurons (dots) migrate past early-produced neurons (vertical lines) and end up in more superficial layers.

Precursors of pyramidal neurons, the major projections neurons of cerebral cortex, are thought to move from the ventricular zone to the pia along radial glial fibers (Fig. 2.3). This primitive lamination of the neocortex proceeds in an inside-out pattern in that new cells take more superficial positions whereas old cells are positioned in deeper layers of the cortical plates (Rakic, 1988). During cerebellar development, two different neuronal precursors employ radial migration for their final destination. In the embryonic cerebellum, Purkinje cells, the principal output neurons, migrate along radial glial fibers towards the surface from the neuroepithelium of cerebellar primordium. In the post-natal cerebellum of rodents, cells in the external germinal layer migrate inwards along the fibers of Bergmann glia to form the internal granular layer (Yamada and Watanabe, 2002). Like in the cortex, this migratory behavior induces an inside-out pattern in the neuronal populations.

2.3.1.1. Role of the *reelin* gene in radial migration

A key insight into radial migration came from studies of *reeler* mice, one of the founding members of the behavioural mutants reported in the first database of mutations affecting the development of the CNS (Sidmand et al, 1965). These mice were recognized to exhibit widespread neuroanatomical defects in several structures of the brain and spinal cord. In the *reeler* cortex, the positions of neurons are inverted, such that the layers are generated in an outside-in manner. Moreover, the characteristic appearance of the radial glia scaffold is disturbed during late stages of corticogenesis, and radial fibers are deployed at oblique angles (Mikoshiba et al., 1983; Hunter-Schaedle, 1997). It was also shown that radial glia differentiate less extensively and disappear early in development, being replaced by astrocytes sooner that in normal cortex (Hunter-Schaedle, 1997).

The neuroanatomical disruptions in the *reeler* brain suggested that the mutation affected a gene that is critical for controlling cell positioning in the developing CNS. Recently, mutations in Reelin were also reported in humans displaying autosomal recessive lissencephaly and cerebral hypoplasia (Hong et al., 2000). Lissencephaly is a condition of severe neuronal migration alteration that results in a smooth appearance of the brain surface in humans. Thus, migration disorders result in similar misplacements of neurons in laminated brain regions in both mice and humans.

The gene disrupted in *reeler* mice encodes Reelin, a large extracellular protein (385 kDa) (D'Arcangelo et al., 1995). The N-terminal part shares similarity with F-spondin, a protein secreted by floor plate cells that directs neural crest cell migration and neurite outgrowth (Klar et al., 1992). The central part of Reelin consists of eight internal repeats of 350-390 amino acids. Theses domains are related to those found in extracellular proteins such as Tenascin and Restrictin and in the integrin family of receptors. Most Reelin is expressed in the Cajal-Retzius cells in the marginal zone of the neocortex and the cerebellum. It is secreted precisely at the location where neurons stop migrating and detach from radial glia. Therefore Reelin was suggested to provide positional information to migrating neurons that instructs them to stop and detach from their guides.

Reelin is able to bind two transmembrane receptors, the very low-density lipoprotein receptor (VLDLR) and the apolipoprotein E receptor 2 (ApoER2) present on migrating neurons (D'Arcangelo et al., 1999; Hiesberger et al., 1999). In the mouse cortex, VLDLR is selectively expressed in the migrating neurons that will make contact with Reelin in the marginal zone, consistent with a role of VLDLR as a receptor for a stop signal (Fig. 2.4). In contrast, ApoER2 is more ubiquitously expressed throughout the developing brain (Trommsdorff et al., 1999). Mice lacking either VLDLR or ApoER2 do not show abnormal phenotypes, but mice lacking both genes exhibit anatomical defects almost identical to those found in *reeler* mice (Trommsdorff et al., 1999). Taken together, these findings suggest that VLDLR and ApoER2 function in a coordinated and partially overlapping fashion. Binding of Reelin to these receptors induces an intracellular cascade that instructs neurons to occupy the proper location in the developing CNS.

Mice defective for the *scrambler* gene show a phenotype similar to that found in the *reeler* mutants (Goldowitz et al., 1997). *scrambler* corresponds to the *disabled* (Dab-1) gene encoding a tyrosine phosphorylated cytoplasmic protein that can bind the intracellular region of VLDLR and ApoER2 (Trommsdorff et al., 1999). Dab-1 is expressed in the Reelin responsive cortical plate neurons as well as in the Purkinje cells, with a pattern similar to those of VLDLR and ApoER2. Moreover, tyrosine phosphorylation of Dab-1 is increased by extracellular application of Reelin and the level of basal tyrosine phosphorylation in *reeler* mice is lower than in wild type mice (Howell et al., 1999). Mutations in the phosphorylation sites of Dab-1 cause ataxia and abnormalities in cell positioning in the cerebral and cerebellar cortices (Howell et al., 2000). There is thus strong evidence to support a pathway from the secreted protein Reelin to the transmembrane receptors VLDLR and ApoER2 to Dab-1 phosphorylation (Fig. 2.4). Other genes have been implicated in the Reelin pathway, although their role is not fully understood (Rice and Curran, 2001).

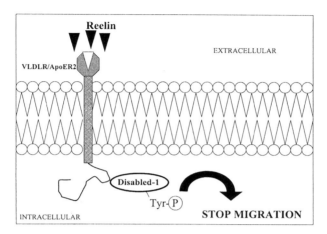

Figure 2.4. Mode of action of Reelin. Reelin is able to bind two transmembrane receptors, the very low-density lipoprotein receptor (VLDLR) and the apolipoprotein E receptor 2 (ApoER2), both present on migrating neurons. After receptor activation, the cytoplasmic protein Disabled-1 is phosphorylated on a tyrosine residue leading to the activation of an intracellular cascade. Then, neurons stop migrating and detach from the radial glial fibers to occupy their final place in the brain.

2.3.2. Glial migration

One of the major functions of vertebrate glia is to myelinate axons, which is successfully achieved in central and peripheral nervous systems upon glial migration. This complex and timed process requires glial cells to initiate migration, to find the direction of movement and to stop migrating as cells reach the final destination. This entails several steps: changes in cell adhesion, reorganization in the actin cytoskeleton and cell polarization. *In vitro* and *in vivo* studies have identified cell adhesion as well as secreted molecules (chemoattractants and chemorepellents) as migratory cues. Most molecules are expressed in neurons and/or astrocytes, underscoring the importance of neuron-glia interactions during development. The intracellular pathway responding to the external cues starts being elucidated and seems to require the same molecules that control axonal growth and navigation.

The study of a dynamic process such as migration has been often limited by two factors. On one side, most commonly used techniques for labelling cell types rely on the fixation of samples, on the other, real time analyses have been realised in cell culture and/or in slice tissues, due to nervous system complexity. The recent development of green fluorescent protein (GFP) based tools has opened new perspectives in the analysis of dynamic processes in real time and in whole animals. This non invasive approach will certainly shed new and important insights in the field of glial migration.

2.3.2.1. Oligodendrocyte migration

The optic nerve constitutes a relatively simple system for studying vertebrate glial migration, since it only contains axons and glial cells. Oligodendrocyte precursors (OLPs) originate within the brain and migrate along the optic nerve in a chiasmal-to-retinal direction. Optic nerve explant and cell culture studies have shown a role of secreted molecules such as semaphorins and netrins as guidance cues for OLP migration (Sugimoto et al., 2001; Spassky et al., 2002). The expression profile of these molecules is consistent with their role as ligands in the migration of OLPs. These chemotactic factors also control axonal guidance by attracting or repelling growth cones, suggesting a common path in guiding axons and glia.

2.3.2.2. Migration in the zebrafish lateral line

The group of Nüsslein-Volhard has realised a developmental analysis of axon-glia interactions in living zebrafish (Gilmour et al., 2002). Glial cells associated with the sensory system called lateral line migrate along the sensory axon bundle in a rostral to caudal manner. By laser ablation, genetic manipulations and time-lapse analysis, they have shown that glial cells require axons to migrate (Gilmour et al., 2002). High-resolution movies of glia and axons during fish development demonstrate that glial cells never go ahead of axons during development. Moreover, in mutants that show an abnormal migration of the nerve, (*sonic you, you-too, fused somites*) glial cells follow the abnormal nerve trajectory. Finally, laser ablation of the neuronal cell bodies that send those axons indeed leads to nerve degeneration and to glial stalling.

2.3.2.3. Glial migration in the fly PNS

The fly eye develops from an epithelial group of cells called eye imaginal disc. Photoreceptors (R) differentiate within the disc in a posterior-to-anterior progression and send axons towards the first visual ganglion, the lamina, which is part of the optic lobe. Retinal basal glia or subretinal glia differentiate within the optic lobe and then move into the disc using the optic stalk (Choi and Benzer, 1994; Rangarajan et al., 1999). Glial migration does not require photoreceptor axons as substratum (Rangarajan et al., 1999). In fact, it precedes the differentiation of such axons and is necessary to direct them towards the lamina. Once in the disc, subretinal glial cells migrate anteriorly onto the basal surface of the eye epithelium until they reach the front of photoreceptor differentiation, there they migrate in response to signals coming from the environment. The Gilgamesh casein kinase, which stops migration, is expressed in the eye epithelium (Hummel et al., 2002) and seems to control *hedgehog*, which has also been shown to affect glial migration (Rangarajan et al., 2001) (Fig. 2.5). Although these data strongly suggest that subretinal glia are guided by chemoattractants and/or repellents, it will be interesting to determine whether such cells send far reaching extensions that contact the differentiating photoreceptors.

Wing glial cells arise from sensory organ lineages, each lineage producing a glial precursor endowed with limited proliferative potential (Van De Bor et al., 2000). Such glial precursor migrates as it proliferates, its progeny following the direction taken by the growing axon (Giangrande et al., 1993). As in the zebrafish lateral line, glial cells are never seen ahead of axons (Fig. 2.5), in addition, mutants in which axons stop navigating also show glial migration arrest. Finally, mutants in which axons take ectopic directions are covered by glial cells. All these data suggest that wing glia use axons as a migratory substratum.

The different glial migratory behaviours observed so far underscore the diversity of developmental strategies used in time and space to make cells reach their final destination. Combined with the genetic approach, real time analyses will be instrumental in unravelling the molecular and cellular mechanisms underlying glial migration. This will also help us understanding the rational for using specific cues.

2.4. Axon guidance

After neuronal differentiation, polarized extensions grow towards specific targets by using distinct cellular and molecular cues. In many cases, glial cells provide such cues that allow axons to orient their growth and/or to select the appropriate target.

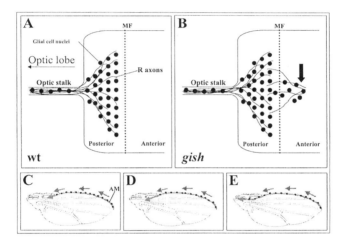

Figure 2.5. Migration in the fly PNS. In the wild-type eye disc, photoreceptor axons project posteriorly away from the morphogenetic furrow (MF) into the optic stalk and then into the optic lobe (A). In *gilgamesh* (*gish*) mutant eye discs, glial cells are abnormally present anteriorly to the MF (B) in comparison with the wild-type (A). In these discs, photoreceptor axons go in the opposite direction, crossing the MF under the influence of glial cells (see arrow in B). During wing development, sensory neurons located along the anterior margin (AM) send axons that fasciculate into a single nerve (green in C-E), navigate proximally and find targets in the CNS. Glial cells (red ovals indicate the glial nuclei) follow the nerve and migrate in the same direction (blue arrows). No glial nucleus is ever found proximal to nerve terminals while axons are still navigating.

2.4.1. Evolutionary conservation at the midline

Bilaterally symmetric animals are able to transmit information between the left and the right sides of their body to integrate sensory input and to coordinate motor output. Thus, many neurons in the CNS project so-called commissural axons across the midline. Interestingly, these axons are never observed to recross the midline. On the other hand, some neurons project axons that remain on the ipsilateral side of the CNS, without ever crossing the midline. Several studies demonstrate that specialized cells that reside at the ventral midline of the developing vertebrate spinal cord and Drosophila ventral nerve cord play critical roles in regulating the guidance of both crossing and non-crossing axons. Work over the past several years has demonstrated that many, if not most, of the fly navigational cues are provided by glia and their precursors. The molecular mechanisms that control midline guidance appear to be evolutionarily conserved (Kaprielian et al., 2000).

2.4.1.1. Guidance at the Drosophila midline

In the ventral nerve cord of Drosophila, some neurons stay along the ipsilateral longitudinal connectives whereas others cross the midline in one of two distinct tracts, the anterior or the posterior commissure, turn orthogonally and project into one of the longitudinal connectives (Fig. 2.6A). A set of glial cells pioneer and then populate the CNS midline (Granderath and Klambt, 1999). These midline glia (MG) and their processes constitute the cellular environment that commissural axons encounter as they make their way from one side of the ventral nerve cord to the other. Genetic and biochemical experiments suggest that two dual-function secreted cues are especially important to this process-netrin (Serafini et al., 1994; Mitchell et al., 1996) and slit (Rothberg et al., 1990; Kidd et al., 1999). Both of these cues are the products of MG (Rothberg et al., 1990; Mitchell et al., 1996; Hummel et al., 1999).

Netrins are required for the guidance of commissural growth cones to the midline of the developing Drosophila CNS. During the initial period of commissure formation, midline cells express two netrins: netrin-A and netrin-B (Harris et al., 1996; Mitchell et al., 1996). Later, these two genes are expressed only in MG cells. In netrin-A/netrin-B double mutant embryos, commissures are thin or completely absent (Harris et al., 1996; Mitchell et al., 1996). This phenotype is rescued when either Netrin-A or B is expressed in MG, indicating that the localized glial expression of netrins at the midline is important for correct axon guidance. Such chemoattractive activity for Netrins is in agreement with vertebrate data (see below and Chisholm and Tessier-Lavigne, 1999). frazzled, a gene encoding the netrin receptor (Kolodziej et al., 1996), is expressed in central and in peripheral axons. The phenotypes of frazzled mutant embryos strongly resemble those of the netrin-A/netrin-B double mutant embryos and can be rescued by expressing frazzled specifically in neurons (Kolodziej et al., 1996). Attraction by Netrins is essential for at least some commissural axons to grow across the midline, but does not appear to dictate the choice of a contralateral versus ipsilateral pathway.

slit was initially identified in a large scale screen for mutants affecting midline crossing. In slit mutant embryos, both ipsilateral and commissural axons enter the midline but never leave it, resulting in a collapsed commissure phenotype (Rothberg et al., 1990; Battye et al., 1999; Kidd et al., 1999) (Fig. 2.6B). Slit is a large extracellular matrix protein that is secreted by midline glial cells and found associated with the surface of axons (Rothberg et al., 1990). The screen also led to the identification of roundabout (robo) and commissureless (comm), which show opposite phenotypes, namely multiple midline crossing (Seeger et al., 1993) and no crossing at all, respectively (Fig. 2.6C,D).

Slit repels axons that express Robo. Repulsion prevents ipsilaterally projecting axons from entering the midline and contralaterally projecting axons from re-entering the midline once they have crossed it (Kidd et al., 1998). Three Robo proteins have recently been identified in *Drosophila*. While *Robo1* mutations display the typical multiple midline crossing phenotype, loss of the three products mimics the commissure-collapsed phenotype observed in *slit* embryos (Fig. 2.6D). This result and the expression profile of the three proteins indicate overlapping functions in the establishment of proper guidance at the midline (Rajagopalan et al., 2000). *Robo1, 2* and *3* encode proteins belonging to the Ig-CAM family (Kidd et al., 1998). Axons extending toward or across the midline express very low levels of Robo proteins (Fig 2.6F). In contrast, crossed segments of commissural axons as well as ipsilaterally projecting axons express high levels of Robo proteins (Fig. 2.6E,G). This permits to suggest that Robo proteins normally prevent midline crossing and function as receptors for the Slit inhibitory ligand localized to the midline (Brose et al., 1999; Kidd et al., 1999).

The transmembrane protein Commissureless is normally required for axons to cross the midline and behaves as a powerful negative regulator of Robo proteins (Tear et al., 1996; Kidd et al., 1998). Overexpression of *comm* in neurons leads to a decrease in the level of Robo 1 and phenocopies the *robo 1* phenotype (Kidd et al., 1998). Moreover, in *comm* embryos, the levels of Robo1 are increased (Kidd et al., 1998). The groups of Tear and Dickson have shown that Comm function is required in CNS neurons for Robo axon targeting (Georgiou and Tear, 2002; Keleman et al., 2002). Moreover, they demonstrate that Comm is expressed in contralaterally but not ipsilaterally projecting neurons and that its expression is temporally regulated. *comm* mRNA is detected in contralaterally projecting neurons for a short time, while their axons cross the midline. Axon guidance at the CNS midline is thus controlled by the levels of Robo, which in turn depends on the precisely regulated expression of Comm (Keleman et al., 2002).

Tissue culture experiments have shown that coexpression of Comm and Robo alters Robo's subcellular localization. In the absence of Comm, Robo protein accumulates at the cell surface (Fig. 2.6H); however, when both proteins are present, Robo colocalizes with Comm to intracellular compartments, which are probably late endosomes (Fig. 2.6I). Moreover, Comm needs to interact with Robo to affect Robo's localization (Keleman et al., 2002). These findings suggest that Comm prevents Robo from reaching the cell surface by binding and targeting it directly to endosomes.

How does Comm alter Robo trafficking? The Comm protein contains a LPSY motif that is necessary for protein endosomal sorting (Keleman et al., 2002). This motif is the one recognized and ubiquitinated by the ubiquitin-protein ligase DNedd4 (Myat et al., 2002). Mutagenizing the LPSY motif perturbs Comm/DNedd4 interaction thereby interfering with Comm regulation of Robo localization. Moreover, such mutation also interferes with Comm gain of function activity at the midline.

One model suggested by these findings is that ubiquitination of Comm by DNedd4 allows Comm to sequester Robo protein away from the cell surface by directing Robo from the Golgi to the endosomes (Fig. 2.6I). Therefore, changes in axonal sensitivity to external cues during pathfinding across the midline make use of ubiquitin-dependent mechanisms to regulate transmembrane protein levels.

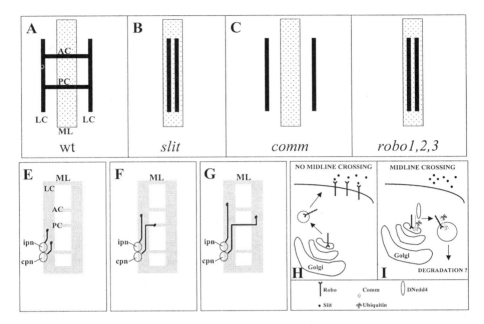

Figure 2.6. Role of the *slit-robo-comm* pathway in axon guidance at the fly midline. In wild-type embryos, the ventral cord displays two longitudinal connectives (LC) running parallel on each side of the midline (ML), an asymmetric structure that is crossed by the anterior and the posterior commissures (AC and PC, respectively). In *slit* embryos, all axons enter the midline but never leave it, resulting in a collapsed commissure phenotype (B). An opposite phenotype is seen in *comm* embryos in which axons never cross the midline (C). *robo1,2,3* triple mutant embryos show the same phenotype as that observed in *slit* embryos, i.e., collapsed commissures (D). Initially, both growth cones of ipsilateral (ipn) and contralateral (cpn) axons express Robo (in red) (E). Comm is specifically expressed in the cpn while they are crossing the midline. This results in a loss of Robo at the cpn growth cone membrane (F). Once cpn axons have crossed the midline, Comm expression is downregulated and Robo is present again at the cpn growth cone membrane (G). This allows repulsion by Slit, which prevents a new cross. The ipn axon never expresses Comm and never crosses the midline (E-G). Neurons only expressing Robo (ipn and cpn after midline crossing), accumulate it at the membrane. Axons can then respond to the Slit repellent signal and do not cross the midline (H). Neurons expressing Comm and Robo do not accumulate Robo at the membrane. Axons are unable to respond to Slit and cross the midline (I). In these axons, Slit/Robo signaling is blocked by a mechanism involving ubiquitination of Comm by DNedd4. This ubiquitination step facilitates the sorting of Comm and Robo in late endosomes (I). Once cpn has crossed the midline, Comm expression is downregulated and Robo is present again at the membrane.

2.4.1.2. Guidance at the vertebrate midline

During early stages of spinal cord development, two classes of interneurons can be distinguished based on whether or not their axons cross the midline. Commissural interneurons located at dorsolateral positions on either side of the spinal cord extend axons that project ventrally toward the floor plate (Colamarino and Tessier-Lavigne, 1995). After reaching the ventral midline, commissural axons cross through the ventral most third of the floor plate (Bovolenta and Dodd, 1990). At the contralateral margin of the floor plate, most of these axons turn orthogonally and project within longitudinally oriented ventral axon bundle adjacent to the floor plate (Colamarino and Tessier-Lavigne, 1995). These axons do not recross the midline and could be compared to the commissure axonal pathway of *Drosophila*.

Association interneurons, a second early developing population of dorsolaterally positioned spinal neurons, also extend axons towards the floor plate. However, before encountering the floor plate, these axons extend parallel to the ventral midline along the ipsilaterraly projecting lateral axon bundle (Colamarino and Tessier-Lavigne, 1995). These axon tracts are similar to the longitudinal connectives of *Drosophila*.

The floor plate expresses axonal chemoattractants and is required for commissural axons to cross the midline and to properly execute subsequent guidance decisions. These findings indicate that vertebrate floor plate and *Drosophila* midline might be considered equivalent structures. Indeed, netrins are floor plate-derived molecules and *deleted in colorectal cancer* (DCC), the vertebrate ortholog of the *frazzled* receptor, is present on commissural axons (Serafini et al., 1994; Keino-Masu et al., 1996). Loss of Netrin1 (Serafini et al., 1996) or DCC (Fazeli et al., 1997) in mice results in aberrant commissural axon pathfinding. Actually, the glial or neuronal origin of Netrin1 is not known.

As in invertebrates, proper pathfinding at the midline requires that growth cones integrate both positive and negative environmental guidance cues. Mammalian orthologs of Robo and Slit have been identified, their expression profiles being consistent with a guidance role (Brose and Tessier-Lavigne, 2000). *In vitro* studies have shown that rodent Slit proteins can repel axons, as well as migrating neurons (Brose et al., 1999; Hu, 1999; Li et al., 1999; Nguyen Ba-Charvet et al., 1999; Wu et al., 1999; Ringstedt et al., 2000; Chen et al., 2001; Shu and Richards, 2001). Tessier-Lavigne and collaborators have generated mice deficient in two of the three mouse *slit* genes (*slit1* and *slit2*) and found striking defects in several major CNS tracts in the forebrain (Bagri et al., 2002) and also during development of the visual system (Plump et al., 2002). In the forebrain, *robo1, robo2, slit1* and *slit2* mRNAs expression correlates with the development of cortical and thalamic projections (Bagri et al., 2002). *slit1/slit2* double mutant mice show abnormal midline crossing in several pathways (Bagri et al., 2002; Plump et al., 2002) making it likely that a Robo/Slit based repulsive guidance system regulates midline crossing in the developing spinal cord. However, the apparent absence of a clear *commissureless* ortholog suggests that comm-facilitated down-regulation of Robo expression on midline crossing axons may not be required in mammals (Tear et al., 1996; Kidd et al., 1998).

2.4.2. Drosophila eye development: *nonstop* and photoreceptor axon targeting

Once axons have navigated through permissive or repulsive environment, they must establish their correct synaptic contacts. The visual system of *Drosophila melanogaster* provides a powerful genetic system to analyse the cellular and molecular mechanisms regulating axon target selection. Using the developing *Drosophila* compound eye model, Zipursky and collaborators have shown that glial cells play a vital role in target layer selection of retinal axons (Poeck et al., 2001).

The *Drosophila* compound eye comprises around 800 ommatidia, each containing eight photoreceptors (R) belonging to two subgroups: six outer R cells (R1-R6) and two inner R cells (R7, R8). The eight axons of each ommatidium project together as a fascicle in a topographic fashion into one of the brain lobes. In the fly visual system, each R subgroup projects to a different synaptic layer into the brain. R1-R6 axons stop in the lamina, while R7 and R8 axons pass the lamina and stop in the medulla. The growth cones of R1-R6 terminate in the lamina between two distinct glial cell layers, the epithelial and the marginal glial cells. A third glial cell sheath provided by the medulla glial cells is found deeper in the brain demarcating the boundary between the lamina and the medulla. Growth cones of R1-R6 pause between the epithelial and the marginal glial cell layers for about four days before they start to form synaptic connections with specific lamina neurons.

Recently, the Zipursky laboratory has identified a gene called *nonstop*, encoding an ubiquitin-specific protease required in glial cells for correct axon guidance. In *nonstop* mutants, the outer R axons do not stop their growth in the lamina but instead continue to advance into the medulla (Poeck et al., 2001) (Fig. 2.7). Moreover, they have shown that the development of the epithelial, marginal and medulla glial cells is severely affected, leading to a strong reduction of the cell number. Finally, they have shown that loss of glial cells but not of neurons at an early stage of lamina development results in R1-R6 mistargeting. Therefore, the presence of glial cells is necessary to inform the growth cones about their final targets. This example is a good illustration of the neuron-glia interactions that are necessary to establish a precise and correct organisation of the neural network that composes the nervous system.

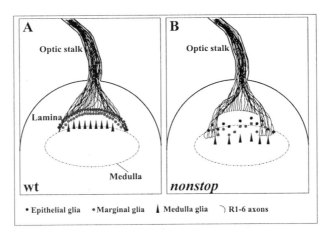

Figure 2.7. Role of glia in fly axons target selection. In the wild-type larval optic lobe, R1-6 axons terminate into the lamina, between the epithelial and the marginal glia (A). In *nonstop* mutants, epithelial, marginal and medulla glial cells fail to develop normally and are reduced in number. As a consequence, many R1-6 axons fail to terminate into the lamina and project into the medulla (B). Axons in the center of the projection field frequently stop within the lamina (B).

2.5. Nerve regeneration

Axonal regeneration is one of the clearest examples of the specificity of glial-neuronal interactions. In fact, axonal growth after wounding strictly depends on the glial environment (e.g. CNS vs. PNS).

It is well known that PNS axons are able to regenerate whereas axons of the adult mammalian CNS are capable of only a limited amount of regrowth after injury. Why do the axons of the mature mammalian PNS regenerate after injury while CNS axons do not? The main obstacles to regeneration are considered to be damaged myelin and subsequent exposure to myelin-associated inhibitors along with formation of the glial scar (for a review see Fawcett and Asher, 1999). Indeed neutralising at least some myelin inhibitors leads to improved growth in the CNS. A number of individual proteins that inhibit axon growth have been identified: myelin-associated glycoprotein (MAG), Nogo, and, most recently, oligodendrocyte-myelin glycoprotein (OMgp) (Kottis et al., 2002; Wang et al., 2002b) (Fig. 2.8). Although distinct in molecular structure, these proteins share a number of common attributes, including their expression and localization in the myelin membrane directly adjacent to the axon.

In the PNS, only MAG seems to be expressed. Moreover, regeneration takes place only after myelin debris have been cleared (a process called Wallerian degeneration) and Schwann cells have reverted to a non myelinating phenotype, when they downregulate expression of some myelin proteins (Fawcett and Keynes, 1990).

2.5.1. Role of NOGO, MAG and OMgp in growth inhibition

Myelin-associated glycoprotein (MAG) is present in the CNS and in the PNS (Tang et al., 1997). The Filbin group has shown that CHO cells transfected with MAG inhibit neurite growth from both developing cerebellar and adult dorsal root ganglion (DRG) neurons. The finding of a MAG proteolytic product supports the hypothesis that MAG works as an extracellular ligand (Mukhopadhyay et al., 1994). To study the function of MAG *in vivo* during development and regeneration after injury, MAG-deficient mice have been generated (Li et al., 1994; Montag et al., 1994). In these mutant mice, essentially normal myelin is formed. These mutant mice display only a rather small increase in axon regeneration in the CNS, although there is enhanced regeneration in peripheral nerves (Fitch and Silver, 1997; Schafer et al., 1996).This indicates the complexity of action of MAG, and also the presence of many inhibitory molecules in the injured CNS in comparison with the PNS. However, mutant mice older than 8 months revealed extensive PNS demyelination and axonal regeneration, suggesting that MAG is required for the maintenance of a stable myelin/axon interface (Fruttiger et al., 1995). Taken together, these results demonstrate the inhibitory activity of MAG during axon regeneration.

The Nogo gene produces three different splice variants, one of which, NogoA, is specifically expressed in the CNS. NogoA is present on the cell surface of OLs and has two functional domains: Nogo66 and Amino-Nogo. Nogo66 contains the extracellular loop region, while Amino-Nogo contains the N-terminal domain. While Nogo66 specifically contributes to myelin-derived inhibition of neurite growth, the Amino-Nogo fragment inhibits spreading and migration of non-neuronal cells, as well as neurite growth (Fournier et al., 2001).

OMgp is the most recently identified of the inhibitory components of myelin (Kottis et al., 2002; Wang et al., 2002b). OMgp was found to be highly enriched in Phospholipase C-released fractions of myelin and shown to have potent growth cone collapsing and neurite outgrowth inhibitory activities.

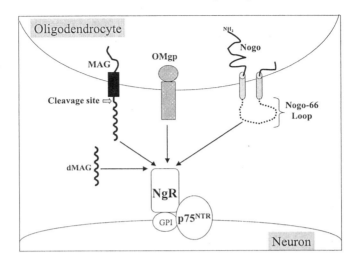

Figure 2.8. Inhibitors of axonal regeneration. Myelin-associated protein (MAG), oligodendrocyte-myelin glycoprotein (OMgp) and Nogo66 are ligands for the Nogo66 receptor (NgR) that is localized to the membrane via a glycosylphosphatidylinositol (GPI) linkage. MAG, OMgp and Nogo66 are expressed by oligodendrocytes and bind neuronal NgR. These ligands do not present any homology amongst them. Only the Nogo66 region of NogoA binds NgR (Nogo66 loop). The p75 neurotrophin receptor (p75NTR) interacts with NgR and represents a coreceptor of NgR for MAG, OMgp and Nogo signaling. dMAG constitutes an extracellular product arising from proteolytic cleavage (arrow) in the MAG protein.

All three proteins (MAG, Nogo and OMgp) have a similar distribution in the myelin sheath, suggesting that all contribute to growth inhibition in the adult CNS. The ability of these proteins to affect axonal growth implies that a signal is transduced to the neuron and that these proteins behave as ligands. The Strittmatter group followed up on the initial cloning of Nogo to identify the receptor for the Nogo66 domain, using an expression cloning strategy to isolate binding proteins. A single receptor, NgR, was identified and found to encode a protein that is associated with the cell membrane by a glycosylphosphatidylinositol (GPI) linkage (Fournier et al., 2001). Mutated forms of the receptor eliminated growth inhibition by Nogo66, supporting its importance as a receptor for Nogo. NgR is highly expressed in brain, and *in situ* hybridization experiments show that NgR is predominantly expressed by neurons (Fournier et al., 2001). The NgR is also able to bind and mediate the inhibitory activities of Nogo66 (Fournier et al., 2001), OMgp (Wang et al., 2002a) and MAG (Domeniconi et al., 2002; Liu et al., 2002).

The GPI anchored nature of NgR indicates the requirement for additional transmembrane proteins to transduce the inhibitory signals into the neurons. Recently, it was shown that the p75 neurotrophin receptor (p75NTR) interacts with NgR and corresponds to a coreceptor of NgR for MAG, Nogo and OMgp signalling (Wang et al., 2002a; Wong et al., 2002). Using a neurite outgrowth assay, He and collaborators have shown that neurons from p75NTR mutant mice are insensitive to the inhibition of CNS myelin supporting the idea that MAG, Nogo and OMgp account for most of the inhibitory activities associated with CNS myelin (Wang et al., 2002a). Thus, playing with NgR- p75^{NTR} signalling after CNS axonal injury may help to block the myelin-dependent inhibition of axonal regeneration.

2.6. Cell death

The acquisition and the maintenance of the appropriate cell number are often controlled at the level of cell death. Glial-neuronal interactions are pivotal for the homeostasis of the nervous system by controlling glial and neuronal survival. The intimacy of such interactions is demonstrated by the finding that neurons send signal that control glial cell number and glial cells send signals that control neuronal cell number.

2.6.1. Neuronal control of glial survival: neurotrophins and the EGF pathway

The axonal-derived Neuregulin-1 (NRG-1), a member of the Early Growth Factor (EGF) family, acts as a survival-promoting factor on Schwann cells in the mammalian nervous system (Garratt et al., 2000). Indeed, NRG-1 is one of the most important trophins that central and peripheral neurons provide to Schwann cells, the glial cells of peripheral nerves and ganglia. Multiple isoforms of NRG-1, some transmembrane and some secreted, are generated by alternative splicing; these are produced by many types of neurons, including motor, sensory, and sympathetic neurons, very soon after they are born (Marchionni et al., 1993; Corfas et al., 1995; Falls, 2003). NRG-1 proteins are then transported down the length of axons, where they are presented to axon-associated Schwann cells and to peripheral targets, including muscles (Yang et al., 1998). NRG-1 signaling is transduced through the cell surface receptors ErbB2, ErbB3, and ErbB4, which are structurally and functionally related to the EGF receptor (Carraway et al., 1994; Lemke, 1996; Burden and Yarden, 1997).

Recently, two different members of the EGF family were shown to function as gliatrophins in *Drosophila*. Indeed, two distinct groups have shown that the neuregulin homolog Vein maintains survival of a subpopulation of longitudinal glia (Hidalgo et al., 2001), while the TGFα homolog Spitz maintains survival of midline glia (Bergmann et al., 2002). In both cases, the trophic ligands are secreted by adjacent axons at concentrations sufficient for the survival of only a subset of the target glial population.

Fly longitudinal glia (LG) move medially after their birth to contact the pioneering axons of the longitudinal fascicles and then migrate together with the growth cones, eventually extending on and ensheathing the longitudinal nerve tracts. Longitudinal glial cells are produced in excess before axon-glia contact is established and apoptosis is visible in not connected cells just after contact is established. The authors have shown that apoptosis of LG is increased in *vein* mutant embryos, suggesting that this gene is able to control glial cell death (Hidalgo et al., 2001). To test this hypothesis, the authors use the neuronally targeted RNAi to specifically inhibit Vein synthesis in the pioneer axons. A loss of LG is observed in this case. Moreover, a dominant-negative DER (Drosophila EGF Receptor) expressed by glial cells is also able to increase apoptosis. Finally, expression of a Vein transgene in pioneer neurons rescues the glial cell death phenotype. In conclusion, Vein is secreted by neurons to provide trophic support required by glial cells. In *vein/spitz* double mutant embryos, there is an increase of LG loss suggesting that additional factors contribute to glial survival.

The midline glia (MG) undergoes important cell death during development. MG survival is directly correlated with MAP kinase (MAPK) activity levels and requires direct phosphorylation of the pro-apoptotic protein Hid by MAPK (Bergmann et al., 2002). Expression of the dominant-negative DER in MG increases the amount of cell death. Similar results were obtained in *spitz* mutant embryos showing that the Spitz/DER pathway is involved in MG survival. This cell death can be rescued after expression of Spitz in neurons but not in MG. Moreover, overexpression of activated Spitz leads to rescue of additional MG, indicating that physiological levels of Spitz are limiting, as one would expect from a trophic factor. All these results show that neurons provide signals for glia survival (Bergmann et al., 2002). In *spitz/hid* double mutant embryos, there is also a decrease of apoptosis, suggesting that MG survival is regulated by Spitz signal that suppresses Hid. To summarise, a cascade from the extracellular ligand Spitz, through cell surface EGFR and the ras/MAPK pathway suppresses a default death pathway dependent on Hid to regulate the death of MG cells during development (Bergmann et al., 2002).

2.6.2. Glial control of neuronal survival: *dropdead, repo, swisscheese*

Like in mammals, insect neurons are dependent upon glial extrinsic trophic support for survival. Since many years, it was suggested that glial-neuronal interactions are necessary for neuronal survival during *Drosophila* development (Buchanan and Benzer, 1993; Xiong and Montell, 1995). The *repo* gene is expressed and required in all fly glial cells (Halter et al., 1995). In flies homozygous for a viable allele of *repo*, neurodegeneration is observed in the eye, showing that alteration of glial cell function leads to neuronal death (Xiong and Montell, 1995). Similar results were described in other glia-affecting mutants like *drop-dead* or *swiss-cheese* (Buchanan and Benzer, 1993; Kretzschmar et al., 1997). These two genes are expressed by glial cells and in homozygous mutant flies for each of these genes, glial cell differentiate abnormally leading to important neuronal death. Finally, when almost all glia are missing in *glide/gcm* embryos, important neuronal apoptosis occurs during development (Hosoya et al., 1995; Jones et al., 1995; Vincent et al., 1996). Taken together, this implies that glial cell function is required for neuronal survival during development and at adult stage.

2.7. Concluding remarks

The nervous system represents the most complex tissue in our organism. The sophisticated network of neurons and glia generated by the stem cells allows us to respond and adapt to the numerous internal and external stimuli we constantly encounter during life. Although neurons and glia have very distinct roles, it is clear from past and recent results that their development, function and survival are tightly linked via cell interactions that use multiple molecular pathways. These symbiotic interactions require fine tuning and constant readjustments to accommodate the plastic requirements of the nervous system.

The challenge for the next generations of neurobiologists will be to devise non invasive approaches to characterize such interactions and to understand their specificity in time and space.

A better knowledge of such interactions has a twofold goal. It will allow us to understand how complex tissues are built during development and preserved during ontogenesis. In the long term, it will also likely have therapeutical implications in repair strategies after brain damage or in demyelinating diseases. For example, the identification of factors controlling neuron-glia interactions could be used to guide endogenously generated or transplanted cells at the site of demyelination.

Acknowledgements. Work in the laboratory was supported by the Institut National de la Santé et de la Recherche Médicale, the Centre National de la Recherche Scientifique, the Hôpital Universitaire de Strasbourg, the Association pour la Recherche contre le Cancer and by EEC grant (Contract QLG3-CT-2000-01224). LS was supported by an ARC fellowship.

2.8. References

Akiyama Y, Hosoya T, Poole AM, Hotta Y (1996) The gcm-motif: a novel DNA-binding motif conserved in Drosophila and mammals. Proc Natl Acad Sci U S a 93:14912-14916.

Akiyama-Oda Y, Hosoya T, Hotta Y (1998) Alteration of cell fate by ectopic expression of Drosophila glial cells missing in non-neural cells. Dev Genes Evol 208:578-585.

Alfonso TB, Jones BW (2002) gcm2 promotes glial cell differentiation and is required with glial cells missing for macrophage development in Drosophila. Dev Biol 248:369-383.

Altshuller Y, Copeland NG, Gilbert DJ, Jenkins NA, Frohman MA (1996) Gcm1, a mammalian homolog of Drosophila glial cells missing. FEBS Lett 393:201-204.

Anson-Cartwright L, Dawson K, Holmyard D, Fisher SJ, Lazzarini RA, Cross JC (2000) The glial cells missing-1 protein is essential for branching morphogenesis in the chorioallantoic placenta. Nat Genet 25:311-314.

Bagri A, Marin O, Plump AS, Mak J, Pleasure SJ, Rubenstein JL, Tessier-Lavigne M (2002) Slit proteins prevent midline crossing and determine the dorsoventral position of major axonal pathways in the mammalian forebrain. Neuron 33:233-248.

Bao ZZ, Cepko CL (1997) The expression and function of Notch pathway genes in the developing rat eye. J Neurosci 17:1425-1434.

Battye R, Stevens A, Jacobs JR (1999) Axon repulsion from the midline of the Drosophila CNS requires slit function. Development 126:2475-2481.

Beatus P, Lendahl U (1998) Notch and neurogenesis. J Neurosci Res 54:125-136.

Bergmann A, Tugentman M, Shilo BZ, Steller H (2002) Regulation of cell number by MAPK-dependent control of apoptosis: a mechanism for trophic survival signaling. Dev Cell 2:159-170.

Bernardoni R, Miller AA, Giangrande A (1998) Glial differentiation does not require a neural ground state. Development 125:3189-3200.

Bovolenta P, Dodd J (1990) Guidance of commissural growth cones at the floor plate in embryonic rat spinal cord. Development 109:435-447.

Brose K, Tessier-Lavigne M (2000) Slit proteins: key regulators of axon guidance, axonal branching, and cell migration. Curr Opin Neurobiol 10:95-102.

Brose K, Bland KS, Wang KH, Arnott D, Henzel W, Goodman CS, Tessier-Lavigne M, Kidd T (1999) Slit proteins bind Robo receptors and have an evolutionarily conserved role in repulsive axon guidance. Cell 96:795-806.

Buchanan RL, Benzer S (1993) Defective glia in the Drosophila brain degeneration mutant drop-dead. Neuron 10:839-850.

Burden S, Yarden Y (1997) Neuregulins and their receptors: a versatile signaling module in organogenesis and oncogenesis. Neuron 18:847-855.

Buzanska L, Spassky N, Belin MF, Giangrande A, Guillemot F, Klambt C, Labouesse M, Thomas JL, Domanska-Janik K, Zalc B (2001) Human medulloblastoma cell line DEV is a potent tool to screen for factors influencing differentiation of neural stem cells. J Neurosci Res 65:17-23.

Carraway KL, 3rd, Sliwkowski MX, Akita R, Platko JV, Guy PM, Nuijens A, Diamonti AJ, Vandlen RL, Cantley LC, Cerione RA (1994) The erbB3 gene product is a receptor for heregulin. J Biol Chem 269:14303-14306.

Chen JH, Wen L, Dupuis S, Wu JY, Rao Y (2001) The N-terminal leucine-rich regions in Slit are sufficient to repel olfactory bulb axons and subventricular zone neurons. J Neurosci 21:1548-1556.

Chisholm A, Tessier-Lavigne M (1999) Conservation and divergence of axon guidance mechanisms. Curr Opin Neurobiol 9:603-615.

Choi KW, Benzer S (1994) Migration of glia along photoreceptor axons in the developing Drosophila eye. Neuron 12:423-431.

Colamarino SA, Tessier-Lavigne M (1995) The role of the floor plate in axon guidance. Annu Rev Neurosci 18:497-529.

Corfas G, Rosen KM, Aratake H, Krauss R, Fischbach GD (1995) Differential expression of ARIA isoforms in the rat brain. Neuron 14:103-115.

D'Arcangelo G, Miao GG, Chen SC, Soares HD, Morgan JI, Curran T (1995) A protein related to extracellular matrix proteins deleted in the mouse mutant reeler. Nature 374:719-723.

D'Arcangelo G, Homayouni R, Keshvara L, Rice DS, Sheldon M, Curran T (1999) Reelin is a ligand for lipoprotein receptors. Neuron 24:471-479.

de la Pompa JL, Wakeham A, Correia KM, Samper E, Brown S, Aguilera RJ, Nakano T, Honjo T, Mak TW, Rossant J, Conlon RA (1997) Conservation of the Notch signalling pathway in mammalian neurogenesis. Development 124:1139-1148.

Domeniconi M, Cao Z, Spencer T, Sivasankaran R, Wang K, Nikulina E, Kimura N, Cai H, Deng K, Gao Y, He Z, Filbin M (2002) Myelin-associated glycoprotein interacts with the Nogo66 receptor to inhibit neurite outgrowth. Neuron 35:283-290.

Falls DL (2003) Neuregulins: functions, forms, and signaling strategies. Exp Cell Res 284:14-30.

Fawcett JW, Keynes RJ (1990) Peripheral nerve regeneration. Annu Rev Neurosci 13:43-60.

Fawcett JW, Asher RA (1999) The glial scar and central nervous system repair. Brain Res Bull 49:377-391.

Fazeli A, Dickinson SL, Hermiston ML, Tighe RV, Steen RG, Small CG, Stoeckli ET, Keino-Masu K, Masu M, Rayburn H, Simons J, Bronson RT, Gordon JI,

Tessier-Lavigne M, Weinberg RA (1997) Phenotype of mice lacking functional Deleted in colorectal cancer (Dcc) gene. Nature 386:796-804.

Fitch MT, Silver J (1997) Glial cell extracellular matrix : boundaries for axon growth in development and regeneration. Cell Tissue Research 290: 379-384

Fournier AE, GrandPre T, Strittmatter SM (2001) Identification of a receptor mediating Nogo-66 inhibition of axonal regeneration. Nature 409:341-346.

Fruttiger M, Montag D, Schachner M, Martini R (1995) Crucial role for the myelin-associated glycoprotein in the maintenance of axon-myelin integrity. Eur J Neurosci 7:511-515.

Furukawa T, Mukherjee S, Bao ZZ, Morrow EM, Cepko CL (2000) rax, Hes1, and notch1 promote the formation of Muller glia by postnatal retinal progenitor cells. Neuron 26:383-394.

Gaiano N, Nye JS, Fishell G (2000) Radial glial identity is promoted by Notch1 signaling in the murine forebrain. Neuron 26:395-404.

Garratt AN, Britsch S, Birchmeier C (2000) Neuregulin, a factor with many functions in the life of a schwann cell. Bioessays 22:987-996.

Georgiou M, Tear G (2002) Commissureless is required both in commissural neurones and midline cells for axon guidance across the midline. Development 129:2947-2956.

Giangrande A, Murray MA, Palka J (1993) Development and organization of glial cells in the peripheral nervous system of Drosophila melanogaster. Development 117:895-904.

Giesen K, Hummel T, Stollewerk A, Harrison S, Travers A, Klambt C (1997) Glial development in the Drosophila CNS requires concomitant activation of glial and repression of neuronal differentiation genes. Development 124:2307-2316. '

Gilmour DT, Maischein HM, Nusslein-Volhard C (2002) Migration and function of a glial subtype in the vertebrate peripheral nervous system. Neuron 34:577-588.

Goldowitz D, Cushing RC, Laywell E, D'Arcangelo G, Sheldon M, Sweet HO, Davisson M, Steindler D, Curran T (1997) Cerebellar disorganization characteristic of reeler in scrambler mutant mice despite presence of reelin. J Neurosci 17:8767-8777.

Granderath S, Klambt C (1999) Glia development in the embryonic CNS of Drosophila. Curr Opin Neurobiol 9:531-536.

Gunther T, Chen ZF, Kim J, Priemel M, Rueger JM, Amling M, Moseley JM, Martin TJ, Anderson DJ, Karsenty G (2000) Genetic ablation of parathyroid glands reveals another source of parathyroid hormone. Nature 406:199-203.

Halter DA, Urban J, Rickert C, Ner SS, Ito K, Travers AA, Technau GM (1995) The homeobox gene repo is required for the differentiation and maintenance of glia function in the embryonic nervous system of Drosophila melanogaster. Development 121:317-332.

Harris R, Sabatelli LM, Seeger MA (1996) Guidance cues at the Drosophila CNS midline: identification and characterization of two Drosophila Netrin/UNC-6 homologs. Neuron 17:217-228.

Hatten ME (1999) Central nervous system neuronal migration. Annu Rev Neurosci 22:511-539.

Henrique D, Hirsinger E, Adam J, Le Roux I, Pourquie O, Ish-Horowicz D, Lewis J (1997) Maintenance of neuroepithelial progenitor cells by Delta-Notch signalling in the embryonic chick retina. Curr Biol 7:661-670.

Hidalgo A, Kinrade EF, Georgiou M (2001) The Drosophila neuregulin vein maintains glial survival during axon guidance in the CNS. Dev Cell 1:679-690.

Hiesberger T, Trommsdorff M, Howell BW, Goffinet A, Mumby MC, Cooper JA, Herz J (1999) Direct binding of Reelin to VLDL receptor and ApoE receptor 2 induces tyrosine phosphorylation of disabled-1 and modulates tau phosphorylation. Neuron 24:481-489.

Hojo M, Ohtsuka T, Hashimoto N, Gradwohl G, Guillemot F, Kageyama R (2000) Glial cell fate specification modulated by the bHLH gene Hes5 in mouse retina. Development 127:2515-2522.

Hong SE, Shugart YY, Huang DT, Shahwan SA, Grant PE, Hourihane JO, Martin ND, Walsh CA (2000) Autosomal recessive lissencephaly with cerebellar hypoplasia is associated with human RELN mutations. Nat Genet 26:93-96.

Hosoya T, Takizawa K, Nitta K, Hotta Y (1995) glial cells missing: a binary switch between neuronal and glial determination in Drosophila. Cell 82:1025-1036.

Howell BW, Lanier LM, Frank R, Gertler FB, Cooper JA (1999) The disabled 1 phosphotyrosine-binding domain binds to the internalization signals of transmembrane glycoproteins and to phospholipids. Mol Cell Biol 19:5179-5188.

Howell BW, Herrick TM, Hildebrand JD, Zhang Y, Cooper JA (2000) Dab1 tyrosine phosphorylation sites relay positional signals during mouse brain development. Curr Biol 10:877-885.

Hu H (1999) Chemorepulsion of neuronal migration by Slit2 in the developing mammalian forebrain. Neuron 23:703-711.

Hummel T, Schimmelpfeng K, Klambt C (1999) Commissure formation in the embryonic CNS of Drosophila. Development 126:771-779.

Hummel T, Attix S, Gunning D, Zipursky SL (2002) Temporal control of glial cell migration in the Drosophila eye requires gilgamesh, hedgehog, and eye specification genes. Neuron 33:193-203.

Hunter-Schaedle KE (1997) Radial glial cell development and transformation are disturbed in reeler forebrain. J Neurobiol 33:459-472.

Jacobs JR (2000) The midline glia of Drosophila: a molecular genetic model for the developmental functions of glia. Prog Neurobiol 62:475-508.

Jacobs JR, Hiromi Y, Patel NH, Goodman CS (1989) Lineage, migration, and morphogenesis of longitudinal glia in the Drosophila CNS as revealed by a molecular lineage marker. Neuron 2:1625-1631.

Jones BW, Fetter RD, Tear G, Goodman CS (1995) glial cells missing: a genetic switch that controls glial versus neuronal fate. Cell 82:1013-1023.

Kageyama R, Ohtsuka T (1999) The Notch-Hes pathway in mammalian neural development. Cell Res 9:179-188.

Kageyama R, Ishibashi M, Takebayashi K, Tomita K (1997) bHLH transcription factors and mammalian neuronal differentiation. Int J Biochem Cell Biol 29:1389-1399.

Kammerer M, Giangrande A (2001) Glide2, a second glial promoting factor in Drosophila melanogaster. Embo J 20:4664-4673.

Kammerer M, Pirola B, Giglio S, Giangrande A (1999) GCMB, a second human homolog of the fly glide/gcm gene. Cytogenet Cell Genet 84:43-47.

Kanemura Y, Hiraga S, Arita N, Ohnishi T, Izumoto S, Mori K, Matsumura H, Yamasaki M, Fushiki S, Yoshimine T (1999) Isolation and expression analysis of a novel human homologue of the Drosophila glial cells missing (gcm) gene. FEBS Lett 442:151-156.

Kaprielian Z, Imondi R, Runko E (2000) Axon guidance at the midline of the developing CNS. Anat Rec 261:176-197.

Keino-Masu K, Masu M, Hinck L, Leonardo ED, Chan SS, Culotti JG, Tessier-Lavigne M (1996) Deleted in Colorectal Cancer (DCC) encodes a netrin receptor. Cell 87:175-185.

Keleman K, Rajagopalan S, Cleppien D, Teis D, Paiha K, Huber LA, Technau GM, Dickson BJ (2002) Comm sorts robo to control axon guidance at the Drosophila midline. Cell 110:415-427.

Kidd T, Bland KS, Goodman CS (1999) Slit is the midline repellent for the robo receptor in Drosophila. Cell 96:785-794.

Kidd T, Brose K, Mitchell KJ, Fetter RD, Tessier-Lavigne M, Goodman CS, Tear G (1998) Roundabout controls axon crossing of the CNS midline and defines a novel subfamily of evolutionarily conserved guidance receptors. Cell 92:205-215.

Kim J, Jones BW, Zock C, Chen Z, Wang H, Goodman CS, Anderson DJ (1998) Isolation and characterization of mammalian homologs of the Drosophila gene glial cells missing. Proc Natl Acad Sci U S A 95:12364-12369.

Klar A, Baldassare M, Jessell TM (1992) F-spondin: a gene expressed at high levels in the floor plate encodes a secreted protein that promotes neural cell adhesion and neurite extension. Cell 69:95-110.

Kolodziej PA, Timpe LC, Mitchell KJ, Fried SR, Goodman CS, Jan LY, Jan YN (1996) frazzled encodes a Drosophila member of the DCC immunoglobulin subfamily and is required for CNS and motor axon guidance. Cell 87:197-204.

Kottis V, Thibault P, Mikol D, Xiao ZC, Zhang R, Dergham P, Braun PE (2002) Oligodendrocyte-myelin glycoprotein (OMgp) is an inhibitor of neurite outgrowth. J Neurochem 82:1566-1569.

Kretzschmar D, Hasan G, Sharma S, Heisenberg M, Benzer S (1997) The swiss cheese mutant causes glial hyperwrapping and brain degeneration in Drosophila. J Neurosci 17:7425-7432.

Lemke G (1996) Neuregulins in development. Mol Cell Neurosci 7:247-262.

Lewis J (1996) Neurogenic genes and vertebrate neurogenesis. Curr Opin Neurobiol 6:3-10.

Li C, Tropak MB, Gerlai R, Clapoff S, Abramow-Newerly W, Trapp B, Peterson A, Roder J (1994) Myelination in the absence of myelin-associated glycoprotein. Nature 369:747-750.

Li HS, Chen JH, Wu W, Fagaly T, Zhou L, Yuan W, Dupuis S, Jiang ZH, Nash W, Gick C, Ornitz DM, Wu JY, Rao Y (1999) Vertebrate slit, a secreted ligand for the transmembrane protein roundabout, is a repellent for olfactory bulb axons. Cell 96:807-818.

Lindsell CE, Boulter J, diSibio G, Gossler A, Weinmaster G (1996) Expression patterns of Jagged, Delta1, Notch1, Notch2, and Notch3 genes identify ligand-receptor pairs that may function in neural development. Mol Cell Neurosci 8:14-27.

Liu BP, Fournier A, GrandPre T, Strittmatter SM (2002) Myelin-associated glycoprotein as a functional ligand for the Nogo-66 receptor. Science 297:1190-1193.

Lu QR, Sun T, Zhu Z, Ma N, Garcia M, Stiles CD, Rowitch DH (2002) Common developmental requirement for Olig function indicates a motor neuron/oligodendrocyte connection. Cell 109:75-86.

Lu QR, Yuk D, Alberta JA, Zhu Z, Pawlitzky I, Chan J, McMahon AP, Stiles CD, Rowitch DH (2000) Sonic hedgehog--regulated oligodendrocyte lineage genes encoding bHLH proteins in the mammalian central nervous system. Neuron 25:317-329.

Marchionni MA, Goodearl AD, Chen MS, Bermingham-McDonogh O, Kirk C, Hendricks M, Danehy F, Misumi D, Sudhalter J, Kobayashi K, et al. (1993) Glial growth factors are alternatively spliced erbB2 ligands expressed in the nervous system. Nature 362:312-318.

Marquardt T, Pfaff SL (2001) Cracking the transcriptional code for cell specification in the neural tube. Cell 106:651-654.

Mehler MF, Mabie PC, Zhang D, Kessler JA (1997) Bone morphogenetic proteins in the nervous system. Trends Neurosci 20:309-317.

Mikoshiba K, Nishimura Y, Tsukada Y (1983) Absence of bundle structure in the neocortex of the reeler mouse at the embryonic stage. Studies by scanning electron microscopic fractography. Dev Neurosci 6:18-25.

Miller AA, Bernardoni R, Giangrande A (1998) Positive autoregulation of the glial promoting factor glide/gcm. Embo J 17:6316-6326.

Mitchell KJ, Doyle JL, Serafini T, Kennedy TE, Tessier-Lavigne M, Goodman CS, Dickson BJ (1996) Genetic analysis of Netrin genes in Drosophila: Netrins guide CNS commissural axons and peripheral motor axons. Neuron 17:203-215.

Mizuguchi R, Sugimori M, Takebayashi H, Kosako H, Nagao M, Yoshida S, Nabeshima Y, Shimamura K, Nakafuku M (2001) Combinatorial roles of olig2 and neurogenin2 in the coordinated induction of pan-neuronal and subtype-specific properties of motoneurons. Neuron 31:757-771.

Montag D, Giese KP, Bartsch U, Martini R, Lang Y, Bluthmann H, Karthigasan J, Kirschner DA, Wintergerst ES, Nave KA, et al. (1994) Mice deficient for the myelin-associated glycoprotein show subtle abnormalities in myelin. Neuron 13:229-246.

Morrison SJ, Perez SE, Qiao Z, Verdi JM, Hicks C, Weinmaster G, Anderson DJ (2000) Transient Notch activation initiates an irreversible switch from neurogenesis to gliogenesis by neural crest stem cells. Cell 101:499-510.

Mukhopadhyay G, Doherty P, Walsh FS, Crocker PR, Filbin MT (1994) A novel role for myelin-associated glycoprotein as an inhibitor of axonal regeneration. Neuron 13:757-767.

Myat A, Henry P, McCabe V, Flintoft L, Rotin D, Tear G (2002) Drosophila Nedd4, a ubiquitin ligase, is recruited by Commissureless to control cell surface levels of the roundabout receptor. Neuron 35:447-459.

Nguyen Ba-Charvet KT, Brose K, Marillat V, Kidd T, Goodman CS, Tessier-Lavigne M, Sotelo C, Chedotal A (1999) Slit2-Mediated chemorepulsion and collapse of developing forebrain axons. Neuron 22:463-473.

Novitch BG, Chen AI, Jessell TM (2001) Coordinate regulation of motor neuron subtype identity and pan-neuronal properties by the bHLH repressor Olig2. Neuron 31:773-789.

Nye JS (1999) The Notch proteins. Curr Biol 9:R118.

Park HC, Mehta A, Richardson JS, Appel B (2002) olig2 is required for zebrafish primary motor neuron and oligodendrocyte development. Dev Biol 248:356-368.

Parnavelas JG, Nadarajah B (2001) Radial glial cells. are they really glia? Neuron 31:881-884.

Patten I, Placzek M (2000) The role of Sonic hedgehog in neural tube patterning. Cell Mol Life Sci 57:1695-1708.

Plump AS, Erskine L, Sabatier C, Brose K, Epstein CJ, Goodman CS, Mason CA, Tessier-Lavigne M (2002) Slit1 and Slit2 cooperate to prevent premature midline crossing of retinal axons in the mouse visual system. Neuron 33:219-232.

Poeck B, Fischer S, Gunning D, Zipursky SL, Salecker I (2001) Glial cells mediate target layer selection of retinal axons in the developing visual system of Drosophila. Neuron 29:99-113.

Rajagopalan S, Nicolas E, Vivancos V, Berger J, Dickson BJ (2000) Crossing the midline: roles and regulation of Robo receptors. Neuron 28:767-777.

Rakic P (1972) Mode of cell migration to the superficial layers of fetal monkey neocortex. J Comp Neurol 145:61-83.

Rakic P (1988) Specification of cerebral cortical areas. Science 241:170-176.

Rangarajan R, Gong Q, Gaul U (1999) Migration and function of glia in the developing Drosophila eye. Development 126:3285-3292.

Rangarajan R, Courvoisier H, Gaul U (2001) Dpp and Hedgehog mediate neuron-glia interactions in Drosophila eye development by promoting the proliferation and motility of subretinal glia. Mech Dev 108:93-103.

Rao MS (1999) Multipotent and restricted precursors in the central nervous system. Anat Rec 257:137-148.

Ramon y Cajal S (1911) *Histology of the Nervous System of Man and Vertebrates.* Transl. L Swanson, N Swanson. Oxford, UK : Oxford Univ. Press (From Spanish) (1995)

Reifegerste R, Schreiber J, Gulland S, Ludemann A, Wegner M (1999) mGCMa is a murine transcription factor that overrides cell fate decisions in Drosophila. Mech Dev 82:141-150.

Rice DS, Curran T (2001) Role of the reelin signaling pathway in central nervous system development. Annu Rev Neurosci 24:1005-1039.

Ringstedt T, Braisted JE, Brose K, Kidd T, Goodman C, Tessier-Lavigne M, O'Leary DD (2000) Slit inhibition of retinal axon growth and its role in retinal axon pathfinding and innervation patterns in the diencephalon. J Neurosci 20:4983-4991.

Rothberg JM, Jacobs JR, Goodman CS, Artavanis-Tsakonas S (1990) slit: an extracellular protein necessary for development of midline glia and commissural axon pathways contains both EGF and LRR domains. Genes Dev 4:2169-2187.

Schafer M, Fruttiger M, Montag D, Schachner M, Martini R (1996) Disruption of the gene for the myelin-associated glycoprotein improves axonal regrowth along myelin in C57BL/Wlds mice. Neuron 16:1107-1113.

Schreiber J, Sock E, Wegner M (1997) The regulator of early gliogenesis glial cells missing is a transcription factor with a novel type of DNA-binding domain. Proc Natl Acad Sci U S A 94:4739-4744.

Schreiber J, Riethmacher-Sonnenberg E, Riethmacher D, Tuerk EE, Enderich J, Bosl MR, Wegner M (2000) Placental failure in mice lacking the mammalian homolog of glial cells missing, GCMa. Mol Cell Biol 20:2466-2474.

Seeger M, Tear G, Ferres-Marco D, Goodman CS (1993) Mutations affecting growth cone guidance in Drosophila: genes necessary for guidance toward or away from the midline. Neuron 10:409-426.

Serafini T, Kennedy TE, Galko MJ, Mirzayan C, Jessell TM, Tessier-Lavigne M (1994) The netrins define a family of axon outgrowth-promoting proteins homologous to C. elegans UNC-6. Cell 78:409-424.

Serafini T, Colamarino SA, Leonardo ED, Wang H, Beddington R, Skarnes WC, Tessier-Lavigne M (1996) Netrin-1 is required for commissural axon guidance in the developing vertebrate nervous system. Cell 87:1001-1014.

Shu T, Richards LJ (2001) Cortical axon guidance by the glial wedge during the development of the corpus callosum. J Neurosci 21:2749-2758.

SidmandRL, Green MC, Appel SH (1965) *Catalog of the Neurological Mutants Mouse*. Boston: Harvard Univ. Press

Spassky N, de Castro F, Le Bras B, Heydon K, Queraud-LeSaux F, Bloch-Gallego E, Chedotal A, Zalc B, Thomas JL (2002) Directional guidance of oligodendroglial migration by class 3 semaphorins and netrin-1. J Neurosci 22:5992-6004.

Sugimoto Y, Taniguchi M, Yagi T, Akagi Y, Nojyo Y, Tamamaki N (2001) Guidance of glial precursor cell migration by secreted cues in the developing optic nerve. Development 128:3321-3330.

Takebayashi H, Yoshida S, Sugimori M, Kosako H, Kominami R, Nakafuku M, Nabeshima Y (2000) Dynamic expression of basic helix-loop-helix Olig family members: implication of Olig2 in neuron and oligodendrocyte differentiation and identification of a new member, Olig3. Mech Dev 99:143-148.

Tang S, Woodhall RW, Shen YJ, deBellard ME, Saffell JL, Doherty P, Walsh FS, Filbin MT (1997) Soluble Myelin-Associated Glycoprotein (MAG) Found in Vivo Inhibits Axonal Regeneration. Mol Cell Neurosci 9:333-346.

Tanigaki K, Nogaki F, Takahashi J, Tashiro K, Kurooka H, Honjo T (2001) Notch1 and Notch3 instructively restrict bFGF-responsive multipotent neural progenitor cells to an astroglial fate. Neuron 29:45-55.

Tear G, Harris R, Sutaria S, Kilomanski K, Goodman CS, Seeger MA (1996) commissureless controls growth cone guidance across the CNS midline in Drosophila and encodes a novel membrane protein. Neuron 16:501-514.

Trommsdorff M, Gotthardt M, Hiesberger T, Shelton J, Stockinger W, Nimpf J, Hammer RE, Richardson JA, Herz J (1999) Reeler/Disabled-like disruption of neuronal migration in knockout mice lacking the VLDL receptor and ApoE receptor 2. Cell 97:689-701.

Turner DL, Cepko CL (1987) A common progenitor for neurons and glia persists in rat retina late in development. Nature 328:131-136.

Udolph G, Rath P, Chia W (2001) A requirement for Notch in the genesis of a subset of glial cells in the Drosophila embryonic central nervous system which arise through asymmetric divisions. Development 128:1457-1466.

Umesono Y, Hiromi Y, Hotta Y (2002) Context-dependent utilization of Notch activity in Drosophila glial determination. Development 129:2391-2399.

Van De Bor V, Giangrande A (2001) Notch signaling represses the glial fate in fly PNS. Development 128:1381-1390.

Van De Bor V, Walther R, Giangrande A (2000) Some fly sensory organs are gliogenic and require glide/gcm in a precursor that divides symmetrically and produces glial cells. Development 127:3735-3743.

Van De Bor V, Heitzler P, Leger S, Plessy C, Giangrande A (2002) Precocious expression of the Glide/Gcm glial-promoting factor in Drosophila induces neurogenesis. Genetics 160:1095-1106.

Vetter ML, Moore KB (2001) Becoming glial in the neural retina. Dev Dyn 221:146-153.

Vincent S, Vonesch JL, Giangrande A (1996) Glide directs glial fate commitment and cell fate switch between neurones and glia. Development 122:131-139.

Wang KC, Kim JA, Sivasankaran R, Segal R, He Z (2002a) P75 interacts with the Nogo receptor as a co-receptor for Nogo, MAG and OMgp. Nature 420:74-78.

Wang KC, Koprivica V, Kim JA, Sivasankaran R, Guo Y, Neve RL, He Z (2002b) Oligodendrocyte-myelin glycoprotein is a Nogo receptor ligand that inhibits neurite outgrowth. Nature 417:941-944.

Weinmaster G (1997) The ins and outs of notch signaling. Mol Cell Neurosci 9:91-102.

Wong ST, Henley JR, Kanning KC, Huang KH, Bothwell M, Poo MM (2002) A p75(NTR) and Nogo receptor complex mediates repulsive signaling by myelin-associated glycoprotein. Nat Neurosci 5:1302-1308.

Wu W, Wong K, Chen J, Jiang Z, Dupuis S, Wu JY, Rao Y (1999) Directional guidance of neuronal migration in the olfactory system by the protein Slit. Nature 400:331-336.

Xiong WC, Montell C (1995) Defective glia induce neuronal apoptosis in the repo visual system of Drosophila. Neuron 14:581-590.

Yamada K, Watanabe M (2002) Cytodifferentiation of Bergmann glia and its relationship with Purkinje cells. Anat Sci Int 77:94-108.

Yang JF, Zhou H, Pun S, Ip NY, Peng HB, Tsim KW (1998) Cloning of cDNAs encoding xenopus neuregulin: expression in myotomal muscle during embryo development. Brain Res Mol Brain Res 58:59-73.

Zhou Q, Anderson DJ (2002) The bHLH transcription factors OLIG2 and OLIG1 couple neuronal and glial subtype specification. Cell 109:61-73.

Zhou Q, Wang S, Anderson DJ (2000) Identification of a novel family of oligodendrocyte lineage-specific basic helix-loop-helix transcription factors. Neuron 25:331-343.

Zhou Q, Choi G, Anderson DJ (2001) The bHLH transcription factor Olig2 promotes oligodendrocyte differentiation in collaboration with Nkx2.2. Neuron 31:791-807.

2.9. Abbreviations

AM	Anterior margin
bHLH	Basic helix-loop-helix
BMPs	Bone morphogenetic proteins
CNS	Central nervous system
cpn	Contralateral axon
DER	*Drosophila* EGF receptor
DRG	Dorsal root ganglion
EGF	Early growth factor

EGFR	Early growth factor receptor
GBS	Glide-binding site
GFAP	Glial fibrillary acidic protein
GFP	Green fluorescent protein
Glide\Gcm	Glia cell deficient\ Glia cell missing
GPI	Glycosylphosphatidylinositol
ipn	Ipsilateral axon
LG	Longitudinal glia
MAG	Myelin associated glycoprotein
MAPK	MAP kinase
MF	Morphogenetic furrow
MG	Midline glia
Notch1 IC	Notch1 intracellular domain
NRG-1	Neuregulin-1
OLs	Oligodendrocytes
Omgp	Oligodendrocyte myelin glycoprotein
OLPs	Oligodendrocyte precursors
$p75^{NTR}$	p75 neurotrophin receptor
pMN domain	Motor neuron progenitor domain
PNS	Peripheral nervous system
R	Photoreceptor

Chapter 3

Structural association of glia with the various compartments of neurons

Andreas Reichenbach[1*], Amin Derouiche[2], Jens Grosche[1] and
Menachem Hanani[3]

[1] Paul Flechsig Institute for Brain Research, Leipzig University, Leipzig, Germany,
[2] Anatomical Institute, Cologne University, Germany, and
[3] Laboratory of Experimental Surgery, Hadassah University Hospital, Jerusalem, Israel

*Corresponding author: reia@server3.medizin.uni-leipzig.de

Contents

3.1. The first player: Neurons - polarized cells with several specialized compartments

Neurons are cells that receive, transform and propagate information. For this purpose, they are endowed with a variety of processes or other cellular compartments, dedicated to one or more of these tasks. Generally, neurons are polarized in that one pole is optimized to receive information, and the other to transmit it to targets such as other neurons, muscles, glands, or to the circulating blood. The receptor pole may consist of a sensory process, which probably has been present from the most primitive origin of the neurons (Hanström, 1928; Lenz, 1968; Kanno, 1989; Lacalli, 1990). The sensory apparatus usually involves a sensory organelle, often consisting of one or more modified cilia which are sensitive to a distinct 'adequate' type of stimulus (an exception may be multimodal 'free nerve endings' of nociceptors). In phylogenetically higher animals, most neurons are no longer capable of direct sensory reception; rather, they receive information from specialized sensory cells, and/or from other neurons. In these cases, the sensory process has been replaced by a dendritic tree, which receives information via synaptic contacts. That is, dendrites are modified sensory processes adapted to the 'measurement' of neurotransmitter molecules. Some vertebrate neurons still possess both a sensory process *and* dendrites (Vigh-Teichmann and Vigh, 1974) (Fig. 3.1). The effector pole usually consists of an axon, and its main feature is the presynaptic terminal, capable of transmitting signals (usually, in the form of secreted neurotransmitter molecules) to other cells. These distinct neuronal compartments are characterized by specific, 'optimized' morphological and functional properties, such as the expression of certain ion channels, ligand receptors, etc. The generation of regenerative Na^+ currents (i.e., action potentials) is not a distinctive feature of any of the compartments. The axon (usually) as well as the sensory processes and/or the dendrites (frequently) may be able to generate action potentials. These all-or-nothing responses are necessary for the propagation of information along processes that are too long for an effective propagation of amplitude-coded signals. The action potentials are initiated at or close to the initial segment (or adjacent to the sensory terminal in the case of dorsal root ganglion cells), and may be either continuous or saltatory; in the latter case, the cell process is usually myelinated. It should be mentioned here that Ca^{2+}-carried action potentials may occur as well (often simultaneously with the Na^+-carried action potentials); these cause a Ca^{2+} influx into the cells and are probably involved in intracellular second-messenger signal cascades.

3.2. The other player: Glia - polarized cells with several specialized compartments

Astroglial cells (astrocytes, Bergmann glial cells, tanycytes, and retinal Müller glial cells) are characterized by endfeet contacting a basal lamina around blood vessels, the pia mater (or the vitreous body of the eye), or both (type II process: Reichenbach, 1989). Radial glial cells (tanycytes and Müller cells) are bipolar, and additionally contact the ventricular surface (or the subretinal space, respectively) (type I process). Astrocytes may display a radial orientation (like Bergmann glia) but they never contact the ventricular system. Both type II and type I processes are thought to enable the cells to exchange molecules with large extracellular compartments such as the perivascular space or the cerberospinal fluid, as well as with blood vessels (for review, see Reichenbach, 1989). In addition, all astroglial cells display another type of cell process which contacts neuronal elements (type III process). These processes and contacts are responsible for structural and functional glia-neuron interactions (Fig. 3.2), and will be subject of this chapter.

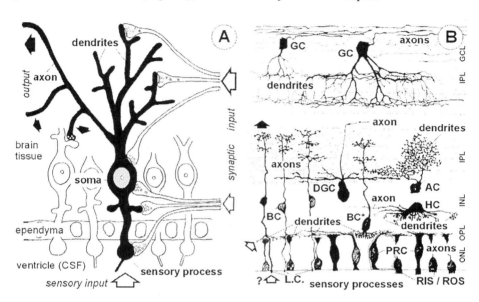

Figure 3.1. Neurons and their compartments. **A:** The cerebrospinal fluid (CSF) contact neurons (Vigh-Teichmann and Vigh, 1974) may be regarded as a model of specialized neuronal compartments, as it displays a sensory process (primarily for *sensory input*), a soma and dendritic tree (primarily for *synaptic input*), and an axon (primarily for *synaptic output*). **B:** Neurons of the frog retina (Ramón y Cajal, 1972). Two views of the inner plexiform layer (IPL) are separately shown on top of one another, to show the cell processes more clearly. In lower vertebrates, most of the bipolar cells (BP) retain features of 'universal neurons' by displaying both a sensory process (ending with a Landolt's club, LC, in the subretinal space) and a dendritic arborization, in addition to an axon [ending with elaborate branching in the inner plexiform layer (IPL)]. Other frog bipolar cells (BP*) - like all bipolar cells in mammalian retinae and like the other types of vertebrate retinal neurons - show cellular specialization, which means a loss of diversity of cellular compartments. Thus, photoreceptor cells (PRC) possess sensory processes (inner (RIS) and outer segments (ROS)) and axons; most neurons possess dendrites and axons. Some types of horizontal cells and amacrine cells do not possess an axon; their processes may be both pre- and postsynaptic. GC - retinal ganglion cells, DGC - displaced ganglion cell; AC - amacrine cell; HC - horizontal cell. GCL - ganglion cell layer, INL - inner nuclear layer, OPL - outer plexiform layer; ONL - outer nuclear layer. White arrows - sensory/synaptic inputs, black arrows - output from neurons. It remains to be elucidated whether Landolt's clubs have a role in sensory reception. Slightly modified, with permission from Vigh-Teichmann and Vigh, 1974 (A) and Ramón y Cajal, 1972 (B).

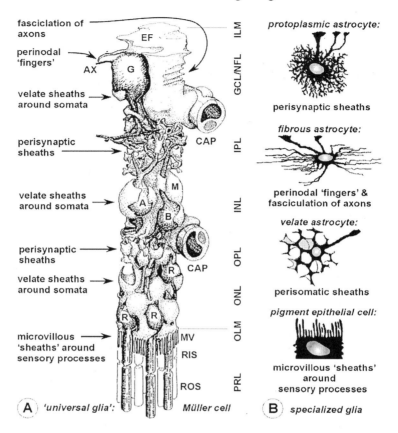

Figure 3.2. Astroglial cells and their structural associations with neuronal compartments. **A:** The retinal radial glial (Müller) cell may be considered as a model of specialized glial compartments, as it displays virtually all known types of perineuronal contacts. **B:** Specialized types of glial cells display only one predominant distinct type of glio-neuronal associations. As in the case of neurons, cellular specialization means loss of diversity of cellular compartments. ILM – inner limiting membrane; G - ganglion cell, A - amacrine cell; B – bipolar cell; M - Müller cell soma; R - photoreceptor cell somata; EF - Müller cell endfoot; MV - Müller cell microvilli; RIS - inner segments of photoreceptor cells; ROS - outer segments of photoreceptor cells; CAP - retinal capillaries. GCL/NFL - ganglion cell and nerve fiber layers, IPL - inner plexiform layer, INL - inner nuclear layer, OPL - outer plexiform layer; ONL - outer nuclear layer, OLM – outer limiting membrane, PRL - photoreceptor layer. With permission, from Reichenbach et al., 1993 (**A**); original drawings by AR (**B**). Oligodendrocytes and peripheral glial cells are not shown here.

Other macroglial cells are polarized, and display specialized associations with neuronal compartments, as well. In the central nervous system (CNS), the oligodendrocytes are associated with many axons; in the peripheral nervous system (PNS), myelinating and non-myelinating Schwann cells are responsible for such associations with neurites. Specialized Schwann cells, so-called 'teloglia', are associated with the axon terminals on muscle cells (i.e., the motor endplates) and with the sensory endings of neurites. Furthermore, satellite glial cells surround the somata of neurons in sensory ganglia, and supporting or sustentacular cells are associated with the sensory processes of receptor cells. In the peripheral autonomic ganglia neurons are surrounded by an envelope of satellite glial cells, but in the enteric nervous system, glial cells are similar to astrocytes (Hanani and Reichenbach, 1994). Another astroglia-like cell type, the olfactory ensheathing cell, is found in the olfactory nerve and in the superficial layers of the olfactory bulb (Doucette, 1984; Valverde and Lopez-Mascaraque, 1991). Most of these cells will be introduced in the following sections, and can be found in the summarizing Figure 3.16.

It is believed that glial cells mediate an indirect exchange of molecules between neuronal compartments and blood vessels (or extracellular spaces such as the cerebrospinal fluid). This might occur within a single glial cell (e.g., in an astrocyte which possesses both type II and type III processes) or via gap-junctional coupling of populations of glial cells (e.g., between oligodendrocytes and astrocytes (Robinson et al., 1993)).

3.3. The sites of the interplay: 'peripheral astrocyte processes' (PAPs) as specific 'peripheral glial processes' (PGPs)

The CNS consists of three main compartments, neurons (about 50% of total volume, e. g., in rat brain), glia (about 20% of volume), and blood vessels (less than 10% of volume) in addition to a variable extracellular space. Therefore, a close association of glial and neuronal elements must frequently occur even if the elements were randomly distributed. In lower invertebrates, presumptive glial cells are merely identified by their structural relationship to neuronal elements (Lacalli, 1990). The aim of this chapter is to highlight glio-neuronal associations that can be considered by the nature of their morphology or physiological properties to have functional significance.

Most glio-neuronal associations are formed, on the glial side, by specialized terminal protrusions or end-branches of the glial cytoplasm. These structures are characterized - and discriminated from the thicker 'stem' processes, side branches, and/or somata from which they arise – by their paucity in cytoplasmic organelles. Generally, they appear as thin membrane out-foldings which may assume lamellar or finger-like shapes. Based on their variable shape in astrocytes, they have been given various names, such as 'lamellipodia and filopodia' (Chao et al., 2002), 'lamellae and finger-like extensions' (Wolff, 1968), or, 'peripheral astroglial processes' (PAPs; Derouiche and Frotscher, 2001) which makes no assumption concerning shape.

The PAPs, but not the thicker astroglial cell processes or somata, were shown to contain actin-binding ERM molecules such as ezrin (Derouiche and Frotscher, 2001; Derouiche et al., 2002), which are probably involved in the generation and maintenance of their complex shapes and the creation of high surface-to-volume ratios (up to more than 30 $\mu m^2/\mu m^3$). Although individual PAPs usually are small structures, due to their large number they may constitute about half of the astroglial volume and about 80% of the surface area (Chao et al., 2002). The large surface area is thought to give space for the insertion of membrane proteins such as ion channels, ligand receptors, and carrier molecules, necessary for functional interactions with the neuronal compartments contacted by the PAPs (section 3.10.).

In addition the PAPs, there exists a wealth of glio-neuronal associations involving most non-astrocytic cells in the CNS and PNS. These are of diverse shapes but generally are formed by fine terminal processes similar to the PAPs. For example, this includes the microvillous processes of ependymoglial cells adjacent to photoreceptor cells (section 3.4.1.), the trophospongia of satellite cells (section 3.5.4.), and even the myelin sheaths on PNS and CNS axons, as extremely specialized elements (section 3.6.3.). We propose here the term 'peripheral glial processes' (PGPs), in analogy to the PAPs. Many of the following paragraphs review these types of glio-neuronal associations, in relation to specific neuronal compartments.

It should also be mentioned that the actual interface between neurons and PGPs is constituted by an extracellular cleft. The width of this cleft may vary considerably, depending on the developmental and/or functional state, or on local specializations. Furthermore, this cleft contains an extracellular matrix that also may vary in its abundance and molecular composition, and which is thought to contribute crucially to the wealth of structural and functional neuro-glial interactions.

3.4. Glio-neuronal associations at the receptor pole

The tasks and structural adaptations of the associated glial cells vary depending on whether the receptor pole of a neuron consists of a true sensory process or of a dendritic tree, specialized to measure the concentration of transmitter molecules. Furthermore, the length and diameter of a given neuronal process may require specific adaptations of the associated glial elements.

3.4.1. Sensory processes / organelles

Within the central nervous system (CNS) of vertebrates, sensory neurons occur in the walls of the third ventricle (cerebrospinal fluid - CSF - contact cells; cf. Fig. 3.1) and in the retina of the eye (and, in non-mammalian vertebrates, of the pineal, parapineal and/or frontal organ). Generally, the sensory processes of these cells (located in the ventricular cavity or in the subretinal space) are associated with the microvilli of neighboring ependymoglial cells. In the retina, the microvilli of Müller cells are inserted in the interspaces between the photoreceptor cell inner segments (Figs. 3.2A, 3.3A-C). The outer segments of the photoreceptor cells are embedded in rather complex microvillar sheaths extending from the pigment epithelium. These may contain either melanin pigment granules (to absorb surplus photons at daylight) and/or guanine crystals (to reflect not-yet-absorbed photons in dark environments) (Fig. 3.3B, C). There is evidence that, facilitated by the large surface area of the microvilli, the ependymocytes / Müller cells / pigment epithelial cells perform an intense exchange of molecules with the sensory processes of the neurons; for instance, the clearance of excess extracellular K^+ ions, the delivery of lactate/pyruvate to fuel the Krebs cycle of the photoreceptor inner segments, and the transport of photopigment metabolites have been described (for reviews, see Steinberg, 1985; Newman and Reichenbach, 1996).

It has been pointed out that, like Müller cells that ensheathe the sensory processes of retinal photoreceptor cells, the sustentacular or supporting cells ensheathe the sensory processes of olfactory sensory cells in fish and mouse (Breipohl et al., 1974).

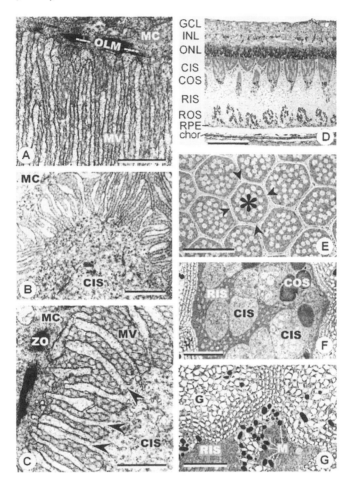

Figure 3.3. Glial microvilli surround the sensory processes of photoreceptor cells. **A-C:** Microvilli (MV) of Müller cells (MC) surround cone inner segments (CIS) in the tree shrew retina. **A:** Radial section at the level of the outer limiting membrane (OLM). **B:** Tangential section slightly distal of the OLM; a CIS is surrounded by palisades of microvilli. **C:** Higher magnification of a section close to (**B**); the CIS extends flat 'fins' between the rows of Müller cell microvilli (arrowheads). ZO - zonulae occludentes of the OLM. With permission, from Reichenbach et al., 1995b. **D-F:** Microvilli of pigment epithelial cells form cup-like structures surrounding the inner and outer segments of photoreceptor cells in the elephant nose fish (*Gnathonemus petersi*). **D:** Semi-thin tangential section through the posterior pole of the eye; the retina proper is relatively thin but there are bundles of very long inner and outer segments of photoreceptor cells, ensheathed by very long processes from the retinal pigment epithelium (RPE). **E:** Transverse section at the level of the cone inner segments (CIS). The bundles of RIS (asterisk) are enveloped by cytoplasmic sheaths (arrowheads). **F:** Electron micrograph at the level of the transition between cone inner (CIS) and outer segments (COS); the rod inner segments (RIS) run deeper towards the pigment epithelium. **G:** Another electron micrograph

just proximal to the level of the transition between rod inner and outer segments. Whereas layered arrays of light-reflecting guanine crystals (G) help the photoreceptors within a bundle to absorb a maximum of photons, light scattering into adjacent bundles of photoreceptors is further diminished by melanin granules (M); both structures are generated by the pigment epithelium. GCL - ganglion cell layer, INL - inner nuclear layer, ONL - outer nuclear layer, ROS - rod outer segments, chor - choroid. Calibration bars, 1 μm (**A**, **B**), 0.5 μm (**C**), 100 μm (**D**), 50 μm (**E**), and 5 μm (**F**, **G**). Original photographs; courtesy of E. Ulbricht (**D**, **E**) and F. Makarov and M. Francke (**F**, **G**).

In the PNS of vertebrates, the dorsal root ganglion (DRG) cells extend long processes which end in their target organs, forming specialized sensory organelles. For example, mechanoreceptors (Pacinian corpuscles, etc) may involve specialized structures derived from the associated glial cells ('teloglia') and also from epidermal structures (Fig. 3.4A, B). The associated glial structures may contribute to the properties of sensory transduction. Even the so-called 'free nerve endings' (the receptors for pain and temperature) have been shown to be enwrapped by accompanying Schwann cells, which only leave some free areas where the axonal membrane directly abuts the surrounding environment, and is undercoated by a typical fine filamentous substructure (called 'receptor matrix'). It is assumed that these exposed areas contain the membrane receptors, and constitute the receptive sites (Messlinger, 1996).

As the sensory processes of the DRG cells are very long, an effective signaling requires the conduction of action potentials. This conduction may be non-saltatory (in the case of slowly-conducting nociceptive and thermoreceptive fibers, which are enwrapped by cytoplasmic tongues of nonmyelinating Schwann cells) or saltatory (in most mechanoreceptive fibers). In this latter case, the fibers are myelinated by myelinating Schwann cells (sections 3.4.2., 3.6.3, 3.6.4.). Thus, these sensory processes display most of the ultrastructural and functional features of axons, and are usually termed 'axons' although they are ontogenetically and even electrophysiologically (Bowe et al., 1985; Kocsis et al., 1986) distinct entities.

In invertebrates, various sensory organs consist of one or a few neurons, and accompanying glial cells (Keil, 1997; Gho et al., 1999) (Fig. 3.4B). As in the case of the sensory endings of the DRG neurons, these glial structures may be involved in sensory transduction.

3.4.2. Dendrites

For most neurons, dendrites are the main sites of synaptic input. For this purpose, the dendritic tree possesses a large surface membrane area which is generated by multiple branching of the stem dendrite. Much of the non-synaptic surface of the stem dendrites may be covered by glial sheaths; the processes of several adjacent glial cells may contribute to the sheath around one stem dendrite (Fig. 3.5A,B). As the dendrites are major constituents of the neuropile (gray matter), their sheaths are provided by the glial cells of the gray matter, i.e., by protoplasmic astrocytes, or - in the cerebellum - by Bergmann glial cells which are a subtype of radial astrocytes. Another component of a subpopulation of peridendritic sheaths are the perineuronal nets, which consist of a particular extracellular matrix (sections 3.5.1., 3.8., Fig. 3.14A-C) and are covered by net-like PGPs. It can be speculated that both the peridendritic glial sheaths and the perineuronal nets serve for the buffering and clearance of ions and bioactive molecules in the adjacent extracellular clefts.

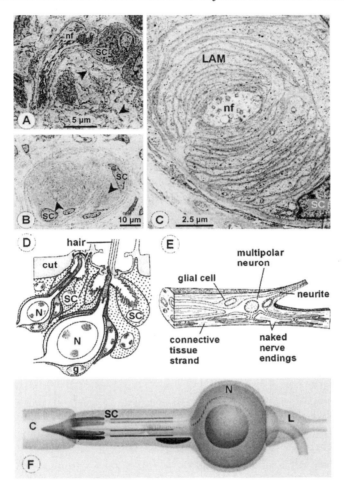

Figure 3.4. Specialized glial cells are integral parts of peripheral mechanoreceptors. **A-C:** Vertebrate cutaneous receptors. **A:** A Ruffini ending in rat peridontium, consisting of nerve fibers (and their endings) (nf) and associated Schwann cells (SC), both embedded in dense collagen bundles of the peridontal ligament (arrowheads). **B, C:** "Simple" coiled corpuscles of the monkey lip. An entire corpuscle is shown in **B**; it contains two nerve fibers (arrowheads) and several Schwann cells (SC). **C:** At higher magnification it becomes obvious that the central nerve fiber (nf) is enveloped in glial lamellae (LAM) constituting the inner core. With permission, from Munger and Ide (1988). **D-F:** Insect mechanoreceptors. **D:** Schematic drawing of a campiniform hair sensile of the cricket. Around the sensory hair and the sensory neurons (N), a very complex arrangement of sheath cells (SC) is placed; the soma and axon of the nerve cells is embedded in a glial sheath (g); cut, cuticula. With permission, from Gnatzy and Schmidt (1971). **E:** Schematic drawing of a stretch receptor ('strand receptor'). The sensory neuron and its ensheathing glial cell are embedded in a connective tissue strand. Note that a basal lamina envelops the glial cells but is not shown here. With permission, from

Osborne (1970). **F:** Semi-schematic drawing of a chordotonal organ in *Drosophila*. The sensory neuron (N) is associated with three specialized glial cells, cap cell (C), scopolale cell (SC), and ligament cell (L) of which the latter contacts the axon of the sensory neuron. Ligament and cap cells are many times longer than shown; they span, with some tension, the scopolale cell-nerve cell pair. With permission, from Carlson et al. (1997).

In some instances, the dendrites are very long, and may not allow electrotonic signal propagation to the soma. It has been shown that the dendrites of Purkinje neurons in the cerebellum possess "hot spots" in their membrane where Ca^{2+}-mediated action potentials can be generated (Llinas et al., 1969; Llinas, 1975). Action potentials are generated in the dendritic membrane of many other types of neurons (reviewed by Häusser et al., 2000). This fits with the idea that these action potentials serve as an auxiliary aid to convey distal information along long 'dendritic cables' (e.g., of neocortical pyramidal cells) towards the soma. Once these action potentials arrive at the soma they are attenuated (Stuart et al., 1997a) such that they do not predominate the other synaptic inputs. Such long dendrites, or parts of them, may even be myelinated by oligodendrocytes (Pinching, 1971) (Fig. 3.5C,D). On the other hand, it has been suggested that dendrite-initiated spikes may amplify multiple simultaneous synaptic input (Häusser et al., 2000). This dendritic spike generation must be distinguished from active back-propagation of axon-derived action potentials which also occurs in many types of neurons (reviewed by Häusser et al., 2000) and which may provide a feedback signal of neuronal output, inducing dendritic responses such as local rises of $[Ca^{2+}]_i$ or dendritic transmitter release, as observed in dopaminergic cells of the substantia nigra and mitral cells of the olfactory bulb (reviewed by Häusser et al., 2000).

3.5. Glio-neuronal associations at the neuronal soma

Depending on the size of a given neuronal soma, its glial sheath may be provided by one or more glial cells. Large neurons may be ensheathed by velate terminal processes of several astrocytes (e.g., in mammalian neocortex) or by the flat somata of several satellite glial cells (e.g., in the sensory ganglia; Fig. 3.7). By contrast, several densely packed small neuronal somata (often termed granule cells) may be ensheathed by the velate processes of one or a few glial cells, such as cerebellar granule cells (by velate astrocytes: Chan-Palay and Palay, 1972; Fig. 3.2B), retinal photoreceptor and bipolar cells (by Müller cells: Reichenbach et al., 1989; Figs. 3.2A, 3.6A-C), or the granule cells of the hippocampal fascia dentata (Fig. 3.6D, E). Irrespective of these differences, in most neurons the somata and the stem dendrites share the same glial sheaths. This coincides with the fact that the soma is another main site of synaptic input to most neurons. It can thus be assumed that the perisomatic sheaths serve similar purposes as the peridendritic ones, viz. the homeostasis of the surrounding extracellular space, and the metabolic exchange between neurons and glial cells.

An exception are the myelinated somata of some neurons (e.g., in vestibular ganglia) (section 3.5.4.).

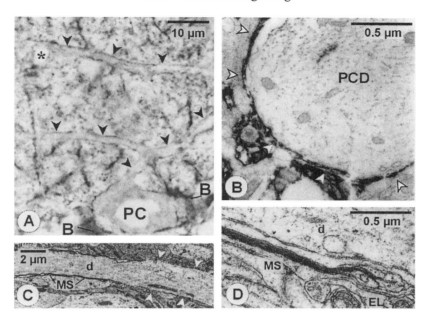

Figure 3.5. Ensheathing of dendrites. **A:** Rat cerebellar cortex. A Purkinje cell and its dendrites are more or less completely outlined by glial processes. Note the perpendicular dark lines representing the main processes of Bergmann glial cells. Two of their perikarya (B) can be seen attached to that of the Purkinje cell (PC). The horizontal and oblique light structures are dendrites demarcated by the fine glial processes (arrowheads), which have been labeled by anti-Merlin. The asterisk labels a capillary. (A. Derouiche and O. Carpèn, unpublished observations). **B:** Astroglial sheath around a Purkinje cell stem dendrite (PCD) in the rat cerebellum; glial cytoplasm (arrowheads) is labeled for S-100 (photoconversion). The sheath is almost complete (although it is provided by more than one individual Bergmann glial cell: Grosche et al., 2002). Original electron micrograph by Martin Rickmann, Göttingen. **C:** Myelinated mitral cell dendrite (d) in the monkey brain. The myelin sheath (MS) is present only along a part of the dendrite; other parts are devoid of myelin (arrowheads). **D:** Another myelinated dendrite at higher magnification. The myelin sheath is embedded into two glial cytoplasmic tongues, and terminates in cytoplasmic end lamellae (EL). With permission, from Pinching (1971).

3.5.1. Velate sheaths

Perisomatic velate glial sheaths may be formed by retinal Müller cells, astrocytes including Bergmann glial cells, olfactory ensheathing cells, and enteric glial cells. Usually, such sheaths cover the soma surface almost completely (Fig. 3.6 A-E), with the exception of "holes" where a direct apposition of neuronal membranes occurs at synaptic sites. These holes are also visible in the perineuronal nets that fill the interfaces between neuronal membranes and glial sheaths but leave space for synaptic contacts (section 3.8.). Several astroglial cells may contribute to the sheath around one large neuronal soma, such as found in Purkinje cells of the cerebellum (Fig. 3.6 F,G). It should be noted, however, that groups of neuronal somata without individual glial sheaths (i.e., with direct apposition of their membranes) can be found in some brain stem nuclei.

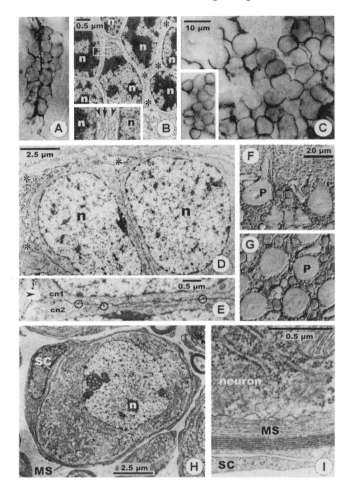

Figure 3.6. Velate sheaths of neuronal somata. **A-C:** Complete ensheathing of photoreceptor cell somata by Müller cell processes in the outer nuclear layer of a rabbit retina. **A:** Golgi-impregnated Müller cell process in the outer nuclear layer; radial section. There are many honeycomb-like velate sheaths around individual photoreceptor cell somata (also visible in the inset of **C**). **B:** Electron micrograph of the outer nuclear layer; each photoreceptor cell nucleus (n) is surrounded by a thin rim of its own cytoplasm, and by a thin velate tongue of Müller cell cytoplasm (asterisks). The inset shows the boxed area at higher magnification; there are three cytoplasmic lamellae (two photoreceptors - arrowheads; Müller cell - arrow). **C:** Flat-mounted rabbit retina; the processes of several neighboring Golgi-labeled Müller cells form a 'network' of velate sheaths on neuronal cell somata in the inner nuclear layer; inset: flat-mounted outer nuclear layer. The calibration bar is valid also for (**A**). With permission, from Reichenbach et al., 1989 (**A, C**) and original micrograph, courtesy of H. Wolburg (**B**). **D-G:** In the rat hippocampus and cerebellum, the somata of neurons are surrounded by glial cell processes. **D, E :** Rat hippocampus. **D:** Two granule neurons (n), very closely apposed within the granule cell layer of the fascia dentata. They are ensheathed and separated by extremely fine astrocytic lamellae which are identified by silver grains revealing glutamine synthetase immunoreactivity (silver-intensified DAB). Note the glia process (asterisks) ensheathing the cells at left and on top. **E:** The glial process separating the cells (arrowhead) can be identified

only at higher magnification, by the overlaying silver grains (some are encircled). cn1, cytoplasm one neuron; cn2, cytoplasm of the other neuron. **F, G:** Also the somata of Purkinje cells (P) in the cerebellar cortex are almost completely embedded in cytoplasmic sheaths arising from the adjacent Bergmann glial cells (small somata, surrounded by cytoplasm immunolabeled for glutamine synthetase). **F:** Radial section, **G:** tangential section; the calibration bar is valid also for (**G**). With permission, from Reichenbach et al. (1995a). **H, I:** Myelinated soma of a neuron in the murine spiral ganglion; the lamellae of the myelin sheath (MS) are shown at higher magnification in (**I**). SC - Schwann cell, n – nucleus of the neuron. With permission, from Romand and Romand (1987).

3.5.2. Myelinated somata

Some sensory ganglia are characterized by two specific features, (i) synaptic information processing does not take place in them, and (ii) the information propagation needs to be very rapid (e.g., in the vestibular and acoustic pathways). In these cases, the neuronal somata may be considered as mere "bulgings of a continuous information transport cable" (dendrite - soma - axon), necessary to maintain the cell processes. All compartments of the cable, including the soma, may be myelinated (Fig. 3.6H,I) (e.g., Romand and Romand, 1987). A mathematical model of action potential conduction across myelinated somata of mammalian auditory-nerve neurons has been provided (Colombo and Parkins, 1987). Myelination has also been observed on granule cells in the cerebellum of the monkey (Cooper and Beal, 1976). Whereas the perisomatic velate sheaths are formed by astrocytic cells, myelination of neuronal somata is provided by oligodendrocytes (CNS) or myelinating Schwann cells (PNS).

3.5.3. Satellite sheaths

In peripheral ganglia of vertebrates, with the exception of enteric ganglia, the neuronal somata are covered by satellite glial cells (Fig. 3.7A), whose number increases with the size of the neuron (Pannese, 1981; Matsumoto and Rosenbluth, 1986). These cells are rather flat and are devoid of long elaborate processes. They are mutually coupled by gap junctions (Hanani et al., 2002; Hanani et al., 1999; Pannese, 1981; Pomeroy and Purves, 1988) (Fig. 3.7B). Satellite glial cells have transporters for amino acid neurotransmitters (Schon and Kelly, 1974; Berger and Hediger, 2000), and thus may regulate the neuronal environment. It has been proposed that in some ganglia these cells function as a barrier for the diffusion of substances between the blood and the perineuronal space (Ten Tusscher et al., 1989), but this was not supported by a later study (Allen and Kiernan, 1994). There is evidence for functional signaling via NO between neurons and satellite cells in DRG (Thippeswammy and Morris, 2002.)

3.5.4. Trophospongia

In many invertebrate ganglia, a central "neuropilar" region (containing the dendrites and axons of the neurons, and neuropile glial cells) is surrounded by a "cortex" that contains the neuronal somata and their ensheathing cells (Hanström, 1928). Within this cortex, the situation resembles that in vertebrates, in that neurons are covered by glial sheaths. An intriguing finding in many invertebrate ganglia is the formation of so-called trophospongia (Coggeshall, 1967; Saint Marie et al., 1984; Hoyle et al., 1986). These consist of extensive elaborate interdigitations of small PGPs that enter the neuronal somata (Fig. 3.7E,F). It has been speculated that these structures provide large surface areas for an intense glio-neuronal exchange of molecules. Although such extensive trophospongia have never been found in vertebrates, in vertebrate sensory ganglia it has been observed that neurons may send fine projections into satellite cells (Pannese, 2002).

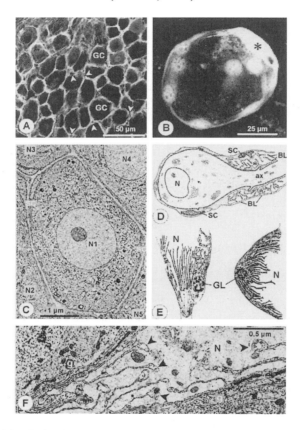

Figure 3.7. Glial cell sheaths on neuronal somata. **A-D:** Complete ensheathing of trigeminal ganglion neuronal somata by satellite cells. **A:** Immunocytochemical demonstration of glutamine synthetase in the satellite glial cells (some of their small nuclei are labeled by arrowheads) which form envelopes on the neurons (GC). **B:** Dye-coupling among perineuronal satellite cells enveloping an individual ganglion cell in a murine lumbar DRG; the dye-injected cell is labeled by an asterisk. Original data (M.H.). **C:** Electron micrograph of a gecko DRG, showing a nerve cell body (N1) and its glial sheath (SC). The satellite glial cell is clearly separated from others encircling adjacent neurons (N2-N5) by a connective tissue space. **D:** Semi-schematic drawing of a neuron (N) in bullfrog DRG, together with its ensheathing satellite cells (SC). Around the initial segment of the axon (ax), the satellite sheath is split into two layers, separated by a connective tissue space (asterisks); the satellite glial cells extend lamellar cytoplasmic tongues into this space, which are covered by basal laminae (BL). (**C**) and (**D**) with permission from Pannese (1981). **E, F:** So-called trophospongium in invertebrate ganglia. **E:** Drawings of glial cells (GL) surrounding a

neuronal soma (right) and the soma and the initial segment of a neuron (left) in metathoracic ganglia of the locust, based upon reconstructions from serial section electron microscopy. Many finger-like protrusions extend into the neuronal cytoplasm. With permission, from Hoyle (1986). F: Electron micrograph of the glial trophospongium (arrowheads) entering the cytoplasm of a neuron (N) in *Leucophaea*; g - satellite glial cells. With permission, from Scharrer and Weitzman (1981).

3.6. Glio-neuronal associations at the effector pole: the axon

The efferent processes of neurons may differ greatly in length and diameter, as well as in functional parameters; all these processes will be termed 'axons' here, as a precise definition of this term is still missing. Short axons such as those of retinal photoreceptors and bipolar cells (rarely exceeding some 50 μm in length) do not generate action potentials, whereas the long axons of the projection neurons in brain and retina conduct information by means of action potentials. As a general rule in vertebrates, axons with a diameter of more than 0.3 μm (CNS) or 2 μm (PNS) perform a saltatory conduction of action potentials. In these axons action potential-generating Na^+ channels are not randomly distributed in the membrane but are focused within small areas ("hot spots") along the axon. Such neurites are covered by myelin sheaths between these hot spots. The myelin sheaths are provided by oligodendrocytes (CNS) or myelinating Schwann cells (PNS) (section 3.6.3.).

Specialized periaxonal sheaths are found in many invertebrates. For instance, in the giant axons of the earthworm such sheaths are formed by many flat glial cells, resembling the satellite cells of vertebrate ganglia (Scharrer and Weitzman, 1980). Among the invertebrates, true myelin sheaths were only found in crustaceans (Heuser and Doggenweiler, 1966; Kusano and LaVail, 1971).

Generally, the axon arises from the soma at a funnel-shaped area termed the axon hillock. In some cases, however, the axon may arise from a common stem process which also gives rise to a dendritic tree (e.g., Fig. 3.1 A), or even from a dendrite. This is frequently observed in neurons of invertebrates. It is noteworthy in this context that not every neuron has a definite axon. Some types of retinal horizontal cells and amacrine cells, for instance, possess 'dendrite-like' processes that may be both pre- and postsynaptic. Another case is the hair cells of the inner ear. At the effector pole of their rod-like somata, they possess presynaptic specializations that are contacted by cup-like postsynaptic elements formed by the dendrites of neurons in the acoustic ganglion (see Fig. 3.12 D).

3.6.1. Unmyelinated axons / axon bundles

In the CNS, short non-spiking axons, although lacking specialized glio-neuronal contacts, are closely associated with glial cells. For instance, the axons of retinal photoreceptor cells run in parallel to the outer stem processes of Müller cells. In the Henle fiber layer of the primate parafoveal retina the two types of cell processes share a rather long common path (up to several hundred micrometers) along which they are closely associated (Fig. 3.8 A). Generally in the CNS, thin unmyelinated axons have no individual glial sheaths; rather, bundles of such axons are enwrapped by the processes of Müller cells (retina) or astrocytes (retina and optic nerve; Fig. 3.8B). It might be speculated that in these cases, the extracellular space is large enough to buffer activity-related increases in the K$^+$ ion concentration without any intervention from glial cells.

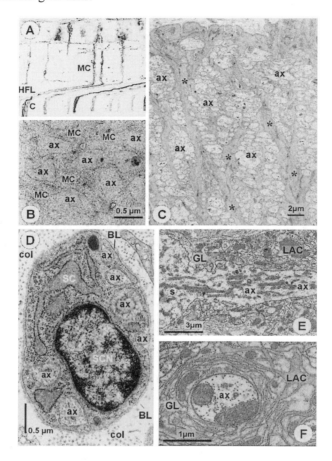

Figure 3.8. Glial associations with unmyelinated fibers. **A-C:** Vertebrate CNS. **A, B:** Henle's fiber layer of the human perifoveal retina. **A:** Golgi-impregnated preparation (Courtesy of B.B.Boycott and H. Waessle). Müller cell processes (MC) and cone axons (C) run in parallel through Henle's fiber layer (HFL). **B:** Electron microscopy reveals no specific associations between the tightly packed cone photoreceptor axons (ax) and Müller cell processes (cross section). **C:** Optic nerve of the goldfish. Several fascicles of unmyelinated optic axons are surrounded by astrocytic processes (asterisks). **D:** Vertebrate PNS; sciatic nerve of the rat. Six individual axons are embedded in cytoplasmic tongues / tunnels of a Schwann cell (SC). Note that the Schwann cell, together with ensheathed axons, is completely embedded within a basal lamina (BL) such that neither the axons nor the Schwann cell membrane is in direct contact with the collagen fibers (col). SCN - Schwann cell nucleus. **E, F:** Invertebrate PNS. Origin of the axon (ax) of a sensory cell of a cercus of the cricket (*Acheta domesticus*); the soma (s) is located at the left side of **E**. Complex glial lamellae (GL) envelop both the axon hillock and the axon. In both the longitudinal (**E**) and the transverse sections (**F**), large lacunae (LAC) are visible between the glial lamellae. Original micrographs, courtesy of H. Wolburg (**B-D**) and of Th. Keil (**E, F**).

In peripheral nerves, however, even individual non-myelinated fibers may be enwrapped in transcellular "tunnels" or "grooves" of non-myelinating Schwann cells (Fig. 3.8C), which are completely enveloped by a basal lamina. This may be caused by the necessity to avoid a direct contact between the axons and the collagen fibrils which are abundant in peripheral nerves. The transition zone between peripheral nerves and the spinal cord is characterized by an abrupt change of the glia-neuron associations along individual fibers (Berthold and Carlstedt, 1977a, b).

In invertebrates, the non-myelinated axons are often enveloped in rather complex (even multilamellar) glial sheaths, which also contact large lacunae of extracellular clefts probably serving as buffer spaces for ions (Fig. 3.8E, F).

3.6.2. Initial segment / axon hillock

In spike-generating neurons, the initial segment (arising from the axon hillock) is traditionally thought to be the site of action potential generation (Catterall, 1984). Depending on the type of neuron, it may or may not be the target of synaptic innervation, probably modulating the excitability of the local or adjacent membrane (*cf.* Stuart et al., 1997b). More recently, experimental evidence has been accumulated showing that the axon proper (i.e., the first heminode and/or the first few nodes of Ranvier in myelinated axons) is the site of action potential initiation (Stuart et al., 1997a, 1997b; Colbert and Pan, 2002), rather than the initial segment. These authors suggest that the initial segment plays a critical role in isolating the axon from electrical load of the soma (i.e., preventing an inactivation of axonal sodium channels by sub-threshold somatic depolarizations) and in facilitating the back-propagation of axonal action potentials onto the soma (Colbert and Pan, 2002) (cf. section 3.4.2.).

The glio-neuronal associations at the initial segment are strikingly variable. In some cases such as retinal ganglion cells, elaborate multiple astroglial sheaths may be wrapped around the initial segment (Holländer et al., 1991; Stone et al., 1995) (Fig. 3.10A). In other cases such as cortical pyramidal cells or motoneurons, an abundant extracellular matrix may cover this area (Fig. 3.16), with accompanying "simple" glial cell processes similar to the peridendritic and perisomatic nets (Brückner et al., 1996b). Rather large extracellular spaces (Brückner et al., 1996b) may provide an additional buffering capacity for ions.

Unlike the relatively simple glial sheath around the soma of the DRG neuron, the axon hillock and initial segment of these cells are wrapped with an elaborate cover of glial membranes. The glial cells form a double (split) layer, with a large extracellular cleft and a basal lamina between the two layers (Pannese, 1981; Matsumoto and Rosenbluth, 1986) (Fig. 3.7D). The action potentials are clearly initiated near the peripheral sensory ending, rather than at the soma, which supports the above-mentioned view that the initial segment - and its coverage by glial cell processes and extracellular matrix - may serve purposes other than the initiation of action potentials.

It is obvious that focused research is required to elucidate the neuronal and glial properties of this functionally important structure.

3.6.3. Myelinated internodal segments of axons

It has already been mentioned that saltatory conduction of action potentials requires the presence of hot spots with a high density of spike-generating Na^+ channels. The distance between these hot spots increases with increasing diameter of the axons (Remahl and Hildebrand, 1990a, b; Hildebrand et al., 1993). The interposed ('internodal') axon membrane in such neurites is covered by high-resistance, high capacitance myelin sheaths, in order to prevent shunt currents before the next hot spot (i.e., node of Ranvier) is reached by the excitation. Generally, not only the internodal distance but also the thickness of myelin sheath increases with the diameter of the myelinated axon (Remahl and Hildebrand, 1990a, b; Hildebrand et al., 1993).

In CNS white matter, adjacent internodes of several small-diameter axons (up to 50) may be myelinated by one oligodendrocyte; such type I oligodendrocytes (Fig. 3.9B) are frequently found in the optic nerve. The thicker the axons, the fewer internodes are myelinated by one oligodendrocyte (Fig. 3.9 B). In the case of extremely thick axons in the spinal cord, one type IV oligodendrocyte may myelinate just one internode. This resembles the situation in the PNS where generally one internode is myelinated by one Schwann cell (Fig. 3.9 C, D).

During ontogenesis, an elaborate interplay between the maturing axons and the ensheathing glial cells is required to establish correct myelination. Once an internode is myelinated, it normally maintains the myelin sheath provided by the very same oligodendrocyte or Schwann cell. This requires a high degree of remodeling of the sheath, because both the diameter and the length of the internode, and thus the length and thickness of the myelin sheath, increase dramatically when the nerve grows in length up to 100-fold from embryo to adult. For more details on myelination see Hildebrand et al. (1993).

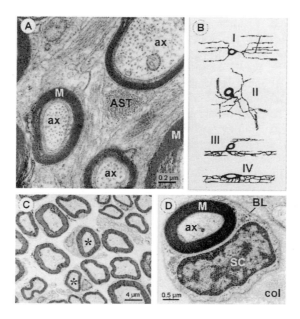

Figure 3.9. Myelinated internodes. **A:** Optic nerve of the tree shrew; the internodes of several axons (ax) are enveloped by oligodendrocyte-derived myelin sheaths (M). Processes of astrocytes (AST) are intermingled. **B:** Semi-schematic drawing of distinct types of oligodendrocytes (original drawings of A.R., after Hortega, 1956). Type I cells may myelinate the internodes of several small-diameter axons in white matter tracts such as the optic nerve; type II cells myelinate less (and thicker) internodes, often in the gray matter; type III cells are associated with the internodes of only a few thick axons, and type IV cells with just one very thick internode. **C:** Sciatic nerve of the rat. Internodes are each myelinated by a single Schwann cell (visible in two cases - asterisks on the axons); thin unmyelinated fibers are also present. **D:** Same preparation at higher magnification, showing one axon (ax) with its myelin sheath (M), the ensheathing Schwann cell (SC), and the surrounding basal lamina (BL). The interspaces are filled with collagen fibrils (col). Original micrographs, courtesy of H. Wolburg (**A, C, D**).

3.6.4. Nodes of Ranvier and node-like specializations of axons

In myelinated axons of vertebrates, the nodes of Ranvier are devoid of a myelin sheath but not of glial contacts: assemblies ('coronae') of small, finger-like PGPs of the fibrous astrocytes contact the nodal membrane (Waxman, 1983; Raine, 1984; Hildebrand et al., 1993; Butt et al., 1994) (Fig. 3.10A, B). These PGPs express the J1 glycoprotein, an adhesion-modulating protein presumably involved in axon-glial interactions modulating the assembly and/or maintenance of nodes of Ranvier (ffrench-Constant et al., 1986). At the axon-glial contact areas, the interposed extracellular clefts are extremely narrow (about 6 µm: Waxman, 1983). However, the adjacent perinodal space contains an abundant extracellular matrix, comparable to that of the perineuronal nets (Raine, 1984; Hildebrand et al., 1993) (Fig. 3.10C). It has been proposed that this matrix buffers the large increases of K^+ ions near the sites of action potential generation (Treherne et al., 1982; Härtig et al., 1999) (section 3.8.).

In peripheral nerves, the nodal neuronal membranes are contacted by similar finger-like PGPs arising from the myelinating Schwann cell itself (reviewed by Raine, 1984). In the transition zones between CNS and PNS (e.g., within the dorsal and ventral roots of the spinal nerves) the "borderline nodes" are abutted by PGPs from both the distal Schwann cell and a proximal astrocyte (Berthold and Carlstedt, 1977b; Fig. 3.10C, D).

Within the mammalian retina (with the exception of hares and rabbits), all optic axons are unmyelinated although the thicker fibers become myelinated in the optic nerve. Nevertheless, the optic axons provide a saltatory conduction of action potentials from the very (intraretinal) origin at the initial segments of retinal ganglion cells; for this purpose, they are endowed with "node-like specializations", i.e., hot spots with high Na^+ channel densities (Hildebrand and Waxman, 1983) in their membrane. Although the missing myelination seems to require rather short internodal distances (Reichenbach et al., 1994), this situation may be a compromise between the need for rapid information transmission on the one hand, and a reasonable optical quality of retinal images on the other hand (myelinated fibers reflect and scatter light). At the node-like specializations, similar coronae of finger-like PGPs are found as at the nodes of Ranvier; they may arise from both astrocytes and Müller cells (Hildebrand and Waxman, 1983; Reichenbach et al., 1988a; Holländer et al., 1991; Fig. 3.10.A).

In the axons of the prawn where the internodes are myelinated by ensheathing glia, rather large perinodal extracellular spaces are partially filled (and sealed at their margins by tight junctions) with fine PGPs from specialized glial cells, termed 'nodal cells' (Heuser and Doggenweiler, 1966; Fig. 3.10G).

The function of the perinodal glial cell processes has been a matter of much speculation. A glio-neuronal exchange of molecules (including the delivery of Na^+ channel molecules (Bevan et al., 1985; Shrager et al., 1985) has been proposed. It has also been speculated that the glial fingers might be sensors of axonal action potentials. Strong depolarizations of the glial membrane could be induced by ephaptic current transmission, and might then trigger metabolic reactions of the glial cells (Chao et al., 1994; Fig. 3.10H).

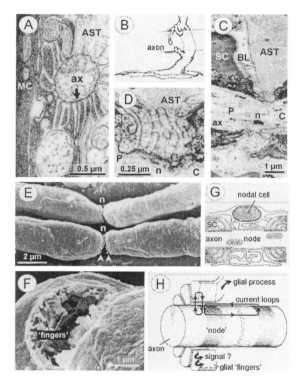

Figure 3.10. Glial associations with nodes of Ranvier and node-like specializations. **A:** Node-like axonal specializations of intraretinal axons (ax) (arrow: electron-dense undercoating of the axonal membrane) are contacted by coronae of finger-like PGPs. These may stem from both Müller cells (MC, electron-dark cytoplasm) and astrocytes (AST, electron-lucent cytoplasm); cat retina. With permission, from Holländer et al., 1991. **B:** Similar PGPs are found at true nodes of Ranvier, e.g., in the optic nerve (with permission, from Butt et al., 1994). **C:** Axon (ax) in the transition zone between CNS (C, *right side*) and PNS (P, *left side*) in the dorsal root of the cat. The axonal membrane at the node of Ranvier (n) is contacted by glial fingers from both a Schwann cell (SC) and an astrocyte (AST). The basal lamina (BL) covers the Schwann cell and the astrocytic endfoot continuously. The internodal sections of the axon are myelinated by the Schwann cell (*left side*) and by an oligodendrocyte (*right side*). **D:** Perinodal space of the same axon, at higher magnification. With permission, from Berthold

and Carlstedt, 1977b. **E:** Scanning electron micrograph of two myelinated fibers in the mouse sciatic nerve; at the nodes of Ranvier (n), the Schwann cells extend finger-like protrusions (arrow). **F:** Closer view of a myelinated nerve fiber in the same nerve, broken at the node. Finger-like projections of the Schwann cell arise from the circumferential collar of the cytoplasm. With permission, from Ushiki and Ide, 1987. **G:** Similar relationships as in the vertebrate CNS are found in some invertebrates: 'Sheath cells' (SC) and 'nodal cells' on the myelinated axon of the prawn (Heuser and Doggenweiler, 1966). **H:** The perinodal PGPs might be sensors of axonal action potentials. Strong depolarizations of the glial membrane could be induced by ephaptic current transmission, and might then trigger metabolic reactions of the glial cells (Chao et al., 1994).

3.7. Glio-neuronal associations at the synapses

In analogy to the synapses, which are the main sites of neuron-to-neuron signaling, the perisynaptic glial sheaths are considered to be the prototypic sites of glio-neuronal interactions. This view has been challenged by the observation that certain synapses, or even large groups of synapses, are devoid of apparent glial contacts (for review, see Chao et al., 2002). Nevertheless, most synapses of the vertebrate CNS are endowed with elaborate glial sheaths, and there is no doubt that the latter constitute a crucial "third element" of the typical synapse, in addition to the presynaptic terminal and the postsynaptic area (Volterra et al., 2002).

3.7.1. Gap junctions

In the adult vertebrate nervous system, neuron-to-neuron signaling via electrical synapses (gap junctions) is the exception rather than the rule. Nevertheless, important signaling pathways such as the scotopic (i.e., rod-driven) retinal information processing, involve transmission via gap junctions (Famiglietti and Kolb, 1975; Vaney, 1991). At present, however, no distinct glial associations to electrical neuronal synapses have been identified.

By contrast, glial cells are known to be extensively coupled by gap junctions in many instances (Fig. 3.11D). This has been demonstrated by dye coupling experiments in both CNS (Gutnick et al., 1981) and PNS (Hanani et al., 1989; Pomeroy and Purves, 1988) (e.g., Fig. 3.7B). Even unidirectional coupling has been reported between different types of retinal glial cells (Robinson et al., 1993). The glial coupling may be modified by neuronal activity.

For a detailed discussion of this topic see Chapter 13.

3.7.2. Chemical synapses

Most synapses are ensheathed by lamellar PGPs (Fig. 3.11), but the degree (or even the presence) of ensheathing may vary considerably even within the same area of the CNS (see Chao et al., 2002). In rat neocortex for example, about 56% of all synaptic perimeters are covered by astroglia while astroglial membranes make up only 22% of all membranes in the neuropil (Landgrebe et al., cited in Chao and Wolff, 2002). In particular, most synaptic clefts are "sealed" at their margins by PGPs (Fig. 3.11A-D), which may even be multilamellar (Fig. 3.11C). However, the situation is different in specialized subcortical structures where multiple synaptic junctions are enclosed in a common glial sheath, termed 'synaptic glomeruli' or 'complex synapses'. Glial coverage in these structures is very high (often there are multilamellar sheaths), and does not penetrate the interior of the complexes, and thus, cannot seal individual synaptic clefts (Fig. 3.11G). As an extreme case, there are even astroglia-free neuropil compartments, e.g., in Rolando's substantia gelatinosa of the spinal cord and in the cochlear nucleus, where thin sensory axons terminate in "synaptic nests" that lack intrinsic glia. More details about brain region- and synapse type-dependent variations in perisynaptic astroglial sheaths can be found in Chao et al. (2002).

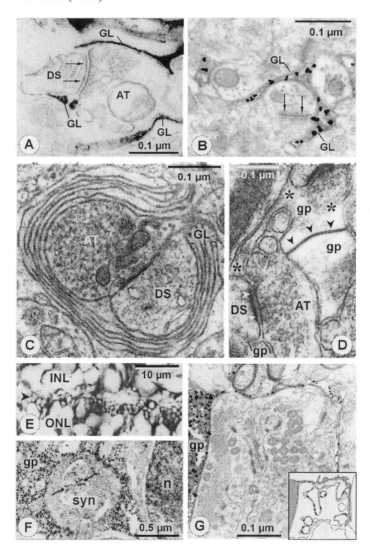

Figure 3.11. Glia-neuron associations at synapses in the vertebrate CNS. **A:** Ensheathing of parallel fiber-Purkinje cell synapses by Bergmann glial cell processes; murine cerebellum. A Bergmann glial cell had been injected by Lucifer yellow, and the dye was then converted into

an electron-dense label. The synaptic clefts (arrows) between the axon terminals /AT) and the dendritic spines (DS) are sealed by glial lamellae (GL) from the injected cell. With permission, from Grosche et al., (2002). **B:** Rat hippocampus. Fine, perisynaptic PGPs are identified by silver grains indicating immunoreactivity for the astrocyte-specific enzyme, glutamine synthetase; one synaptic cleft is labeled by arrows. Original micrograph (A.D.). **C:** In the pontine nuclei of the cat, multilamellar glial sheaths have been observed on spine synapses. With permission, from Narlieva (1988). **D:** Whereas the neuronal elements (axon terminal, AT, and dendritic spine, DS) transmit information via a chemical synapse (postsynaptic density labeled by white arrowheads), the enveloping glial cell processes (gp, asterisks) are coupled by gap junctions. Gap junctions are a common feature of astrocytic profiles easily identified by the parallel appearance of membranes (black arrowheads) enclosing a white line that is narrower than the extracellular space. Original micrograph (A.D.). **E, F:** Rat retina. **E:** Retinal Müller cell processes visualized by glutamine synthetase immunoreactivity (DAB). Level of the outer plexiform layer, between the inner (INL) and the outer nuclear (ONL) layers. The photoreceptor terminals (at the level of the arrowhead) are fully embedded by Müller cell processes, their typical "spherule" shape can be recognized at the light microscopical level. **F:** At the ultrastructural level, a rod spherule (syn) is typically engulfed by Müller glial cell processes (gp), containing glutamine synthetase immunoreactivity (silver-intensified DAB). n, neuronal cell nucleus. Original micrographs (A.D.). **G:** Rat hippocampus. A main glial process (gp; left margin) extends a fine glial process encircling a mossy fibre bouton, which forms several synapses (compare sketch in inset). Glial profiles are identified by silver grains (silver-intensified immunoreactivity for glutamine synthetase). Note that the astrocytic processes do not contact individual synapses but a synaptic arrangement (see inset), in analogy to synaptic glomeruli.

In the PNS, synapses occur not only among neurons but also at non-neuronal targets such as muscle and gland cells. In the case of neuromuscular synapses (Fig. 3.12 A-C), the gap between two tissue compartments of different embryonic origin (neuro-ectoderm and mesoderm) must be bridged. These two compartments are generally separated by a basal lamina, and similarly the synaptic cleft between the (neuro-ectodermal) presynapse and the (mesodermal) postsynapse contains a basal lamina (Fig. 3.12.C). It is likely that bridging of this gap may have been a non-trivial problem in phylogeny. In the ancestors of vertebrates (e.g., represented by the recent lancelet *Branchiostoma*), for example, the presynaptic terminals of the motor axons abut the basal lamina enveloping the neural tube (corresponding to the pia mater in vertebrates); the muscle cells extend neurite-like processes towards the neural tube where they form postsynaptic elements (Flood, 1966; Holland, 1996) (Fig. 3.12 E). In vertebrates, motor nerves run towards the innervated muscles where they form specific synapses on skeletal muscle cells, termed 'motor endplates'. These structures are the best-studied synapses of the body; many of the basic physiological properties of excitatory synaptic transmission have been first studied in these 'model synapses' (for review, see Katz, 1966). Nevertheless, it should be kept in mind that they represent a very specialized type of synaptic contact. In addition to going beyond the borders of the nervous system (e.g., involving a basal lamina as mentioned above), they operate at nearly 100% synaptic efficacy - that is, as a rule every presynaptic action potential evokes a postsynaptic action potential, and a motor response. A similar situation is found in several types of neuro-neuronal synapses in peripheral autonomic ganglia, where a presynaptic action potential elicits a postsynaptic spike (Crowcroft and Szurszewski, 1971). Such synapses are defined as 'strong', and allow high fidelity in signal propagation, but low ability to integrate information. In contrast, many neuro-neuronal synapses in CNS, where information processing involves integration of excitatory and inhibitory inputs, usually require summation of several excitatory postsynaptic potentials to generate a novel spike. This necessity of high synaptic efficacy at motor endplates may require the complex infolding of their synaptic clefts (Fig. 3.12 B,C), in order to enhance the membrane areas available for transmitter release and binding. Furthermore, the motor endplate is not very typical in the transmitter substance used, i.e., acetylcholine. Although important cholinergic systems exist also in autonomic nervous system and even in the brain (Klein and Löffelholz, 1996), most CNS neurons use other molecules (e.g., glutamate or GABA) as messenger molecules. The perisynaptic glial elements of such CNS synapses are involved in the uptake and recycling of these amino acid transmitters (Chapter 9). As acetylcholine is degraded extracellularly by acetylcholine esterase, the motor endplate cannot be used as a model for these glio-neuronal interactions. Nevertheless, it is tightly enveloped by a terminal Schwann cell (Fig. 3.12 A,B) which may be involved in other functional interactions. Indeed, Robitaille and his co-workers (Castonguay et al., 2001) showed that perisynaptic glial cells in the motor endplate actively participate in synaptic transmission.

The characteristics of neuromuscular transmission in smooth muscles are less well understood than those of the skeletal muscles. It is widely accepted that these junctions do not show clear structural specializations and that the synaptic gap is much wider than at the motor endplate. However, in some cases there is evidence for close contacts between nerves and smooth muscle membranes. For example Gabella (1995) has shown that in the rat urinary bladder axonal varicosities, which contain synaptic vesicles, can be as close as 10 nm to the muscle. At these locations the nerve is devoid of a Schwann cell sheath. This forms a 'window', which allows fast diffusion of neurotransmitter, and can be regarded as a neuromuscular junction.

The functional interactions between synaptic elements and their glial sheaths are not yet fully elucidated. An 'insulation' of individual synapses (or groups of them; section 3.7.3) against their microenvironment may prevent the uncontrolled spread of neuronal excitation. For instance, it is now generally accepted that perisynaptic glial membranes may be dominant sites of transmitter transporters, and that glial uptake of released neurotransmitter molecules is crucial for maintaining the spatial and temporal specificity of synaptic transmission (Sarantis and Mobbs, 1992; Oliet et al., 2001). It is noteworthy that the glutamate-neutralizing enzyme, glutamine synthetase, is present in the perisynaptic glial cytoplasm (Derouiche, 1997; Derouiche and Frotscher, 1991; Derouiche and Rauen, 1995; Fig. 3.11.B,E-G). Furthermore, glial receptors for neurotransmitters may be assembled in these membrane areas. Stimulation of these receptors may initiate glial metabolic reactions, beneficial for the activated neuronal compartments (Volterra et al., 2002). It is commonly assumed, but not yet demonstrated, that glutamate which is released from astrocytes (and which may modulate synaptic transmission: Parpura et al., 1994; Kang et al., 1998) originates from perisynaptic glial processes. Release from PGPs would seem logical, but the few physiological data (Kang et al., 1998; Porter and McCarthy, 1995) on slice preparations have not been conclusive. The 'slow' neuronal response to glial glutamate (Kang et al., 1998; Porter and McCarthy, 1995) would also be compatible with a paracrine release away from the synapse, involving the activity of the entire astrocyte. This prompts the question whether the SNARE proteins described in astrocytes (Araque et al., 2000) are predominantly located in their perisynaptic

PGPs.

Perisynaptic PGPs may also be crucially involved in the maintenance and/or degradation of synapses and, thus, in synaptic plasticity (section 3.9.).

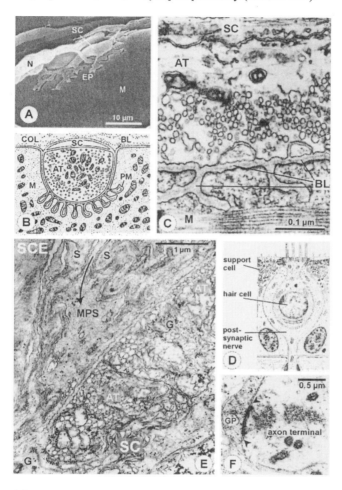

Figure 3.12. Glia-neuron associations at synapses in the vertebrate PNS and in invertebrates, and axo-glial synaptoid contacts. **A-C:** Motor endplate of the frog. **A:** Scanning electron microscopic demonstration of the Schwann cell (SC) covering the neuromuscular synapse (endplate, EP) between a nerve (N) and a muscle fiber (M) of a Chinese hamster. The overlying collagen fibers and basal laminae were removed by pre-treatment with HCl. With permission, from Fujita et al. (1986). **B:** Semi-schematic cross-section through a motor endplate. The axon terminal (AT) is covered by the Schwann cell (SC), and is inserted into the muscle (M). The postsynaptic membrane (PM) is folded in a complex manner, and contains a basal lamina (BL). The entire endplate complex is overlaid by collagen fibers (COL). With permission, from Couteaux (1958). **C:** Ultrastructurally, the synaptic cleft between the axon terminal (AT) and the muscle fiber (M) contains a basal lamina (BL). The endplate is covered by a Schwann cell (SC). With permission, from Heuser and Reese (1977). **D:** Giant calyx synapse on a type-II vestibular hair cell; almost the entire sensory cell, acting as the

presynaptic element, is embedded in the large postsynapse; both are enveloped by support cells. With permission, from Wersäll (1956). **E:** Atypical axo-muscular synapses ('central endplates') in the lancelet (*Branchiostoma*). The motor axon terminals (AT) end under the surface of the spinal cord (SC) where they are contacted by muscular (!) postsynaptic terminals (MPS). Within the spinal cord, the axon terminals are enveloped by glial cell processes (G); the motor postsynaptic endings are ensheathed by sheath cells (S). SCE - envelope of the spinal cord (collagen). With permission, from Flood (1966). **F:** Axoglial contact in the area postrema of the cat; the axon terminal makes a specific contact (arrowheads) with a glial cell process (GP) extending from an ependymoglial cell. With permission, from D'Amelio et al. (1986).

3.7.3. The concept of glial "microdomains"

In Bergmann glial cells, the existence of so-called microdomains has been demonstrated (Grosche et al., 1999; 2002). They occur as repetitive units on the stem processes, or as appendages of another microdomain. Each microdomain consists of a thin stalk and a cabbage-like, very complex head structure that bears the lamellar perisynaptic sheaths for about 5 synapses (Fig. 3.13B, C). It has been shown that these microdomains may interact with "their" synapses, independent of other microdomains and also of the stem process. Stimulation of the axons ending in the ensheathed synapses causes transient intracellular Ca^{2+} rises in individual microdomains (Grosche et al., 1999) (Fig. 3.13D). Furthermore, mathematical simulation of the cable properties reveals that even large (e. g., glutamate-induced) depolarizations of the perisynaptic membranes are not conducted over the stalks towards neighboring microdomains, or towards the stalk (Grosche et al., 2002). The energetic demands of each individual microdomain may be supported by the mitochondria found in the "head" structures (Grosche et al., 1999; 2002). The glial microdomains overlap; in every given volume unit of the molecular layer, at least two microdomains, originating from different Bergmann glial cells, interdigitate. This may fit with the observation that Purkinje cells express two functionally distinct populations of synaptic spines, and that individual spines are capable of independent activation (Denk et al., 1995), as the glial microdomains may be adjusted to meet this functional diversity of Purkinje cell synapses. In addition to the perisynaptic sheaths, the heads of the microdomains were shown to extend numerous "glial thimbles", forming complete caps on small neuronal protrusions (Fig. 3.13E), which may represent dying or growing synapses (cf. section 3.9.2.).

Similar microdomains may also exist in other areas of the brain where they may be formed, as complex PGPs, by protoplasmic astrocytes.

3.7.4. Neurosecretory terminals

A special case of a neuronal effector pole are neurosecretory 'presynapses' on basal laminae at blood vessels, such as in the stalk of the hypophysis. All abluminal areas of this basal lamina that are not abutted by neurosceretory nerve endings are covered by glial cell processes (Knowles and Anand Kumar, 1969; Lichtensteiger et al., 1978). The neuronal *vs.* glial coverage ratio may greatly vary in dependence on the functional state of the neurosecretory system (Fig. 3.15E, F).

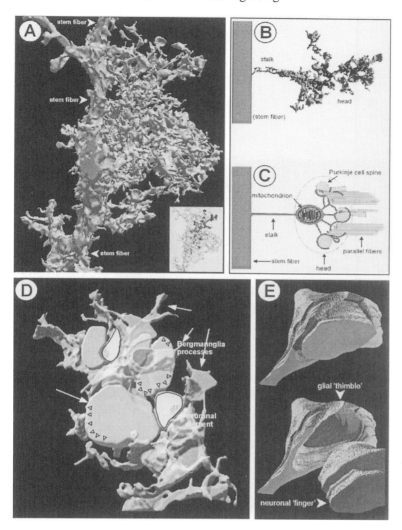

Figure 3.13. Microdomains of Bergmann glial cell processes in the murine cerebellum. **A:** 3-D reconstruction of a part of a Bergmann glial cell process. The living cell was dye-injected in a perfused cerebellar slice; then, after fixation and dye-conversion, about 600 consecutive serial ultrathin sections were photographed in the electron microscope, and the images of the dye-labeled profiles were reconstructed by a computer program. The inset shows a substructure labeled in blue; this part was quantitatively analyzed (see **B, C**). With permission, from Grosche et al. (1999). **B:** Glial microdomain as part of the 3-D reconstruction shown in **A**. **C:** Schematic drawing of such a glial microdomain and its relationships to the neuronal elements. **D:** 3-D reconstruction of a group of neighboring cerebellar synapses (yellow-green; synaptic clefts: orange) together with the surrounding leaflets provided by the injected Bergmann glia (blue-grey). The arrowheads point to neuronal surfaces not covered by glial sheaths from the labeled cell. **E:** 3-D reconstruction of a glial "thimble" and the neuronal "finger" covered by it; shown in apposition (*top*) and separated for better discrimination between the two compartments (*bottom*). With permission, from Grosche et al. (1999) (**A, B**) and from Grosche et al. (2002) (**C-E**).

3.7.5. A special case: neuro-glial synapses

In the developing CNS, the occurrence of neuro-glial synapse-like contacts has been described (e.g., Okado and Yokota, 1982), and has been accounted for by either erroneous growth of neurites, or by unknown developmental interactions. In some instances, presynaptic neuronal terminals abut glial cells even in the mature nervous system. Such axo-glial synapses have been described in the cerebellum of the adult frog (Palacios-Prü et al., 1983). Another type of 'synaptoid junctions' involves ependymoglial cells as postsynaptic elements, e.g., in the hypophysis and in the median eminence (Wittkowski, 1967, 1973; Rafols, 1986) but also in other brain regions (Leonhardt and Backhus-Roth, 1969). An example from the area postrema of the cat is shown in Figure 3.12 F (D'Amelio et al., 1986). Possibly such neuro-glial 'synapses' are involved in the control of glial secretory activity but clear-cut evidence for that remains to be shown.

3.8. Perineuronal nets and perinodal extracellular matrix

It has been mentioned above that a special extracellular matrix may cover neuronal somata, dendrites, and initial segments (perineuronal nets), as well as the nodes of Ranvier (Fig. 3.14) and the sensory processes of, e.g., photoreceptor cells (Berman, 1969; Hageman and Johnson, 1991). A similar matrix has been found in invertebrates (Treherne et al., 1982). This matrix comprises some basic components such as hyaluronic acid, proteoglycans, and tenascins (Celio and Blümcke, 1994), but may vary considerably among different CNS areas, between different neuron types, and between soma and Ranvier nodes (Brückner et al., 1996a, b; Carlson and Hockfield, 1996). Generally, matrix components can be visualized by the binding of specific lectins, antibodies, or cationic dyes (cf. Fig. 3.14) but the perineuronal nets may also be labeled in Golgi-stained preparations (Brauer et al., 1982). Because astrocytic PGPs may form comparable net-like structures on neuronal somata and dendrites, it is assumed that both the neurons and their ensheathing glia contribute to the formation of the matrix at the spaces between the two cell compartments. (Derouiche et al., 1996) (Fig. 3.14D, E).

A common feature of the various types of extracellular matrix seems to be their anionic character (Rambourg, 1971). It has been hypothesized that the anionic binding sites of the matrix may interact with cations (Na^+ and/or K^+, and perhaps Ca^{2+}) and constitute a buffer system for these ions in the narrow extracellular spaces, challenged by large ionic currents flowing through the excited neuronal membrane (Treherne et al., 1982; Brückner et al., 1993; Härtig et al., 1999) (Fig. 3.14 I). For example, the generation of action potentials involves large Na^+ inward currents through regenerative Na^+ channels, accompanied by large K^+ outward currents through voltage-sensitive K^+ channels. The K^+ currents are delayed and overlap only partially in time course with the Na^+ currents; furthermore, the Na^+ channels may be predominantly inserted in membrane areas distant from the accumulation sites of K^+ channels (e.g., Safronov, 1999; Williams and Stuart, 2000). These spatio-temporal imbalances in inward and outward currents of cations should cause dramatic electric and osmotic forces, and movements of cation-Cl^- pairs, within the narrow extracellular spaces. These may be prevented by the buffering capacities of the anionic binding sites of the extracellular matrix, where Na⁺ may replace K⁺ and vice versa as shown in Figure 3.14 I.

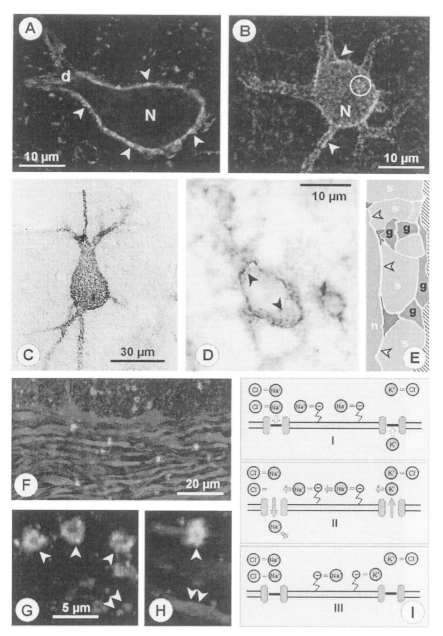

Figure 3.14. Relationships between synapses, glia, and the extracellular matrix of perineuronal nets. **A, B:** The 'holes' of the perineuronal nets are sites of synaptic contacts. **A:** Neuron (N) in the lateral vestibular nucleus of the rat; confocal optic section through the cell.

The soma and dendrites (d) are almost completely surrounded by a net of extracellular matrix (labeled red; soy-bean agglutinin binding) with the exception of the synaptic contact sites; the presynaptic terminals are labeled by parvalbumine immunohistochemistry (green). **B:** Basket interneuron (N) in the cortex of the rat; summarized staple of confocal images through several levels. Soma and dendrites of this cell are covered by a more close-meshed net (visualized by wheat-germ agglutinin, in green) because the synaptic buttons (visualized in red: immunohistochemistry for GABA dehydrogenase) are smaller than those of the cell in (**A**). The encircled area shows that there is no overlap between the net and the presynaptic terminals. Original micrographs; courtesy of G. Brückner, Leipzig. **C:** The matrix surrounds the soma of a non-pyramidal neuron in the upper layer IV of the rat parietal cortex in a virtually complete manner (with the exception of synaptic contact sites). **D :** Rat cortex. A perineuronal net is revealed by lectin staining (brown; soybean agglutinin). Astrocytes (blue) were labelled by anti-glutamine synthetase. The astrocyte in the top left corner extends a process onto the neuron. The top and bottom part of the neuron is covered by net-forming PGPs (arrowheads), which intermingle with the lectin stain. **E:** The glial sheath is less complete, and more distant from the neuronal surface, than the perineuronal net. This is shown on a neuron of the medial cerebellar nucleus of a rat; semi-schematic drawing of the matrix (brown) and the glial sheaths (g; blue) around the surface of the neuron (n) and its synaptic contacts (s; green); the arrowheads point to synaptic contact zones; unidentified structures are hatched. With permission, from Brückner et al., 1996b (**C**) and modified after Fig. 10b of Brückner et al., 1993 (**E**). **F-H:** Demonstration of the extracellular matrix (visualized by means of soy bean agglutinin, green) surrounding nodes of Ranvier in the rat medulla oblongata (trapezoid body). Two crossing fiber tracts are shown, with some fibers running perpendicular to the plane of the optical section (**F:** *top*; **G**) and the others in parallel to it (**F:** *bottom*, **H**). Many fibers express parvalbumin (immunocytochemical labeling; red). The paranodal matrix (arrowheads) is visible as circles in the optical cross-sections (**G**) or as short lines in the longitudinal sections (**H**). The double arrowheads point to internodia which are devoid of extracellular matrix. Original confocal micrographs, courtesy of G. Brückner. **I:** Hypothesis of ion buffering by the extracellular matrix. Anionic binding sites of the matrix may buffer cations moving through spatially separated Na^+ and K^+ channels at high velocity, thus preventing large extracellular osmotic shifts which would be caused by movements of cation-Cl^- pairs. With permission, from Härtig et al. (1999).

This hypothesis fits well with the observed presence of specialized extracellular matrix at sites where high ionic current densities occur, such as the nodes of Ranvier. It may also account for the observation that within a given brain region, not all neurons are endowed with perineuronal nets. In rat cortex, the nets preferentially surround neurons that express the potassium channel Kv3.1b subunit, which are supposed to be fast-spiking neurons (Härtig et al., 1999). It has also been demonstrated that the development of perineuronal nets in culture is stimulated by chronic high K^+-induced depolarization (Brückner and Grosche, 2001). The hypothesized cation buffer capacity of the perinodal matrix may also account for earlier findings of an ongoing spiking activity of isolated frog axons in Na^+ free solutions, which was only maintained when the paranodal glia (and matrix) was intact (Müller-Mohnsen et al., 1975). It is noteworthy that the sites of extracellular matrix accumulation are often accompanied by local enlargements of the extracellular cleft, which may further contribute to the buffer function (Brückner et al., 1996b). It remains to be established why specific types of neurons, and specific compartments of a given neuron, seem to require the presence of such specialized extracellular buffer sites.

3.9. Structural plasticity

The neuron-associated glial cell processes in both CNS and PNS are highly dynamic structures. Much of the functional plasticity of the nervous system, both during embryonic development and in mature processes such as learning and memory, seems to require a contribution of the perisynaptic glial elements.

3.9.1. Development

The type III glial processes in neuropil, particularly the PGPs, develop in mutual dependence on the developing neuronal cell processes and synapses. The number and complexity of side branches increase rapidly during early ontogenesis (Reichenbach and Reichelt, 1986; Hanke and Reichenbach, 1987; Senitz et al., 1995; Grosche et al., 2002) (Fig. 3.15 A, B). It has been pointed out that specialized glia-neuron contacts cannot be elaborated until neurons have completed their differentiation (Waxman et al., 1983; Hildebrand and Waxman, 1984). (For possible mechanisms involved in these developmental adaptations, see section 3.10.).

3.9.2. Remodeling

Morphological variations among perisynaptic glia at a given time-point may largely reflect the plasticity of individual glial processes in response to the recent history of adjacent synaptic activity (Xu-Friedmann et al., 2001). Astrocytes may respond rapidly (i.e., within about 45 minutes: Rohlmann et al., 1994) to axotomy-induced changes of the activity of the ensheathed neuronal elements. The structure of perisynaptic astroglial processes may change due to long-term potentiation (Wenzel et al., 1991) (Fig. 3.15 C, D), kindling (Hawrylak et al., 1998), stimulation of afferents (Güldner and Wolff, 1977), and, in the hippocampus, to changes in estrogen levels (Klintsova et al., 1995). A changed glial coverage of synapses may not only involve an outgrowth of PGPs but also retraction, autophagy, and lysosomal degradation of glial membranes (Landgrebe et al., cited by Chao and Wolff, 2002). It should be kept in mind that even minute changes of the size and/or shape of perisynaptic glial sheaths may cause dramatic changes of the efficacy of a given synapse (Oliet et al., 2001). First, the extracellular volume changes, which modifies the effective concentration and/or availability of neurotransmitters. Secondly, changes of the distance between the synaptic cleft and the perisynaptic glial membrane (and of the exposed surface area of the latter) modify the number of the accessible glial transporters and hence the uptake rate of the transmitter molecules. The same applies to the glial uptake / redistribution of neuronally released K^+ ions, modulating the extracellular K^+ concentration and, thereby, the neuronal excitability. It is noteworthy that the effective concentration of glial cell-derived neuroactive substances may be controlled by the same mechanisms. Furthermore, the connexin-43 mediated gap junctional coupling among astrocytes is also rapidly modified by changes in neuronal activity (Rohlmann et al., 1994; Rouach et al., 2001). This will change the efficacy not only of individual synapses but also of large functional compartments of the neuropil.

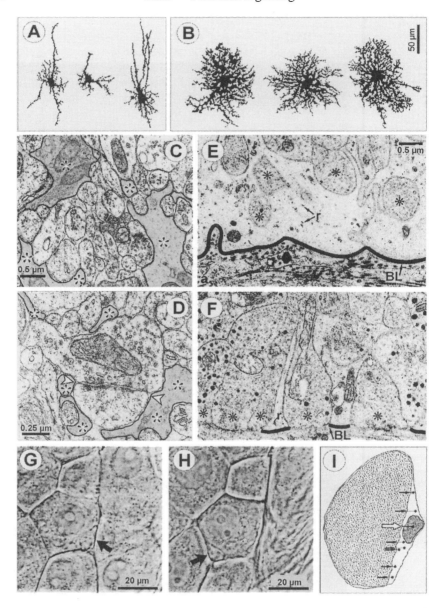

Figure 3.15. Plasticity of perineuronal glial processes. **A, B:** Development-related changes in the complexity of astroglial cell processes in the human neocortex (area 11, layers III-V), Golgi impregnation. **A:** Three representative cells from neonatal brain; **B:** cells from normal adult brain (40 years). With permission, from Senitz et al., 1995. **C, D:** After long-term potentiation (LTP), the perisynaptic astroglial coverage increases in dentate gyrus of adult rats. Whereas in the unstimulated neuropile, many synapses are nearly devoid of astroglial contacts **(C)**, eight hours after LTP induction most of the synaptic clefts (arrowheads), and much of the pre- and postsynaptic elements, are covered by glial sheaths **(D)**. Glial profiles are labeled by shadows and asterisks. With permission, from Wenzel et al. (1991). **E, F:** The coverage of

portal capillaries by glial endfeet is decreased when neurosecretion is induced by the activation of nicotinic acetylcholine receptors. **E:** Under control conditions, much of the pericapillary basal lamina (BL) is covered by the endfeet of tanycytes as identified by the presence of ribosomes (r) and the lack of neurosecretory vesicles in their cytoplasm; the endings of the neurosecretory axons (asterisks) do not contact the basal lamina. **F:** After stimulation, the glial coverage of the basal lamina is dramatically reduced (inked), and many vesicle-containing nerve endings establish direct access to the basal lamina. With permission, from Lichtensteiger et al. (1978). **G-I:** Remodeling of synaptic sites, and their associated satellite glia, on the somata of identified parasympathetic ganglion cells in the adult mouse. **G, H:** Video images of an identified ganglion cell and its associated glial cells observed over a period of several weeks. A glial cell nucleus (arrows) is apparent at a new location after a 21 day interval. **I:** The glial nucleus (large white arrow) is always associated with the sites of synaptic contacts (black arrows). With permission, from Pomeroy and Purves (1988).

It is now well established that in the mature brain, not only the size and shape but even the number of synapses may be modified by changes in neuronal activity. In the normal adult rat cortex at any time, about 1% of all synapses are in the process of regression and remodeling (Wolff et al., 1995). Thus, "synaptic stripping" and phagocytosis of regressive synapses seem to be important functions of perisynaptic astroglial processes not only during ontogenesis (Missler et al., 1993) but also in adulthood (Wolff et al., 1995). This may explain why "atypical synapses" such as "empty presynaptic elements" and vacated postsynaptic densities are usually surrounded by astrocytic profiles (Adams and Jones, 1982); a similar phenomenon may be represented by the glial thimbles in the cerebellum (Grosche et al., 2002) (Fig. 3.13E). Whereas in cases of massive, acute neuronal degeneration the phagocytosis of neuronal debris is mainly performed by microglia, the normal remodeling of individual synapses may be attributed largely to astrocytic cells. Both astrocytes and ependymoglial cells are capable of rapid phagocytosis. In the retina, disc shedding of photoreceptor outer segments occurs with a circadian rhythm, and is reflected by cyclic changes in the phagocytotic metabolism of retinal pigment epithelial cells.

It was shown that astroglia can not only remove "obsolete" synapses but also contribute to the formation and maintenance of new synapses *in vitro* (Pfrieger and Barres, 1996), for instance, by providing cholesterol for the lipoprotein synthesis of the neurons (Mauch et al., 2001), or via specific growth factors (e.g., Lein et al., 2002). It has been shown that visual cortical plasticity (changes of ocular dominance) may be induced even in adult cats if immature astrocytes were implanted (Müller and Best, 1989). As a candidate for the first step in inducing such adaptive changes, long-term potentiation (LTP) has been proposed (Wenzel et al., 1991). It is interesting in this context that LTP may be induced if a sub-threshold stimulation of the synapse is coupled to simultaneous experimental depolarization of the adjacent glial cells (Sastry et al., 1988).

In the PNS too, convincing evidence has been found for an involvement of glial cells in synaptic remodeling. Purves (1989) showed that in parasympathetic ganglia, the synaptic sites on individual neurons may change with time. Generally in these ganglia, the nuclei and perinuclear somata of the ensheathing satellite glial cells are located over neuronal membrane areas that receive many synaptic contacts. With changing sites of the synaptic input, the somata of the satellite cells move towards the new synaptic areas (Pomeroy and Purves, 1988) (Fig. 3.15 G-I). The mechanism(s) of this remodeling remain to be elucidated, as well as a possible active role of the glial cells in this process. The use of current techniques of high-resolution in-vivo microscopy is expected to help in solving these questions.

3.10. Summary and conclusions: molecular basis, 'rules of construction', dynamics, and functional impact of PGPs

On the basis of the description above, it can be generalized that each of the neuronal compartments - from receptor to effector pole - is associated with a specific glial compartment (Fig. 3.16). This organization is not random but appears to be governed by principles of development and plasticity of perineuronal glial structures that maintain glio-neuronal interactions. This topic is discussed briefly below, with particular reference to the astrocytic PAPs.

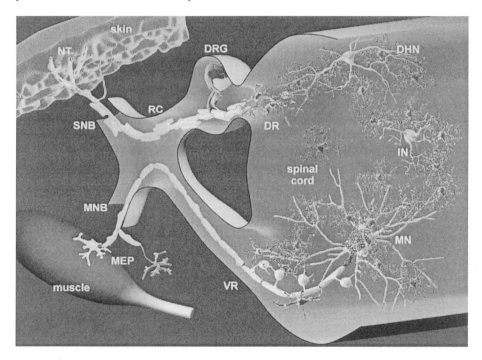

Figure 3.16: Summary of glio-neuronal associations along the signaling pathways from receptor pole to effector pole. As an example, the pain-induced withdrawal reflex arc is given. It should be noted that the neuronal circuit is simplified (e.g., the reflex is actually multisynaptic, and involves more interneurons in the spinal cord than shown). The peripheral pathways are unproportionally shortened in order to maintain clarity. To visualize the ensheathed elements, parts of the covering of neuronal elements by glial sheaths (which actually is virtually complete, with the exception of the nonmyelinated axons in the central part of the dorsal root) have been omitted. The color codes are, yellow - neuronal dendrites and somata, red - axons, pink - sensory processes; white - oligodendrocytes, bluish white - Schwann cells, light blue – satellite glial cells, dark blue - protoplasmic astrocytes, green - fibrous astrocytes; brown - perineuronal nets. NT, nociceptive terminal; SNB, sensory nerve fiber bundle; RC, ramus communis; DRG, dorsal root ganglion; DR, dorsal root; DHN, dorsal

horn neuron; IN, (one of the) interneuron(s); MN, motoneuron; VR, ventral root; MNB, motor nerve bundle; MEP, motor endplate. Original drawing (J.G.) based upon unpublished original data of Gert Brückner and Siegried Mense, and on published data (Carlstedt, 1977; Gobel, 1978; Pannese, 1981; Matsumuto and Rosenbluth, 1986; Sugiura et al., 1986: Hoheisel and Mense, 1987; Mense, 1990; Messlinger, 1996).

It has been shown (Figs. 3.11, 3.13) that the PAPs form flat or lamellar sheaths (see e. g. Wolff, 1968; Chao et al., 2002) that contact or even enclose most of the synaptic structures. In contrast to the stem processes, the lamellae are virtually devoid of organelles and cytoskeletal elements (with the exception of complexes of actin filaments and actin-binding proteins). The microvilli of ependymoglial cells, surrounding the sensory processes of CSF contact neurons and photoreceptor cells, share similar properties. Both terminal lamellae and microvilli contain ezrin and radixin (Derouiche and Frotscher, 2001). These actin-binding proteins link the cell membrane to the actin cytoskeleton, which may maintain the complex, thin side branches with their large surface-to-volume ratios of up to more than 20 μm^{-1} (Wolff, 1968; Grab et al., 1983; Reichenbach et al., 1988b; Grosche et al., 2002) and long microvilli with surface-to-volume ratios of up to 50 μm^{-1} (Reichenbach et al., 1992). Moreover, ezrin and radixin may not only be involved in the maintenance, but also in the growth and remodeling of fine glial end processes. In cell cultures, glial filopodia (comparable to those of neuronal growth cones) are heavily immunoreactive for both molecules (Fig. 3.17 C-E).

The formation of PGPs may be stimulated by the onset of neuronal activity, and the growing glial filopodia (Takahashi et al., 1990) may be attracted (or repelled) by signals from active neurons. For such neuron-derived signals, K^+ ions (Reichelt et al., 1989) and neurotransmitters such as glutamate (Cornell-Bell et al., 1990) (Fig. 3.17 A,B), GABA (Kettenmann et al., 1991; Runquist and Alonso, 2003), and/or serotonin and noradrenaline (Paspalas and Papadopoulos, 1998) have been proposed as candidate molecules. Stimulation of protein kinase A induces the growth of short processes which extend flat membranous sheaths from the glial growth cones, which might be important for ensheathing neuronal elements (Althaus et al. 1990). Furthermore, not only the growth but also the retraction of glial cell processes is thought to be important for the adjustment of glio-neuronal interactions. As a model of this latter mechanism, stellation of cultured astrocytes has been used. Astrocytes in culture are flat, polygonal cells, but under the influence of increased intracellular concentration of cAMP (Kimelberg et al., 1978), and also as a result of various agents, such as phorbol esters (Mobley et al., 1986) and amyloid beta protein (Abe and Saito, 2000), the processes retract and the cells become stellate. Stellation was also observed in peripheral (enteric) glia in the presence of phorbol esters (Hanani et al., 1997). Recently it was found that specific stimuli such as glutamate (Abe and Saito, 2000) or hypoxia (Schmidt-Ott et al., 2001) can reverse stellation. Interestingly, endothelin reversed the action of hypoxia on the cultured astrocytes, suggesting that the retraction of glial cell processes is actively regulated.

Evidence in support of this idea was presented by Iino et al. (2001), who inserted, by means of adenoviral-mediated gene transfer, the Ca^{2+}-impermeable GluR2 subunit into AMPA receptors of Bergmann glia that are normally Ca^{2+} permeable. This caused a retraction of the Bergmann glial cell processes ensheathing synapses on dendritic spines of Purkinje cells, thus retarding removal of synaptically released glutamate. As a further consequence, a multiple innervation of Purkinje cells by climbing fibers was observed (Iino et al., 2001). These findings underline the functional importance of perisynaptic glial sheaths (section 3.7.2). Moreover, they suggest that the ensheathing of synapses by glial cell processes is controlled by physiological signaling molecules released by the synapses. In the case of Bergmann glial cells, stimulation of AMPA receptors by glutamate may modulate Ca^{2+} increases in the ensheathing microdomains of Bergmann glial cells (Grosche et al., 1999) and thus induce mechanisms that stabilize the sheaths. By contrast, (long-term) cessation of synaptic activity (or block of the AMPA receptor-mediated Ca^{2+} influxes: Iino et al., 2001) may cause a withdrawal of the glial sheaths, and consequent changes of the neuronal circuitry.

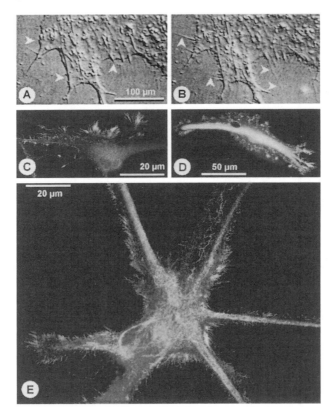

Figure 3.17. Mechanisms of the formation of PGPs, and, thus, of specific glio-neuronal associations. **A, B:** Stimulation of growing filopodia (arrowheads) in cultured rat astrocytes, by application of glutamate (100 µM); **B** was taken 60 sec after **A**. With permission, from Cornell-Bell et al. (1990). **C-E:** Outgrowing filopodia in astroglial cultures. **C:** Complementary labelling of astroglial main processes and filopodia, by antibodies against Ca^{2+}-channels (red) and the actin-binding protein, ezrin (green), respectively. **D, E:** Complementary labelling of astroglial main processes and filopodia, by antibodies against GFAP (red) and the actin-binding protein ezrin (green), respectively, in a "simple" (**D**) and a "complex" (**E**) cell. Original micrographs (A.D.).

This type of mechanisms may act both during ontogeny and in the mature CNS, where they may modify the growth and/or retraction of PGPs even in the short-term range. The actual outcome of this dynamics depends on the strength and pattern of neuronal activity which, in turn, is controlled by sensory inputs and behavioral requirements. For instance, depending on whether rats are kept in enriched environments (Sirevaag and Greenough, 1991) or in complete darkness (Stewart et al., 1986) the complexity of their PAPs may differ significantly.

The following functions have been ascribed to perineuronal glial elements: maintenance of topographic relationships and structural integrity, metabolic interaction including nutrition and transmitter recycling, homeostasis of the extracellular fluid, and short-and long-term modification of synaptic efficacy. It can be stated that the structural prerequisites for all these interactions are provided by the PGPs, located at the appropriate places and endowed with a wealth of versatile molecules. There is also an increasing body of functional evidence for these interactions, which will be presented in the other chapters of this book.

Acknowledgments. The authors thank Gerd Brückner (Paul Flechsig Institute for Brain Research, Leipzig University), Thomas Keil (Max Planck Institute for Biochemistry, München), Felix Makarov (Pavlov Institute of Physiology, University of St. Petersburg), Siegfried Mense (Institute for Anatomy and Cell Biology, Heidelberg University), Thomas Pannicke (Paul Flechsig Institute for Brain Research, Leipzig University), Michael Rickmann (Institute for Anatomy, Göttingen University), Heinz Waessle (Max Planck Institute for Brain Research, Frankfurt/M.), Joachim R. Wolff (Institute for Anatomy, Göttingen University), and Hartwig Wolburg (Institute for Pathology, Tübingen University) for kindly providing preparations, unpublished micrographs or drawings, and for many helpful discussions. AD wishes to thank Andrea Hufschmidt for technical assistance in the preparation of Figures. Original work related to this chapter was supported by the Bundesministerium für Bildung, Forschung und Technologie, interdisciplinary Center for Clinical Research at the University of Leipzig, 01KS9504, Projects C-05 (AR) and Z-10 (JG), and by the Deutsche Forschungsgemeinschaft, RE 849-8/1 (AR) and De 676-2 (AD). MH was supported by the BSF and the Israel Science Foundation

3.11. References

Abe K, Saito H (2000) L-glutamate suppresses amyloid beta-protein-induce stellation of cultured rat cortical astrocytes. J Neurochem 74:280-286.

Adams J, Jones DG (1982) Synaptic remodelling and astrocytic hypertrophy in rat cerebral cortex from early to late adulthood. Neurobiol Aging 3:179-186.

Allen DT, Kiernan JA (1994) Permeation of proteins from blood into peripheral nerves and ganglia. Neuroscience 59:755-764.

Althaus HH, Schwartz P, Klöppner S, Schröter J, Neuhoff V (1990) Protein kinases A and C are involved in oligodendroglial process formation. In: Cellular and Molecular Biology of Myelination. NATO ASI Series. (Jeserich G, Althaus HH, Waehneldt TV, eds.), pp 247-253. Berlin, Springer-Verlag.

Araque A, Li N, Doyle RT, Haydon PG (2000) SNARE-protein dependent glutamate release from astrocytes. J Neurosci 20:666-673.

Berger UV, Hediger MA (2000) Distribution of the glutamate transporters GLAST and GLT-1 in rat circumventricular organs, meninges, and dorsal root ganglia. J Comp Neurol 421:385-399.

Berman ER (1969) Mucopolysaccharides (glycosaminoglycans) of the retina: identification, distribution and possible biological role. Mod Probl Ophthalmol 8:5-31.

Berthold CH, Carlstedt T (1977a) Observations on the morphology of the transition between the peripheral and the central nervous system in the cat. II. General organozation of the transitional region in S₁ dorsal rootlets. Acta Physiol Scan (Suppl) 446:23-42.

Berthold CH, Carlstedt T (1977b) Observations on the morphology of the transition between the peripheral and the central nervous system in the cat. III. Myelinated fibres in S₁ dorsal rootlets. Acta Physiol Scand (Suppl) 446:43-60.

Bevan S, Chiu SY, Gray PTA, Ritchie JM (1985) The presence of voltage-gated sodium, potassium and chloride channels in rat cultured astrocytes. Proc R Soc Lond. B 225:299-313.

Bowe CM, Kocsis JD, Waxman SG (1985) Differences between mammalian ventral and dorsal spinal roots in response to blockade of potassium channels during maturation. Proc R Soc Lond, B 224:355-366.

Brauer K, Werner L, Leibnitz L (1982) Perineuronal nets of glia. J Hirnforsch. 23: 701-708.

Breipohl W, Laugwitz HJ, Bornfeld N (1974) Topological relations between the dendrites of olfactory sensory cells and sustentacular cells in different vertebrates. An ultrastructural study. J Anat 117:89-94

Brückner G, Grosche J (2001) Perineuronal nets show intrinsic patterns of extracellular matrix differentiation in organotypic slice cultures. Exp Brain Res 137: 83-93.

Brückner G, Brauer K, Härtig W, Wolff JR, Rickmann MJ, Derouiche A, Delpech B, Girard N, Oertel WH, Reichenbach A (1993) Perineuronal nets provide a polyanionic, glia-associated form of microenvironment around certain neurons in many parts of the rat brain. Glia 8:183-200.

Brückner G, Bringmann A, Köppe G, Härtig W, Brauer K (1996a) In vivo and in vitro labelling of perineuronal nets in rat brain. Brain Res. 720:84-92.

Brückner G, Härtig W, Kacza J, Seeger J, Welt K, Brauer K (1996b) Extracellular matrix organization in various regions of rat brain gray matter. J Neurocytol. 25: 333-346.

Butt AM, Duncan A, Berry M (1994) Astrocyte associations with nodes of Ranvier: ultrastructural analysis of HRP-filled astrocytes in the mouse optic nerve. J Neurocytol 23: 486-499.

Carlson SD, Hilgers SL, Juang J-L (1997) First developmental signs of the scolopale (glial) cell and neuron comprising the chordotonal organ in the *Drosophila* embryo. Glia 19:269-274.

Carlson SS, Hockfield S (1996) Central nervous system. In: Comper WD (ed) Extracellular Matrix. Volume 1, Tissue Function. Harwood Academic Publishers, Amsterdam, pp. 1-23.

Carlstedt T (1977) Observations on the morphology of the transition between the peripheral and the central nervous system in the cat. IV. Unmyelinated fibers in S1 dorsal rootlets. Acta Physiol Scand (Suppl) 446:61-71.

Castonguay A, Levésque S, Robitaille R (2001) Glial cells as active partners in synaptic functions. Prog Brain Res 132:227-240.

Catterall WA (1984) The molecular basis of neuronal excitability. Science 223:653-661.

Celio MR, Blümcke I (1994) Perineuronal nets - a specialized form of extracellular matrix in the adult nervous system. Brain Res Rev 19: 128-145.

Chan-Palay V, Palay SL (1972) The form of velate astrocytes in the cerebellar cortex of monkey and rat: high-voltage electron microscopy of rapid-Golgi preparations. Z Anat Entw-Gesch 138:1-19.

Chao TI, Skatchkov SN, Eberhardt W, Reichenbach A (1994) Na⁺ channels of Müller (glial) cells isolated from retinae of various mammalian species including man. Glia 10:173-185.

Chao TI, Rickmann M, Wolff JR (2002) The synapse-astrocyte boundary: anatomical basis for an integrative role of glia in synaptic transmission. In: The Tripartite Synapses: Glia in Synaptic Transmission (Volterra A, Magistretti P, Haydon P, eds), pp. 3-23. Oxford: Oxford UP.

Coggeshall RE (1967) A light and electron microscope study of the abdominal ganglion of *Aplysia californica*. J Neurophysiol 30:1263-1287.

Colbert CM, Pan E (2002) Ion channel properties underlying axonal action potential initiation in pyramidal neurons. Nature Neurosci 5:533-538.

Colombo J, Parkins CW (1987) A model of electrical excitation of the mammalian auditory-nerve neuron. Hear Res 31:287-311.

Cornell-Bell A, Thomas PG, Smith SJ (1990) The excitatory neurotransmitter glutamate causes filopodia formation in cultured hippocampal astrocytes. Glia 3:322-334.

Cooper MH, Beal JA (1977) Myelinated granule cell bodies in the cerebellum of the monkey (Saimiri sciurus). Anat Rec 187:249-256.

Couteaux R (1958) Morphological and cytochemical observations on the post-synaptic membrane and motor end-plates and ganglionic synapses. Exp Cell Res Suppl. 5.

Crowcroft PJ, Szurszewski JH (1971) A study of the inferior mesenteric and pelvic ganglia of guinea-pigs with intracellular electrodes. J Physiol (Lond) 219:421-441.

D'Amelio FE, Gibbs MA, Mehler WR, Philpott DE, Savage W (1986) Axoglial contacts in the area postrema of the cat: an ultrastructural study. Anat Rec 215: 407-412.

Denk W, Sugimori, M, Llinas R (1995) Two types of calcium response limited to single spines in cerebellar Purkinje cells. Proc Natl Acad Sci USA 92:8279-8282.

Derouiche A (1997) Coupling of Glutamate Uptake and Degradation in Transmitter Clearance: Anatomical Evidence. In: Neurotransmitter Release and Uptake (Pögün S, ed), pp 263-282. NATO ASI Series: Vol H: Cell Biology Series.

Derouiche A, Frotscher M (1991) Astroglial processes around identified glutamatergic synapses contain glutamine synthetase: evidence for transmitter degradation. Brain Res 552: 346-350.

Derouiche A, Frotscher M (2001) Peripheral astrocyte processes: monitoring by selective immunostaining for the actin-binding ERM proteins. Glia 36:330-341.

Derouiche A, Rauen T (1995) Coincidence of glutamate-aspartate-transporter- (GLAST) and glutamine synthetase- (GS) immunoreactions in retinal glia: evidence for coupling of GLAST and GS in transmitter clearance. J Neurosci Res 42:131-143.

Derouiche A, Härtig W, Brauer K, Brückner G (1996) Spatial relationship of lectin-labelled extracellular matrix and glutamine synthetase-immunoreactive astrocytes in rat cortical forebrain regions. J Anat 189:363-372.

Derouiche A, Anlauf E, Aumann G, Mühlstädt B, Lavialle M (2002) Anatomical aspects of glia-synapse interaction: the perisynaptic glial sheath consists of a specialized astrocyte compartment. J Physiol (Paris) 96:177-182.

Doucette JR (1984) The glial cells in the nerve fiber layer of the rat olfactory bulb. Anat Rec 210:385-391.

Famiglietti EV, Kolb H (1975) A bistratified amacrine cell and synaptic circuitry in the inner plexiform layer of the retina. Brain Res 84:293-300.

ffrench-Constant C, Miller RH, Kruse J, Schachner M, Raff MC (1986) Molecular specialization of astrocytic processes at nodes of Ranvier in rat optic nerve. J Cell Biol 102:844-852.

Flood PR (1966) A peculiar mode of muscular innervation in Amphioxus. Light and electron microscopic studies of the so-called ventral roots. J Comp Neurol 126: 181-218.

Fujita T, Tanaka K, Tokunaga J (1986) Zellen und Gewebe – Ein REM Atlas für Mediziner und Biologen, Gustav Fischer Verlag Stuttgart – New York (p 217).

Gabella G (1995) The structural relations between nerve fibers and muscle cells in the urinary bladder of the rat. J Neurocytol 24:159-187.

Gho M, Bellaiche Y, Schweisguth F (1999) Revisiting the Drosophila microchaete lineage: A novel intrinsically asymmetric cell division generates a glial cell. Development 126:3573-3564.

Gnatzy W, Schmidt K (1971) Die Feinstruktur der Sinneshaare auf den Cerci von *Gryllus bimaculatus* Deg. (Saltatoria, Gryllidae). 1. Faden- und Keulenhaare. Z Zellforsch 122:190-209.

Gobel S (1978) Golgi studies of the neurons in layer I of the dorsal horn of the medulla (trigeminal nucleus caudatus). J Comp Neurol 180:375-394.

Grab D, Reisert I, Pilgrim C (1983). Volumendichte und spezifische Oberflächen neuronaler und gliöser Gewebselemente in verschiedenen Regionen des Rattenhirns. Verh Anat Ges 77:255-256.

Grosche J, Kettenmann H, Reichenbach A (2002) Bergmann glial cells form distinct morphological structures to interact with cerebellar neurons. J Neurosci Res 68:138-149.

Grosche J, Matyash V, Möller T, Verkhratsky A, Reichenbach A, Kettenmann H (1999) Microdomains for neuron-glia interaction: parallel fiber signaling to Bergmann glial cells. Nature Neurosci 2:139-143.

Güldner FH, Wolff JR (1977) Perisynaptic reactions of astroglia in the visual cortex after optic nerve stimulation. Exp Brain Res Suppl. I:343-347.

Gutnick MJ, Connors BW, Ransom BR (1981) Dye coupling between glial cells in the guinea pig neocortical slice. Brain Res 213:486-492.

Hageman GS, Johnson LV (1991) Structure, composition and function of the retinal interphotoreceptor matri2. In: Progr Retinal Res Vol. 10, (Osborne N and Chader J, eds), pp 207-249. Oxford, Pergamon Press.

Hanani M, Reichenbach A (1994) Morphology of HRP-injected glial cells in the myenteric plexus of the guinea-pig. Cell Tissue Res 278:153-160.

Hanani M, Huang TY, Cherkas PS, Ledda M, Pannese E (2002) Glial cell plasticity in sensory ganglia induced by nerve damage. Neuroscience 114:279-283.

Hanani M, Lin Z, Louzon V, Brenner T, Boneh A (1997) Phorbol esters alter the morphology of cultured myenteric glia via a PKC-independent mechanism. Neuroscience Lett 233:61-64.

Hanani, M, Maudlej N, Härtig W (1999) Morphology and intercellular communication in glial cells of the intrinsic ganglia of the guinea-pig urinary bladder. J Auton Nervous System 76:62-67.

Hanani M, Zamir O, Baluk P (1989) Glial cells in the guinea pig myenteric plexus are dye coupled. Brain Res 497:245-249.

Hanke S, Reichenbach A (1987) Quantitative-morphometric aspects of Bergmann glial (Golgi epithelial) cell development in rats. A Golgi study. Anat Embryol 177:183-188.

Hanström B (1928) Vergleichende Anatomie des Nervensystems der wirbellosen Tiere. Berlin, Springer-Verlag.

Härtig W, Derouiche A, Welt K, Brauer K, Grosche J, Mäder M, Reichenbach A, Brückner G (1999) Cortical neurons immunoreactive for the potassium channel Kv3.1b subunit are predominantly surrounded by perineuronal nets presumed as a buffering system for cations. Brain Res 842: 15-29.

Häusser M, Spruston N, Stuart GJ (2000) Diversity and dynamics of dendritic signaling. Science 290:739-744.

Hawrylak N., Fleming JC, Salm AK (1998) Dehydration and rehydration selectively and reversibly alter glial fibrillary acidic protein immunoreactivity in the rat supraoptic nucleus and subjacent glia limitans. Glia, 22: 260-271.

Heuser JE and Doggenweiler CF (1966). The fine structural organization of nerve fibers, sheaths, and glial cells in the prawn, Palaemonetes vulgaris. J Cell Biol 30: 381-403.

Heuser JE, Reese TS (1977) The structure of the synapse. In Handbook of Physiology; The Nervous System. Vol. I, Part I (Kandel ER, ed), pp 261-294. Bethesda, Maryland: American Physiological Society.

Hildebrand C, Waxman SG (1983) Regional node-like specializations in non-myelinated axons of rat retinal nerve fiber layer. Brain Res 58:23-32.

Hildebrand C, Waxman SG (1984) Postnatal differentiation of rat optic nerve fibers: electron microscopic observations of nodes of Ranvier and axoglial relations. J Comp Neurol 224:25-37.

Hildebrand C, Remahl S, Persson H, Bjartmar C (1993) Myelinated nerve fibres in the CNS. Progr Neurobiol 40: 319-384.

Hoheisel U, Mense S (1987) Observations on the morphology of axons and somata of slowly conducting dorsal root ganglion cells in the cat. Brain Res 423:269-278.

Holland LZ (1996) Muscle development in Amphioxus: morphology, biochemistry, and molecular biology. Israel J Zool 42:S-235-S-246.

Holländer H, Makarov F, Dreher Z, van Driel D, Chan-Ling T, Stone J (1991) Structure of macroglia of the retina: sharing and division of labour between astrocytes and Müller cells. J Comp Neurol 313: 587-603.

Hortega P, Del Rio (1956) Variedas morfológicas de oligodendrocitos. Arch Histol (B Aires) 6:239-291.

Hoyle G (1986) Glial cells of an insect ganglion. J Comp Neurol 246:85-103.

Hoyle G, Williams M, Phillips C (1986) Functional morphology of insect neuronal cell-surface/glial contacts: the trophospongium. J Comp Neurol 246:113-128.

Iino M, Goto K, Kakegawa W, Okado H, Sudo M, Ishiuchi S, Miwa A, Takayasu Y, Saito I, Tsuzuki K, Ozawa S (2001) Glia-synapse interaction through Ca^{2+}-permeable AMPA receptors in Bergmann glia. Science 292 :926-929.

Kang J, Jiang L, Goldman SA, Nedergaard M (1998) Astrocyte-mediated potentiation of inhibitory synaptic transmission. Nature Neurosci 1: 683-692.

Kanno T (1989) The physiology and cell biology of paraneurons. Arch Histol Cytol 52, Suppl.:9-12.

Katz B (1966) Nerve, Muscle, and Synapse. New York, McGraw-Hill Book Co.

Keil TA (1997) Comparative morphogenesis of sensilla: A review. Int J Insect Morphol Embryol 26:151-160.

Kettenmann H, von Blankenfeld G, Trotter J (1991) Physiological properties of oligodendrocytes during development. Ann NY Acad Sci 633:64-77.

Kimelberg HK, Narumi S, Bourke RS (1978) Enzymatic and morphological properties of rat brain astrocytic cultures, and enzymatic development in vivo. Brain Res 153:55-77.

Klein J, Löffelholz K (1996) Cholinergic Mechanisms: from Molecular Biology to Clinical Significance. Progr Brain Res 109:1-373.

Klintsova A, Levy WB, Desmond NL (1995) Astrocytic volume fluctuates in the hippocampal CA1 region across the estrous cycle. Brain Res 690:269-274.

Kocsis JD, Bowe CM, Waxman SG (1986) Different effects of 4-aminopyridine on sensory and motor fibers: pathogenesis of paresthesias. Neurology 36:117-120.

Knowles F, Anand Kumar TC (1969) Structural changes, related to reproduction, in the hypothalamus and in the pars tuberalis of the rhesus monkey. Phil Trans Roy Soc Lond. (Biol.) B, 256:357-375.

Lacalli TC (1990) Structure and organization of the nervous system in the actinotroch larva of Phoronis vancouverensis. Phil Trans R Soc Lond B 327:655-685.

Lein PJ, Beck HN, Chandrasekaran V, Gallagher PJ, Chen H-L, Lin Y, Guo X, Kaplan PL, Tiedge H, Higgins D (2002) Glia induce dendritic growth in cultured sympathetic neurons by modulating the balance between bone morphogenetic proteins (BMPs) and BMP antagonists. J Neurosci 22:10377-10387.

Lenz TL (1968) Primitive Nervous Systems. pp. 1-148, New Haven, Yale University Press.

Leonhardt H, Backhus-Roth A (1969) Synapsenartige Kontakte zwischen intraventrikulären Axonendigungen und freien Oberflächen von Ependymzellen des Kaninchengehirns. Z Zellforsch Mikrosk Anat 97:369-376.

Lichtensteiger W, Richards G, Kopp HG (1978) Changes in the distribution of non-neuronal elements in rat median eminence and in anterior pituitary hormone secretion after activation of tuberoinfundibular dopamine neurones by brain stimulation or nicotine. Brain Res 157:73-88.

Llinas R (1975) Electroresponsive properties of dendrites in central neurons. Adv Neurol 12:1-13.

Llinas R, Nicholson C, Freeman JA, Hillman DE (1969) Dendritic spikes versus cable properties. Science 163: 97.

Matsumoto E, Rosenbluth J (1986) Structure of the satellite cell sheath around the cell body, axon hillock, and initial segment of frog dorsal root ganglion cells. Anat Rec 215:182-191.

Mauch DH, Nägler K, Schumacher S, Göritz C, Müller E-C, Otto A, Pfrieger FW (2001) CNS synaptogenesis promoted by glia-derived cholesterol. Science 294: 1354-1357.

Mense S (1990) Structure-function relationships in identified afferent neurones. Anat Embryol 181:1-17.

Messlinger K (1996) Functional morphology of nociceptive and other fine sensory endings (free nerve endings) in different tissues. In: Progress in Brain Research Vol. 113 (Kumazawa T, Kruger L, Mizumura K, eds), pp 273-298. Amsterdam, Elsevier.

Missler M, Wolff A, Merker H-J, Wolff JR (1993) Pre- and postnatal development of the primary visual cortex of the common marmoset. II. Formation, remodelling, and elimination of synapses as overlapping processes. J Comp Neurol 333:53-67.

Mobley PL, Scott SL, Cruz EG (1986) Protein kinase C in astrocytes; a determinant of cell morphology. Brain Res 389:366-369.

Müller CM, Best J (1989) Ocular dominance plasticity in adult cat visual cortex after transplantation of cultured astrocytes. Nature 342:427-430.

Müller-Mohnsen H, Tippe A, Hillenkamp F, Unsöld E (1975) About the importance of paranodal structures of the Ranvier node for the impulse regeneration. Z Naturforsch 30:271-277.

Munger BL, Ide C (1988) The structure and function of cutaneous sensory receptors. Arch Histol Cytol 51:1-34.

Narlieva N (1988) Multilamellar glial envelopes of synapses in the pontine nuclei of the cat. Acta anat 131:227-230.

Newman EA, Reichenbach A (1996) The Müller cell: a functional element of the retina. Trends Neurosci 19:307-312.

Okado N, Yokota N (1982) Axoglial synaptoid contacts in the neural lobe of the human fetus. Anat Rec 202:117-124.

Oliet SH, Piet R, Poulain DA (2001) Control of glutamate clearance and synaptic efficacy by glial coverage of neurons. Science 292: 923-926.

Osborne MP (1970) Structure and function of neuromuscular junctions and stretch receptors. Symp R Entomol Soc London 5:77-100.

Palacios-Prü EL, Mendoza RU, Palacios L (1983) In vitro and in situ formation of neuronal-glial junctions. Exp Neurol 182:541-569.

Pannese E (1981) The satellite cells of the sensory ganglia. Adv Anat Embryol Cell Biology 65:1-111.

Pannese E (2002) Perikaryal surface specializations of neurons in sensory ganglia. Int Rev Cytol 220:1-34.

Parpura V, Basarsky TA, Liu F, Jeftinija K, Jeftinija S, Haydon PG (1994) Glutamate mediated astrocyte neuron signalling. Nature 369:744-747.

Paspalas CD, Papadopoulos GC (1998) Ultrastructural evidence for combined action of noradrenaline and vasoactive intestinal polypeptide upon neurons, astrocytes, and blood vessels of the rat cerebral cortex. Brain Res Bull 45:247-259.

Pfrieger FW, Barres BA (1996) New views on synapse-glia interactions. Curr Opin Neurobiol 6:615-621.

Pinching AJ (1971) Myelinated dendritic segments in the monkey olfactory bulb. Brain Res 29:133-138.

Pomeroy SL, Purves D (1988) Neuron/glia relationships observed over intervals of several months in living mice. J Cell Biol 107:1167-1175.

Porter JT, McCarthy KD (1995) GFAP-positive hippocampal astrocytes respond to glutamatergic neuroligands with increases in [Ca2+]i. Glia 13:101-112.

Purves D (1989) Assessing some dynamic properties of the living nervous system. Quart J Exp Physiol 74:1089-1105.

Rafols JA (1986) Ependymal tanycytes of the ventricular system in vertebrates. In: Astrocytes. Vol. 1. Development, Morphology and Regional Specification of Astrocytes. (Fedoroff S, Vernadakis A, eds), , pp. 131-148, London, Academic Press.

Raine CS (1984) On the association between perinodal astrocytic processes and the node of Ranvier in the C.N.S. J Neurocytol 13:21-27.

Rambourg A (1971) Morphological and histochemical aspects of glycoproetins at the surface of animal cells. Int Rev Cytol 31:57-114.

Ramón y Cajal S (1892) The Structure of the Retina. (Engl. transl., 1972), Springfield, IL, Thomas.

Reichelt W, Dettmer D, Brückner G, Brust P, Eberhardt W, Reichenbach A (1989) Potassium as a signal for both proliferation and differentiation of rabbit retinal (Müller) glia growing in cell culture. Cell Signalling 1:187-194.

Reichenbach A (1989) Attempt to classify glial cells by means of their process specialization using the rabbit retinal Müller cell as an example of cytotopographic specialization of glial cells. Glia 2:250-259.

Reichenbach A, Reichelt W (1986) Postnatal development of radial glial (Müller) cells of the rabbit retina. Neurosci Lett 71:125-130.

Reichenbach A, Schippel K, Schümann R, Hagen E (1988a) Ultrastructure of rabbit nerve fibre layer - neuro-glial relationships, myelination, and nerve fiber spectrum. J Hirnforsch 29:481-491.

Reichenbach A, Hagen E, Schippel K, Eberhardt W (1988b) Quantitative electron microscopy of rabbit Müller (glial) cells in dependence of retinal topography. Z Mikroskop-Anat Forsch 102:721-755.

Reichenbach A, Schneider H, Leibnitz L, Reichelt W, Schaaf P, Schümann R (1989) The structure of rabbit retinal Müller (glial) cells is adapted to the surrounding retinal layers. Anat Embryol 180:71-79.

Reichenbach A, Siegel A, Senitz D, Smith TG jr (1992) A comparative fractal analysis of various mammalian astroglial cell types. Neuroimage 1:69-77.

Reichenbach A, Stolzenburg J-U, Eberhardt W, Chao TI, Dettmer D, Hertz L (1993) What do retinal Müller (glial) cells do for their neuronal "small silblings"?. J Chem Neuroanat 6:201-213.

Reichenbach A, Siegel A, Rickmann M, Wolff JR, Noone D, Robinson SR (1995a) Distribution of Bergmann glial somata and processes: implications for function. J Brain Res 36:509-517.

Reichenbach A, Frömter C, Engelmann R, Wolburg H, Kasper M, Schnitzer J (1995b) Müller glial cells of the tree shrew retina. J Comp Neurol 360:257-270.

Remahl S, Hildebrand C (1990a) Relation between axons and oligodendroglial cells during initial myelination. I. The glial unit. J Neurocytol 19:313-328.

Remahl S, Hildebrand C (1990b) Relation between axons and oligodendroglial cells during initial myelination. II. The individual axon. J Neurocytol 19:883-898.

Robinson SR, Hampson ECGM, Munro MN, Vaney DI (1993) Unidirectional coupling of gap junctions between neuroglia. Science 262:1072-1074.

Rohlmann A, Laskawi R, Hofer A, Dermietzel R, Wolff JR (1994) Astrocytes as rapid sensors of peripheral axotomy in the facial nucleus of rats. NeuroReport 5: 409-412.

Romand MR, Romand R (1987) The ultrastructure of spiral ganglion cells in the mouse. Acta Otolaryngol (Stockh) 104:29-39.

Rouach N, Glowinski J, Giaume C (2001) Activity-dependent neuronal control of gap-junctional communication in astrocytes. J Cell Biol 149:1513-1526.

Runquist M, Alonso G (2003) Gabaergic signaling mediates the morphological organization of astrocytes in the adult rat forebrain. Glia 41:137-151.

Safronov BV (1999) Spatial distribution of Na^+ and K^+ channels in spinal dorsal horn neurones: role of the soma, axon and dendrites in spike generation. Prog Neurobiol 59:217-241.

Saint Marie RL, Carlson SD, Chi C (1984) The glial cells of insects. In: Insect Ultrastructure. (King RC, Akai R, eds), pp. 435-475, Plenum.

Sarantis M, Mobbs P (1992) The spatial relationship between Müller cell processes and the photoreceptor output synapse. Brain Res 584:299-304.

Sastry BR, Goh JW, May PBY, Chirwa SS (1988) The involvement of nonspiking cells in long-term potentiation of synaptic transmission in the hippocampus. Can J Physiol Pharmacol 66:841-844.

Scharrer B, Weitzman M (1980) Die Glia der wirbellosen Tiere. In: Neuroglia I (Oksche A, ed), pp. 157-175, Berlin, Springer-Verlag.

Schmidt-Ott KM, Xu AD, Tuschick S, Liefeldt L, Kresse W, Verkhratsky A, Kettenmann H, Paul M (2001) Hypoxia reverses dibutyryl-cAMP-induced stellation of cultured astrocytes via activation of the endothelin system. FASEB J 15:1227-1229.

Schon F, Kelly JS (1974) Autoradiographic localization of (^{3}H)GABA and (^{3}H)Glutamate over satellite glial cells. Brain Res 66:275-288.

Shrager P, Chiu SY, Ritchie JM (1985) Voltage-dependent sodium and potassium channels in mammalian cultured Schwann cells. Proc Natl Acad Sci USA 82:948-952.

Senitz D, Reichenbach A, Smith TG jr (1995) Surface complexity of human neocortical astrocytic cells: changes with development, aging, and dementia. J Brain Res 36:531-537.

Sirevaag AM, Greenough WT (1991) Plasticity of GFAP-immunoreactive astrocyte size and number in visual cortex of rats reared in complex environments. Brain Res 540:273-278.

Steinberg RH (1985) Interactions between the retinal pigment epithelium and the neural retina. Doc Ophthalmol 60:327-346.

Stewart MG, Bourne RC, Gabbott PLA (1986) Decreased levels of an astrocytic marker, glial fibrillary acidic protein, in the visual cortex of dark-reared rats: measurement by enzyme-linked immunosorbent assay. Neurosci Lett 63:147-152.

Stone J, Makarov F, Holländer H (1995) The glial ensheathment of the soma and axon hillock of retinal ganglion cells. Vis Neurosci 12:273-279.

Stuart G, Schiller J, Sakmann B (1997a) Action potential initiation and propagation in rat neocortical pyramidal neurons. J Physiol 505:617-632.

Stuart G, Spruston N, Sakmann B, Häusser M (1997b) Action potential initiation and backpropagation in neurons of the mammalian CNS. Trends NeuroSci 20:125-131.

Sugiura Y, Lee CL, Perl ER (1986) Central projections of identified, unmyelinated © afferent fibers innervating mammalian skin. Science 234:358-361.

Takahashi T, Misson J-P, Caviness jr VS (1990) Glial process elongation and branching in the developing murine neocortex: a qualitative and quantitative immunohistochemical analysis. J Comp Neurol 302:15-28.

Ten Tusscher MP, Klooster J, Vrensen GF (1989) Satellite cells as blood-ganglion cell barrier in autonomic ganglia. Brain Res 490:95-102.

Thippeswamy T, Morris R. (2002) The roles of nitric oxide in dorsal root ganglion neurons. Ann NY Acad Sci 962:103-110.

Treherne JE, Schofield PK, Lane NJ (1982) Physiological and ultrastructural evidence for an extracellular anion matrix in the central nervous system of an insect (Periplaneta americana). Brain Res 16:255-267.

Ushiki T, Ide C (1987) Scanning electron microscopic studies of the myelinated nerve fibres of the mouse sciatic nerve with special reference to the Schwann cell cytoplasmic network external to the myelin sheath. J Neurocytol 16:737-747.

Valverde F, Lopez-Mascaraque L (1991) Neuroglial arrangements in the olfactory glomeruli of the hedgehog. J Comp Neurol 307: 658-674.

Vaney DI (1991) Many diverse types of retinal neurons show tracer coupling when injected with biocytin or neurobiotin. Neurosci Lett 125:187-190.

Vigh-Teichmann I, Vigh B (1974) The infundibular cerebrospinal fluid contacting neurons. Adv Anat Embryol Cell Biol 50:1-91.

Volterra A, Magistretti P, Haydon P (eds) The Tripartite Synapses: Glia in Synaptic Transmission. Oxford University Press, pp. 1-272. 2002

Waxman SG (1983) The astrocyte as a component of the node of Ranvier. Trends Neurosci 9:250-253.

Waxman SG, Black JA, Foster RE (1983) Ontogenesis of the axolemma and axoglial relationships in myelinated fibers: electrophysiological and freeze-fracture correlates of membrane plasticity. Int Rev Neurobiol 24:433-484.

Wenzel J, Lammert G, Meyer U, Krug M (1991) The influence of long-term potentiation on the spatial relationship between astrocyte processes and potentiated synapses in the dentate gyrus neuropil of rat brain. Brain Res 560:122-131.

Wersäll J (1956) Studies on the structure and innervation of the sensory epithelium of the cristae ampullares in the guinea pig. Acta oto-laryngologia (Stockh) Suppl 126:1-85.

Williams SR, Stuart GJ (2000) Action potential backpropagation and somato-dendritic distribution of ion channels in thalamocortical neurons. J Neurosci 20:1307-1317.

Wittkowski W (1967) Synaptische Strukturen und Elementargranula in der Neurohypophyse des Meerschweinchens. Z Zellforsch 82:434-458.

Wittkowski W (1973) Elektronenmikroskopische Untersuchungen zur funktionellen Morphologie des tubero-hypophysären Systems der Ratte. Z Zellforsch 139:101-148.

Wolff J (1968) The role of astroglia in the brain tissue. Acta Neuropathol Suppl IV:33-39.

Wolff JR, Laskawi R, Spatz WB, Missler M (1995) Structural dynamics of synapses and synaptic components. Behav Brain Res 66:13-20.

Xu-Friedmann MA, Harris KM, Regehr WG (2001) Three-dimensional comparison of ultrastructural characteristics at depressing and facilitating synapses onto Purkinje cells. J Neurosci 21:6666-6672.

3.12. Abbreviations

AMPA	α-amino-3-hydroxy-5-methyl-4-isoxazole propionate
cAMP	Cyclic adenosine monophosphate
CNS	Central nervous system
CSF	Cerebrospinal fluid
DRG	Dorsal root ganglion
GABA	γ-aminobutyric acid
GluR	Glutamate receptors
IPL	Inner plexiform layer
LC	Landolt's club
LTP	Long-term potentiation
NO	Nitric oxide
PAPs	Peripheral astroglial processes
PGPs	Peripheral glial processes
PNS	Peripheral nervous system
PRC	Photoreceptor cells
RIS	Rod inner segments
ROS	Rod outer segments
SNARE	Soluble N-ethyl maleimide-sensitive factor attachment protein receptor

Chapter 4

Morphological plasticity of astroglial/neuronal interactions: functional implications

Glenn I. Hatton

Department of Cell Biology and Neuroscience
University of California, Riverside, CA 92521 USA

Corresponding author: glenn.hatton@ucr.edu

Contents

4.1. Introduction

Structure and function are inextricably wedded, a principle extending far beyond studies of nervous systems. Nowhere is this principle more profoundly and consistently exemplified than it is in nervous systems, however. It is clear, for example, from the diversity of cell types, the specializations of portions of cells, as well as the various contacts and intercellular juxtapositions, that functional diversity can be predicted from structural specialization. Thus, it is easy to understand that spinal motoneurons, with their long myelinated axons, carry out a different set of functions than do neurons that are devoid of axons, such as retinal amacrine cells. The former are engaged in high-speed transfer of information over long distances; the latter are not. Still, these two cell types remain neurons that integrate and process the information that they are specialized to receive and transmit. More subtle variations in neuron types than those gross differences seen between motoneurons and amacrine cells have been appreciated for some time now, of course. The presence or absence of spines on dendrites is an immediate clue to functional diversity among otherwise similar neurons, as is the presence or absence of microvesicles in dendrites, or whether the cell's axon arises from the soma or from a proximal dendrite. This tight structure-function relationship holds not only for the individual cells themselves, but also for the larger structures formed by cell aggregates, e.g., the juxtapositions of cells within a nucleus in the brain. Such juxtapositions are known to be dynamic, even in the mature animal.

4.1.1. Glial associations with different parts of neurons

Similar to neuronal structures, and as discussed in Chapter 3, glial cells come in a variety of types, sizes and shapes, each type having recognized (although not yet completely understood) special functions. There are astroglia, ependymoglia, microglia and oligodendroglia, and at least some variation within each of these types. Heavily committed to an insulating function, oligodendroglia associate chiefly with the axonal portions of central neurons as myelinating cells, although in the olfactory bulb there are myelinated dendrites (Peters et al., 1991, p. 97). Microglia wander around among the neurons performing their phagocytic tasks and secreting bioactive agents as needed, and may become antigen-presenting cells when conditions demand. Ependymoglia line the walls of the ventricles and the spinal canal and contribute to the production of cerebrospinal fluid, but are not a homogeneous cuboidal cell population as they are so often labeled, as they, too, can have processes that extend into the subependymal layer (Mercier et al., 2002). A newly suspected role for ependymoglia is providing a microenvironment for the production of central nervous system stem cells (see Chapter 5). In general, ependymoglia have limited direct associations with mature neurons. A fourth major glial cell type, astrocytes, is morphologically and thus, apparently in some measure functionally distinct from the other three types. Astroglia are also distinct in that they are found to associate with all portions of neurons, from the tips of the dendrites to the axon terminals.

Just within the class of astrocytes, the main focus of this chapter, there is a considerable degree of heterogeneity that implies correspondingly diverse functional characteristics. Heterogeneity as a characteristic of the cells termed astroglia has long been well recognized (Wilkin et al., 1990; Batter et al., 1992). Typical astrocyte markers, such as glial fibrillary acidic protein (GFAP) or glutamine synthetase, are expressed by cells as morphologically diverse as the Bergmann glia of the cerebellum, the fibrous astrocytes of the optic tract and the small star-shaped astroglia of the hippocampus. These cell types all qualify as astrocytes, but their functional roles in their respective brain areas are predicted, on structure-function principles, to be closely related to their morphological specializations. Bergmann glia are huge, polarized cells, which in rat extend from the cerebellar pial surface to the Purkinje cell body area, i.e., spanning the outer molecular layer, the entire expanse of Purkinje cell dendritic tree and the soma, usually stopping just short of the axon initial segment. This arrangement puts Bergmann glial processes in close apposition to most synapses on the Purkinje neuron, and these number in the tens of thousands (Reichenbach et al., 1995, see also Chapter 3). One predicted functional implication of this one-astrocyte-to-many-synapse structural arrangement is that there is some degree of coordination of the neuronal/glial bi-directional signaling for each part of the Purkinje cell dendritic tree. Other, so-called vellate, not obviously polarized astrocytes are much smaller and occupy the more internal zones of the cerebellar cortex gray matter (Palay and Chan-Palay, 1974). These are likely to perform functions that are somewhat different from those executed by the Bergmann glia. See Chapters 3 and 12 for discussions of some of these functions. We return later in this chapter to a consideration of specific ways in which astrocytes associate and may alter their association with the dendrites, somata and terminals of the same neurons.

4.1.2. Numbers and space-filling capacity of astrocytes

Commonly accepted estimates of the numbers of neurons in the human brain run in the area of 10^{12}, a number that seems to grow with each successive attempt to count the brain's granule cells (Nauta and Feirtag, 1986). To this one must add that there are about nine or ten glial cells for every neuron. While these astronomical numbers are dazzlingly difficult to comprehend, they are highly consistent with the emerging concepts of the multitude of functions that are being attributed to this non-neuronal cell class, many of which are covered in subsequent chapters of this volume. Glia are estimated to account for about 40-50% of the cellular volume in brains of mammals and a somewhat lower percentage in non-mammalian vertebrates. Since a large proportion of the total number of glial cells consists of astroglia, it follows that these glia occupy much of the brain's parenchymal space that is not devoted to neurons. Important to note here is that this astrocyte occupation is not mere random space filling, as the old concept of the neuroglia as "neural glue" suggested. Although astroglia do generally interpose themselves between neighboring neurons, insinuating their fine processes into even tiny interneuronal clefts in a seemingly random fashion, they also consistently serve as interface cells between brain elements of neural and non-neural origin. For instance, astrocytes occupy an overwhelming proportion of the basal lamina that separates the pial surface from the brain parenchyma (see Fig. 2 in Mercier and Hatton, 2001). Virtually all of the basal lamina surrounding the brain's vasculature (i.e., endothelial and smooth muscle cells, pericytes and macrophages) is completely occupied by astroglial endfeet. Figure 4.1 shows an example of GFAP immunoreactivity (-ir) in astrocytic processes investing a blood vessel that is entering the brain from the ventral surface. Astrocytic occupation of the area adjacent to the pial surface is also evident in Figure 4.1. GFAP-ir is commonly the way astrocytes are viewed at the light microscopic (LM) level, but recent work has suggested that the picture of astrocyte morphology derived from GFAP-ir is incomplete at best and may be misleading as discussed below.

4.2. Astrocyte morphology - a closer look

4.2.1. Astrocyte domains and volume estimates

GFAP and vimentin are intermediate filament proteins (8-10 nm diameter) that form part of the cytoskeletal structure of astrocytes. Often, but not always, only one of these proteins is expressed by any given cell, with vimentin being generally found

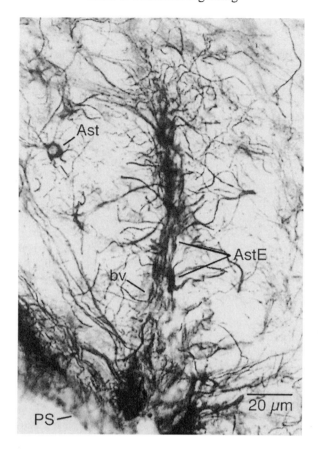

Figure 4.1. Glial fibrillary acidic protein immunoreactivity (GFAP-ir) in a coronal section from rat ventral hypothalamus. A large blood vessel (bv) entering the brain through the pial surface (PS) is covered by astrocyte endfeet (AstE). Long immunostained processes from ventral glial lamina astrocytes are seen coursing dorsolaterally on the left side of the vessel. A smaller, more stellate-shaped astrocyte in indicated (Ast). Antibody visualized with 3, 3'-diaminobenzidine.

more frequently in astroglia of immature brains, and GFAP being more often expressed in mature brains. For an example of individual astrocytes from adult brain staining with antibodies against both vimentin and GFAP, see Mercier and Hatton (2000, Fig. 6). In any case, there are many other structural elements that make up the astrocyte cytoskeleton besides these two intermediate filament proteins. Not surprisingly therefore, recent work has determined that immunostaining for GFAP, for example, often reveals only a small portion of the astrocyte's actual cellular volume. Cell volume estimates based on GFAP-ir were only ~15% of the cell volumes estimated from filling astrocytes with a fluorescent dye (Bushong et al., 2002). These measurements were made on hippocampal astroglia, and the estimates may not be exactly the same for astrocytes from all other brain areas, but they may not be grossly different. Clearly, one important implication of this work is that the most frequently presented view of astrocytes in brain rather seriously underestimates the volumes of these cells and thus their actual space-filling capacity. An illustration of the difference between what is visualized with GFAP-ir and the actual cell area contained within the plasma membrane is presented in Figure 4.2. This illustration comes from neocortical astrocytes in culture, from which it can be seen that even in two-dimensional space much that is astrocytic is not conveyed by the GFAP-ir of the cell. One must ever be prepared, then, to mentally supply the missing 70-85% of the actual volume when viewing astrocytes in GFAP-ir.

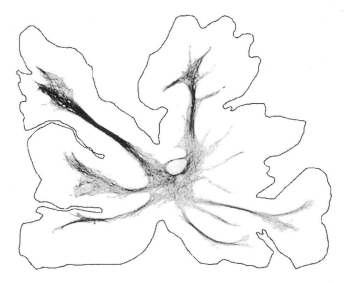

Figure 4.2. Estimated space-filling capacity of an isolated cultured neocortical astrocyte in two dimensions given by outlining plasma membrane. Cytoskeletal elements shown here are revealed by GFAP immunostaining.

Misleading also was the picture of astrocyte domains derived solely from GFAP staining. Earlier models of how the space not occupied by neurons was partitioned by the astroglia suggested that there was a considerable degree of interdigitation among neighboring astrocytes in brain. By filling hippocampal astrocytes with fluorescent dyes, Bushong et al. (2002) were able to discern, at the LM level, that there appeared to be minimal overlap between the domains of adjacent astrocytes. Confirmation of this was gained with electron microscopy (EM) when the fluorescent dye, Lucifer Yellow (LY) was injected and photo-oxidized in the presence of diaminobenzidine to yield an electron dense product. Under these conditions, little encroachment was seen by one astrocyte into a neighbor's domain. Before deciding that this is a general principle, it will be necessary to determine whether astrocytes in other brain areas obey these same rules. To the extent that these rules of eminent domain generally apply to astrocytes, we will need to alter our current conceptualization of the structural plan for brain astroglia. Until now and despite some evidence to the contrary (see below), this concept has been based rather casually on the assumption of random space filling.

4.2.2. Mechanisms of astrocyte morphological plasticity

That astrocytes and other glial-like cells undergo shape changes in response to activation of second messenger cascades has been known for some time (reviewed by van Calker and Hamprecht, 1980). In particular, activation of adenylyl cyclase (AC) and the subsequent cAMP - protein kinase A cascade leads to changes in the shapes of cells in culture. Serum-containing culture media usually induce flattened, relatively amorphous appearances in cultured cells. An example of this appearance in a primary culture of astroglia from adult rat pituitary neural lobe (NL) is shown in Figure 4.3A. Activation of β-adrenergic receptors (βARs), which in turn stimulates AC, or application of membrane permeant cAMP analogues that bypass the receptors and activate protein kinase A, are capable of transforming, within minutes at room temperature, most of the cells in the culture into process-bearing forms that are phase-bright and somewhat stellate in shape (Fig. 4.3B). Such conversions in morphology are slowly reversed. The mechanisms of shape change in these cells are thought to involve actin and actin binding proteins that are attached to both the glial plasma membrane and to the filamentous and other cytoskeletal structures, both microfilaments and intermediate filaments as well as to microtubules (Matsunaga et al., 1999; Miyata et al., 1999). That is, activation of receptors linked the eventual activation of protein kinase A (e.g., β-adrenergic) induces a retraction of the plasma membrane toward the main cytoskeleton of the astrocyte, as seen in Figure 4.3 (Hatton et al., 1991).

4.3. Astrocyte/neuronal juxtapositions

As illustrated in Chapter 3 and here alluded to above, mammalian astroglia are found in association with all major neuronal substructures: dendrites, somata, axons and axon terminals. Often individual astrocytes make simultaneous alliances with more than one of these neuronal substructures, e.g., dendritic spines and/or shafts receiving synaptic terminal contacts may be enveloped by one or more processes of the same astrocyte (e.g., see Chapter 3, Fig. 3.11A, C; Peters et al., 1991, p. 165). Somata of even the most densely packed neuronal nuclei are likely to be seen separated from one another only by fine glial processes, at least under certain physiological conditions (Fig. 4.4A). Dendrites and dendritic extensions are often observed to be conspicuously ensheathed by astrocytic processes that appear to isolate and insulate them from their dendritic neighbors and from other neuronal elements (Fig. 4.4B). Astroglial processes tend also to insinuate themselves between the unmyelinated axons of the mammalian brain, and are well documented to associate closely with the exposed axonal membrane at the Nodes of Ranvier or at node-like specializations (Chapter 3, Fig. 3.10A; Peters et al., 1991, p. 253). Astrocytes of the rat neurohypophysis are known to surround and engulf both the neurosecretory axons and axon terminals that have found their way there from the hypothalamus. Figure 4.5 provides a clearly discernable example of this arrangement, in which the cytoplasm of one astrocyte is engulfing at least four neurosecretory axons and two terminals. Engulfed terminals are so identified by their small size and the presence of both dense core and clear vesicles (Miyata et al., 2001). Note that the cytoplasm of a second astrocyte (lower right) does not appear to interdigitate extensively, if at all, with that of the upper one.

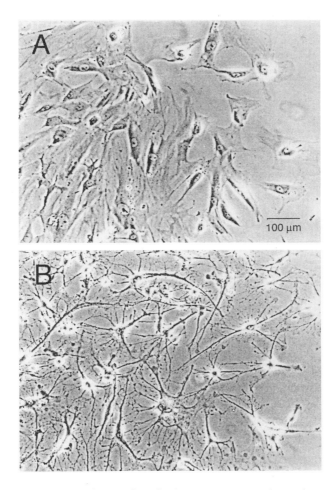

Figure 4.3. Phase-contrast micrographs of primary astrocyte cultures immunostained for GFAP. *A*. Flattened confluent control culture. *B*. Process-bearing appearance was produced by 60 min treatment of this culture with 500 nM isoprenaline in the absence of serum. Such effects are blocked by β–adrenergic antagonists. Data from Bicknell et al., 1989.

Given the ability of transmitters or other neuroactive substances to effect shape changes and process withdrawal in astroglia, one must at least entertain the idea that many, if not all of these illustrated relationships are merely snapshots in time. That is, observations under different sets of conditions or physiological states may yield varied relationships, such as neuronal membrane directly adjacent to membrane of a neighboring neuron instead of next to that of an astrocytic process as is usually the case. Indeed, decades ago Green and Maxwell (1961) were puzzled to find such neuron-neuron juxtapositions in the hippocampus and dentate gyrus. Although not yet known for the hippocampus, in other systems we are beginning to understand some of the mechanisms involved and the functional consequences ensuing from these plastic changes in neuron/astrocyte juxtaposition.

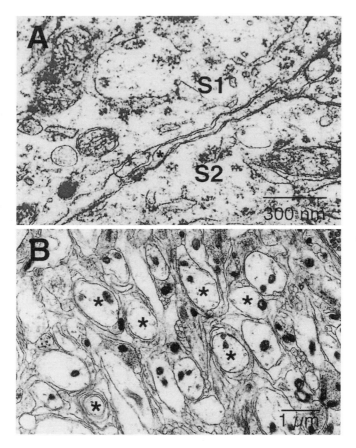

Figure 4.4. Electron micrographs of supraoptic nucleus, showing astrocyte space-filling capacity (i.e., astroglial occupation of interneuronal spaces) under basal conditions. *A*. Two magnocellular somata (S1 and S2) are separated by a fine astrocytic process (*).*B*. In the dendritic zone, dendrites (*) are individually wrapped by astrocytic processes that separate most adjacent dendrites from their neighbors.

4.4. Function-related neuronal/glial plasticity

4.4.1. An illustrative model

Reversible plastic changes in astrocyte morphology and juxtapositions with neighboring neurons in response to physiological stimuli were first described in the *in vivo* magnocellular hypothalamo-neurohypophysial system (mHNS) of the rat over two decades ago (Tweedle and Hatton, 1977). In light of its precedence in this regard and its continuing contributions to our understanding of the processes and implications of function-related morphological plasticity, this model system is used here as a prime illustrative example of glial-neuronal bi-directional signaling. As background for appreciating the physiological meaning and functional importance of the plastic changes discussed, a brief overview of the relevant structural and functional characteristics of the mHNS follows in this and the next two sections. More extensive recent reviews of important aspects of the mHNS are available to the interested reader (Miyata and Hatton, 2002; Theodosis, 2002).

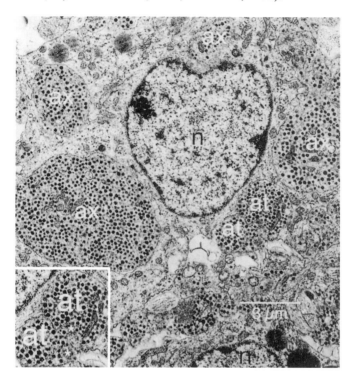

Figure 4.5. Electron micrograph of two neural lobe astrocytes with prominent nuclei (n) from a rat maintained under basal conditions. The upper astrocyte is engulfing at least four neurosecretory axons (ax) and two axon terminals (at), so identified by the presence of both large dense core vesicles and clear microvesicles. The latter are indicated (*) in the inset.

A three-dimensional representation of a rat brain is diagrammed in Figure 4.6. The brain is cut away at the level of the supraoptic (SON) and paraventricular (PVN) nuclei in the anterior hypothalamus, revealing the parvocellular PVN axonal projections to the median eminence and the projections of the magnocellular neurons, via the pituitary stalk, to the neurohypophysis. It was in the supraoptico-neurohypophysial portion of the mHNS that glial/neuronal plasticity and functional interactions were first discovered, and it is this area that has been most extensively studied. To the limited extent that it has been studied in this context, the PVN has been found to show morphological plasticity similar to that reported for the SON.

4.4.2. Morphological plasticity in the supraoptic nucleus

Production of either oxytocin (OT) or vasopressin (VP) is the responsibility of the two SON magnocellular neuron populations. Released in response to physiological challenges, such as dehydration, parturition and suckling of the young, OT and VP have well known actions on peripheral tissues of the kidney, uterus, myoepithelial cells of the mammary glands and certain vascular beds. Under basal conditions (i.e., in the absence of such physiological challenges), SON neurons are spontaneously active, though relatively quiescent. Physiological activation of the system leads to the development of two distinct, largely intrinsically generated firing patterns that characterize the two cell types, as was first exquisitely shown by Brimble and Dyball (1977; for review see Armstrong, 1995). As discussed below, astrocyte signaling appears to play roles in both the maintenance of quiescence under basal conditions and the production and maintenance of the activated states.

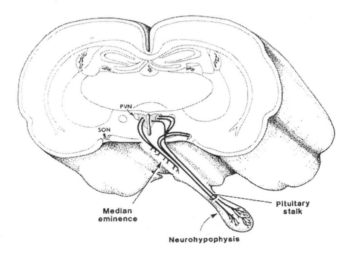

Figure 4.6. Diagram of rat brain cut away at the level of the supraoptic (SON) and paraventricular (PVN) nuclei showing the principal axonal projections of the magnocellular neurons to the neurohypophysis.

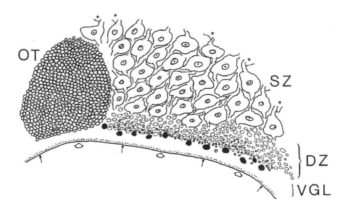

Figure 4.7. Diagram of rat SON and the pial-glial limitans in coronal plane. Profiles representing somata are lateral to the myelinated fibers of the optic tract (OT) in the somatic

zone (SZ). Dendrites projecting dorsally and ventrally from the somata have been truncated for simplicity, as have the axons arising from the dorsally projecting dendrites (*). Ventral to the SZ are the parallel-projecting dendrites (unfilled small circles), depicted in cross section, and constituting the dendritic zone (DZ). Mingling with only the most ventral dendrites are the astroglial cell nuclei (larger filled circles), whose ventrally projecting processes (shown in Fig. 4.8A) fill the clear space between the basal lamina (small arrows) and the most ventral dendrites. These astroglial cell bodies and processes constitute the ventral glial lamina (VGL). Dorsally projecting processes from these glia fill most of the space not occupied by the somata and dendrites. Open arrows indicate pia mater.

Neurons in the rat SON are large (15-25 μm diameter) and densely packed, when compared to hypothalamic neurons in general. Also when compared to that reference group, the SON displays a higher degree of organization, a factor contributing to its model system status. Depicted diagrammatically in Figure 4.7 are some of the essential features of the SON that are involved in its plastic capabilities. Positioned immediately lateral to the optic chiasm and optic tract, the SON consists of somatic and dendritic zones and a row of astrocytes that makes up the ventral glial lamina (VGL). SON somata generally give rise to a dorsally projecting dendrite from which the parent axon usually arises (* in diagram, and see Fig. 4.8B) and one to three ventrally projecting dendrites (truncated here for simplicity). Since these latter dendrites turn to run rostrocaudally in parallel with one another, they are seen in cross section as the dendritic zone (DZ) in this coronal plane diagram. Filled ovoid shapes representing the astrocyte nuclei are seen at the dorsal aspect of the VGL. As is the case in virtually all areas where brain parenchyma meets extraparenchymal tissue, there is a basal lamina (small arrows) separating the astrocytes of the VGL from the pia mater (solid line; open arrows). Under basal conditions, the VGL astrocytes project long processes dorsally throughout the DZ and the somatic zone (SZ), wrapping the dendrites and insinuating themselves between adjacent somata (e.g., see Fig. 4.4). Astrocytic membrane that is not involved in the dorsal projections fills the space between the DZ and the pial surface (Fig. 4.8A). Visualized with GFAP immunostaining, dorsally projecting processes from the VGL astrocytes are shown wending their way through the OT neuronal dendrites and somata (Fig. 4.8B). Unstained are the VP neurons that comprise the other 50% of SON nerve cells. Also unseen in this GFAP immunostain is the remaining ~ 70-85% of each astrocyte (see Fig. 4.2) that fills the apparently open spaces between the neighboring dendrites or cell bodies, as is clearly visible in the top portion of Figure 4.8A.

Electron micrographs reveal the close relationships of the SON neurons to their associated astrocytes. Readily seen at the EM level are the fine astrocytic processes that are interposed between these magnocellular neurons of a normally hydrated animal (Fig. 4.4). Strikingly different is the picture presented by the SONs of either dehydrated or lactating animals (Fig. 4.9A), in which large areas of neural membrane are closely apposed to (but not in actual contact with) other neural, rather than glial membrane. These intercellular distances are estimated to be ~ 10 nm. Correlated with this glial withdrawal is an increase in the number of multiple synapses (i.e. one terminal forming synapses with two or more postsynaptic elements). An example of such a synapse from a dehydrated rat SON is shown in Figure 4.9B, in which one terminal (arrows) is making axo-somatic synapses with two somata (S1 and S2). Individual terminals may also make multiple synapses with both somata and dendrites or with two or more dendrites. Using serial thin sectioning methods, as many as seven postsynaptic elements have been observed being synaptically contacted by one terminal in the activated SON (Modney and Hatton, 1989). It is noteworthy that, under the aforementioned conditions, (1) multiple synapses increase in number while single conventional synapses decrease, (2) there is no ingrowth of new terminals (i.e., no observed growth cones), and (3) the time course of multiple synapse formation has been observed to be too rapid for axonal sprouting to occur. These are factors that have forced the interpretation that multiple synapses in this system arise from single ones. The way in which this might occur is easily imagined from the other synapse in Figure 4.9B, where a conventional single synapse is evident with S1, but the terminal is separated from S2 by fine astrocyte processes (arrowheads). Retraction of these fine astrocytic processes would allow a second synapse to be made with S2. Similarly, astroglial process retraction in the DZ results in dendritic bundling, in which two or more dendrites are apposed without intervening glial membrane (Fig. 4.9C). Increased also are axo-dendritic multiple synapses, one of which is labeled with an asterisk.

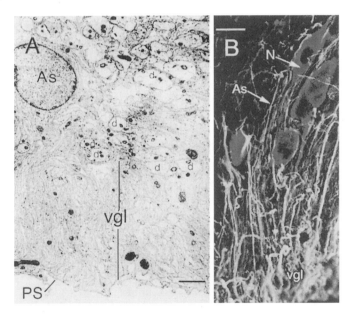

Figure. 4.8. Micrographs of the supraoptic nucleus. *A*. Electron micrograph showing the extensive astroglial membrane that fills the ventral glial lamina (vgl). Dendrites (d), some of which are in bundles, are cut in cross section. As: astrocyte nucleus. PS: pial surface. Bar = 2 μm. *B*. Astrocyte (GFAP, green)-neuronal (red) appositions in the SON, under conditions of low demand for the release of peptides. N: magnocellular OT neuron; As: astrocytic process. Bar = 20 μm.

Important to note at this juncture is that the plastic changes, discussed herein, that are induced by activation of the mHNS, are largely reversed when the physiological conditions revert to something akin to the *status quo ante*. Rehydration of a previously dehydrated animal results in reinsertion of astroglial processes into the spaces between somata, rewrapping of the dendrites, sharp decline in the number of multiple synapses, etc. (Tweedle and Hatton, 1984; Perlmutter et al., 1985). Similarly reversed in the postweaning mother are the changes wrought in the SON by the ordeals of parturition and suckling of the offspring (Theodosis and Poulain, 1984).

Another plastic change that accompanies activation of this system is an increase in gap junctional intercellular communication (as measured by dye coupling) among SON neurons. As with interneuronal gap junctions in many other brain areas, conventional transmission EM has not been a tool effective in revealing them in the SON dendritic zone, probably because there are too few connexons per junction for clear resolution. Thus, gap junctions in the SON have been inferred from dual intracellular recordings (Yang and Hatton, 1988), dye and tracer coupling studies (Hatton et al., 1987; Hatton and Yang, 1994) as well as from *in situ* hybridization for connexin mRNA (Micevych et al., 1996) and immunocytochemical labeling for connexin protein (Miyata and Hatton, 1997). Such coupling is dendrodendritic and is exclusively observed between cells expressing the same peptide (i.e., either OT or VP). Since dendrites that are wrapped by glia and isolated from one another, the way they are under basal conditions (e.g. Fig. 4.4B), could not readily come into close apposition for connexin docking, the glial retraction must play at least a permissive role in interneuronal gap junction formation. Support for this hypothesis, of course, comes from the positive relationship between glial retraction and increased coupling among the neurons.

4.4.3. Morphological plasticity in the neurohypophysis

As indicated in Figure 4.6, parent axons from the magnocellular neurons of both the PVN and the SON terminate in the neurohypophysis. One of the singular advantages of this mHNS model system is that one can investigate the somata and dendrites in the hypothalamus and the terminals in the neurohypophysis of the same neurons, along with their associated astrocytes. That plastic changes, parallel to those described in the SON, occur at the level of the terminals when physiological conditions activate the mHNS has been known for many years (Tweedle and Hatton, 1980; 1982). Contrary to assertions commonly made about these "neurovascular" terminations (and others such as exist in the median eminence), the axonal endings of neurosecretory neurons do not terminate "on the blood vessels" of the NL, but on or near the basal lamina lining the pial surface, beyond which are the perivascular spaces surrounding the NL's fenestrated capillaries. Neurosecretory materials released from terminals abutting the basal lamina have relatively unfettered access to these capillaries. Under basal conditions, the terminals, many of which are engulfed by the pituicytes (Fig. 4.5), are thereby allowed to occupy a relatively smaller portion of the basal lamina, while a larger portion is occupied by pituicyte membrane. With physiological activation of the mHNS, the pituicytes in situ undergo dramatic shape changes from rounded spheroids to a process-bearing and somewhat stellate morphology, quite similar to that seen in primary cultures of adult pituicytes (Fig. 4.3). During this process of morphological transformation, the pituicytes release many, but not all, of the engulfed axons and terminals and retract from their dominant occupation of the basal lamina. This results in increased basal lamina occupation by neurosecretory terminals (Tweedle and Hatton, 1987) and, obviously also, in the removal of a potential diffusion barrier to released secretory materials

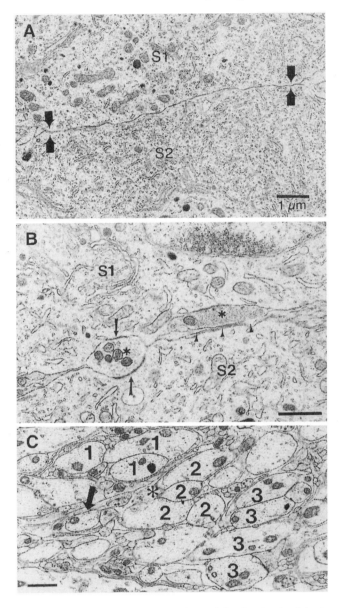

Figure. 4.9. Electron micrographs of supraoptic nuclei of animals dehydrated by saline drinking. *A.* Extensive membrane apposition (membrane length between pair of arrows) between two magnocellular somata (S1 and S2). *B.* Synaptic bouton (*, left) making multiple synapses (arrows) with two somata (S1 and S2). On the right, an elongated terminal (*) synapses with S1, but is separated from S2 by a thin astrocytic process (arrowheads), which upon retraction would allow formation of a new synapse with S2. *C.* Dendritic bundling upon retraction of astrocyte processes (arrow). Dendrites in apposition with no intervening astroglial processes (i.e., bundles) are labeled with like numbers (e.g., a bundle of three, marked with #1s, etc.). An axo-dendritic multiple synapse is indicated (*). All scale bars = 1 μm.

entering the blood. Interestingly, there is an enlargement of the terminals that are allowed to contact the basal lamina, while those that remain primarily in contact with the astrocytes do not enlarge (Miyata et al., 2001). Since terminal size is positively related to efficacy of release (Pierce and Lewin, 1994), the implication of this plastic change seems clear. Like the plastic changes seen in the SON, those in the NL are reversed with a return to basal conditions.

4.5. Functional significance of plastic changes

4.5.1. Astroglia-to-neuron signaling under basal conditions

Although many of the morphological changes mentioned here have been long recognized, recent work has contributed much to our understanding of the functional properties of glial/neuronal bi-directional signaling in the mHNS. Both astroglia-to-neuron and neuron-to-astroglia signaling have been demonstrated in the mHNS, as they have in some other brain regions. The mHNS, however, appears to be the first in which there is clear evidence for astroglial-to-neuron signaling that is initiated by systemic events, rather than by neuronally generated transmitters. Astroglia in many brain regions as well as the SON and NL (Reymond et al., 1996; Decavel and Hatton, 1995; Miyata et al., 1997), synthesize and express the inhibitory amino acid taurine (2-aminoethanesulfonic acid). Taurine is well known as an osmolyte that is released though anion channels (see Chapters 8 and 16) in response to a number of stimuli, including stretch or swelling that accompanies high $[K^+]_o$ (Vitarella et al., 1994) or low osmolality (Pasante-Morales et al., 2002), but can also be released via receptor-mediated actions (Martin and Shain, 1993). Taurine is an endogenous agonist at either glycine or γ-aminobutyric acid type A receptors (glyRs or GABA$_A$Rs, respectively), with higher affinities at glyRs.

4.5.1.1. Astroglia-to-neuron signaling in the SON

In a well-hydrated animal, when the extracellular fluid compartment is normo- to hypo- osmotic and glial coverage of SON neurons is most extensive (e.g., as in Fig. 4.10A), it has been shown that there is a continuous low level of taurine release from the astrocytes (Deleuze et al., 1998). This taurine is sufficient to tonically inhibit firing of VP neurons via activation of strychnine-sensitive glyRs (Hussy et al., 1997). Acutely raising the plasma osmolality quickly reduces or abolishes the glial release of taurine and blockade of the SON glyRs in water loaded animals increases VP neuronal excitability. Removal of the glial source of taurine also raised neuronal excitability (Deleuze et al., 1998). Thus, it appears that the systemic hypotonicity signal received by the SON astrocytes is volume-transmitted (Agnati et al., 1995) to the VP neurons in the form of an inhibitory amino acid input to high affinity glyRs that are probably located extrasynaptically. From the data in Figure 4.10A, it appears that the glial-generated taurine signals might also influence the presynaptic terminals contacting SON dendrites, to the extent that these terminals express glyRs or GABA$_A$Rs, which has not yet been determined.

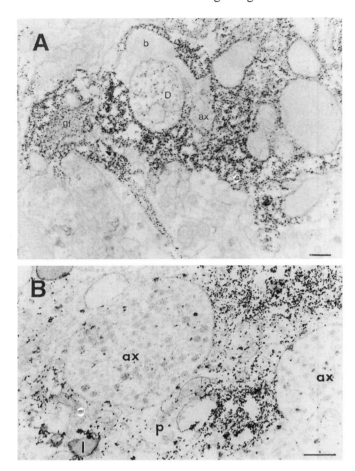

Figure. 4.10. Electron micrographs of taurine-expressing astroglia. *A*. Taurine-immunoreactive astrocyte completely surrounding an axon (ax) and its bouton (b) making contact with a supraoptic dendrite (D). Visible in this astrocyte are glial filaments (gf). Note that although the astrocyte is replete with taurine-ir, the dendrite and the afferent process contain little or none. Scale bar = 290 nm. *B*. Neurosecretory axons (ax) in the neural lobe containing dense core vesicles. Taurine-ir fills the surrounding pituicyte (P) cytoplasm, which also contains a lipid body (l), characteristic of pituicytes. Scale bar = 500 nm. Taurine-ir visualized with gold substituted silver periodate in both *A* and *B*. Data in *A* from Decavel and Hatton, 1995; in *B* from Miyata et al., 1997

4.5.1.2. Astroglia-to-neuron signaling in the NL

Taurine is abundantly expressed in the astroglia but not in the terminals of the NL (Fig. 4.10B), and its selective release is evoked by lowering the extracellular fluid osmolality (Miyata et al., 1997). While this stimulus released taurine in increasing amounts with time, it did not affect release of GABA (not shown) or glutamate, and actually reduced the release of glutamine (Fig. 4.11). Furthermore, high $[K^+]_o$-evoked release of VP from isolated NLs was reduced via glyR activation by taurine from the pituicytes (Hussy et al., 2001). By contrast, taurine has the opposite effect on basal release from isolated NLs, enhancing release of both OT and VP. This is apparently accomplished by opening Cl⁻ channels in these terminals, which then *depolarize* the membrane potential because of their high resting $[Cl^-]_i$ (Song and Hatton, 2003). Therefore, the glial-generated taurine signal at the level of the somata and dendrites under basal conditions reduces excitability of SON neurons, but at the level of the terminals this same signal maintains some regulated amount of hormone release. Both of these are accomplished by opening Cl⁻ channels.

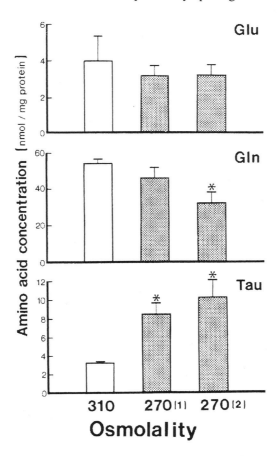

Figure 4.11. Effect of hypoosmotic perfusion on amino acid release from isolated neurohypophysis *in vitro.* Neural lobes were pre-incubated in isosmotic aCSF, superfused with control medium and a control sample collected after 20 min. They were then superfused with hypoosmotic (270 mOsm/kg) aCSF. Two collection times are shown: 270(1), 20 to 40 min and 270(2), 40 to 60 min. *Significant differences from isosmotic aCSF at $p < 0.05$ by using paired t-test. The bars are mean concentrations (± s.e.m.) from five samples of six pituitaries each. Glu, glutamate; Gln, glutamine; Tau, taurine. Data from Miyata et al., 1997.

4.5.2. Barrier function of astroglia under basal conditions

As mentioned above, by engulfing the neurosecretory axons and occupying large areas of the basal lamina, the NL astrocytes provide a partial barrier to any released substances entering the perivascular spaces. SON astrocytes likely serve a similar function under conditions of low demand for peptide release, as they wrap the dendrites and cover much of the somatic membrane. It is of some interest here that axons and terminals in the NL are not the only peptide release sites from SON neurons. That there is intra-SON release of both OT and VP has been known since the pioneering physiological studies of Moos et al. (1984) and the anatomical work of Pow and Morris (1989). Any peptide released during those times when astroglia are interposed between adjacent somata or dendrites would first come into contact with glial rather than neuronal membrane. Due to the increased tortuosity, extracellular matrix protein expression and perhaps increased amounts of endopeptidases within the extracellular space at such times, the released neuropeptides may never reach other neuronal targets. Thus, the astrocytes can present an effective, but movable barrier to this type of neuron-neuron interaction. One implication might be that glial movement is essential for proper functioning under activated conditions.

4.5.3. Implications of astrocyte withdrawal

Retraction of astrocytic processes from portions of the neuronal membranes rather radically changes the neuronal microenvironment in several ways. First, a most proximal source of effective K^+ uptake is no longer nearby. Since this glial withdrawal occurs at a time of mHNS activation via, for instance, osmotic stimuli, excitatory synaptic and perhaps other inputs, it is accompanied by increased neuronal firing. The K^+ that is extruded with each action potential has one less source for its rapid removal from the immediate vicinity of the neuronal membrane. In addition, the neighboring neuron, formerly at least one astrocytic process away (i.e., two glial membranes plus astrocyte cytoplasm; Fig. 4.4), is now adjacent, as little as 10 nm away (Fig. 4.9), and its enhanced electrical activity is also contributing to the elevated $[K^+]_o$ in the reduced space. Such increased $[K^+]_o$ should not only contribute to the membrane depolarization of the magnocellular neurons but also to the depolarization of their presynaptic inputs, both excitatory and inhibitory. Perhaps more importantly, astroglial retraction from the areas around glutamatergic synapses will allow prolonged glutamate action, due to reduced capacity for uptake (Oliet et al., 2001). Enhanced excitation is the net overall result observed. Additionally, the source of inhibitory influence by taurine is less ubiquitous after astrocyte withdrawal. If the glial retraction was evoked by dehydration, the glial taurine release would have already been inhibited osmotically. This would not be the case in the lactating animal, however, where the extracellular fluids are low- to normo- osmotic. As alluded to above, once the astrocyte processes retract from the spaces between the neuronal membranes, peptides released from somata and dendrites can more freely reach target receptors on the nearby neurons. Such peptide release within the SON has been shown to modulate the activity of both OT and VP neurons (Moos et al., 1984; Gouzenes et al., 1998) and to occur in response to systemic stimuli (Neumann et al., 1993; 1996).

Increased gap junction formation between the dendrites of the mHNS neurons is another accompaniment and implied consequence of astrocyte retraction in the DZ. The further implication here is that increased gap junctional communication somehow reorganizes, at least subtly but perhaps profoundly, the circuitry among mHNS neurons with prolonged activation. Since no clear functional consequences of increased gap junctional communication have yet been demonstrated, this idea is controversial and still under investigation.

4.6. Astroglial/neuronal bi-directional signaling in the mHNS

4.6.1. Neurotransmitter release may target both neurons and glia

Once it was established that astroglia could express receptors (as well as transporters) for various neurotransmitters, not only in culture but also in situ in the adult brain, the concept of signaling from neurons to glia was accepted. That this communication is bi-directional is now becoming clear, and is discussed in several chapters in this volume. Not yet part of the thinking of most neuroscientists, however, is the idea that neuronal inputs to particular brain areas might be targeting both the neuronal and the glial elements of the region. Yet, data relevant to this concept have long been available. For example, although still somewhat controversial, apparently due to more to an unwillingness to part with established concepts than to any flaws in the supporting data, there is much evidence for non-synaptic release sites for certain neurotransmitters such as acetylcholine and noradrenaline (Umbriaco et al., 1994; Descarries and Umbriaco, 1995). Moreover, the work of Buma and colleagues (Buma et al., 1984; Buma and Nieuwenhuys, 1988) and of Morris and Pow (1988; Pow and Morris, 1989) strongly suggests that neuroeffector molecules can be released from many more sites than simply axon terminals at conventional synapses. Now that it has been demonstrated that even synaptically released transmitters reach the astrocytes surrounding the synapse, it is certainly not disputable that transmitters released at non-synaptic sites are targeted for more than one cell type (e.g., neurons, glia and perhaps even perivascular and vascular cells). A particular case in point here involves the release of noradrenaline (or adrenaline) from varicosities that do not appear at the ultrastructural level to make conventional synapses (Descarries and Umbriaco, 1995). That there are many noradrenergic varicosities in the ventral portion of the SON was revealed long ago (McNeill and Sladek, 1980), and often erroneously interpreted as indicting a selective noradrenergic input to the VP neurons whose somata tend to occupy the more ventral SON regions (for review see Hatton, 1990). A more reasonable interpretation in light of later work is that the non-synaptic release of catecholamines into the ventral SON reaches both the VP and the OT dendrites that inhabit this zone, and the presynaptic terminals from neurons carrying other transmitters. Released catecholamines in this region appear to modulate neuronal activity via activation of α_1- and α_2- adrenoceptors (Armstrong et al., 1982; Khanna et al., 1993). In addition, the astrocytes of the region express β-adrenergic receptors (βARs) (Lafarga et al., 1992), the activation of which evokes retraction in of mHNS astrocyte processes both in primary cultures and in acutely isolated tissue (Bicknell et al., 1989; Luckman and Bicknell, 1990; Smithson et al., 1990; Hatton et al., 1991).

Catecholaminergic (Descarries and Umbriaco, 1995) and cholinergic (Theodosis and Mason, 1989; Umbriaco et al., 1994) terminals do not appear to be unique in forming presynaptic release sites in the relative absence of postsynaptic specializations. Axons from the histaminergic cell groups in the tuberomammillary nucleus innervate the SON (Inagaki et al., 1988). Ultrastructural examination of a large number of histaminergic terminals in the SON revealed an abundance of boutons that were immunopositive for L-histidine decarboxylase (the synthetic enzyme for histamine). These terminals made extensive appositions, particularly with SON dendrites, but also both with unlabeled boutons that were synapsing on the dendrites and with the local astrocytes (Decavel and Hatton, unpublished observations). Collectively, these observations suggest that paracrine release of transmitter/modulator molecules is intended to target, via volume transmission, more than one cell type in the region. In addition to the glial shape changes, mentioned above, that can be evinced by catecholamines activating βARs, non-synaptically released neural signals to these astrocytes may also evoke elevations in $[Ca^{2+}]_i$. Regardless of the avenue by which $[Ca^{2+}]_i$ is raised, there is the potential for this signal to release transmitters, such as glutamate (Parpura and Haydon, 2000) that further modulate intercellular communication. Astrocytes of various types have been found to respond to receptor activation by histamine and noradrenaline with elevations in $[Ca^{2+}]_i$ (Kirischuk et al., 1996; Jung et al., 2000). As for acetylcholine, recent work has shown that astrocytes express α7 nicotinic receptors, the activation of which raises $[Ca^{2+}]_i$ both by fluxing large amounts of Ca^{2+} through the channel and by calcium-induced calcium release from internal stores. (Sharma and Vijayaraghavan, 2001; 2002).

4.6.2. Bi-directional signaling in the neurohypophysis

At present, the clearest evidence for two-way signals between the neural and astroglial compartments in the mHNS exists for the NL. This signaling probably involves both paracrine release, such as that apparent in the SON, and release of transmitters and modulators at synaptoid contacts between nerve terminals and pituicytes. Such contacts have been known since the early work of Wittkowski and Brinkmann (1974) who showed that they varied in number with dehydration. Termed "synaptoid" because they lack one essential feature of synaptic contacts (Fig. 4.12), the postsynaptic membrane specialization, these contacts are one route of communication among all of the various neural and glial elements in the NL (Boersma and Van Leeuwen, 1994) but particularly involve the OT and VP terminals (Boersma et al., 1993). NL astroglia release taurine in response to systemic signals of hypotonicity, and taurine modulates peptide release from VP and OT terminals (see section 4.5.1.2). That the peptides released from the terminals can also affect the glia has been demonstrated. Primary cultures of adult rat NL pituicytes respond to low nanomolar concentrations of VP with sharp rises (> 400 nM) in $[Ca^{2+}]_i$. Similar responses were obtained with OT at one order of magnitude higher concentrations, but responses to both peptides were blocked by vasopressin V_1 antagonists (Hatton et al., 1992). If these calcium responses trigger release of neuroactive substances (e.g., glutamate or taurine, etc.), then there would be short loop feedback information flowing between the neural and glial compartments. In the case of glutamate, the release of which has already been demonstrated in response to $[Ca^{2+}]_i$ rises, then the feedback would likely be positive, facilitating peptide release. This positive feedback would, of course, be interrupted during the time it takes to refill internal calcium stores. Therefore, since it would be intermittent, the positive feedback would not produce instability. If, on the other hand, taurine were to be released (this has not been shown), then the feedback might be either negative or positive depending upon the conditions under which the peptide was released (see section 4.5.1.2). In either case, the bi-directional signaling possibilities in the NL are clearly established.

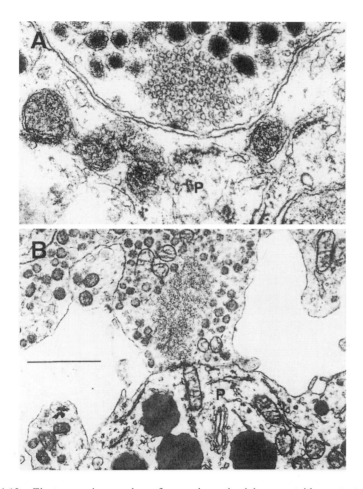

Figure 4.12. Electron micrographs of neurohypophysial synaptoid contacts between neurosecretory axons and astroglia. *A*. Basal conditions. High power micrograph of a neurosecretory axon containing both dense core vesicles and clear microvesicles, making a synaptoid contact with a pituitary astrocyte (P). Note complete absence of electron dense "postsynaptoid" membrane specialization. *B*. Dehydrated by saline drinking. Lower magnification micrograph similar to *A*, but in which the extracellular space is expanded, as is typical of neural lobes from stimulated rats. Scale bar = 660 nm in *A* and 1 μm in *B*.

4.7. Concluding remarks

Astrocytes appear to play important functional roles in the physiology of the mammalian central nervous system. These roles are expressed in part through plastic changes in morphology of astroglia in response to systemic signals (such as those arising from increased or decreased extracellular fluid osmotic pressure) as well as through responding to neurotransmitters emanating from neural terminals. In both cases, the astroglia have the capability to retract or extend their processes, thereby altering glia-neuron and neuron-neuron juxtapositions. Also, in either case the astroglia can release neuroeffector molecules that may modulate synaptic and non-synaptic transmission. Whether the relationships that have been documented in the mHNS will eventually be found expressed wholly or only partly in other brain systems remains to be determined.

Acknowledgements. The author's research is supported by NIH grant NS09140. Thanks are due P.J. Hatton, V. Parpura and T. A. Ponzio for helpful comments on an earlier draft of the manuscript.

4.8. References

Agnati LF, Zoli M, Stromberg I, Fuxe K (1995) Intercellular communication in the brain: wiring versus volume transmission. Neuroscience 69:711-726.

Armstrong WE (1995) Morphological and electrophysiological classification of hypothalamic supraoptic neurons. Prog. Neurobiol. 47:291-339.

Armstrong WE, Sladek CD, Sladek JR (1982) Characterization of noradrenergic control of vasopressin release by the organ-cultured rat hypothalamo-neuro-hypophyseal system. Endocrinology 111:273-279.

Batter DK, Corpina RA, Roy C, Spray DC, Hertzberg EL, Kessler JA (1992) Heterogeneity in gap junction expression in astrocytes cultured from different brain regions. Glia 6:213-221.

Bicknell RJ, Luckman S, Inenaga K, Mason WT, Hatton GI (1989) β-Adrenergic and opioid receptors on pituicytes cultured from adult rat neurohypophysis: regulation of cell morphology. Brain Res. Bull. 22:379-388.

Boersma CJC, Sonnemans MAF, van Leeuwen FW (1993) Immunoelectron microscopic demonstration of oxytocin and vasopressin in pituicytes and in nerve terminals forming synaptoid contacts with pituicytes in the rat neural lobe. Brain Res. 611:117-129.

Boersma CJC, van Leeuwen FW (1994) Neuron-glia interactions in the release of oxytocin and vasopressin from the rat neural lobe: The role of opioids, other neuropeptides and their receptors. Neuroscience 62:1003-1020.

Brimble M, Dyball REJ (1977) Characterization of the responses of oxytocin- and vasopressin- secreting neurones in the supraoptic nucleus to osmotic stimulation. J. Physiol. 271:253-271.

Buma P, Nieuwenhuys R (1988) Ultrastructural characteristics of exocytotic release sites in different layers of the median eminence of the rat. Cell Tiss. Res. 252:107-114.

Buma P, Roubos E, Buijs R (1984) Ultrastructural demonstration of exocytosis of neural, neuroendocrine and endocrine secretions with an in vitro tannic acid (TARI) method. Histochemistry 80:247-256.

Bushong E, Martone M, Jones Y, Ellisman M (2002) Protoplasmic astrocytes in CA1 stratum radiatum occupy separate anatomical domains. J. Neurosci. 22:183-192.

Decavel C, Hatton GI (1995) Taurine immunoreactivity in the rat supraoptic nucleus: Prominent localization in glial cells. J. Comp. Neurol. 354:13-26.

Deleuze C, Duvoid A, Hussy N (1998) Properties and glial origin of osmotic-dependent release of taurine from the rat supraoptic nucleus. J. Physiol. 507:463-471.

Descarries L, Umbriaco D (1995) Ultrastructural basis of monoamine and acetylcholine function in CNS. Sem. Neurosci. 7:309-318.

Gouzenes L, Desarmenien M, Hussy N, Richard P, Moos F (1998) Vasopressin regularizes the phasic firing pattern of rat hypothalamic magnocellular vasopressin neurons. J. Neurosci. 18:1879-1885.

Green JD, Maxwell DS (1961) Hippocampal electrical activity I. Morphological aspects. EEG Clin. Neurophysiol. 13:837-846.

Hatton GI (1990) Emerging concepts of structure-function dynamics in adult brain: the hypothalamo-neurohypophysial system. Prog. Neurobiol. 34:437-504.

Hatton GI, Bicknell RJ, Hoyland J, Bunting R, Mason WT (1992) Arginine vasopressin mobilises intracellular calcium via V1-receptor activation in astrocytes (pituicytes) cultured from adult rat neural lobes. Brain Res. 588:75-83.

Hatton GI, Luckman S, Bicknell RJ (1991) Adrenalin activation of β2-adrenoceptors stimulates morphological changes in astrocytes (pituicytes) cultured from adult rat neurohypophyses. Brain Res. Bull. 26:765-769.

Hatton GI, Yang QZ (1994) Incidence of neuronal coupling in supraoptic nuclei of virgin and lactating rats: estimation by neurobiotin and Lucifer Yellow. Brain Res. 650:63-69.

Hatton GI, Yang QZ, Cobbett P (1987) Dye coupling among immunocytochemically identified neurons in the supraoptic nucleus: increased incidence in lactating rat. Neuroscience 21:923-930.

Hussy N, Bres V, Rochette M, Duvoid A, Alonso G, Dayanithi G, Moos F (2001) Osmoregulation of vasopressin secretion via activation of neurohypophysial nerve terminals glycine receptors by glial taurine. J. Neurosci. 21:7110-7116.

Hussy N, Deleuze C, Pantaloni A, Desarmenien MG, Moos F (1997) Agonist action of taurine on glycine receptors in rat supraoptic magnocellular neurones: possible role in osmoregulation. J. Physiol. 502:609-621.

Inagaki N, Yamatodani A, Ando-Yamamoto M, Tohyama M, Watanabe T, Wada H (1988) Organization of histaminergic fibers in the rat brain. J. Comp. Neurol. 273:283-300.

Jung S, Pfeiffer F, Deitmer J (2000) Histamine-induced calcium entry in rat cerebellar astrocytes: evidence for capacitative and non-capacitative mechanisms. J. Physiol. 527:549-561.

Khanna S, Sibbald J, Day TA (1993) α-Adrenoceptor modulation of A1 noradrenergic neuron input to supraoptic vasopressin cells. Brain Res. 613:164.

Kirischuk S, Tuschick S, Verkhratsky A, Kettenmann H (1996) Calcium signalling in mouse Bergmann glial cells mediated by α 1-adrenoreceptors and H1 histamine receptors. Eur.J. Neurosci. 8:1198-1208.

Lafarga M, Berciano M, Delolmo E, Andres MA, Pazos A (1992) Osmotic stimulation induces changes in the expression of β-adrenergic receptors and nuclear volume of astrocytes in supraoptic nucleus of the rat. Brain Res. 588:311-316.

Luckman S, Bicknell RJ (1990) Morphological plasticity that occurs in the neurohypophysis following activation of the magnocellular neurosecretory system can be mimicked in vitro by beta-adrenergic stimulation. Neuroscience 39:701-709.

Martin DL, Shain W (1993) β-Adrenergic-agonist stimulated taurine release from astroglial cells is modulated by extracellular [K+] and osmolarity. Neurochem. Res. 18:437-444.

Matsunaga W, Miyata S, Kiyohara T (1999) Redistribution of MAP2 immunoreactivity in the neurohypophysial astrocytes of adult rats during dehydration. Brain Res. 829:7-17.

McNeill TH, Sladek JR (1980) Simultaneous monoamine histofluorescence and neuropeptide immunocytochemistry: II. Correlative distribution of catecholamine varicosities and magnocellular neurosecretory neurons in the rat supraoptic and paraventricular nuclei. J. Comp. Neurol. 193:1023-1033.

Mercier F, Hatton GI (2000) Immunocytochemical basis for a meningeo-glial network. J. Comp. Neurol. 420:445-465.

Mercier F, Hatton GI (2001) Connexin 26 and basic fibroblast growth factor are expressed primarily in the subpial and subependymal layers in the adult brain parenchyma: roles in stem cell proliferation and morphological plasticity? J. Comp. Neurol. 431:88-104.

Mercier F, Kitasako JT, Hatton GI (2002) Anatomy of the brain neurogenic zones revisited: fractones and the fibroblast/macrophage network. J. Comp. Neurol. 451:170-188.

Micevych P, Popper P, Hatton GI (1996) Connexin 32 mRNA levels in the rat supraoptic nucleus: Up-regulation prior to parturition and during lactation. Neuroendocrinology 63:39-45.

Miyata S, Furuya K, Nakai S, Bun H, Kiyohara T (1999) Morphological plasticity and rearrangement of cytoskeletons in pituicytes cultured from adult rat neurohypophysis. Neurosci. Res. 33:299-306.

Miyata S, Hatton GI (1997) Connexin-32 protein in magnocellular neurons of the rat hypothalamus: light and electron microscopic immunocytochemistry. Soc. Neurosci. Abstr. 23:420.

Miyata S, Hatton GI (2002) Activity-related, dynamic neuron-glial interactions in the hypothalamo-neurohypophysial system. Microsc. Res. Tech. 56:143-157.

Miyata S, Matsushima O, Hatton GI (1997) Taurine in posterior pituitary: Localization in astrocytes and selective release by hypoosmotic stimulation. J. Comp. Neurol. 381:513-523.

Miyata S, Takamatsu H, Maekawa S, Matsumoto N, Watanabe K, Kiyohara T, Hatton GI (2001) Plasticity of neurohypophysial terminals with increased hormonal release during dehydration: ultrastructure and biochemical analyses. J. Comp. Neurol. 434:413-427.

Modney BK, Hatton GI (1989) Multiple synapse formation: a possible compensatory mechanism for increased cell size in rat supraoptic nucleus. J. Neuroendocrinol. 1:21-27.

Moos F, Freund-Mercier M, Guerne Y, Guerne J, Stoeckel M, Richard P (1984) Release of oxytocin and vasopressin by magnocellular nuclei in vitro: specific facilitatory effect of oxytocin on its own release. J. Endocrinol. 102:63-72.

Morris JF, Pow DV (1988) Capturing and quantifying the exocytotic event. J. Exp. Biol. 139:81-103.

Nauta WJH, Feirtag M (1986) Fundamental Neuroanatomy. New York: W. H. Freeman & Co.

Neumann I, Douglas A, Pittman Q, Russell J, Landgraf R (1996) Oxytocin released within the supraoptic nucleus of the rat brain by positive feedback action is involved in parturition-related events. J. Neuroendocrinol. 8:227-233.

Neumann I, Ludwig M, Engelmann M, Pittman Q, Landgraf R (1993) Simultaneous microdialysis in blood and brain: oxytocin and vasopressin release in response to central and peripheral osmotic stimulation and suckling in the rat. Neuroendocrinology 58:637-645.

Oliet SHR, Piet R, Poulain DA (2001) Control of glutamate clearance and synaptic efficacy by glial coverage of neurons. Science 292:923-926.

Palay SL, Chan-Palay V (1974) Cerebellar cortex, cytology and organization. Berlin: Springer Verlag.

Parpura V, Haydon PG (2000) Physiological astrocytic calcium levels stimulate glutamate release to modulate adjacent neurons. Proc. Nat. Acad. Sci. USA 97:8629-8634.

Pasante-Morales H, Franco R, Ochoa L, Ordaz B (2002) Osmosensitive release of neurotransmitter amino acids: relevance and mechanisms. Neurochem. Res. 27:59-66.

Perlmutter LS, Tweedle CD, Hatton GI (1985) Neuronal/glial plasticity in the supraoptic dendritic zone in response to acute and chronic dehydration. Brain Res. 361:225-232.

Peters A, Palay SL, Webster H (1991) The fine structure of the nervous system. New York: Oxford University Press.

Pierce J, Lewin G (1994) An ultrastructural size principle. Neuroscience 58:441-446.

Pow DV, Morris JF (1989) Dendrites of hypothalamic magnocellular neurons release neurohypophysial peptides by exocytosis. Neuroscience 32:435-439.

Reichenbach A, Siegel A, Rickmann M, Wolf J, Noone D, Robinson S (1995) Distribution of Bergmann glial somata and processes: implications for function. J. Hirnforsch. 36:509-517.

Reymond I, Almarghini K, Tappaz M (1996) Immunocytochemical localization of cysteine sulfinate decarboxylase in astrocytes in cerbellum and hippocampus: A quatitative double immunofluorescence study with glial fibrillary acidic protein and S-100 protein. Neuroscience 75:619.

Sharma G, Vijayaraghavan S (2001) Nicotinic cholinergic signaling in hippocampal astrocytes involves calcium-induced calcium release from internal stores. Proc. Nat. Acad. Sci. USA 98:4148-4153.

Sharma G, Vijayaraghavan S (2002) Nicotinic receptor signaling in nonexcitable cells. J. Neurobiol. 53:524-534.

Smithson KG, Suarez I, Hatton GI (1990) β-Adrenergic stimulation decreases glial and increases neural contact with the basal lamina in rat neurointermediate lobes incubated in vitro. J.Neuroendocrinol. 2:693-699.

Song Z, Hatton GI (2003) Taurine and the control of basal hormone release from rat neurohypophysis. Exp. Neurol. in press.

Theodosis DT (2002) Oxytocin-secreting neurons: a physiological model of morphological neuronal and glial plasticity. Front. Neuroendocrinol. 23:101-135.

Theodosis DT, Mason WT (1988) Choline acetyltransferase immunocytochemical staining of the rat supraoptic nucleus and its surroundings. A light-and electron- microscopic study. Cell Tiss. Res. 254:119-124.

Theodosis DT, Poulain DA (1984) Evidence for structural plasticity in the supraoptic nucleus of the rat hypothalamus in relation to gestation and lactation. Neuroscience 11:183-193.

Tweedle CD, Hatton GI (1977) Ultrastructural changes in rat hypothalamic neurosecretory cells and their associated glia during minimal dehydration and rehydration. Cell Tiss. Res. 181:59-72.

Tweedle CD, Hatton GI (1980) Evidence for dynamic interactions between pituicytes and neurosecretory axons in the rat. Neuroscience 5:661-667.

Tweedle CD, Hatton GI (1982) Magnocellular neuropeptidergic terminals in neurohypophysis: rapid glial release of enclosed axons during parturition. Brain Res. Bull. 8:205-209.

Tweedle CD, Hatton GI (1984) Synapse formation and disappearance in adult rat supraoptic nucleus during different hydration states. Brain Res. 309:373-376.

Tweedle CD, Hatton GI (1987) Morphological adaptability at neurosecretory axonal endings on the neurovascular contact zone of the rat neurohypophysis. Neuroscience 20:241-246.

Umbriaco D, Watkins K, Descarries L, Cozzari C, Hartman B (1994) Ultrastructural and morphometric features of the acetylcholine innervation in adult rat parietal cortex: an electron microscopic study in serial sections. J. Comp. Neurol. 348:351-373.

van Calker D, Hamprecht B (1980) Effects of neurohormones on glial cells. In: Advances in Cellular Neurobiology pp 31-67. New York: Academic Press.

Vitarella D, DiRisio DJ, Kimelberg HK, Aschner M (1994) Potassium and taurine release are highly correlated with regulatory volume decrease in neonatal primary rat astrocyte cultures. J. Neurochem. 63:1143-1149.

Wilkin GP, Marriott DR, Cholewinski AJ (1990) Astrocyte heterogeneity. Trends Neurosci. 13:43-46.

Yang QZ, Hatton GI (1988) Direct evidence for electrical coupling among rat supraoptic nucleus neurons. Brain Res. 463:47-56.

4.9. Abbreviations

AC	Adenylyl cyclase
aCSF	Artificial cerebrospinal fluid
βARs	β-adrenergic receptors
EM	Electron microscopy
GABA$_A$Rs	γ-aminobutyric acid type A receptors
glyRs	Glycine receptors
GFAP	Glial fibrillary acidic protein
-ir	Immunoreactivity
LM	Light microscopy
LY	Lucifer Yellow
mHNS	Magnocellular hypothalamo-neurohypophysial system
NL	Pituitary neural lobe or neurohypophysis
OT	Oxytocin
PVN	Paraventricular nucleus of the hypothalamus
SON	Supraoptic nucleus
VGL or vgl	Ventral glial lamina
VP	Vasopressin
$[X^{\pm}]_i$	Intracellular concentration of ion X
$[X^{\pm}]_o$	Extracellular concentration of ion X

Chapter 5

Astroglia as a modulation interface between meninges and neurons

Frederic Mercier

Laboratory of Matrix Pathobiology
Biomedical Research Center T408
University of Hawaii, 1993 East-West Rd, Honolulu, HI 96822 USA

Corresponding author: fmercier@pbrc.hawaii.edu

Contents

5.1 Introduction

The current view is that glial cells play important roles in brain functions. Previous authors have shown that glial cells (primarily astrocytes) are connected by gap junctions and functionally cooperate to form a network and coordinate interactions with neurons (see Chapter 13). On the basis of newly revealed anatomical data (Mercier and Hatton, 2000; 2001, Mercier et al., 2002; 2003) and re-analysis of the literature, it is here proposed that the glial network is an anatomical and functional interface between the neuronal compartment and meninges. Meninges are widely thought to be merely protective membranes that do not serve any important physiologically relevant function during adulthood. However, meninges produce numerous cytokines and growth factors (GF) throughout adulthood. Numerous of these signaling molecules bind to heparan sulfate proteoglycans (HSPG) and/or interact with other extracellular matrix proteins contained in the basal lamina (BL) that is systematically interposed between meningeal cells and astrocytes of the glia limitans (GL). Therefore, meningeal-produced cytokines and GF can directly influence glial cell functions. Similar mechanisms have been demonstrated during development between the connective tissues and parenchymal tissues or epithelia (mesodermo-neuroectodermal or mesodermo-epithelial induction). Astrocytes produce cytokines and GF, likely in response to the information they receive from meningeal and vascular cells. This may form the basis of signaling cascades from the meninges to neurons via astrocytes. Reciprocally, neurons may respond to the information they receive from astrocytes by producing signaling molecules that may in turn influence glial and meningeal-vascular cells. Thus, the entire astrocytic compartment may represent a modulation interface between meninges and neurons.

The first part of this review provides anatomical data supporting this view. The second part of the review focuses on examples suggesting a role for astrocytes as a functional interface between neurons and the connective tissue cells. It is hypothesized that astrocytes, after integrating information from the meningeal/vascular cells, promote brain plasticity and permit creation and maintenance of neuronal circuitry. Three examples are examined. The first one, discussed in a previous review (Mercier and Hatton, 2004), illustrates the role of astrocytes in the morphological and functional plasticity of the neuroendocrine system. The second example highlights the immune and inflammatory roles of astrocytes and meningeal cells, and speculates on the multi-cellular cooperation that ultimately may lead to brain circuitry protection. The third example describes recent advances in the biology of neural stem cells (NSC) in the adult brain, and presents data supporting the idea that astrocytes may serve as a source of NSC and the generation of new neurons and glial cells. A conclusion focuses on future directions that may arise from considering astrocytes and glial cells in general, as a functional interface between neurons and brain connective tissue.

5.2 Astroglial structure

5.2.1. Definitions

Glial cells are the resident non-neuronal cells of the brain parenchyma. The parenchyma of any tissue is defined as "the essential elements" of the tissue and the extraparenchyma as connective and vascular tissue. The "essential elements" of the tissue is a vague term. Fortunately, a BL, which is a mat of extracellular matrix, is interposed between the parenchyma and extraparenchyma of every organ and tissue (Fahrquar, 1991; Mercier and Hatton, 2004). The BL, is electron-dense, therefore visible without staining by transmission electron microscopy (however, the use of post-staining with uranyl acetate and lead citrate does enhance the electron density). Because of its multiple antigenic properties, the BL is also easily labeled at the light microscopic level (Mercier and Hatton, 2000; 2001; Mercier et al., 2002; 2003). The cells located beyond the BL are extraparenchymal cells (endothelial cells, smooth muscle cells, pericytes, fibroblasts, macrophages and mast cells). The non-neuronal resident parenchymal cells (glial cells) represent a heterogeneous population in the central nervous system (CNS). Except in neurogenic zones (subjacent to the ependyma of the ventricles), one distinguishes unambiguously the different glial cell types in adult mammalian brain by their location and ultrastructural characteristics (Peters et al., 1991). The list of glial cell types in the adult mammalian CNS is as follows: astrocytes, oligodendrocytes, microglial cells, ependymocytes, epithelial cells of the choroid plexus, tanycytes, ensheathing glia of the olfactory bulb (Ramon-Cueto and Avila, 1998; Au and Roskam, 2002), retinal Müller cells, and Bergmann glia of the cerebellum. Because of the morphology of their processes, the last four cell types may be classified as "adult radial glial cells". However, because of their poorly branched elongated processes, one might classify the astrocytes of the GL as radial glial cells. The issue of glial cell classification in the neurogenic zones is complex. NSC, progenitor cells, and trans-differentiating neural cells with transient phenotypes populate the ventricle walls, and are numerous within the walls of the lateral ventricles (Doetsch et al., 1997; Mercier et al., 2002). Moreover, the identity of NSC is controversial (see later sections).

In addition to neurons and glial cells, the brain parenchyma contains immune system derived-cells migrating from both blood and meninges: Kolmer cells, epiplexus (supraependymal) cells, migrating perivascular macrophages (all these cells belong to the macrophage/monocyte lineage), and T and B lymphocytes. These cells easily cross border zones and associated BL (Hickey et al., 1991; Silverman et al., 2000; Bechmann et al., 2001). The issue of trans-differentiation of immune cells into glial cells, for example of macrophages into microglial cells, is controversial and is discussed in a later section.

The ultrastructural characteristics of the different glial cell types will not be analyzed here. The reader is invited to consult the excellent descriptions provided by Peters et al., (1991), but information about gross morphology and identity of astrocyte specific markers, is detailed in later sections.

5.2.2. Morphology and location

Although morphologically heterogeneous, astrocyte cell populations possess common structural characteristics that allow their identification. Astrocytes usually have a 4-5 µm circular nucleus surrounded by a narrow band of cytoplasm and display several elongated and rarely branched processes. Astrocyte subtypes are commonly distinguished from each other on the basis of their process morphology, and their location in brain. Stellate astrocytes are star shaped and possess moderately elongated processes radiating from the cell body (Fig. 5.1D). These astrocytes are found everywhere in brain except at border zones, i.e., pial and blood vessel (BV) surfaces. The stellate astrocytes separate neuronal cell bodies, dendrites and axons, via their processes. These astrocytes are typical in brain gray matter, but are also found in white matter. The processes of adjacent stellate astrocytes contact each other to form a loose meshwork in which neurons are inserted. The meshwork of stellate astrocytes is usually not visible with glial fibrillary acidic protein (GFAP) immunostaining because the terminal processes rarely contain this intermediate filament. Conversely, radial astrocytes are usually grouped and have their cell bodies in proximity to border zones (meninges) (Fig. 5.2B, 5.3C). Radial astrocytes possess numerous short processes that are intermingled and directed towards adjacent radial astrocytes and commonly display only one thick and poorly branched process measuring up to 200 μm that deeply penetrates the gray matter, separating neuronal somata and processes. Radial astrocytes form lines in brain border zones, delineating a zone termed the GL (Fig. 5.2B, 5.3). The GL is found at the brain surface, at the surface of major brain subdivisions, and at the periphery of large BV penetrating the brain. The GL faces meningeal (connective tissue) cells. Thus, proximity to connective tissue cells seems to correlate with radial morphology. The connective tissue facing the radial astrocytes consists of fibroblasts, macrophages, and an abundant extracellular matrix rich in collagen fibers primarily consisting of collagen-1. Interestingly, collagen-1 is known to influence the morphology of astrocytes in vitro, inducing a radial morphology with long processes (Goetschy et al., 1987). Ultrastructural evidence for collagen fibers in labyrinthine BL structures between astrocyte and fibroblast processes at the GL/pia interface suggests functional interactions between pial cells and GL astrocytes (Mercier et al., 2003). Moreover, macrophages and fibroblasts produce diverse GF and cytokines that may locally induce (inductive microenvironment) and control astrocyte morphology (Mercier and Hatton, 2004). Transforming growth factor β–1 (TGFβ–1), a molecule primarily produced by meningeal cells in the adult brain, is known to prevent branching and stabilize pre-formed branched structures in both embryonic and adult tissues (Gilbert, 1994). The mechanisms underlying the inductive microenvironment for radial morphology may involve the BL joining GL astrocytes and pial cells, because BL concentrate, activate, and present GF and cytokines to the cells to which they are apposed (Gilbert, 1994).

5.2.3. Intermediate filaments

Astrocytes are usually identified immunocytochemically and ultrastructurally by their intermediate filaments (IF). The electron-dense IF, which measure 8-9 nm in diameter and several μm long, are organized in bundles that are easily detected by transmission electron microscopy in the perinuclear cytoplasm and in the astrocyte processes (Fig. 5.6A). Other glial cells (ependymocytes, tanycytes, and microglia) possess intermediate filaments, but astrocytes are the only brain cells that express GFAP upon non-pathological conditions. This characteristic is widely used to identify astrocytes by immunocytochemistry. However, subpopulations of astrocytes express vimentin, another IF, instead of GFAP (Fig. 5.3C). Figure 5.1A shows astrocytes in culture, visualized by GFAP immunoreactivity. Because astrocyte processes bearing little or no GFAP extend far beyond the large GFAP bearing processes, light microscopic images using this marker are misleading (Bushong et al., 2002; see Chapter 4). Astrocytes extend thin lamellate processes that can be visualized by immunostaining for ezrin, a molecule anchoring microfilaments to the plasma membrane (Derouiche and Froetscher, 2001). These immunoreactive lamellate processes, which have been confirmed by ultrastructure, have a preferential location in the perisynaptic microenvironment in situ. Lamellate processes are likely to contribute to the dynamic properties of synapses (Derouiche and Froetscher, 2001, Chapter 4). GFAP immunoreactivity in situ is primarily found in large astrocyte processes abutting BV (Fig. 5.1B-C), ependyma (Figs. 5.1D, 5.2A), large processes of stellate astrocytes (Fig. 5.1D, arrowhead), elongated processes of radial-like astrocytes, running tangentially to brain borders (Figs. 5.2B, 5.3B), and the surface of large BV. The tightly packed astrocytes found in brain borders form the GL. The dramatic morphological changes that astrocytes undergo upon physiological stimuli or pharmacological manipulations require subcellular redistribution of most cytoskeletal proteins, including GFAP (Safavi-Abbasi et al., 2001). Interestingly, GFAP expression is regulated by basic fibroblast growth factor (bFGF) and TGFβ–1 (Reilly et al., 1998). Although TGFβ–1may be found in neuronal and astrocyte extracts (Spohr et al., 2002), this does not mean that this GF is produced by neurons and astrocytes. In situ hybridization studies have shown that TGFβ–1 mRNA is primarily localized in meningeal cells (Unsicker et al., 1991). Thus, the targeted action of this GF on astrocytes may not reflect neuron-glia interactions but meningeal-glia interactions. In addition, bFGF is also primarily produced by meningeal cells (Gonzalez et al., 1995, reviewed in Mercier and Hatton, 2004). Together, these data suggest that meningeal cells may control the intermediate filament production of the GL astrocytes.

5.2.4. Gap junctional network

Astrocytes, which are highly coupled to each other by gap junctions throughout the brain, form a potential gigantic syncytium (Mugnaini, 1986; Chapter 13). Gap junctions are intercellular channels that allow adjacent cells to communicate by exchanging cytoplasmic molecules such as metabolites, ions, and second messengers (Evans and Martin, 2002). Gap junctions consist of clusters of connexin (Cx)-made channels that span the plasma membranes of two adjacent cells. Their structural and functional heterogeneity is due to the possibility of combining different types of Cx molecules in the same channel. Gap junctions are expressed in all organs and tissues (except blood and striated skeletal muscle) during development and throughout life. Gap junctions have been implicated in diverse roles, during both development (morphogenic events) and adulthood (synchronous activity between excitable cells such as myocytes and endocrine cells). However, their functions in most organs and tissues remain to be determined. In common with other tissues, the brain expresses multiple Cx isoforms (Rash et al., 2001). Throughout adulthood, brain gap junctions are preponderant among astrocytes and among meningeal and perivascular cells (Mercier and Hatton, 2001). Gap junctions are also found to connect adjacent neurons. It is believed that interneuronal communication is complementary to the signal transfer created by synapses (Sutor, 2002). Additionally, in vitro experiments suggest that gap junctions contribute to the propagation of injury signals (Frantseva et al., 2002). It is not known exactly what functions the syncytium of coupled astrocytes serves. Interestingly, the most numerous Cx43 immunoreactivity, an indication of the number of astrocytic gap junctions, is found in the GL facing the brain surface (Fig. 5.3A, B) and BV surface (Fig. 5.3 A, arrow). The high density of astrocytic processes in proximity to the meninges permits these important inter-astrocytic connections. However, the functional significance of potentially high inter-astrocytic coupling via gap junctions in the brain surface is unknown (but see Chapter 13). Along the brain surface, the thickness of the GL is correlated with the thickness of the underlying meninges. In figure 5.3A, the ventral GL, facing the thick ventral meninges (enclosing the arteries of the Circle of Willis) consists of a 50-70 μm thick Cx43 immunoreactive GL. The GL of the dorsal or lateral cortex is thinner, and displays less meningeal coverings (not shown). A thin layer of astrocytes covers the thin perivascular connective tissue layer of arterioles (Fig. 5.3A, arrow). These anatomical characteristics suggest functional interactions between astrocytes and meningeal cells.

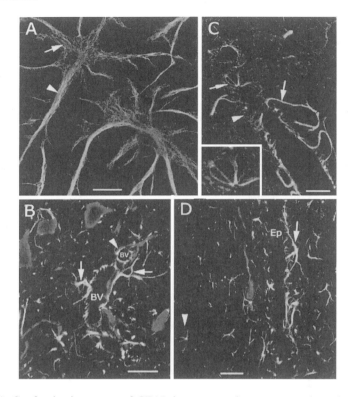

Figure 5.1. Confocal microscopy of GFAP immunoreactive astrocytes (green). **A**: Typical morphology of supraoptic nucleus astrocytes after 3 days in cell culture. The cultured astrocytes are large, express a network of GFAP-ir intermediate filaments in the perinuclear cytoplasm (arrow), and display thick ramified immunoreactive processes (arrowhead). **B**: In situ, astrocytes are smaller and have a narrow perinuclear cytoplasm (arrows). Astrocytes are shown here in the paraventricular nucleus. Brain BV are enveloped by GFAP-ir astrocytes. Some processes of oxytocin-ir neurons (red) envelop perivascular astrocytes (arrowhead). **C**: Detail of perivascular astrocytes showing numerous Cx43-ir puncta (red, arrow), an indication of numerous gap junctions in the astrocytic zone. The inset shows a 2x magnification of the areas indicated by a thin arrow (rosette). **D**: Stellate astrocytes (arrow) in the walls of the third ventricle. Note the decreasing gradient of GFAP immunoreactivity from the subependymal layer to deeper zones (arrowhead). Ep: ependyma of the third ventricle. Scale bars. A: 5 μm; B, C: 10 μm; D: 20 μm.

As mentioned above, meningeal cells express a high density of gap junctions (Mercier and Hatton, 2001), which, like astrocytic gap junctions, are functional (Spray et al., 1991). Immunoreactivity for Cx26, Cx30, and Cx43, and all combinations of these Cxs, are found at cell-to-cell appositions among meningeal cells (primarily fibroblasts) throughout pia, arachnoid, dura, choroid plexus stroma, and BV sheaths (Mercier and Hatton, 2001; unpublished observation). Macrophages are quantitatively the second most frequent cell type in the superficial meninges, but outnumber fibroblasts in the sheaths of small BV. Macrophages and fibroblasts contact each other by their processes to form a network throughout the meninges and projections in brain (Mercier and Hatton, 2001; Mercier et al., 2002). The evidence for Cx26, Cx30 and Cx43 immunoreactivity throughout meninges, BV sheaths and choroid plexus stroma further supports the existence of a functional network throughout the brain connective tissue (unpublished observation).

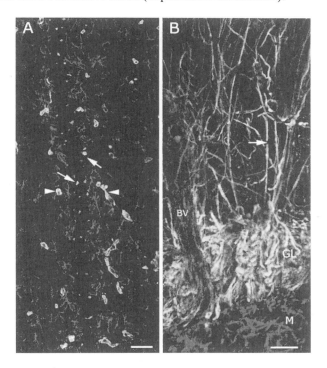

Figure 5.2. Confocal microscopy of astrocytes. **A**: Walls of the third ventricle. The GFAP-ir (red) astrocytes linearly arranged along the subependymal layer face specialized laminin-ir (green) BL structures (fractones, arrows). Arrowheads: BV. **B**: GL of the supraoptic nucleus. The somata and intertwined short processes of brain-surface astrocytes are located in the GL. However, they possess long processes spanning the neuron-containing zone (arrow). Brain-surface astrocytes express both GFAP (green) and vimentin (red), particularly in the GL zone, which appears yellowish. Meningeal cells (M) and vascular cells (BV) express only vimentin. Scale bars: A: 50 μm; B: 20 μm.

5.2.5. Contacts with extraparenchyma

5.2.5.1. Basal laminae

BL are mats of extracellular matrix interfacing parenchymal cells with extraparenchymal cells (Farquhar, 1991). In brain, a BL delineates the interface between the astrocytes of the GL and extraparenchymal cells. The principal extraparenchymal cells abutting this BL are macrophages, fibroblasts, endothelial cells and pericytes. Alternatively to extraparenchymal cells, the BL abutting the GL astrocytes eventually face the Virchow Robin space (Fig. 5.8A) and the meningeal subarachnoid space. A BL also exists between vascular cells (Fig. 5.6). Folding and branching of the BL between astrocyte endfeet permits numerous astrocytes to contact the BL, at the BV surface (Fig. 5.7), brain surface (Fig. 5.10) and subependymal layer of ventricles (Fig.5.8). Location, structure and ultrastructure of brain BL in the adult rat are described in Mercier and Hatton, (2000; 2001) and in Mercier et al., (2002; 2003) for the neurogenic zones. Collagens, laminins, HSPG, and chondroitin sulfate proteoglycans (CSPG), and fibronectin, are among the most important BL components (Farquhar, 1991). All of these matrix components play important roles for transducing signals between the cells that abut the BL. Due to their ability to bind and activate families of GF and cytokines promoting proliferation and differentiation, the HSPG are particularly important (Roberts et al., 1988). Laminins, fibronectin, and CSPG are important in defining pathways in which immature neurons proliferate and migrate. For example, the neuroblasts (A cells, see Doetsch et al., 1997) migrate from the subependymal layer to the olfactory bulb via the rostral migratory stream (RMS) (Lois et al., 1996), a pathway rich in CSPG and other extracellular matrix components (Brannon-Thomas et al, 1996; Steindler et al., 1998). Studies have also shown that laminins and fibronectin are effective in promoting migratory pathways for growth cones. Overall, it has been shown that BL are actively involved in morphogenic events, including neurogenesis during development, but we are far from a complete understanding of their role and function in the adult tissue. It has been demonstrated in vitro that collagens and fibronectin directly influence proliferation and morphological changes of astrocytes (Goetschy et al., 1987). Other potential functions of BL and their proteoglycan components throughout adulthood are reviewed by Sherman et al., (2002). It is likely that the extracellular matrix proteins of the BL interfacing astrocytes with meningeal cells may play important roles in transmitting information that ultimately leads to morphological and functional changes in the neural tissue compartment (see later sections). Throughout life, both astrocytes and meningeal/vascular cells are major sources and targets of GF and cytokines (reviewed in Althaus and Landsberg, 2000; Benn et al., 2001; Mercier and Hatton, 2004). Additionally, following injury within the CNS system, reconstitution of the BL at the GL astrocyte/connective tissue interface (Abnet et al., 1991) is one of the essential steps towards successful recovery of structure and function, including positioning of new neurons (Choi, 1994). However, some components of the BL prevent full recovery after injury (Stichel et al., 1999). The high density of astrocytes endfeet abutting or entering in the folds of the specialized BL (fractones) in the subependymal layer of ventricles (Fig. 5.8B) may reflect inductive mechanisms related to neurogenesis or neuroendocrine regulation (Mercier et al., 2002; 2003).

5.2.5.2. Vascular cells

Contrary to common belief, the contact surface between astrocytes and endothelial cells is restricted. Pericapillary astrocytes primarily contact macrophages, and pericytes, located respectively in the adventitia and media. Figure 5.4 shows three representative brain capillaries. The endothelium of the first capillary is primarily covered by a pericyte and its enveloping processes that prevent an important surface contact between the astrocyte endfeet and the endothelial cells (Fig. 5.4A, see also Fig. 5.5). This capillary does not show any adventitial layer. The second capillary displays an even more restricted contact zone (15 %) between endothelial cells and astrocytes (Fig. 5.4B). The macrophages present in the adventitia of this capillary cover 57 % of the astrocyte/vascular contact zone. The third capillary is entirely covered by the perivascular macrophage layer, preventing any contact between astrocytes and endothelial cells (Fig. 5.4C). Endothelial cells, pericytes, and macrophages, can be contacted by the same astrocyte endfoot, all cells contacting each other via BL (Fig. 5.5).

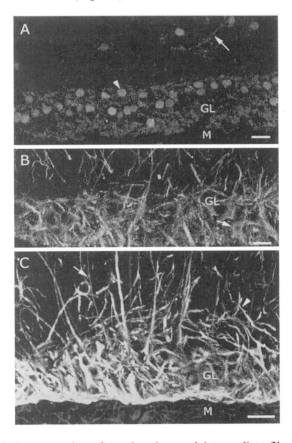

Figure 5.3. Particular expression of gap junctions and intermediate filaments in the GL. Images of the ventral cortex. **A:** The somata (arrowhead) of GL astrocytes are strongly bFGF-ir (green). The numerous Cx43-ir puncta (red) indicate how extensively the processes of GL astrocytes are interconnected by gap junctions. Cx43-ir puncta (arrow) and bFGF-ir somata indicate the presence of perivascular astrocytes. M: meninges. **B:** Another view of the GL showing GFAP (green) and Cx43 (red). Note the location of astrocyte somata (arrow). **C:** While most of the intertwined processes of the GL astrocytes are immunoreactive for both GFAP (green) and vimentin (red) (consequently appearing yellow), the long astrocyte processes spanning the neuron-containing zone are primarily vimentin-ir (arrow) or GFAP-ir (arrowhead). Scale bars: 10 μm.

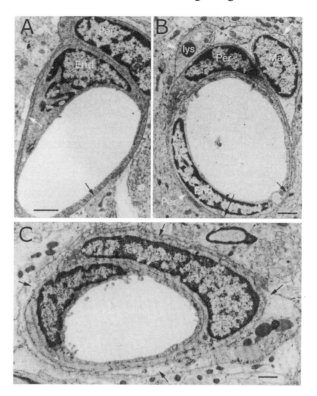

Figure 5.4. Pial (adventitial) sheath of capillaries. **A**: A pericyte (Per) with a long process (white arrow) covers the endothelium (End) of this capillary. There is an important contact zone between the astrocytes and the End (black arrow). **B**: This capillary displays two perivascular macrophages (Mac) (white arrows), identified by their location (perivascular layer), lysosomes (lys), and electron-lucent cytoplasm. The contact zone between astrocytes and the endothelium is narrow (between the black arrows), representing 15% of the astrocytic/extraparenchymal cell contact zone. Macs and Per respectively represent 57 % and 28 % of the astrocytic/extraparenchymal cell contact zone. **C**: The Mac layer (arrows) covers 100% of the vascular cells. Astrocytes face macrophages. Scale bars: 1 μm.

The literature relating functional interactions between astrocytes and extraparenchymal cells refers to astrocytes/endothelium interactions. Endothelial cells are the main targets of finger-like repeated geometrical units (rosettes) formed by astrocyte endfeet (Kacem et al., 1998). One rosette is shown here (Fig. 5.1C, inset). These authors suggest that this organization could allow direct metabolic exchanges between astrocytes and endothelial cells. Astrocytes and endothelial cells may also mutually influence their fate and function via production of GF and cytokines that may bind and be activated in the BL located at their interface. For example, it has been shown in vitro that purified endothelial cells induce the differentiation of astrocytes precursor cells (Mi et al., 2001). The endothelial cells are also a central component of the blood brain barrier, which allows immune cell migration and restrict molecule diffusion (Rubin and Staddon, 1999). The properties of endothelial cells contributing to the barrier are themselves subject to regulation by signals derived from both immune cells and astrocytes (Prat et al., 2001). The fate of astrocytes and endothelial cells is also closely related during development, astrocytes evolving concurrently with brain vasculature (Zerlin and Goldman, 1997). Finally, throughout life, both cell types may cooperate and contribute to the proper functioning of neuronal networks, participating in synapse formation and plasticity, participating in neuronal metabolism, and providing blood-borne information. In addition to endothelial cells, astrocytes directly contact pericytes (Fig. 5.4A, B). The function of pericytes is not clearly understood (Thomas, 1999).

5.2.5.3. Perivascular and meningeal cells

Macrophages and fibroblasts of the brain connective tissue (meninges, perivascular sheaths, stroma of the choroid plexus) are the most frequent extraparenchymal cells contacting astrocytes. The brain connective tissue deeply penetrates the brain (Mercier et al., 2002; Mercier and Hatton, 2001; 2004). Most brain BV have connective tissue sheaths that represent extensions of the pia-arachnoid (Mercier et al., 2002). Macrophages outnumber fibroblasts in capillaries, but fibroblasts outnumber macrophages in large BV and in the meninges. Macrophages and fibroblasts connect to each other by their elongated processes to form a network along the longitudinal axis of the vessel, both along the vasculature and pia-arachnoid (Mercier et al., 2002). In addition, the presence of gap junctions and Cx immunoreactivity at cell-to-cell junctions in the meninges, perivascular layer, and choroid plexus stroma (Mercier and Hatton, 2001) suggests the existence of a general brain connective tissue network, made of fibroblasts and macrophages. Because meningeal cells are functionally coupled by gap junctions (Spray et al, 1991), it is possible that the macrophage/fibroblast network forms a functional syncytium throughout the CNS.

Macrophages are located beneath the outer vascular BL, within the third vascular layer (tunica adventitia) (Fig. 5.4B, C, 5.6, 5.7). Thus, one can easily distinguish these cells from parenchymal macrophages (microglial cells). Microglial cells located in the periphery of BV are not separated from astrocytes by a BL (Fig. 5.10B). It is usually thought that the "pial sheath" of BV only covers large BV like arteries and arterioles. In fact, the pial sheath extends to capillaries (Mercier et al., 2002; Mercier and Hatton, 2004, illustrated here in Figs. 5.4 and 5.6). Some capillaries, usually the smallest ones, do not show any perivascular (adventitial) layer (Fig. 5.4A). However, most capillaries possess a perivascular layer, containing primarily macrophages (Figs. 5.4B,C, 5.6). Perivascular macrophages are distinguished from pericytes either anatomically by their location in the third layer, adventitia, of the vessel wall, and/or ultrastructurally because they possess large lysosomes and are less electron-dense than pericytes (Fig. 5.4B,C) (see also Bechmann et al., 2001). In addition, perivascular macrophages are immunocytochemically detected via their specific cell surface antigen CD163 (also termed ED2) (Graeber et al., 1989). Neither pericytes nor macrophages normally fully cover the endothelial layer of the capillary, allowing astrocytes to directly contact the endothelium (Fig. 5.5). The macrophage layer entirely covers the smooth muscle layer in arterioles (Fig. 5.6). In both arterioles and arteries, macrophages and fibroblasts bathe in an extension of the subarachnoid space, termed Virchow Robin space (Fig. 5.8). At the brain surface and between major brain structures, the GL astrocytes also face macrophages and fibroblasts (Fig. 5.10).

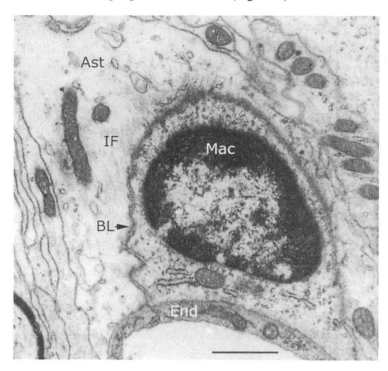

Figure 5.5. Astrocyte coverings capillaries. In this capillary, the astrocyte endfeet are apposed to the endothelium (End). Note the astrocyte endfoot completely covering the perivascular macrophage (Mac). There is no pericyte at this level of the BV. A BL interfaces the astrocyte with the Mac. IF: intermediate filaments. Scale bar: 1 μm.

What is the function of macrophages? In brain, it is widely accepted that these cells are instrumental in the initiation of the immune response (Thomas, 1999). Perivascular macrophages are antigen-presenting cells, producing inflammatory cytokines and GF (reviewed in Hickey, 2001). These cells are highly migratory, can accumulate at sites of injury, and are constantly renewed from the bone marrow/monocyte lineage (Shelper and Adrian , 1986; Hickey and Kimura, 1988). Although not investigated for their immune functions *per se*, meningeal and choroid plexus macrophages may play similar roles, and are likely to be constantly renewed from the bone marrow/monocyte lineage (Hickey and Kimura, 1988).

Figure 5.9 recapitulates the anatomical interactions between astrocytes and extraparenchymal cells. Astrocytes primarily face macrophages and fibroblasts, but also contact pericytes, and endothelial cells. In brain, neurons and their processes never directly contact extraparenchymal cells (although partial contact exists in circumventricular organs). Thus astrocytes represent anatomically an obligatory interface between neurons and extraparenchymal cells.

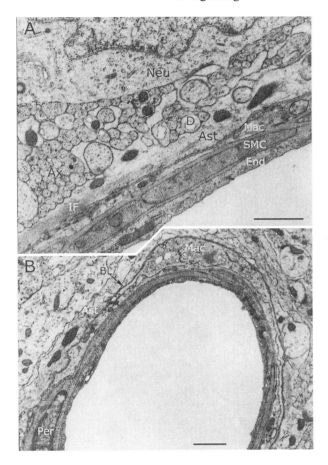

Figure 5.6. Perivascular cytoarchitectonics. **A**: Astrocyte endfeet (Ast), usually displaying intermediate filaments (IF), are always interposed between the different neuronal components (axons (Ax), dendrites (D) and somata (Neu)) and the vascular components. The BV wall consists of three cell layers, which respectively comprise macrophages (Mac) (and eventually fibroblasts), pericytes (Per) or smooth muscle cells (SMC), and endothelial cells (End). **B**: Astrocytes and macrophages face each, both apposed to the perivascular BL. The macrophage processes entirely cover pericytes and endothelial cells, preventing contacts between these cells and the astrocytes. Scale bars: 1 μm.

5.3. Astroglial function

5.3.1. Summary of currently recognized astrocytic functions

Astrocytes regulate K^+ levels and extracellular pH, contribute to the metabolism of neurotransmitters, are sources and targets of cytokines and GF that affect neuronal and vascular functions (Althaus and Landsberg, 2000), undergo morphological changes ultimately leading to neuroendocrine regulation in the hypothalamus (Hatton, 2002), intervene in maintenance and formation of synapses (Ullian et al.,

2001), influence the blood brain barrier properties (Rubin and Staddon, 1999), participate in the immune response and inflammation, produce chemokines attracting inflammatory cells, are involved in apoptosis and phagocytosis of inflammatory cells, influence the differentiation of immune cells and the proliferation of most brain cell types, and may serve as NSC to replace glia and neurons throughout adulthood (Doetsch et al., 1999).

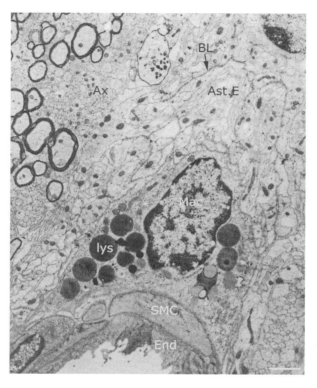

Figure 5.7. Multiple astrocyte/macrophage contacts along the astrocyte coverings of arterioles. A projection of the perivascular BL encloses densely packed astrocyte endfeet (Ast.E). These endfeet terminate on the BL covering a huge perivascular (adventitial) macrophage (Mac). Ax: axons; End: endothelium; lys: lysosome; SMC: smooth muscle cell. Scale bar: 2 μm.

Providing compelling evidence for bi-directional communication between astrocytes and neurons, it has been shown that astrocytes can respond to synaptically released neurotransmitters by intracellular Ca^{2+} signals that propagate among astrocytes, which in turn release neuroactive substances modulating synaptic transmission (Haydon, 2001, Chapter 15).

Moreover, astrocytes of the hypothalamic neuroendocrine system are likely to participate in neuroendocrine regulation via different mechanisms involving morphological plasticity and production of signaling molecules that directly or indirectly influence neurosecretory neurons (see Section 5.3.2.1. below).

As detailed above, the GL astrocytes, at the brain surface, and the astrocytes that enwrap BV, face macrophages and fibroblasts. The BL delineating the GL may serve as an interface of communication, regulating the activity of GF, cytokines produced on both sides of the BL. This structural and functional organization strongly suggests the existence of interactions between astrocytes and connective tissue cells. Macrophages and fibroblasts strongly express cytokines and GF (Franzen et al., 1999, reviewed in Mercier and Hatton, 2004). Moreover, astrocytes are both targets and producers of GF and cytokines (Althaus and Landsberg, 2000; Benn et al., 2001). It is known that cytokines are powerful regulators of glial cell activation (John et al, 2003). Particularly interesting in the context of this review, it has been shown that macrophages produce cytokines that directly affect astrocyte proliferation (Khan and Wigley, 1994).

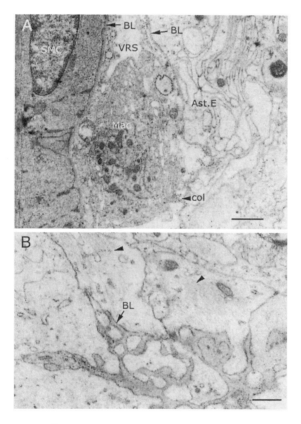

Figure 5.8. Other astrocyte/BL contacts. **A**: Astrocytes enveloping BV of large diameter. Numerous astrocyte endfeet (Ast.E) contact the perivascular BL, which delineates the parenchymal/extraparenchymal interface. Perivascular (adventitial) cells, primarily macrophages (Mac, only a portion of the perinuclear cytoplasm is visible here) and fibroblasts, bathe in the Virchow-Robin space (VRS), an extension of the subarachnoid space. col: collagen fibers; SMC: smooth muscle cells. **B**: Astrocytes in the ventricle wall. Most astrocyte endfeet (containing intermediate filaments, arrowheads) contact the specialized BL (fractones) in the subependymal layer. Scale bars: 1 μm.

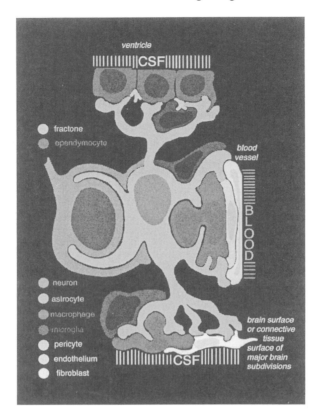

Figure 5.9. Brain cytoarchitectonics. Astrocytes interface with neurons and vascular/meningeal cells. At the surface of BV, GL astrocytes primarily contact macrophages (connective tissue macrophages), and to a lesser extent, pericytes and endothelial cells. At the brain surface, and between major brain subdivisions delineated by meningeal projections, GL astrocytes contact pial macrophages and fibroblasts. On the parenchymal side, astrocytes contact neurons, microglial cells (parenchymal macrophages), and ependymocytes. Because astrocytes systematically interface, there are no direct contacts between neurons and connective tissue/vascular cells in the brain. Astrocytes, together with macrophages, fibroblasts, and vascular cells are in key locations to modulate the information between neurons and the fluid (blood and CSF) carriers of signals.

5.3.2. Astrocytes interfacing with neurons and meninges

It is now established that astrocytes actively participate in brain plasticity. Brain plasticity encompasses events as different as maintenance of neuron integrity and circuitry, synapse formation and maintenance, neural stem cell proliferation, differentiation, and migration, and tissue integration of new neurons, glial cells, vascular and meningeal cells, neuronal apoptosis, astrocytes morphological changes that modify neural tissue architecture and function, immune surveillance, and response to injury/repair. The following sections examine the literature supporting the view that astrocytes may function as an interface between neurons and meningeal/perivascular cells throughout the brain, serving diverse functions.

Neuronal-astrocytic interactions are beyond the scope of this review, which focuses more on meningeal/astrocytic interactions, and considers the possibility that astrocytes play a role of intermediary between neurons and meningeal cells.

5.3.2.1. Meningeal/astrocytic interactions and neuroendocrine secretion

Reversible morphological changes involving astrocytes and pituicytes (modified astrocytes in the neurohypophysis) occur in the magnocellular hypothalamo-neurohypophysial system (mHNS) under physiological conditions or pharmacological conditions that induce or mimic osmotic changes (see Chapter 4). These astrocytic morphological changes, which occur throughout the entire mHNS, i.e. in the supraoptic nucleus, paraventricular nucleus, accessory nuclei, and neural lobe of the hypophysis, lead to reorganization of the astrocyte-magnocellular neuron interactions and associated modulation of the neuronal secretory activity. The magnocellular neurons produce the neurohormones vasopressin and oxytocin, involved among other functions in the regulation of osmolarity and lactation. Indeed, mHNS is a model system that illustrates neuron-astrocyte interactions and morpho-functional plasticity. Detailed morphological description of the mHNS system, and potential mechanisms of interactions between astrocytes and magnocellular neurons, are reviewed in Hatton (1999; 2002), Hussy (2002) and Mercier and Hatton, (2004). The focus here is not to review the morphological and functional reversible changes occurring in the mHNS upon dehydration and rehydration but to highlight the possibility that astrocytes may represent an anatomical and functional interface between meningeal cells and neurons in this model of plasticity. The anatomical organization of the hypothalamic portion of the mHNS is schematically illustrated in figure 5.11A (coronal view). Astrocytes display intimate contacts with the magnocellular neurons at every level of the neuronal organization (see structure in Mercier and Hatton, (2000) and ultrastructure in Hatton, (2002). The most impressive anatomical portion of the mHNS organization illustrating meningeal-neuronal-astrocytic interactions is the supraoptic nucleus. In this nucleus, most of the astrocytes display a radial-like morphology, with somata located in the GL (Figs. 5.2B), intertwined basal processes beneath the somata (Fig. 5.10), and radial processes that span the entire nucleus (Fig. 5.2B), insinuating between adjacent neuronal somata (see Chapter 4 and Fig. 6B in Mercier and Hatton, 2000).

In the ventral part of the nucleus, the numerous basal processes of astrocytes terminate on the BL that is interfacing with the GL and meninges (Fig. 5.10). The BL is often folded, forming labyrinthine structures that permits more contact surface between the processes and somata of meningeal cells and the astrocyte endfeet (see figure 8 in Mercier et al., 2003). Collagen fibers are usually interposed between astrocyte endfeet and meningeal cell endfeet in these labyrinthine structures (Mercier et al., 2003).

When physiological conditions such as dehydration, lactation arouse the mHNS, morphological and functional changes occur in the supraoptic nucleus (Hatton, 2002). The plastic changes in the core and dendritic zone (more ventral portion) of the supraoptic nucleus consist of astrocytic retraction. This leads to more appositions between neuronal elements, an increase in the number of synapses, an increase in gap junctional intercellular communication, a stimulatory effect on the firing of magnocellular neurons, and the release of neurohormones (Hatton, 2002). Correlated with these changes is a drastic reorganization of the astrocytic basal processes in the ventral GL (Bobak and Salm, 1996). This is illustrated in Figure 5.10. In this experiment, dehydration was obtained in adult rats by substitution of a 2% saline solution for tap water for 5 days. Electron microscopy revealed a reorientation of individual astrocytes processes from a direction perpendicular (vertical) to the pial surface (Fig. 5.10A, control animal), to one parallel (horizontal) to this region (Fig. 10B, dehydrated animal). The plastic changes were reversible, the astrocyte processes being vertical in rats allowed to rehydrate.

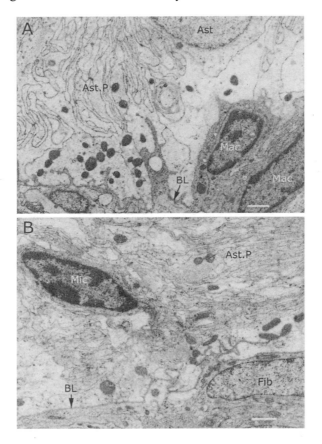

Figure 5.10. Ultrastructural changes of supraoptic nucleus astrocytes upon dehydration. **A**: Upon normal conditions of hydration, the individual astrocyte processes (arrow) are perpendicular to the pial surface. Pial macrophages (Mac) are visible beneath the BL delineating the GL ventrally. Ast: astrocyte nucleus. **B**: After dehydration by substitution of 2% saline for tap water for 5 days, individual astrocyte processes are reoriented, and become parallel to the pial surface (arrow). A microglial cell (Mic) is inserted between the numerous astrocyte endfeet. A pial fibroblast (Fib) is visible beneath the BL. Scale bars: 1 μm.

Interestingly, one can observe an increase in the numbers of macrophages in the pia subjacent to the supraoptic nucleus after dehydration (unpublished observation). Numerous microglial cells were also observed in the GL after dehydration (Fig. 10B).

A possibility is that these microglia have been recruited from pial macrophages, after translocating through the BL. This would be in agreement with recent data suggesting the meningeal origin of microglia (reviewed in Hickey, 2001). The factors that contribute to the induction of the morphological and functional changes in the supraoptic nucleus are far from being totally understood (Hussy, 2002). However, it has been shown that interleukin-1β (IL-1β influences the secretion of vasopressin and oxytocin (Christensen, 1990). Astrocytes in brain, as well as pituicytes in the pituitary neural lobe express IL-1β receptors (Christensen et al., 1999; reviewed in Mercier and Hatton, 2004). It is widely recognized that macrophages are the principal source of IL-1β (Lin et al., 2000). Thus, a possible scenario in the regulation of the mHNS would be that meningeal macrophages, which are highly migratory cells, are recruited from the pia-arachnoid surrounding the anterior cerebral artery after "sensing" osmolarity changes in the cerebrospinal fluid (CSF) or arterial blood. Then, some of these macrophages would infiltrate through the BL and enter among astrocytes of the GL. Both meningeal macrophages and microglia would deliver GF and cytokines such as IL-1β to astrocytes. Other potent meningeal cytokines and GF, such as bFGF, oncostatin M (Tamura et al., 2003), growth differentiation factor-15/Macrophage inhibitory cytokine-1 (GDF-15/MIC-1) (Schober et al., 2001), tumor necrosis factor-α (TNF-α, transforming growth factor-α (TGF-α, TGFβ-1, and amphiregulin (a new member of the epidermal growth factor family that is highly immunoreactive in the pia subjacent to the supraoptic nucleus, unpublished observation), are also worth considering as potential candidates for macrophage/astrocyte interactions.

The GF produced by the macrophage/microglial cells may, in turn, influence the expression of the amino acid taurine by astrocytes (reviewed in Hussy, 2002; Hatton, 2002). It has been shown that taurine is constantly released from the astrocytes of the mHNS under basal osmotic conditions and efflux is inhibited by dehydration (Deleuze et al., 2000). Taurine is a known agonist for glycine receptors, which are expressed by magnocellular neurons in the supraoptic nucleus (Hussy, 2000). Release of taurine from astrocytes in the hydrated animal leads to glycine receptor activation and ultimately has an inhibitory effect on the firing of vasopressin neurons. This scenario, diagrammatically illustrated in figure 5.11B, is supported by recent findings showing that tyrosine kinase inhibition reduces the basal level of taurine from isolated supraoptic nuclei perfused with hypoosmotic solutions (Deleuze et al, 2000). Because intracellular action of IL-1β are mediated via protein kinase interactions, it is interesting to speculate on the possibility that the cells responsible for controlling the production and release of taurine by the astrocytes of the GL are the meningeal macrophages located just beneath the GL. The same scenario may occur at every level of the magnocellular organization, macrophages being omnipresent in the mHNS, in the pia underlying the supraoptic nucleus (Fig. 5.10, see also Fig. 8A in Mercier et al., 2003), in the BV sheaths irrigating the supraoptic nucleus (see Fig. 7 in Mercier et al., 2003), in the pituitary neural lobe, in the paraventricular nucleus, and in the BV sheaths that are central to the organizations of the magnocellular accessory nuclei (not shown). Thus, the microglial cells, which are regularly arranged along the wall of the third ventricle in the magnocellular periventricular area (Fig. 4 in Mercier et al., 2003), may play a role in neuroendocrine regulation. Macrophages may also regulate neuroendocrine secretion

via production of nitric oxide (NO). Macrophages express the inducible form of
nitric oxide synthase (iNOS), and also express CD8, a stimulator of NO production
(Lin et al., 2000). NO can have inhibitory effects on neurohormone secretion (Lutz-
Becher and Koch, 1994). Supporting their implication in the regulation of the mHNS,
numerous macrophages infiltrate the GL of the supraoptic nucleus after dehydration
(Fig. 5.10B). Another possible interaction between meningeal cells and astrocytes
may be mediated by TGFβ–1, a molecule that is expressed primarily by meningeal
cells, and that regulates GFAP expression (Reilly et al., 1998).

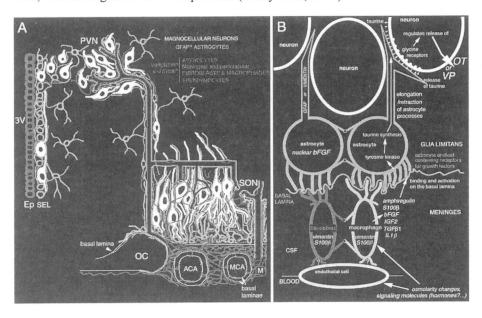

Figure 5.11. A model for meningeal-astrocytic-neuronal morphological and functional
interactions. **A**: Structural organization of the hypothalamic portion of the hypothalamo-
neurohypophysial system. Astrocytes are located between connective tissue (meningeal and
perivascular) cells and magnocellular neurons in both supraoptic nucleus (SON) and
paraventricular nucleus (PVN). The meningeal and perivascular cells themselves interface
astrocytes with the fluids (blood and CSF). ACA: anterior cerebral artery; MCA: medial
cerebral artery; M: meninges; OC: optic chiasm. **B**: Functional scenario leading to the
regulation of neurohormone release after hydration or dehydration. In this scenario, the
osmotic changes or signaling molecules present in the fluids (CSF and blood) lead to the
production of cytokines and GF by meningeal and perivascular macrophages and fibroblasts.
The cytokines and GF bind and are activated in the BL interfacing meningeal cells and
astrocytes. The astrocytes, which possess receptors for cytokines and GF, are activated via
tyrosine kinase mechanisms that ultimately lead to the production of the amino acid taurine.
Taurine is released at the astrocytic-neuronal interface, binds to glycine receptor, and regulates
the production and release of neurohormones vasopressin (VP) or oxytocin (OT).

In conclusion, it is likely that the role of the meningeal tissue in mHNS function
has been underestimated. The mHNS is one of the brain structures possessing the
most developed contacts with the connective tissue (meninges and BV sheaths)
(Mercier and Hatton, 2000; 2004). The specialized astrocytes of the hypothalamus,

and their homologues in the neural lobe, pituicytes, may represent both an anatomical and functional interface between meningeal cells and the magnocellular neurosecretory neurons.

5.3.2.2. Response after injury

All types of CNS injuries (chemical, mechanical, and immunological) are systematically associated with astrogliosis. Astrogliosis is characterized by the presence of large numbers of reactive astrocytes, distinguished from normal astrocytes by their large size, their long processes, and the high expression of GFAP (reviewed in Norton et al., 1992; Chen and Swanson, 2003). However, it has been shown that most of the cells that proliferate after brain injury are not astrocytes but inflammatory cells, endothelial cells, and microglial cells (reviewed in Norton et al., 1992). Based on multiple pulse-labeling of [H^3] thymidine incorporation, it has been shown that the limited number of astrocytes that proliferate after injury are vimentin$^+$ astrocytes, which later co-express GFAP or switch to GFAP$^+$ astrocytes. The reactive astrocytes, in concert with meningeal cells, secrete a variety of growth inhibitory molecules such as tenascin-C, proteoglycans, and ephrins, into the extracellular matrix and BL surrounding the lesion

It is well known that meningeal/perivascular cells and astrocytes cooperate and coordinate their response after injury. Reflecting this coordination, the increase of GFAP expression observed after injury correlates with the onset of infiltration of inflammatory cells (primarily macrophages and lymphocytes). Although the precise mechanisms are not elucidated, meningeal and perivascular macrophages participate in the initiation of the response to injury by releasing diverse cytokines that, in turn, activate astrocytes (Norton et al., 1992). The cytokines produced by these cells, play an important role in triggering astrogliosis and structural/functional astrocytic changes (Khan and Wigley, 1994). A common response to CNS insult is the localized increase of TNF-α, and IL1-β, both of which are primarily produced by macrophages (Wong et al., 1996; Aloe et al., 1999), and both can induce gliosis (Balasingam et al., 1994). Because there is no barrier that prevents the passage of GF and cytokines from the brain connective tissue to the neural side of the brain (the blood brain barrier is primarily defined by endothelial cells, not by connective tissue cells, see Mercier and Hatton, 2004) these factors can influence the fate and function of glial cells and neurons. In addition, the extracellular matrix molecules comprising the BL that is interposed between meningeal and glial cells, bind and activate GF and cytokines released by the vascular and connective tissue cells. In the BL, HSPG-bound GF and cytokines interact with other extracellular matrix (ECM) molecules such as collagens, laminins, and matrix metalloproteinases, to mediate their actions on the adjacent neural tissue. Because of their location, the astrocytes of the GL (including perivascular astrocytes) are likely to be the prime targets for the factors activated in the BL. For example, IL-1β a cytokine primarily produced by the macrophages present in the meninges and perivasculature serve to promote repair of the CNS (Mason et al., 2001). The ECM molecules and associated GF and cytokines also serve as a stimulus for induction of astrogliosis, cell migration, proliferation, differentiation, apoptosis, wound healing, and immune surveillance (Martins-Green, 2000). Immune surveillance of the brain involves the infiltration of immune cells, including macrophages, lymphocytes, dendritic cells, and mast cells into the meninges, perivasculature (Virchow Robin space), and brain parenchyma (T lymphocyte and macrophage infiltration). Thus, these cells have ample opportunity to influence the fate and function of glial cells and neurons via the multiple factors they release in the CSF and intercellular space bathing neurons and glial cells. Resident microglial cells and infiltrating macrophages that differentiate into microglial cells when entering the neural compartment also represent an important source of (and target for) cytokines (Hanisch, 2002).

In addition to their participation in the immune surveillance of the brain, connective tissue cells and immune cells may participate in morphological and functional plasticity of the neural tissue. T lymphocytes foster repair of the nervous system (reviewed in Schwartz and Cohen, 2000). Here again, the brain connective tissue-astrocyte interface may play a crucial role. After injury, astrocytes and meningeal cells interact to form a new BL (Abnet et al., 1991). The role of meningeal cells in repairing neural tissue is controversial. Regenerative processes after stab wound or chemical injury involve axonal growth and reconnection, gliogenesis, proliferation and migration of meningeal cells, and angiogenesis. Ishikawa et al., (1995) demonstrated that meningeal cells promote repair of magnocellular axons after hypophysectomy. At least tanycytes support this regeneration (Chauvet et al., 1995). However, meningeal cells are also considered as preventing regeneration. Failure of regenerative process of the nervous system is partly due to meningeal-produced semaphorins, chemorepulsive axon guidance cues expressed throughout life, which form barriers to the re-growing neural tissue (Pasterkamp and Verhaagen, 2001). Although complex and poorly investigated, these data highlight possible interactions involving meningeal cells, glial cells, and neurons. Although the mechanisms remain to be investigated, they may involve cytokine cascades, with signals primarily originating from the meninges, and relayed by astrocytes. For example, IL-1β produced by meningeal/perivascular macrophages may induce the production of interleukin-6 (IL-6) by astrocytes, and IL-6 induces functional changes at the neuronal level. As mentioned in the previous section IL-6 stimulates vasopressin and oxytocin release (Yasin et al., 1994).

5.3.2.3. Immune system

Although not the basic cells of the brain immune system, it has been recently recognized that astrocytes intervene in brain immune functions. The immunological surveillance of the brain is a complex concept. The brain is constantly monitored by migrating cells responsible immune functions, such as lymphocytes, hematopoetic-derived macrophages, mast cells that populate the meninges, perivascular layer (Virchow-Robin space) and choroid plexus stroma, and by microglial cells in the parenchyma. Because cells of the immune system are highly migratory, pass through the CNS (Hickey et al., 1991; Silverman et al., 2000; Bechmann et al., 2001), and easily trans-differentiate, one cannot distinguish so clearly what are the respective involvements of the general immune and local immune systems. It is not clear whether microglial cells arrive in brain parenchyma before birth (reviewed in Hickey, 2001), or are slowly repopulated from meningeal/perivascular macrophages (Ling and Wong, 1993). It is more widely recognized that perivascular and meningeal macrophages are themselves bone marrow derived cells, and are continuously being repopulated from blood monocytes (Hickey et al., 1988, Bechmann et al., 2001).

Thus, it is possible that microglial cells derive from the hematopoietic cells. Supporting this concept, Eglitis and Mezey (1997) have shown that hematopoietic cells could differentiate into both macroglia and microglia. The cell lineages of brain immune cells, and brain cells in general, including those of astrocytes and neurons, are discussed further in the next section. The basic principles of immunological surveillance of T and B-lymphocytes, macrophages and microglia are reviewed by Hickey (2001) and are not the focus of this review.

The ability of astrocytes to function as immunocompetent cells in the CNS is discussed in detail by Dong and Benveniste (2001). Briefly, astrocytes can be induced to express major histocompatibility complex (MHC) class II molecules by interferon γ (IFN-γ), TNF-α and other cytokines. MHC class II molecules are required for normal immune responses, being essential for lymphocyte development, antigen presentation, and antigen presenting cells (primarily macrophages in brain) and T lymphocyte activation. Although controversial, it has been shown that astrocytes could function as antigen presenting cells for activation of T lymphocytes. In addition, astrocytes produce numerous immunologically relevant cytokines and GF such IL-6 and monocyte chemoattractant protein-1 (MCP-1). IL-6 regulates immunoglobulin synthesis in activated lymphocytes B, and plays a role in T lymphocyte maturation and activation. But IL-6 is also a potent differentiating factor, controlling monocyte-macrophage conversion, astrocytes proliferation, and neuronal survival (reviewed in Dong and Benveniste, 2001). Astrocytes are the major source of MCP-1, a potent monocyte chemoattractant that is secreted in response to IL1-β, TGF-β, and IFN-γ, molecules that are primarily expressed in brain by meningeal and choroid plexus cells. MCP-1 receptor is expressed on monocytes and activated T lymphocytes. In rats with experimental autoimmune encephalomyelitis (EAE), apoptotic inflammatory cells associate more closely with astrocytes than with microglial cells (reviewed in Pender and Rist, 2001). In addition, astrocytes can phagocytose apoptotic lymphocytes, but microglial cells are more efficient than astrocytes in removing apoptotic lymphocytes (Magnus et al., 2002). In another review, Becher et al., (2000) highlighted the role of microglial, astrocytic and vascular/perivascular cell cooperation in the immune response. Communication between the cells of the immune system occurs either via direct cell-cell contacts or via cytokines and GF. The macrophages and dendritic cells are usually recognized as the professional cells that capture and process antigens as a result of their ability to endocytose pathogens and cellular debris (reviewed in Becher et al., (2000). There are also the antigen presenting cells that interact with T lymphocytes, being important for homing these cells in the CNS (Hickey and Kimura, 1988). Endothelial cells, microglial cells, and astrocytes are also potential antigen presenting cells. Becher et al., (2000) discussed the notion that infiltration of immune cells is a response to processes that occur in the nervous system, and that the interactions between the different brain cell types participating in immune functions ultimately lead to the CNS defense, removal of apoptotic cells and cellular debris.

Interestingly, and reflecting another potential role in the immune defense, astrocytes synthesize the three forms of NOS, and produce NO, which is involved in necrotic killing of cells and invading pathogens, apoptosis, and tissue remodeling (Murphy, 2000). Benn et al., (2001) discuss the production of other cytotoxic mediators by astrocytes. Moreover, it has been shown that chemokines produced by perivascular astrocytes contribute to the properties of the blood brain barrier and the entry of immune cells (Prat et al., 2001).

A complex interplay between migrating T lymphocytes, meningeal and perivascular macrophages, microglial cells, and astrocytes will dictate the final immune response. Because they also express cytokines and GF (Mercier and Hatton, 2004), mast cells, fibroblasts, and neurons, may also indirectly intervene in the immune response. Astrocytes, which are both targets and producers of cytokines and GF, may play a central role in mediating cross-communication between immune cells and neurons. Future investigations will likely establish the respective roles of brain cells in the coordinated interplay for an efficient immune response.

5.3.2.4. Neural stem cell biology

5.3.2.4.1. Astrocytes as neural stem cells throughout adulthood

New neurons and glial cells are produced throughout adulthood in the mammalian brain (Altman, 1963; Goldman and Nottebohm, 1983), including human brain (Eriksson et al., 1998). The new neural cells originate from NSC that proliferate and differentiate, primarily along the ventricle walls, and then migrate to replace (at least to some extent) glial cells and neurons lost throughout adulthood in brain. However, neither the NSC, nor the mechanisms leading to proliferation and differentiation of these cells, have been clearly identified.

Some individual cells (a low percentage of the total number of cells) extracted from the ventricle walls, defined as stem cells, are capable of generating neurospheres, which are clusters of cells that contain potential neurons, astrocytes and oligodendrocytes, because they express specific markers of these cells (Reynolds and Weiss, 1992; Weiss et al., 1996). A stem cell by definition is a cell that is capable of self-renewing, and is pluripotent, i.e. capable of generating different cell types.

Although controversial, the leading current view is that astrocytes, or a subpopulation of these cells located in the ventricle walls (primarily the lateral ventricle), NSC throughout adulthood (Doetsch et al, 1999; Laywell et al., 2000; Seri et al., 2001; Alvarez-Buylla et al., 2002; reviewed in Alvarez-Buylla et al, 2001). Other studies have implicated ependymocytes, the cells that line the ventricle walls, as candidates for NSC (Johansson, 1999). The experiments supporting the current views are based on the capabilities of isolated astrocytes (Laywell et al., 2000), and of astrocyte trans-differentiated from oligodendrocytes (Kondo and Raff, 2000), to generate neurospheres in vitro in response to epidermal growth factor (EGF) or bFGF. These two GF are mitotic for a single population of NSC originating from the subependymal layer (Gritti et al., 1999). These observations show that astrocytes can behave as NSC *in vitro*.

Other experiments support the view that astrocytes can also behave as NSC *in vivo*. Astrocytes of the subependymal layer divide to generate different precursor cells, among them amplifying precursor cells (C cells), which in turn generate A cells, after ablation of both A and C cells by antimitotic agents (Doetsch et al., 1999). After migration along the rostral migratory stream (RMS), A cells infiltrate the olfactory bulb, a structure that is (for unknown reason) constantly renewing its neurons (Alvarez-Buylla and Garcia-Verdugo, 2002). Other investigations have shown that choroid plexus epithelial cells can transdifferentiate into astrocytes in vivo (Kitada et al., 2001). In fact, more and more data suggest that numerous cells, even cells originating from peripheral organs and tissues, are capable of transdifferentiating into neural-like cells (Bjornson et al., 1999; Woodburry et al., 2000; Zhao et al., 2000). In addition, a series of experiments suggests a continuing influx of bone marrow-derived cells throughout the adult mammalian brain (Ling, 1979; Ling and al., 1980; Leong and Ling, 1992, Ling and Wong, 1993, Lassmann et al., 1993, Azizi et al., 1998). According to these authors, bone marrow-derived circulating monocytes extravasate, engraft in the brain connective tissue, replacing meningeal, perivascular, and choroid plexus macrophages, and further generate microglial cells after a transitory phenotype as ameboid microglia. Additionally, Azizi et al., (1998) have shown that after engrafting, bisbenzimide-labeled bone marrow cells migrate through the brain, survive for a long period of time, following migratory pathways of A cells. Although this is controversial (Wagers et al., 2002) and merits further investigation, recent studies even suggest that some of the bone marrow-derived cells may become astrocytes (Eglitis and Mezey, 1997) and neurons after their infiltration and integration in brain, in both adult rats and humans (Mezey et al., 2000; 2003; Brazelton et al., 2000). In these experiments, transplanted bone marrow cells from male donors infiltrate the brain and differentiate into neural cells. For humans, Mezey et al. analyzed post-mortem brain tissue of female patients whose bone marrow had been totally irradiated and transplanted with male bone marrow donor cells: in every case, the brain contained thousands of neurons (detected by immunocytochemistry) still bearing the Y chromosome (detected by in situ hybridization). A potential problem, however, is that bone marrow cells can "fuse" spontaneously with stem cells, a phenomenon termed cell fusion (Terada et al., 2002; Vassilopoulos et al., 2003; Wang et al., 2003). Mezey et al. argue that the fusion phenomenon is minimal, potentially concerning a very restricted number of cells. Another problem for the theory of bone marrow-derived neural cells in the adult is that some authors were unable find astrocytes or neurons (except one), after injecting green florescent protein (GFP)- labeled purified bone marrow stem cells (GFP$^+$HSC) into lethally irradiated nontransgenic recipients (Wagers et al., 2002). One may believe all groups of scientists if one considers that non-purified bone marrow extracts or cultured marrow cells were used in one case (Mezey et al.; Brazelton et al.), and that purified hematopoietic stem cells were used in the other case (Wagers et al.). Indeed, it is possible that a second pool of bone marrow stem cells, for example mesenchymal stem cells (derived from the bone marrow connective tissue (stroma)?) or even differentiated cells from either the bone marrow hematopoietic lineage or the bone marrow stroma (for example fibroblasts or macrophages) may behave as NSC after their integration in the brain connective tissue (meninges, perivascular layer, or choroid plexus stroma). It is widely accepted that routes of entry of bone marrow −derived immune cells exist in the adult mammalian brain (reviewed in Williams and Hickey; 2002). In addition, it is clear that stem cells express characteristics of differentiated cells in several mature tissues, including the brain (Coulombe et al., 1989; Hu et al., 1997; Alvarez-Buylla et al, 2001). Further work is required to clarify whether the circulating monocytes or other bone marrow-derived cells (stromal or parenchymal), infiltrate the brain only to repopulate the pool of meningeal and perivascular macrophages, Kolmer cells of the choroid plexus, and epiplexus cells lining the ependyma of ventricles, eventually microglia, or if newborn neurons and glial cells also originate from these immune cells after their translocation and trans-differentiation into the brain parenchyma. Interestingly, differentiated macrophages are present in both stroma of the bone marrow (as connective tissue cell) and as a fully differentiated terminal lineage in the hematopoetic lineage. Furthermore, the macrophage-like epiplexus cells lining the ependyma are likely to infiltrate to the ependyma (reviewed in Ling and Wong, 1993), a characteristic that one can interestingly correlate with the location of the potential astrocytes that serve as NSC in the adult brain (Alvarez-Buylla et al., 2001). Tanycytes also possess also extend a long cilium into the CSF of the lateral ventricle (for references, see Mercier et al., 2002; 2003). Here again, further work is required to clarify the lineage relationships of all these cell types.

Also controversial, Woodburry et al., (2000; 2002) have highlighted a trans-differentiation potential of bone marrow cells. These cells change morphology to become neuron-like cells expressing neuronal markers after a few hours in vitro upon application of inducing media containing GF and dimethylsulfoxide.

The resulting picture is quite confusing. Does the adult NSC represent a pool of quiescent cells that derive from the primitive neuroepithelium, waiting for cues to multiply and differentiate into mature form? Contradicting the dogma that stem cells are quiescent inactive cells, it has been shown that hematopoietic stem cells strongly interact with connective tissue cells to deform, branch, and extend motile pseudopodial membrane extensions in direction of stromal cells under the influence of stromal derived factor-1 (Frimberger et al., 2000). Does the pool of adult NSC constantly repopulate from the bone marrow and blood cell lineages? Do differentiated neural cells (including astrocytes) de-differentiate into stem cells upon application microenvironment cues present in the ventricle wall? There are currently no clear answers to these questions. However, that only few cells of the brain neurogenic zones pass the "neurosphere test" is informative. This means that a small fraction of the astrocytes behave as stem cells. Astrocytes represent more than 80% of the brain cells, and are also the most numerous cells in the subependymal layer of ventricles (neurogenic zones). Which astrocyte subpopulation may behave as stem cells?

5.3.2.4.2. Radial glial cells as neural stem cells throughout adulthood

Astrocytes, oligodendrocytes and neurons are thought to derive from neuroepithelial progenitor cells, and microglia from the myeloid cells of the hematopoetic lineage. In the adult ventricle walls exists a subpopulation of vimentin-expressing glial cells, of radial morphology, termed tanycytes. These cells may be considered as radial glia persisting throughout adulthood. They are plastic cells, which also exist in the walls of the third ventricle where they intervene in morphological plasticity and repair after injury (Chauvet et al., 1995). Embryonic radial glial cells are particularly interesting because they are believed to be either neuronal precursors (Noctor et al., 2001) and to guide the migration of new neurons during brain morphogenesis (Rakic, 1988; Liour and Yu , 2003). The issues surrounding the regulation of the radial glial cell phenotype, and the role of radial glial cells as precursor cells during development, have been reviewed by Gregg et al., (2002). Briefly, radial glial cells have been first identified in the neuroepithelium lining the ventricles (reviewed in Bentivoglio and Mazarello, 1999). These cells, whose somata are located in the ependyma or subependymal layer (subventricular zone) are easily identified by their radial appearance, the cells bearing a long process that reaches the pia, and a short one that reaches the ventricular lumen (this is also true for tanycytes, and a subpopulation of astrocytes that may behave as NSC in adulthood (Avarez-Buylla, 2001; Alves et al., 2002). Radial glial cells are the earliest cells to differentiate from the neuroepithelium, and are primarily known as cells that scaffold and support migration of newly generated neurons during development (reviewed in Gregg and al., 2002; Bentivoglio and Mazzarello, 1999). However, some radial glial cells persist postnatally and even throughout adulthood as tanycytes lining the third and lateral ventricles, and cerebellar Bergmann glia. The astrocytes of the supraoptic nucleus and periamygdaloid cortex (Mercier and Hatton, 2000) may be also considered to be surviving radial glia, possessing long processes spanning the nuclei, and other small processes contacting the pia. All radial glial cells, including the adult types, express the intermediate filament vimentin. In addition, they may or may not express GFAP (Mercier and Hatton, 2000), depending of their location and physiological conditions.

Soon after birth, radial glia initiate a process of transformation into GFAP astrocytes (reviewed in Alves et al., 2002). However, the restricted commitment of radial glia to glial lineage has been recently challenged. It has been demonstrated that subpopulations of radial glia can give rise to glia, neurons, or both glia and neurons (Noctor et al., 2001; reviewed in Gaiano and Fishell, 2002; Gregg et al., 2002). Noctor et al. injected a GFP-labeled retrovirus into the ventricle of E16 rat embryos. One day after injection, vimentin immunoreactive cells with radial glia morphology were infected with the virus and labeled with GFP. Three days after injection, the authors observed arrayed clones. Each of these clones contained neuron-like cells expressing specific neural markers and one vimentin immunoreactive cell. The authors also used time-lapse videomicrography to show that the infected radial glia divided asymmetrically to produce neuroblasts that migrated into the cortex, along the radial process of the cell that produced them. Identity of radial glia and their neuronal progeny were assessed by electrophysiology. Moreover, isolation of radial glia by fluorescent cell sorting, revealed a neuronal lineage (Malatesta et al., 2000). Nothing similar has been established during adulthood. However, it has been recently shown that proliferating cells in neurogenic zones are closely associated with radial-glia like astrocytes expressing both vimentin and GFAP (Alonso, 2001). Interestingly, mature astrocytes can transform into transitional radial glia that support directed migration of transplanted immature neurons within the adult mouse neocortex (Leavitt et al., 1999). Further investigations are required to determine whether or not the vimentin-positive radial-glia-like tanycytes of the ventricle wall may serve as NSC throughout adulthood.

5.3.2.4.3. Meningeal cells as inducers and/ or source of neural stem cells in
          adulthood

The mechanisms controlling cell proliferation, differentiation, and migration in the ventricle wall remains shrouded in mystery. We are at an early stage of discovering and characterizing the signaling molecules that operate in the ventricle wall to ultimately induce and control neurogenesis and gliogenesis. It has been shown, both in vivo and in vitro, that GF and cytokines are involved in the proliferation and differentiation processes (Tao et al., 1996; Weiss et al., 1996; Falk and Frisen 2002). However, the mechanisms orchestrating expression, release, and activation of these signaling molecules are unknown. An important characteristic to remember is that adult neurogenesis occurs only in restricted zones, primarily the ventricle walls. In addition, the rate of neurogenesis and the type of cells produced differ along the ventricle wall. Neurogenesis in adult mammals is more intense in the lateral ventricles than other ventricles. The anterior portion of lateral ventricle primarily generates neurons, and the posterior portion more glial cells. This suggests that different inductive microenvironmental cues exist in different brain zones and within the subependyma. Steindler et al., (1998) highlighted the role of boundary ECM molecules in neurogenesis during development. These authors introduced the concept of "cordones" to reflect the existence of specific pathways or structural organizations, usually delineating boundaries, along which neural cells multiply, differentiate, and migrate. These dense accumulations of ECM molecules are likely to correspond to BL, and adjacent meningeal cells as BV sheaths and other pial projections interfacing different brain zones. Meninges, which are neural crest and/or mesodermic derivatives, already exist during early neurogenesis, covering the neuroepithelium (O'Rahilly and Muller, 1986; Choi, 1994). During development, the meninges and overlying BL participate in brain scaffolding and morphogenesis (Sievers et al., 1993). There is no reason to think that postnatal and adult neurogenesis fundamentally differs from neurogenesis during development. Meningeal cells still express GF and cytokines (reviewed in Mercier and Hatton, 2004). HSPG are highly expressed in BL, and play a crucial role in binding and activating GF (reviewed in Iozzo, 1998). bFGF is a prototype of a family of heparin binding GF that regulate cell proliferation and differentiation (Roberts et al., 1988, Reiland and Rapraeger, 1993). HSPG are expressed virtually in all zones delineated by the meninges and its multiple projections in brain. It is worth repeating that, via the vasculature, the meninges, systematically covered by BL, penetrate virtually every brain zone (Mercier and Hatton, 2004).

The recent characterization of a dense BL network in the subependyma presents new perspectives. These BL, termed fractones, harbor the processes of neuroblasts, astrocytes, microglia, and the basal processes of ependymocytes (Mercier et al., 2002). The fractones exist in the lateral ventricle, where they are abundant and particularly well connected to local BV, but fractones are also encountered in the subependymal layer of other ventricles (Mercier et al., 2003) and the subependyma of the spinal cord (unpublished observation). The fractones, just beneath the ependyma, are connected at their base to local perivascular macrophages that belong to "the fibroblast/macrophage network" throughout the meninges and its projections in brain (Mercier et al., 2002; Mercier and Hatton, 2000; 2004). Although the properties and functional potential of perivascular macrophages have been poorly investigated, it is worth mentioning their known role in immune surveillance (reviewed in Thomas, 1999; Hickey, 2001).

Based on all literature cited in the above section, I suggest that the microenvironmental cues necessary for NSC proliferation and differentiation are produced and controlled by the meninges and its projections in brain. In neurogenic zones of the adult brain (lateral ventricles), the meninges consist of BV sheaths and choroid plexus stroma (Mercier et al., 2002; Mercier and Hatton, 2004). The choroid plexus is known as an important source of entry of GF and cytokines (Johanson et al, 2000;

Stopa et al., 2001). It is also, like meninges and perivasculature (adventitial layer), the compartment of entry for cells originating from the bone marrow (Hickey et al, 1988). Interestingly, amphiregulin, a GF highly expressed in the choroid plexus (Falk and Frisen, 2002) and in the lateral ventricle wall (unpublished observation), induces *in vitro* the production of neurospheres containing neurons and astrocytes (Falk and Frisen, 2002).

The meninges would exert their induction and control mechanisms by producing the appropriate GF and cytokines, after their binding and activation in fractones (in the subependymal layer) or in the BL interfacing with stroma and epithelium of the choroid plexus. Meningeal cells produce GF and cytokines that influence NSC proliferation and differentiation *in vivo* or *in vitro*: bFGF (Gritti et al., 1999), amphiregulin (Falk and Frisen), TNF-α (Wu et al, 2000). Interestingly, BL HSPG such as perlecan and syndecan, and CSPG are associated with progenitors cells (Diers-Fenger et al., 2001; Winkler et al., 2002). A potential 'dual induction pathway' via subependymal vasculature and choroid plexus may appear complex, but is conceivably suitable and favorable for mechanisms of attraction/repulsion by chemokines in between the two structures, to ultimately control the fate and migration of cells, whatever their phenotype. Indeed, the migration processes are required for both A cells, and monocyte-derived macrophages. Macrophages enter the choroid plexus (as circulating monocyte), traverse the choroid plexus stroma and epithelium (as stromal macrophage), then the ventricular lumen (as Kolmer cells), reach the ependyma (as supra-ependymal cells), and infiltrate the subependymal layer. It has been proved by using bone marrow grafted rats after complete irradiation, and tracing techniques of fluorescent cells, that bone marrow-derived monocytes enter the brain via the choroid plexus, BV, and meninges, where they become macrophages (Hickey et al., 1988, Ishihara et al., 1993), and further enter into the brain, becoming ameboid and ramified microglia (Leong and Ling, 1992; Ling et al., 1998). The same authors previously demonstrated that monocytes become "ameboid microglia" and penetrate the ventricle walls and adjacent zones, as well as the meninges (Leong and Ling, 1992; Ling and Wong, 1993). It is also known that after traumatic brain injury, monocytes extravasate, enter brain parenchyma, and take ameboid forms (Tsuchihashi et al., 1981).

A subset of macrophages, phenotypically resembling fibroblasts, and derived from blood monocytes act as pluripotent stem cells, generating neurons or peripheral cell types upon different inducing media (Zhao et al., 2003). In addition to the regular macrophage markers CD14 and CD44, the pluripotent stem cells express CD34, the classical marker of bone marrow stem cells.

Of interest for the role of meningeal cells and glial cells in the neurogenesis process, the cell surface glycoprotein gp130 is expressed by a subset of glial precursors, microglial and meningeal cells (Blass-Kampmann et al., 1997). Gp130 dimerizes with receptors for cytokines regulating NSC self-renewal and differentiation. Chojnacki et al., (2003), demonstrated that gp130, via the Notch1 signaling pathway, is required for the maintenance of and generation of NSC. In the adult, Notch1 is produced by nestin-expressing cells in the subependymal layer and in the dentate gyrus, the sites of neurogenesis and gliogenesis (Irvin et al., 2001). Notch activation can positively determine cell fate and affect neuronal process extension. Activation of the Notch pathway inhibits cell differentiation and maintains cells as progenitors, but also promotes (or restricts) radial glia and astrocyte identity

(Gaiano and Fishell, 2002), cells that might both be the lineal precursors of adult NSC (Alvarez-Buylla et al., 1990), while inhibiting oligodendrocyte differentiation. It has also been shown that the chondroitin sulfate proteoglycan NG2, known as a molecule expressed by oligodendrocyte precursors (Watanabe et al., 2002), is expressed by cells of the microglial lineage (Pouly et al., 1999) and by activated macrophages (Bu et al., 2001). Finally, supporting the idea that adult astrocytes may derive from perivascular/meningeal cells, adult nestin-expressing subependymal cells differentiate into astrocytes in response to brain injury (Holmin et al., 1997). The intermediate filament nestin is a marker of both progenitor stem cells, and a marker of perivascular/meningeal cells.

5.4. The astrocytic hypothesis

The goal of this review was to highlight the possibility that astrocytes might form a functional interface between the brain connective/vascular tissue and neurons. There are several reasons to think that this may be the case.

First, the anatomy of astrocytes is particularly well suited to participate in functional interactions with both neurons and meningeal/perivascular cells. Astrocytes present a developed contact surface with both neurons, and macrophages/fibroblasts. To a lesser extent, astrocytes also directly contact vascular cells.

Second, the BL that systematically interfaces GL/perivascular astrocytes and meningeal/perivascular cells is a potential surface of exchange, binding and activating GF and cytokines produced by cells that abut it. Via this BL, astrocytes and extraparenchymal cells can mutually influence their fate, morphology, and function. Both astrocytes and extraparenchymal cells are major sources of cytokines and GF (Mercier and Hatton, 2004).

Third, the meningeal/perivascular cells are well located to pick up information circulating in blood and CSF. Fibroblasts and macrophages directly bathe in the CSF. These cells also contact vascular cells from which they may pick up information originating from the circulation.

Fourth, the literature strongly suggests that astrocytes and meningeal cells, and the BL located in between, are closely associated in their response to injury (Norton et al., 1992; Choi, 1994). The occurrence of spontaneous meningo-astrocytic interactions in vitro (Struckhoff, 1995) reflects the in vivo phenomena. Both cell types also participate in brain "immune surveillance" and brain inflammation (Dong and Benveniste, 2001; Hickey; 2001).

5.5. Perspectives

The particular anatomical and functional links between astrocytes, neurons, and extraparenchymal cells, suggest that astrocytes may serve as an interface of communication. Astrocytes are ideally located to receive and modulate the signals they receive from both neurons and meningeal/vascular cells. Additionally, meningeal and astrocytic gap junctions may provide pathways of communication for propagating the information over long distances, both in the astrocytic and meningeal compartments. It remains to identify the brain functions and the precise mechanisms that underlie the meningeal/astrocytic interactions. It is suggested here that astrocytes, in cooperation with meningeal/vascular cells, serve to promote and regulate brain plasticity.

Acknowledgements. The author's research is supported by Hawaii Community Foundation grant HCF436-034.

5.6. References

Abnet K, Fawcett JW, Dunnett SB (1991) Interactions between meningeal cells and astrocytes in vivo and in vitro. Dev Brain Res 59:187-196.

Allonso G. 2001. Proliferation of progenitor cells in the adult rat brain correlates with the presence of vimentin-expressing astrocytes. Glia 34:253-266.

Aloe L, Fiore M, Probert L, Turini P, Tirassa P (1999) Overexpression of tumour necrosis factor alpha in the brain of transgenic mice differentially alters nerve growth factor levels and choline acetyltransferase activity. Cytokine 11:45-54.

Altman J (1963) Autoradiographic investigation of cell proliferation in the brain of rats and cats. Anat Rec 145:573-591.

Althaus HH, Landsberg CR (2000) Glial cells as targets and producers of neurotrophins. Int Rev Cytol 197:203-277.

Alvarez-Buylla A, García-Verdugo JM (2002) Neurogenesis in adult subventricular zone. J Neurosci 22:629-634.

Alvarez-Buylla A, Garcia-Verdugo JM, Tramontin AD (2001) A unified hypothesis on the lineage of neural stem cells. Nature Rev Neurosci 2:287-293.

Alvarez-Buylla A, Seri B, Doetsch F (2002) Identification of neural stem cells in the adult vertebrate brain. Brain Res Bull 57:751-758.

Alvarez-Buylla A, Theelen M, Nottebohm F (1990) Proliferation "hot spots" in adult avian ventricular zone reveals radial cell division. Neuron 5: 101-109.

Alves JA, Barone P, Engelender S, Froes MM, Menezes JR (2002) Initial stages of radial glia astrocytic transformation in the early postnatal anterior subventricular zone. J Neurobiol 52:251-265.

Au E, Roskam AJ (2003) Olfactory ensheathing cells of the lamina propria in vivo and in vitro. Glia 41:224-236.

Azizi SA, Stokes D, Augelli BJ, DiGirolamo C, Prockop DJ (1998) Engraftment and migration of human bone marrow stromal cells implanted in the brains of albino rats-similarities to astrocyte grafts. Proc Nat Acad Sci 95:3908-3913.

Becher B, Prat A, Antel JP (2000) Brain immune connections: immuno-regulatory properties of CNS-resident cells. Glia 29:293-304.

Bechmann I, Kwindzinski E, Kovac AD, Simburger E, Horvath T, Gimsa U, Dirnagl U, Priller J, Nitsch R (2001) Turnover of rat brain perivascular cells. Exp Neurol 168:242-249.

Benn T, Halfpenny C, Scolding N (2001) Glial cells as targets for cytotoxic immune mediators. Glia 36:2000-211.

Bentivoglio M, Mazzarello P (1999) The history of radial glia. Brain Res Bul 49:305-315.

Bjornson CR, Rietze RL, Reynolds BA, Magli MC, Vescovi AL (1999) Turning brain into blood: a hematopoietic fate adopted by adult neural stem cells in vivo. Science 283:534-537.

Blass-Kampmann S, Kindler-Rohrborn A, Deissler H, D'urso D, Rajewsky MF (1997) In vitro differentiation of neural progenitor cells from prenatal rat brain: common cell surface glycoprotein on three glial cell subsets. J Neurosci Res 15:95-111.

Bobak JB, Salm AK (1996) Plasticity of astrocytes of the ventral glial limitans subjacent to the supraoptic nucleus. J Comp Neurol 376:188-197.

Brannon-Thomas L, Gates MA, Steindler DA (1996) Young neurons from the adult subependymal zone proliferate and migrate along an astrocyte, extracellular matrix-rich pathway. Glia 17:1-14.

Brazelton TR, RossiFMV, Keshet GI, Blau HM (2000) From marrow to brain: expression of neuronal phenotypes in adult mice. Science 290:1775-1778.

Bu J, Akhtar N, Nishiyama A (2001) Transient expression of the NG2 proteoglycan by a subpopulation of activated macrophages in an excitotoxic hippocampal lesion. Glia 34:296-310.

Bushong EA, Martone ME, Jones YZ, Ellisman MH (2002) Protoplasmic astrocytes in the striatum radiatum occupy separate anatomical domains. J Neurosci 22:183-192.

Chauvet N, Parmentier ML, Alonso G (1995) Transected axons of adult hypothalamo-neurohypophysial neurons regenerate along tanycytic processes. J Neurosci Res 41:129-144.

Chen YM, Swanson RA (2003) Astrocytes and brain injury. J Cereb Blood Flow Metab 23:137-149.

Chojnacki A, Shimazaki T, Gregg C, Weinmaster G, Weiss S (2003) Glycoprotein 130 signaling regulates Notch1 expression and activation in the self-renewal of mammalian forebrain neural stem cells. J Neurosci Res 23:1730-1741.

Choi BH (1994) Role of the basement membrane in neurogenesis and repair of injury in the central nervous system. 28:193-203.

Christensen JD, Hansen EW, Fjalland B (1990) Influence of interleukin-1β on the secretion of oxytocin and vasopressin from the isolated rat neurohypophysis. Pharmacol Toxicol 67:81-83.

Christensen JD, Hansen EW, Frederiksen C, Molris M, Moesby L (1999) Adrenaline influences the release of interleukin-6 from murine pituicytes: role of β2-adrenoreceptors. Eur J Pharmacol 378:143-148.

Coulombe PA, Kopan R, Fuchs E (1989) Expression of keratin K14 in the epidermis and hair follicle: insights into complex programs of differentiation J Cell Biol 109:22952312.

Deleuze C, Duvoid A, Moos FC, Hussy N (2000) Tyrosine phosphorylation modulates the osmosensitivity of volume-dependent taurine efflux from glial cells in the rat suproptic nucleus. J Physiol 523.2:291-299.

Derouiche A, Frotscher M (2001) Peripheral astrocyte processes: monitoring by selective immunostaining for the actin-binding ERM proteins. Glia 36-330-341.

Diers-Fenger M, Kirchhoff F, Kettenmann H, Levine JM, Trotter J (2001) AN2/NG2 protein-expressing glial progenitor cells in the murine CNS: isolation, differentiation, and association with radial glia. Glia 34:213-228.Doetsch F, Caillé I, Lim, DA, García-Verdugo JM, Alvarez-Buylla A (1999) Subventricular zone astrocytes are neural stem cells in the adult mammalian brain. Cell 97:703-716.

Doetsch F, Garcia-Verdugo JM, Alvarez-Buylla A (1997) Cellular composition and three dimensional organization of the subventricular germinal zone in the adult mammalian brain. J Neurosci 17:5046-5061.

Doetsch F, Caille I, Lim DA, Garcia-Verdugo JM, Alvarez-Buylla A (1999) Subventricular zone astrocytes are neural stem cells in the adult mammalian brain. Cell 97:703-716.

Dong Y, Benveniste EN (2001) Immune function of astrocytes. Glia 36:180-190.

Eglitis MA, Mezey E (1997) Hematopoetic cells differentiate into both microglia and macroglia in the brain of adult mice. Proc Nat Acad Sci 94:4080-4085.

Eriksson PS, Perfilieva E, Bjork-Eriksson T, Alborn AM, Nordborg C, Peterson DA, Gage FH (1998) Neurogenesis in the human adult hippocampus. Nat Med 4:1313-1317.

Evans WH, Martin PE (2002) Gap junctions: structure and function. Mol Membr Biol 19:121-136.

Farquhar MG (1991) The glomerular basement membrane. In: Hay HD Editor. Cell Biology of the extacelullar matrix. New York: Plenum Publishing Corp. p. 365-418.

Frantseva MV, Kokarovtseva L, Perze Velazquez JL (2002) Ischemia-induced brain damage depends on specific gap junctional coupling. J Cereb Blood Flow Metab 22:453-462.

Franzen R, Martin D, Daloze A, Moonen G, Schoenen J (1999) Grafts of meningeal fibroblasts in adult rat spinal cord lesion promote axonal regrowth. Neuroreport 10:1551-1156.

Frimberger AE, McAuliffe CI, Werme KA, Tuft RA, Fogarty KE. Benoit BO, Dooner MS, Gaaino N, Fishell G (2002) The role of Notch in promoting glial and neural stem cell fates. Annu Rev Neurosci 25:471-490.

Gilbert SF (1994) In: Developmental Biology, Sinauer Associates Inc., Sunderland, Massachussets, pp 894.

Goetschy JF, Ulrich G, Aunis D, Ciesielski-Treska J (1987) Fibronectin and collagens modulate the proliferation and morphology of astroglial cells in culture. Int J Dev Neurosci 5:63-70.

Goldman SA, Nottebohm F (1983) Neuronal production, migration, and differentiation in a vocal control nucleus of the adult female canary brain. Proc Nat Acad Sci 80:2390-2394.

Gonzalez AM, Berry M, Maher PA, Logan A, Baird A (1995) A comprehensive analysis of the distribution of FGF-2 and FGFR1 in the rat brain. Brain Res 701-201-226.

Graeber MB, Streit WJ, Kreutzberg GW (1989) Identity of perivascular cells in rat brain. J Neurosci Res 22:103-106.

Gregg CT, Chojnacki AK, Weiss S (2002) Radial glial cells as neuronal precursors: the next generation? J neurosci Res 69:708-713.

Gritti A, Frolichsthal-Schoeller P, Galli R, Vescovi AL (1999) Epidermal and fibroblast growth factors behave as mitogenic regulators of for a single multipotent stem-like cell population from the subventricular region of the adult mouse forebrain. J Neurosci 19:3287-3297.

Hanisch UK (2002) Microglia as a source and target of cytokines. Glia 40:140-155.

Hatton GI (1999) Astroglial modulation of neurotransmitter/peptide release from the neurohypophysis: present status. J Chem Neuroanat 16:203-222.

Hatton GI (2002) Glial-neuronal interactions in the mammalian brain. Adv Physiol Educ 26:225-237.

Haydon PG (2001) Glia: listening and talking to the synapse. Nat Rev Neurosci 2:185-193.

Hickey WF (2001) Basic principles of immunological surveillance of the normal central nervous system. Glia 36:118-124.

Hickey WF, Kimura H (1988) Perivascular microglial cells of the CNS are bone marrow derived and present antigen in vivo. Science 239:290-292.

Hickey WF, Hsu BL, Kimura H (1991) T-lymphocyte entry into the central nervous system. J Neurosci Res 28:254-260.

Holmin S, Almqvist P, Lendahl U, Mathiesen T (1997) Adult nestin-expressing subependymal cells differentiate to astrocytes in response to brain injury. Eur J Neurosci 9:65-75.

Hu M, Krause D, Greaves M, Sharkis S, Dexter M, Heyworth C, Enver T (1997) Multilineage gene expression precedes commitment in the hemopoeitic system. Genes Dev 11:774-785.

Hussy N (2002) Glial cells in the hypothalamo-neurohypophyseal system: key elements of the regulation of neuronal electrical and secretory activity. Prog Brain Res 139:95-112.

Iozzo RV (1998) Matrix proteoglycans: from molecular design to cellular function. Annu Rev Biochem 67:609-652.

Irvin DK, Zurcher SD, Nguen T, Weinmaster G, Kornblum HI (2001) Expression patterns of Notch1, Notch2, and Notch3 suggest multiple functional roles for the Notch-DSL signaling system during brain development. J Comp Neurol 436:167-181.

Ishihara S, Sawada M, Chang L, Kim JM, Brightman M (1993) Brain vessels near muscle autografts are sites for entry of isogenic macrophages in brain. Exp Neurol 124:219-230.

Ishikawa K, Kabeya K, Shinoda M, Katakai M, Mori M, Tatemoto K (1995) Meninges play a neurotrophic role in the regeneration of vasopressin nerves after hypophysectomy. Brain Res 677:20-28.

John GR, Lee SC, Brosnan CF (2003) Cytokines: powerful regulators of glial cell activation. Neuroscientist 9:10-22.

Johanson CE, Palm DE, Primiano MJ, Chan P, Knuckey NW, Stopa EG (2000) Choroid plexus recovery after transient forebrain ischemia: role of growth factors and other repair gmechanisms. Cell Mol Neurobiol 20:197-216.

Johansson CB, Momma S, Clarke DL, Risling M, Lendahl U, Frisen J (1999) Identification of a neural stem cell in the adult mammalian central nervous system. Cell 96:25-34.

Kacem K, Lacombe P, Seylaz J, Bonvento G (1998) Structural organization of the perivascular astrocyte endfeet and their and their relationship with the endothelial glucose transporter: a confocal microscopy study. Glia 23;1-10.

Khan S, Wigley C (1994) Different effects of a macrophage cytokine on proliferation in astrocytes and Schwann cells. Neuroreport 5:1381-1385.

Kitada M, Chakrabortty S, matsumoto N, Taketomi M, Ide C (2001) Differentiation of choroids plexus ependymal cells into astrocytes after grafting into the pre-lesioned spinal cord in mice. Glia 36:364-374.

Kondo T, Raff M (2000) Oligodendrocyte precurosr cells reprogrammed to become multipotential CNS stem cells. Science 289:1754-1757.

Laywell ED, Rakic P, Kukekov VG, Holland EC, Steindler DA (2000) Identification of a multipotent astrocytic stem cell in the immature and adult mouse brain. Proc Natl Acad Sci 97:13883-13888.

Leavitt BR, Hernit-Grant CS, Macklis JD (1999) Mature astrocytes transform into transitional radial glia within adult mouse neocortex that supports directed migration of transplanted immature neurons. Exp Neurol 157:43-57.

Leong SK, Ling EA (1992) Amoeboid and ramified microglia: Their interrelationship and response to brain injury. Glia 6:39-47.

Lin TJ, Hirji N, Stenton GR, Gilchrist M, Grill BJ, Schreiber AD, Befus AD (2000) activation of macrophage CD8: pharmacological studies of TNF and IL-1 beta production. J Immunol 164:1783-1792.

Ling EA, Kaur C, Lu j (1998) Origin, nature, and some functional considerations of intraventricular macrophages, with special reference to the epiplexus cells. Microsc Res Tech 41:43-56.

Ling EA, Wong WC (1993) The origin and nature of ramified and amoeboid microglia: a historical review and current concepts. Glia 7:9-18.

Liour SS, Yu RK (2003) Differentiation of radial glia-like cells from embryonic stem cells. Glia 42:109--117.

Lois C, Garcia-Verdugo JM, Alvarez-Buylla A (1996) Chain migration of neuronal precursors. Science 271:978-981.

Malatesta P, Hartfuss E, Gotz M (2000) Isolation of radial glial cells by fluorescent-activated cell sorting reveals a neuronal lineage. Development 127:5253-5263.

Martins-Green M. 2000. Dynamics of cell-ECM interactions. In: Principles of tissue Engineering. Academic Press, Elsevier Bioscience, Amsterdam, pp. 33-55.

Mercier F, Kitasako JT, Hatton GI (2003) Fractones and other basal laminae in the hypothalamus. J Comp Neurol 455: 324-340.

Mason JL, Suzuki K, Chaplin DD, Matsushima GK (2001) Interleukin-1β promotes repair of the CNS. J Neurosci 21:7046-7052.

Mercier F, Hatton GI (2000) Immunocytochemical basis for a meningeo-glial network. J Comp Neurol 420:445-465.

Mercier F, Hatton GI (2001) Connexin 26 and basic fibroblast growth factor are expressed primarily in the subpial and subependymal layers in adult brain parenchyma: roles in stem cell proliferation and morphological plasticity? J Comp Neurol 431:88-104.

Mercier F, Hatton GI (2004) Meninges and perivasculature as mediators of CNS Plasticity. In:Non-neuronal cells in the nervous system: function and dysfunction. EE Bittar, ed., L. Hertz volume ed.; Elsevier Science B.V., Amsterdam; Adv. Mol. Cell Biol 31:215-254.

Mercier F, Kitasako JT, Hatton GI (2002) Anatomy of the brain neurogenic zones revisited: fractones and the fibroblast /macrophage network. J Comp Neurol 451:170-188.

Mezey E, Chandross KJ, Harta G, Maki RA, McKercher SR (2000) Turning blood into brain: cells bearing neuronal antigens generated in vivo from bone marrow. Science 290:1779-1782.

Mezey E, Key S, Vogelsang G, Szalayova I, Lange GD, Cain B (2003) Transplanted bone marrow generates new neurons in human brain. Proc Nat Acad Sci 100:1364-1369.

Mi H, Haeberle H, Barres BA. 2001. Induction of astrocyte differentaition by endothelial cells J Neurosci 21:1538-1547.

Mugnaini E (1986) Cell junctions of astrocytes, ependymal cells and related cells in the mammalian central nervous system, with emphasis on the hypothesis of a generalized functional syncytium of supporting cells. In: Astrocytes, Vol 1, Federov S, Vernadakis A Eds, Orlando Acad Press: pp 329-371.

Murphy S (2000) Production of nitric oxide by glial cells. Glia 29:1-14.

Noctor SC, Flint AC, Weissmann TA, Dammerman RS, Kriegstein AR (2001) Neurons derived from radial glial cells establish radial unita in neocortex. Nature 109:714-720.

Norton WT, Aquino DA, Hozumi I, Chiu FC, Brosnan CF (1992) Quantitative aspects of reactive gliosis: a review. Neurochem Res 17:877-885.

O'Rahilly R, Muller F (1986) The meninges in human development. J Neuropathol Exp Neurol 45:588-608.

Pasterkamp RJ, Verhaagen J (2001) Emerging roles for semaphorins in neural regeneration Brain Res Rev 35:36-54.

Pender MP, Rist MJ (2001) Apoptosis of inflammatory cells in immune control of the nervous system: role of glia. Glia 36:137-144.

Peters A, Palay SL, Webster HD (1991) The fine structure of the nervous system: the neurons and supporting cells. Philadelphia: WB Saunders.

Pouly S, Becher B, Blain M, Antel JP (1999) Expression of a homologue of rat NG2 on human microglia. Glia 27:259-268.

Prat A, Biernacki K, Wosik K, Antel JP (2001) Glial cell influence on the human blood brain barrier. Glia 36:145-155.

Rakic P (1988) Specification of cerebral cortical areas. Science 241:170-176.

Rash JE, Yasumura T, Davidson KG, Furman CS, Dudek FE, Nagy JI (2001) Identification of cells expressing Cx43, Cx30, Cx26, Cx32, and Cx36 in gap junctions of rat brain and spinal cord. Cell Com Adhes 8:315-320.

Ramon-Cueto A, Avila G (1998) Olfactory ensheathing glia: properties and function. Brain Res Bul 46:175-187.

Reilly JF, Maher PA, Kumari VG (1998) Regulation of astrocyte GFAP expression by TGF-β1 and FGF-2. Glia 22:202-210.

Reiland J, Rapraeger AC (1993) Heparan sulfate proteoglycan and FGF receptor target basic FGF to different intracellular destinations. J Cell Sci 105:1085-1093.

Reynolds BA, Weiss S (1992) Generation of neurons and astrocytes from isolated cells of the adult mammalian central nervous system. Science 255:1707-1710.

Roberts R, Gallagher J, Spooncer E, Allen DT, Bloomfield F, Dexter TM (1988) Heparan sulfate bound growth factors: a mechanism for stromal cell mediated haemopoeisis. Nature 332:376-378.

Rubin LL, Staddon JM (1999) The cell biology of the blood brain barrier. Annu Rev Neurosci 22:11-28.

Safavi-Abbasi S, Wolff JR, Missler M (2001) Rapid morphological changes in astrocytes are accompanied by redistribution but not by quantitative changes of cytoskeletal proteins. Glia 36:102-115.

Seri B, Garcia-Verdugo JM, McEwen BS, Alvarez-Buylla A (2001) Astrocytes give rise to new neurons in the adult mammalian hippocampus. J Neurosci 21:7153-7160.

Schwartz M, Cohen I (2000) Autoimmunity can benefit self maintenance. Immunol Today 21:265-268.

Schober A, Bottner M, Strelau J, Kinscherf R, Bonaterra GA, Barht M, Schilling L, Fairlie WD, Breit SN, Unsicker K (2001) Expression of growth differentiation factor-15/macrophage inhibitory ctokie-1 (GDF-15/MIC-1) in the perinatal, adult, and injured rat brain. J Comp Neurol 439:32-45.

Sievers J, Pehleman FW, Gude S, Berry M (1994) Meningeal cells organize the superficial glia limitans of the cerebellum and produce components of both the interstitial matrix and the basement membrane. J neurocytol 23:135-149.

Silverman AJ, Sutherland AK, Wilhelm M, Silver R (2000) Mast cells migrate from blood to brain. J Neurosci 20:401-408.

Spohr TCLDE, Martinez R, da Silva EF, Neto VM, Gomes FCA (2002) Neuro-glia interaction effects on GFAP gene: a novel role for transforming growth factor-beta 1. Eur J Neurosci 16:2059-2069.

Spray DC, Moreno AP, Kessler JA, Dermietzel R (1991) Characterization of gap junctions between cultured leptomeningeal cells. Brain Res 568:1-14.

Steindler DA, Kukekov VG, Brannon Thomas L, Filmore H, Suslov O, Scheffler B, O'Brien TF, Kusakabe M, Laywell ED (1998) Boundary molecules during brain development, injury, and persistent neurogenesis- in vivo and in vitro studies. Prog Brain Res 117:179-196.

Stichel CC, Hermanns S, Luhmann HJ, Lausberg F, Niermann H, D'urso D, Servos G, Hartwig HG, Muller HV (1999) Inhibition of collagenIV deposition promotes regenration of injured CNS axons. Eur J Neurosci 11:632-646.

Stopa EG, Berzin TM, Kim S, Song P, Kuo-Leblanc V, Rodriguez-Wolf M, Baird A, Johanson CE (2001) Human choroid plexus growth factors: what are the implications for CSF dynamics in Alzheimer's disease? Exp Neurol 167: 40-47.

Struckhoff G (1995) Cocultures of meningeal and astrocytic cells. A model for the formation of the glial-limiting membrane. Int J Dev Neurosci 13:595-606.

Struckhoff G, Turzynski A (1995) Demonstration of parathyroid hormone-related protein in meninges and its receptor in astrocytes: evidence for a paracrine meningo-astrocytic loop. Brain Res 676:1-9.

Sutor B (2002) Gap junctions and their implications for neurogenesis and maturation of synaptic circuitry in the developing neocortex. Results Probl Cell Differ 39:53-73.

Terada N, Hamazaki T, Oka M, Hoki M, Mastarlez DM, Nakano Y, Meyer EM, Morel L, Peterson BE, Scott EW (2002) Bone marrow cells adopt the phenotype of other cells by spontaneous cell fusion. Nature 416:542-545.

Thomas WE (1999) Brain macrophages: on the role of pericytes and perivascular cells. Brain Res Rev 31:42-57.

Tsuchihashi Y, Kitamura T, Fujita S (1981) Immunofluorescence studies on the monocytes in the injured rat brain. Acta Neuropathol (Berl) 53:213-219.

Ullian EM, Sapperstein SK, Christopherson KS, Barres BA (2001) Control of synapse number by glia. Science 291:657-661.

Unsicker K, Flanders KC, Cissel DS, Lafyatis R, Sporn MB (1991) Transforming growth factor beta isoforms in the adult rat central and peripheral nervous system. Neuroscience 44: 613-625.

Vassilopoulos G, Wang PR, Russell DW (2003) Transplanted bone marrow regenerates liver by cell fusion. Nature 422:901-904.

Wagers AJ, Sherwood RI, Christensen JL, Weissman IL (2002) Little evidence for developmental plasticity of adult hematopoietic stem cells. Science 297:2256-2259.

Wang X, Willenbring H, Akkari Y, Torimaru Y, Foster M, Al-Dhalimy M, Lagasse E, Finegold M, Olson S, Grompe M (2003) Cell fusion is the principal source of bone-marrow-derived hepatocytes. Nature 422:897-901.

Watanabe M, Toyama Y, Nishiyyama A (2002) differentiation of proliferated NG2-positive glial progenitor cells in a remyelinating lesion. J Neurosci Res 69:826-836.

Weiss S, Dunne C, Hewson J, Wohl C, Wheatley M, Peterson AC, Reynolds BA (1996) Multipotent CNS stem cells are present in the adult mammalian spinal cord and ventricular neuroaxis. J Neurosci 16:7599-7609.

Williams KC, Hickey WF (2002) Central nervous system damage, monocytes and macrophages,and neurological disorders in AIDS. Annu Rev Neurosci 25:537-562.

Winkler S, Stahl RC, Carey DJ, Bansal R (2002) Syndecan-3 and perlecan are differentially expressed by progenitors and mature oligodendrocytes and accumulate in the extracellular matrix. J Neurosci Res 69:477-487.

Wong, ML, Bongiorno PB al-Shekhlee A, Esposito A, Khatri P, Licinio J (1996) IL-1 beat, Il-1 receptor type I and iNOS gene expression in rat brain vasculature and perivascular areas. Neuroreport 7:2445-2448.

Woodburry D, Schwarz EJ, Prockop DJ, Black IB (2000) Adult rat and human bone marrow stromal cells differentiate into neurons. J Neurosci Res 61:364-370.

Woodburry D, Reynolds K, Black IB (2002) Adult bone marrow stromal cells express germline, ectodermal, endodermal, and mesodermal gens prior to neurogenesis. J Neurosci Res 96:908-917.

Wu JP, Kuo JS, Liu YL, Tzeng SF (2000) Tumor necrosis factor-alpha modulates the proliferation of neural progenitors in the subventricular/ventricular zone of adult rat brain. Neurosci Let 292-203-206.

Yasin SA, Costa A, Forsling ML, Grossman A (1994) Interleukin-1β and interleukin-6 stimulate neurohypophyseal hormone release in vitro. J Neuroendocrinol 2:179-184.

Zerlin M, Goldman JE (1997) Interactions between glial progenitors and blood vessels during early postnatal corticogenesis: blood vessel contact represents an early stage of astrocyte differentiation. J Comp Neurol 387:537-546.

Zhao Y, Glesne D, Huberman E (2003) A human peripheral blood monocyte-derived subset acts as pluripotent stem cells. Proc Nat Acad Sci 100:2426-2431.

5.7. Abbreviations

A cells	Pre-migrating neuroblasts
bFGF	Basic fibroblast growth factor
BL	Basal lamina
BV	Blood vessel
CSF	Cerebrospinal fluid
CSPG	Chondroitin sulfate proteoglycans
Cx	Connexin
ECM	Extracellular matrix
GFAP	Glial fibrillary acidic protein
GF	Growth factors
GL	Glia limitans
HSPG	Heparan sulfate proteoglycans
IF	Iintermediate filaments
IFN-γ	Interferon gamma
IL1-β	Interleukin-1-beta
IL-6	Interleukin-6
MHC	Major histocompatibility complex
mHNS	Magnocellular hypothalamo-neurohypophysial system
MCP-1	Monocyte chemoattractant protein-1
NSC	Neural stem cells
NOS	Nitric oxide synthase
RMS	Rostral migratory stream
TGFβ−1	Transforming growth factor beta-1
TNF-α	Tumor necrosis factor-alpha

Chapter 6

Expression and possible functions of glutamate and GABA receptors in glial cells from the hippocampus

Min Zhou and Harold K. Kimelberg[*]

Neural and Vascular Biology Theme, Ordway Research Institute, 150 New Scotland Ave. Albany, NY 12208 USA

*Corresponding author: hkimelberg@ordwayresearch.org

Contents

6.1. Introduction

It is now quite clear that glial cells of all types have receptors. This is hardly surprising since it is the way that all cells sense their environment. However, their first identification some years ago in cultured and isolated glia (Reviewed by Kimelberg 1988; Porter and McCarthy, 1997) were surprising results to neuroscientists who had taken the biologically unsupportable view that only neurons had receptors since this was the way in which one neuron signaled to another. However, the implied perplexity here, why would glia have receptors still remains with us when we are asked the question but what do receptors on glia do? The problem is really that we are putting the cart before the horse, which although horses can push is not the most efficient arrangement for this type of conveyance. We are still trying to find out to a very large extent what glia do and then, although it will not be an epiphany, the functions of glial receptors will likely come into clearer focus. Another general horse and cart problem is that currently in biomedical research we are always asked to come up with a hypothesis for every investigation. This implies that we always know what we are in fact searching for and simply need to test it. This makes for difficulties in glial research where we do not seem to have an adequate database upon which reasonable hypotheses can be proposed. If we admit we are only looking for reliable data we will be criticized for being on a fishing expedition and thus in glial research we have to pretend that we know a lot more than we really do and that our experiments are more precise than they really are. Parenthetically the objective of a fishing expedition is very clear, it is to catch fish and, depending on the tackle, bait and location we will have a pretty good idea which fish we will catch. Only if ichthyology was a new science, perhaps like "glia", would our catch be completely determined by chance aspects of our catching device. For example, in the astrophysicist Eddingtons's fishing-net parable for scientific investigations, a pioneering ichthyologist concludes from his catches that no sea creature is less than two inches long, obviously because his net can't catch anything smaller. Eddington makes the point that the net is analogous to "the sensory and intellectual equipment which we use" for obtaining "the body of knowledge" (Eddington 1939). A related problem is that the classification of glia are also "studies in progress" so often we are not sure what "glia" we are studying, and much like ichthyology or any other scientific field we need to sufficiently systematize before we can analyze.

Because of the considerations mentioned in the preceding paragraph no one can at present write a complete systematic review of the receptors on glia. Nor do we here even attempt a complete review of the work-to-date, because the amount of work done in different experimental systems over the past three decades precludes a reasonable treatment within the space constraints. Also this has been reviewed at several times during the time span of the field (Kimelberg 1995b; Porter and McCarthy, 1997; Verkhratsky and Steinhäuser, 2000), and a broader review covering all regions of the brain makes it even more difficult to relate the data (form) to function. We also believe that the answers to the questions outlined in the first paragraph, what receptors are on glia *in situ* and what do they do, can heuristically better be answered in a more defined region of the brain whose physiology and functions are well characterized. Therefore we focus on a specific region of the rat brain, the hippocampus, and mainly the CA1 region, to ask what glutamate and GABA receptors (GABARs) are present on the glial cells in this region and what could be their functions. The glia present in the CA1 are predominantly glial fibrillary acidic protein (GFAP) immunoreactive positive astrocytes (GFAP(+)) and the more enigmatic GFAP(-)/NG2(+)cells, possibly oligodendrocyte precursors or astrocyte precursors or both and also known as O2-A cells (ffrench-Constant and Raff, 1986; Dawson et al, 2000). We have studied both of these cells electrophysiologically and we have mainly used freshly (acutely) isolated cells, which eschew the problems of recording from individual cells in slices of rapid desensitization of receptors because of slow diffusion, indirect effects from neighboring cells and voltage clamp problems because of the astrocyte syncytium.

Correlative immunocytochemistry is also presented in some cases. The problems of extrapolating from the culture systems, which offer the same experimental advantages as isolated cells and are easier to prepare in much greater quantities and with assured viability, has been investigated or mentioned by several authors (e.g. Kimelberg et al 1997; Porter and McCarthy 1997; Walz 2002).

6.2. Astroglia in freshly isolated preparations

6.2.1. GFAP (+) astrocytes isolated from CA1

We have observed two types of morphologically identical GFAP(+) astrocytes in our isolated preparations which differ in their expression of AMPA receptors (AMPARs) but are similar in their GABARs (Zhou and Kimelberg, 2000, 2001). These also correlate with the presence of predominantly outward K^+ currents plus small Na^+ currents, or outward and inward K^+ currents and no Na^+ currents. We have termed these ORAs (for outwardly rectifying astrocytes) and VRAs (for variably rectifying astrocytes), respectively. There is also heterogeneity in regard to several other properties measured electrophysiologically, such as the presence and absence of glutamate transporter currents. These data are summarized in table 1. The appearance and GFAP staining of the cells, which can be distinguished morphologically, and their typical cation currents are shown in Figs. 6. 1., and 6. 2., respectively.

6.2.2. GFAP(-)/NG2(+) glial cells isolated from CA1

Steinhäuser et al (1994) originally described electrophysiologically "complex" cells in the hippocampus and in isolated cells from the hippocampus which had very similar cation currents to those we later described for ORAs (Zhou and Kimelberg, 2000, 2001, and see Chapter 7). We have found that these "complex" cells are GFAP(-) but express mRNA for GFAP (Zhou et al, 2000). More recently we have also found that these "complex" glial cells are NG2(+) (Schools et al, 2003). The NG2 staining and lack of GFAP staining for these cells is illustrated in Fig. 6.1C. Typical currents for isolated GFAP(-)/NG2(+) cells are shown in Fig. 6.2C and resemble those of ORAs except for the expression of a significantly higher density of K^+_{DR} currents. Also the K^+_A currents typically show less desensitization. These cells were originally termed smooth protoplasmic astrocytes based on their morphology (Levine and Card, 1997). They have been renamed oligodendrocyte precursor cells or O2A cells based on expression of certain marker proteins and lineage studies, particularly in culture but also to a limited extent *in situ* (Dawson et al, 2000). These cells show both glutamate and GABARs (Zhou et al, 2000), but do not express glutamate transporter 1(GLT-1) or L-glutamate/L-aspartate transporter (GLAST) proteins (Schools, Zhou and Kimelberg, unpublished observations, 2003). Some of these data are summarized in table 1 to compare the GFAP(-)/NG2(+) complex cells with ORAs and VRAs.
Bergles et al (2000) have shown that some terminals make synapses on NG2(+) cells *in situ*. Together GFAP(+) astrocytes and the NG2(+) glial cells and their processes fill a large part of the neuropil between interneurons and pyramidal cell processes in the CA1 region (Ogata and Kosaka 2002; Levine and Card 1987).

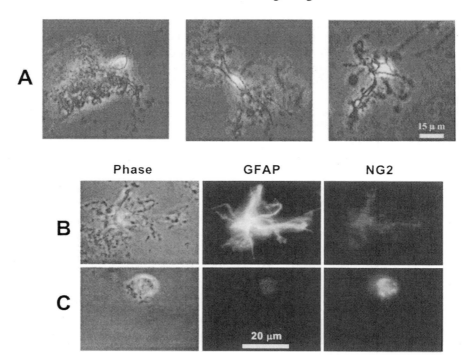

Figure 6.1. Morphology and GFAP/NG2 double staining of freshly isolated astroglia from hippocampal CA1. A, Three examples of phase micrographs of freshly isolated bushy astrocytes from P12 rats (scale bar in the right micrograph applies to all the images on the upper panel, modified from Zhou and Kimelberg, 2000). B and C, are GFAP/NG2 double staining of freshly isolated CA1 cells shows that the bushy and thicker process-bearing glia (B), and the "complex" morphology cell (C) stained for GFAP and NG2, respectively. There was no overlap in GFAP and NG2 immunoreactivities between these two cell populations. The change of morphologies in the fixed cells in B and C as compared to live cells in A, particularly the collapsed processes of the GFAP(-)/NG2(+) cells, could be due to fixation and other steps in the staining procedure. The scale bar in the middle of C applies to all the images in B and C.

6.2.3. Validity of isolated glia

As noted, the isolated glia offer advantages for direct and rapid assessment of the effects of transmitters and other substances without the unknown variable of phenotypic changes induced by culturing. However, the opposite face is to what extent damage occurs, such as proteolytic digestion of surface proteins and loss of fine processes. The evaluation of mRNA by single-cell reverse transcriptase-polymerase chain reaction (SC-RT-PCR) is unlikely to be affected by either of these but, of course, mRNA expression does not mean functional protein is being synthesized. The SC-RT-PCR also allows cell to cell variability to be assessed and a similar advantage, as well as measurement of functional protein by activity, applies to single cell patch-clamp electrophysiology. In terms of comparisons between the isolated cells and cells *in situ,* capacitance measurements of the isolated GFAP(+)

cells reassuringly give similar results to the few measurements done *in situ*. Thus the average value recorded by Bordey and Sontheimer (1997) for astrocyte in hippocampal slices was 27.5 pF (ranging from 7 pF to 100 pF). This average is between the two mean values of 9.5 and 34 pF for ORAs and VRAs, respectively (Zhou and Kimelberg, 2002). This agreement is surprising because the processes of astroglia end in finer and finer velate processes (Kosaka and Hama, 1986; Ogata and Kosaka, 2002; Bushong et al, 2002) and these cannot be detected in phase micrographs of our preparations. It may well be that the capacitance measurements *in situ* are limited by the slow movement of current into the finer processes because of their small cross-sectional areas and therefore high resistances.

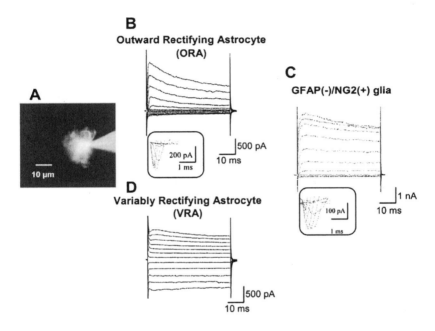

Figure 6.2. A, fluorescence micrograph of a freshly isolated astrocyte filled during recording with Lucifer yellow dye, (0.3% in the pipette), showing bushy processes extending from the cell body. B, C and D, membrane currents in the different cell types induced by 50 ms duration voltage steps from −160 mV to +60 mV in 20 mV increments. GFAP(+) ORAs (B) are characterized by a dominant expression of outward I_{K+A} and I_{K+DR} plus small inward I_{Na+} currents (see inset below B). The ion current profile of NG2(+) glia (C) is qualitatively similar to ORAs in terms of K^+ and Na^+ current expression. However, the outward K^+ currents showed an atypical slower desensitization than expected from the K^+_A component obtained after current subtraction (not shown). Also the density of K^+_A is significantly higher than the ORAs (Schools, Zhou and Kimelberg, unpublished observation, 2003). VRAs (D) are characterized by a symmetric expression of inward and outward K^+ currents that consist of a mixture of predominantly K^+_{OHM} with small contributions by K^+_A and K^+_{DR}, but exhibit no Na^+ currents.

The average membrane capacitance of the NG2(+) complex cells was found to be 11.4 pF for cells from P10 and 9.6 pF for cells from P25 rats (Schools et al, 2002). No values have been published for NG2(+) glia *in situ*. Thus we are led to conclude that electrophysiological measurements will likely give similar results for GFAP(+) astrocytes in the isolated preparations and *in situ* because the patch-clamp technique will not record from the finest processes, and perhaps the same applies to the NG2(+) glia. Whether there are components localized exclusively to the finest velate processes can only be determined by high resolution microscopy *in situ* as has recently been done for the actin binding proteins ezrin and radixin (Derouiche and Frotscher, 2001 and Chapter 3).

Table 6.1. Comparison of properties of GFAP(+) ORAs, VRAs astrocyte subtypes, and GFAP(-)/NG2(+) cells

Properties	VRAs	ORAs	GFAP(-)/NG2(+)
K$^+$ uptake channels	Present	Negligible	Negligible
Sodium current (I_{Na+})	Absent	Present	Present
Glutamate transporter currents	Present	Absent	ND
AMPAR currents	Negligible	Present	Present
GABA$_A$ currents	Present	Present	Present
Swelling activated chloride currents (I_{Swell, Cl^-})	Absent	Present	ND
ClC-2	Present*	Absent*	ND

Data from Zhou and Kimelberg 2000, 2001, 2002, and Zhou et al, 2000. ND: not determined. *: Unpublished observations (Zhou and Kimelberg, 2003).

6.3. Astrocytic glutamate receptors

6.3.1. NMDA receptors

The issue of whether astrocytes express N-methyl-D-aspartate (NMDA) receptors is still unresolved. Early *in situ* patch-clamp recordings from hippocampal slices revealed currents in astrocytes after application of NMDA (Steinhäuser et al, 1994b). However, it is always possible that these were due to secondary activation of astrocyte receptors by substances released from neurons upon activation of their NMDA receptors, as Seifert and Steinhäuser (1995) found no NMDA mediated - currents in astrocytes isolated from the same hippocampal region. In addition, later studies on astrocytes in tissue slices from the spinal cord showed that the effect might not be due to NMDA receptors at all, as the currents were insensitive to changes in glycine and extracellular Mg^{2+} concentrations (Ziak et al, 1998). However, recent studies using Ca^{2+} imaging with confocal microscopy suggest that NMDA receptors may be densely located on the distal processes of astrocytes (Schipke et al, 2001)

6.3.2. Diverse expression of AMPARs by astrocytes

The identification of AMPARs in cultured astrocytes by Bowman and Kimelberg (1984) and Kettenmann and Schachner (1985) provided the initial impetus for exploration of glutamate receptors in astrocyte in slices, which confirmed that astrocytes in a number of brain regions do express AMPARs (see review by Steinhäuser and Gallo, 1996). AMPARs on astrocytes in different regions were found to be composed of different subunits. AMPARs on neurons are generally impermeable to Ca^{2+}, however, the AMPAR expressed by Bergmann glia in cerebellum showed marked Ca^{2+} permeability due to lack of the GluR2 subunit (Muller et al, 1992), and a population of S100β(+) astrocytes in the hippocampus expressed AMPARs with moderate Ca^{2+} permeability (Seifert and Steinhäuser, 1995). Thus, astrocytic AMPARs in different brain regions can be varyingly permeable to Ca^{2+}. As demonstrated by Porter and McCarthy (1995), stimulation of the neuronal afferent Schaffer-collaterals to CA1, resulted in AMPAR and metabotropic glutamate receptor (mGluR) mediated intracellular Ca^{2+} increases and oscillations. Such Ca^{2+} oscillations have been suggested as a mechanism for astrocytic-specific long-range and slow signal transmission (Parri et al, 2001; Aguado et al, 2002 and Chapters 13-15).

For the ionotropic AMPAR expression, it has been clearly shown that functional AMPARs are well-expressed by both GFAP(+) ORAs (Zhou and Kimelberg, 2001) and the GFAP(-)/NG2(+) glia (Seifert and Steinhäuser, 1995; Seifert et al, 1997; Bergles et al, 2000)(see Fig. 6.3). Both cell types also express predominantly voltage-gated outward K^+ and inward Na^+ channels, whereas the GFAP(+) astrocytes lacking or showing far fewer voltage-gated ion channels show a negligible expression (Zhou and Kimelberg, 2001), or are completely devoid of AMPAR currents when measured in excised patches from the astrocyte soma (Bergles and Jahr, 1997). An important caveat here is that, from their whole cell recordings, Bergles and Jahr (1997) recorded from astrocytes that only showed marked voltage- and time- independent inward and outward K^+ currents (i.e. VRA type or completely passive cells showing ohmic K^+ conductances). Although other workers recording from hippocampal GFAP (+) astrocytes *in situ* have shown cells with ORA-type currents (Bordey and Sontheimer , 1997), or dye-coupled hippocampal astrocytes that express Na^+ currents (Carmignoto et al, 1998), the two diverse populations of ORAs and VRAs showing all the differences we find in isolated cells have not yet been identified *in situ*. Our present view is that their different NG2 and GFAP staining shows ORAs and the GFAP(-)/NG2(+) ("complex") cells to be different populations. The postnatal developmental regulation of astrocytic AMPAR has been studied only for GFAP(-)/NG2(+) glia (Seifert et al, 1997; Zhou et al, 2000), which most likely represents the oligodendrocyte progenitor cells (OPCs) as defined by their positive NG2 immunoreactivity (Bergles et al, 2000).

6.3.3. AMPARs change during development

The AMPA receptors of the GFAP(-)/NG2(+) glia show increased current densities, likely attributable to the switch from flop to flip splicing variants, during development (Seifert et al, 1997). Interestingly, these cells also express pronounced voltage-gated outward K^+ currents (I_{K+OUT}) which are down-regulated during postnatal development (Kressin et al, 1995). Other studies have shown that blockade of I_{K+OUT} inhibits the proliferation /differentiation of oligodendrocyte progenitor cells (Gallo et al, 1996; Liu and Almazan 1995; LoTurco et al, 1995) and I_{K+OUT} can be inhibited upon AMPAR activation via a Na^+-dependent mechanism (Borges and Kettenmann 1995; Jabs et al, 1994). The functional significance of these different developmental patterns is presently unknown. It is noteworthy that co-expression of AMPARs with I_{K+OUT} is not a unique feature of NG2(+) glia as we found that GFAP(+) ORAs also show both of them (Zhou and Kimelberg, 2001), and these features persist in freshly isolated ORAs, at least until postnatal day 35. How AMPAR activation may be involved in synaptic transmission and plasticity through release of D-serine is discussed later.

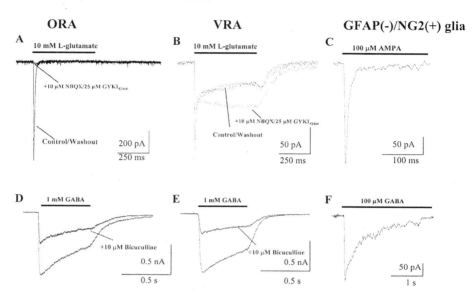

Figure 6.3. Differential expression of glutamate transporter and AMPAR currents, but qualitatively similar expression of GABA$_A$R currents by GFAP(+) ORAs, VRAs and GFAP (-)/NG2(+) glia. A, B, recordings with NO$_3^-$ as the major intracellular anion, 10 mM glutamate (Glu) (at -70 mV) evoked a fast activating and rapidly desensitizing inward current in ORAs (blue trace in A). The response to the same Glu application in VRA showed the initial transient plus a substantial steady-state current during the 0.5 s Glu pulse (blue traces in B). The selective AMPAR antagonists, NBQX (10 μM) + GYKI$_{52466}$ (25 μM), completely blocked the Glu-induced current in an ORA (red trace in A). In the VRA, however, the same antagonists reduced the initial peak current by only 34% and potentiated the steady-state current by 40% (red trace in B). C, AMPAR mediated current induced by the addition of 100 μM AMPA to a GFAP(-) complex glial cell. The cell was clamped at -70 mV with standard (140 mM) KCl electrode solution.   D and E are superimposed traces of recordings from an ORA and a VRA at a holding potential of -70 mV. A 0.5 second 1 mM GABA pulse induced robust inward currents in both of cells with a quite similar desensitization time course (red traces). When the GABA$_A$R antagonist bicuculline (10 μM) was co-applied with 1 mM GABA similar inhibition of GABA-induced currents were found (blue). F, shows a 100 μM GABA-induced current from a GFAP(-)/NG2(+) glia. The duration of GABA exposure was 3 s and the recording condition was the same as for GFAP(+) ORA and VRA in D and E.

Isolated GFAP(-)/NG2(+) "complex "glia (Steinhäuser et al,1994, Zhou et al, 2000) may represent NG2(+) OPCs in the hippocampus (Schools et al 2002). Here another interesting role of the AMPAR is to directly receive glutamatergic inputs, as shown by the measurement of excitatory postsynaptic potentials (EPSPs) upon

Schaffer collateral axon stimulation or the occurrence of spontaneous miniature excitatory postsynaptic potentials (mEPSPs) in OPCs (Bergles et al, 2000). Although the functional significance of neuronal glutamate signaling to OPCs awaits elucidation, the developmental up-regulation in the glutamate current densities (Seifert et al, 1997) suggests an enhanced capability of OPCs to receive neuronal glutamate signaling with maturation. The developmental alternation of splice variants of AMPAR subunits, specifically the switch from flop to flip version, implies a prolonged receptor channel pore opening, which may cause more Ca^{2+} influx at later developmental stages. How the Ca^{2+} rise upon AMPAR activation differs from those commonly seen in GFAP(+) astrocytes and mediated by astrocytic mGluR activation, and whether activation of the AMPARs on OPCs results in OPCs sending back signals to neurons after they are activated by neuronally released glutamate also requires further study is yet to be determined. (also see Chapter 15).

6.3.4. Metabotropic glutamate receptors

A thorough survey of the expression of the different mGluR mRNAs in GFAP mRNA(+) isolated hippocampal astrocytes by single cell RT-PCR showed expression only of the mGluR3 and 5 isoforms (Schools and Kimelberg, 1999 and Fig. 6.4). A good correspondence of these mGluR 3 and 5 mRNAs with their encoded proteins has been demonstrated by a series of follow-up studies. For mGluR3, a confocal immunocytochemisty study revealed that the mGluR3 proteins are present on a population of freshly isolated hippocampus GFAP(+) cells (Schools and Kimelberg 2001, and Fig. 6.5). Cai et al (1997, 2000) examined the developmental profiles of mGluR5 at both the mRNA level by RT-PCR and the functional level by Ca^{2+} imaging studies in freshly isolated GFAP(+) hippocampal astrocytes (Fig. 6.6). These data revealed that both mGluR5 mRNA and Ca^{2+} responses to mGluR5 agonists were down-regulated with increasing age. The significance of mGluR for developmental regulation may involve the formation of astrocyte processes and ensheathment of synapses by astrocytic lamellae, as Cornell-Bell et al (1990) showed that mGluR activation induces increased filopodia formation of the processes of astrocytes in primary culture (also see Chapter 4).

It seems likely that an intracellular Ca^{2+} rise due to mGluR activation is functionally associated with several potential physiological astrocyte functions. For example, it mediates the release of glutamate from astrocytes (Bezzi et al 1998) thereby modulating neuronal plasticity (Kang et al, 1998). An intracellular Ca^{2+} rise can also mediate the release of vasoactive agents thus coupling graded neuronal activities with blood flow supply (Alkayed et al, 1996, 1997). These functions will be covered in the penultimate section of this chapter. However, it should be noted that mGluR5 activation, measured by the intracellular Ca^{2+} rise in acute brain slices from different regions, is produced by a high intensity of neuronal afferent stimulation (Porter and McCarthy, 1996; Pasti et al, 1997, Kang et al, 1998). Thus the conditions under which it occurs *in situ* need to be more precisely defined.

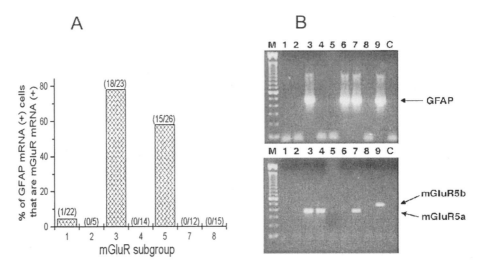

A

B

Figure 6.4.   A. The frequency of expression of mRNAs for the different metabotropic glutamate receptors (mGluR), except mGluR6, in freshly isolated astrocytes which also express mRNA for GFAP.   The ratios on the left (A) refer to the number of the cells expressing each mGluR mRNA over the total number of GFAP mRNA+ cells measured. All the cDNA was obtained after two rounds of PCR except for mGluR3 and 5, which were routinely detectable after one round. Data derived from Schools and Kimelberg (1999). B. Representative gels used for obtaining the data in A. Single cell RT-PCR for GFAP and mGluR5 was performed on single cells from P1-10 hippocampi. The lane aligned vertically in the upper and lower gels are PCR samples from the same cell. M and C represent 100-base pair ladder and media control, respectively.   Most P1-10 mGluR5 cells expressed the 5a alternative splice variant (87%), but 5b was also detected (cell 9).

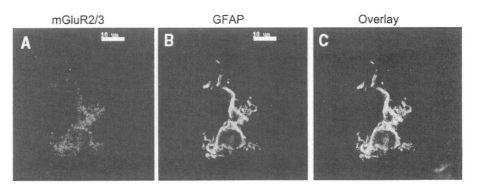

Figure 6.5.   A freshly isolated astrocyte from the hippocampal CA1 was double stained with mGluR 2/3 (red) and GFAP (green) antibodies and their subcellular staining signals were obtained on a laser scanning confocal microscope (Noran; Oz), respectively, based on their distinctive fluorescent excitation spectra.   The 3D images were reconstructed by image software (InterVision software).   The subcellular co-localization was done by overlay of the mGluR 2/3 and GFAP signals. The co-localization gives a yellow color (right panel).

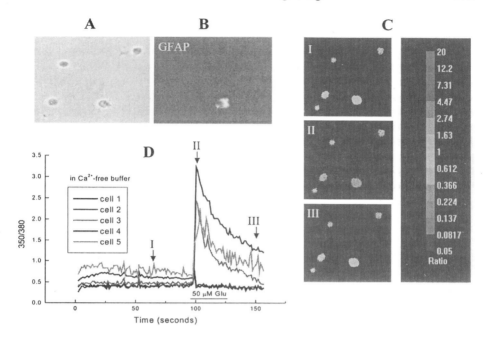

Figure 6.6. Expression of functional mGluR5 by GFAP(+) hippocampal astrocytes. The freshly isolated hippocampal cells were dispersed on poly-D-lysine coated coverslip, then loaded with 4 μM Fura2-AM. The calcium responses were to 50 μM glutamate (Glu) in cells isolated from a P12 rat. A: There are 5 cells in the field of which only cell 4 was positive for GFAP (B). C: 3 ratio images at different times (I-III) are shown. D: time course data derived from imaging data. Arrows mark the times corresponding to the images shown in C. The 350/380 axis refers to the dual excitation ratio.

6.4. Astrocytic GABA receptors

6.4.1. GABA$_A$Rs

The functional examination of GABA$_A$R-mediated currents and their pharmacology led to the clear conclusion that hippocampal glia, including GFAP(+) astrocytes (Fraser et al, 1995; Zhou and Kimelberg, 2001) and GFAP(-)/NG2(+) glia (Zhou et al, 2000) express ionotropic GABA$_A$Rs (Fig. 6. 3). There are a number of other brain regions where GABA$_A$Rs have been identified on glia, as reviewed by Verkhratsky and Steinhäuser (2000). Recent studies in these areas have concentrated on trying to answer two questions. The first question concerns the consequences of membrane potential changes upon GABA$_A$R activation, and the second is related to the possible activation of astrocytic GABA$_A$Rs *in situ*.

The issue of whether activation of GABA$_A$Rs in astrocytes, like neurons, hyperpolarizes, or instead depolarizes the membrane potential is essential to understanding the possible roles that these receptors may have. Cultured astrocytes express a Na$^+$/K$^+$/ 2Cl$^-$ cotransporter and Cl$^-$/HCO$_3^-$ exchanger. These mediate a constant inward transport of Cl$^-$ which maintains [Cl$^-$]$_i$ within a range of 30 to 40 mM (Kimelberg 1981). Because this high intracellular Cl$^-$ concentration gives rise to a rather positive equilibrium Cl⁻ potential (E_{Cl} =~-35 mV at $[Cl^-]_i/[Cl^-]_o$=35/140 mM) as compared to the resting membrane potential governed by E_K (-65 to –75 mV), it has been suggested that under resting membrane conditions GABA$_A$R activation may lead to membrane potential depolarization (see review by Kimelberg, 1990). Very recently, this assumption has been confirmed by a directly electrophysiological approach; perforated-patch recording with anion impermeable gramicidin as the ionophore for the purpose of preventing the $[Cl^-]_i$ being determined by the [Cl⁻] of the pipette solution. By measuring the reversal potential for GABA$_A$R under this condition, Bekar and Walz (2002) estimated that cultured astrocytes have a $[Cl^-]_i$ of 29 mM. Altogether, the results available so far favor a depolarizing role for astrocytic GABA$_A$R in terms of membrane potential changes, but so far this has only been determined for astrocyte in primary cultures. Freshly isolated GFAP(+) astrocytes (Fraser et al, 1995; Zhou and Kimelberg 2001) and astrocytes in hippocampal *in situ* (Steinhäuser et al, 1995; Jabs et al, 1994) also express GABA$_A$R. Using these preparations and the same electrophysiological approach as Bekar and Walz (2002) the issue of the $[Cl^-]_i$ of GFAP(+) astrocytes and the consequences of the activation of GABA$_A$R on the astrocytic membrane potential *in situ* should be resolved.

Another basic question about astrocytic GABA$_A$R function is where these receptors are located in relation to the likely GABA source; the terminals of GABAergic synapses. This concern has been raised since many astrocytic lamellae are relatively far away from postsynaptic sites and the affinity of astrocyte GABA$_A$R for GABA (EC$_{50}$=50μM) is about 3.6 fold lower than that of neurons (EC$_{50}$=14 μM) (Fraser et al, 1995). Moreover, given that astrocytes also express the functional high affinity Na⁺ dependent GABA transporter 1 (GAT-1) and 2/3 (GAT-2/3) (Zhao et al, 2000; Barakat and Bordey, 2002; Kinney and Spain, 2002), GABA diffusing from the synaptic cleft could be quickly removed by the astrocytic GABA transporters, or by GABA transporters located at neuronal postsynaptic sites. Concerning the location of astrocytic GABA$_A$Rs, a recent electron microscopic study revealed that these receptors were located at relatively high densities on the processes of Bergmann glia which enwrap inhibitory synapses (Riquelme et al, 2002). Another study addressed the issue of the functional availability of GABA transporters, measured electrophysiologically, in neocortical astrocytes by stimulating the nearby neocortical tissue ~100 μm away from the recorded astrocyte. Such stimulation resulted in an inward current comprised of both a receptor-mediated current and a GABA transporter current (Kinney and Spain, 2002). Although the stimulating current intensity was greater than is likely to be encountered physiologically, the results suggest that GABA$_A$R activation will occur upon synaptic activity of sufficient intensity.

Lin and Bergles (2001) have recently reported in an abstract that GABA$_A$R may mediate cross-talk between GABAergic neurons and NG2(+) glia as evoked inhibitory postsynaptic potentials (IPSPs) were found after electrical stimulation in the *stratum radiatum*. However, the low frequency of the evoked IPSP and the high intensity stimulation required led them to conclude that there was a low density of such synapses on the NG2(+) glia.

6.4.2. GABA$_B$Rs

Although early studies in cultured astrocytes showed the expression of GABA$_B$Rs (Hosli and Hosli, 1990; Nilsson et al, 1993), examination of astrocytes in slices or in isolated astrocytes did not confirm the existence of astrocytic GABA$_B$Rs *in situ* (Berger et al, 1992; Steinhäuser et al, 1994; Pastro et al, 1995; Fraser et al, 1995). However, a recent study supports the view that hippocampal astrocytes express metabotropic GABA$_B$R and that this receptor plays a critical role in modulation of inhibitory synaptic transmission (Kang et al, 1998).

6.5. Some plausible functions of astrocytic glutamate and GABA receptors

6.5.1. AMPARs and synaptic structure

It has been speculated for a long time that one function of astrocytes is to provide structural and functional support to neurons (see review by Somjen, 1988). Although there has been a relatively large amount of data accumulated on the homeostatic and metabolic roles of astrocytes, the precise mechanisms for how astrocytes interact with neurons and how critical this is to normal neuronal function has only emerged very recently. Astrocytic AMPARs have been suggested to be involved in these processes.

It has been shown that Bergmann glia express AMPARs which are Ca^{2+} permeable due to their lacking the GluR2 subunit (Muller et al, 1992, Burnashev et al, 1992). By converting this Ca^{2+} permeable receptor to a Ca^{2+}-impermeable one via adenoviral-mediated delivery of GluR2 gene into Bergmann glia AMPARs, Iino et al (2001) showed that abolishing Bergmann glia AMPAR Ca^{2+} permeability not only caused substantial withdrawal of Bergmann glia process from synapses but also led to an increased innervation of Purkinje cells by climbing fibers. This strongly suggests that the change in AMPAR Ca^{2+} permeability affects the neuronal-glial morphological relationship. Although a description of the underlying mechanism is not yet available, a possible participation of AMPARs in the regulation of structural synaptic plasticity is evident from this study.

An important question is to what extent the phenomenon observed in Bergmann glia is applicable to other brain regions, like the hippocampus. Astrocytic GluRs in the hippocampus contain GluR2 subunits. Also, unlike the total coverage in the cerebellum (Ventura and Harris, 1999), only around 60% of the synapses in the hippocampus are closely surrounded by astrocytes. Does the low Ca^{2+} permeability of the hippocampal astrocyte AMPAR contribute to this type of hippocampal-specific neuronal-glial anatomy? We presently have no answer to that. Another striking feature of hippocampal astrocytic AMPARs, is that a large population of hippocampal astrocytes express marginal (Zhou and Kimelberg, 2001), or no AMPAR-mediated currents (Bergles et al, 2000, Matthias et al, 2003). The presence of functional astrocytic AMPARs on only one type of hippocampal astrocyte may have implications for hippocampal neuronal–glial architecture formation and plasticity. This needs to be studied in more detail in the hippocampus and its occurrence established for other brain regions.

6.5.2. Astrocytic AMPARs are likely involved in synaptic transmission

The intimate relationship of astrocyte lamellae to synapses has led to considerable discussion regarding the involvement of astrocytes in neuronal transmission. That astrocytes actually express a wide array of neurotransmitter receptors shows clearly the potential abilities of astrocytes to "listen" to neurons (reviewed in Haydon, 2001, and Chapter 15). Thus, the kind of actions that astrocytes may subsequently take to affect neuronal signaling becomes a very interesting question. We will use the example of AMPARs in this context.

In contrast to the high affinity of NMDA receptors to glutamate (EC_{50}=1-10 µM, Chen et al, 2001), the affinity of AMPARs to glutamate is much lower (EC_{50}=342 to 428 µM, Jonas and Sakmann, 1992). Therefore, an immediate question raised is whether the spillover of glutamate from the synaptic cleft to the perisynaptic astrocytic lamellae reaches a concentration high enough to activate astrocytic AMPARs. An elegant study in the cerebellum showed that the extrasynaptic glutamate concentration could reach as high as 160-190 µM (Dzubay and Jahr, 1999) which is sufficient to activate AMPARs. Thus, these data explain the aforementioned study by Porter and McCarthy (1995), where the neuronal afferent stimulation is greater than that used in the study by Dzubay and Jahr (1999).

6.5.3. AMPAR activation likely enhances glutamatergic synaptic transmission by
    releasing D-serine

The finding that D-serine and its converting enzyme, serine racemase, are predominantly located to astrocytes (Schell et al, 1995; Wolosker et al, 1999) opened up an intriguing aspect of astrocytic modulation of neuronal transmission. D-serine exerts a much more potent effect than glycine on the NMDA glycine-binding site and therefore potentiates NMDA receptor activation with a greater sensitivity than glycine (Mothet et al, 2000). The astrocytic AMPAR has been found to serve as a trigger for D-serine release from astrocytes (Schell et al, 1995). Given that AMPARs trigger D-serine release, a critical question here is that in the hippocampus AMPAR currents are predominant features of the ORA type GFAP(+) isolated astrocyte (Zhou and Kimelberg, 2001, 2002). Do ORAs and OPCs, the latter now known receive synaptic input via AMPARs (Bergles et al. 2000), contain serine racemase and D-serine?

6.5.4. GABA$_A$R and K$^+$ channels

Astrocytic GABA$_A$R activation leads to the inhibition of K$^+$ channel conductance and it seems that this inhibition targets more than one K$^+$ channel type (Muller et al, 1994; Steinhäuser et al, 1994b; Pastor et al, 1995; Jabs et al, 1994; Bekar et al, 1999 and Chapter 7). One of the two-pore–domain K$^+$ channels, TASK-1, was found to be densely expressed in the regions where Bergmann glia are located in cerebellum (Kindler et al, 2000). There is evidence showing that the same TASK-1 channel in cerebellar granule cells is inhibited by tonic GABA$_A$ receptor activation (Brickley, 2001). Whether this also occurs in Bergmann glia requires further studies. Hippocampal GFAP(+) astrocytes also express GABA$_A$ receptors and are co-localized with TASK-1 channels (Kindler et al, 2000).

GABA$_A$R activation was also found to inhibit outward K$^+$ currents (Pastor et al, 1995; Jabs et al, 1994; Bekar et al, 1999), and more recent studies in hippocampal astrocytes showed that the inhibition is mainly of the voltage-gated transient outward K$^+$ channel (I_{K+A}) (Bekar and Walz, 2002). Unlike AMPAR-mediated inhibition of both outward (Borges and Kettenmann 1995; Jabs et al, 1994) and inward (Schrode et al, 2002) K$^+$ conductances via a Na$^+$ dependent mechanism, GABA$_A$R- mediated inhibition is caused by the direct decrease of the intracellular chloride concentration ([Cl$^-$]$_i$) (Bekar and Walz, 2002). Thus chloride has been suggested as an intracellular mediator (Walz, 2002).

6.5.5. The role of GABA$_A$Rs in regulation of [Cl$^-$]$_o$ and [pH]$_o$ by astrocytes

Astrocytic GABA$_A$Rs have been proposed as having roles in [Cl$^-$]$_o$ and [pH]$_o$ homeostasis (see review by Fraser et al, 1994). For Cl$^-$, the activation of astrocyte GABA$_A$R-mediated Cl$^-$ efflux is opposite to the functions of GABA transporters which drive Cl$^-$ into astrocytes. How these opposite fluxes may be reconciled spatio-temporally in a single astrocyte is an interesting question. In addition to Cl$^-$ permeability, GABA$_A$Rs are equally permeable to HCO$_3^-$ (Bormann 1988). Thus, their activation could lead to HCO$_3^-$ efflux and increase of [pH]$_o$. Extracellular alkalinization may enhance voltage-gated Ca^{2+} channel activity and consequent synaptic transmission. Thus, it is possible that astrocytic GABA$_A$Rs could be an important source of extracellular HCO$_3^-$, and this would become a feed back mechanism for the enhancement of, for example, inhibitory synaptic transmission (see Chapter 10 for a further treatment of pH regulation in glia).

6.5.6. The role of GABA$_B$R in modulating inhibitory synaptic transmission

The double and triple electrode recording approach taken by Kang et al (1998) made it possible to monitor the cross-talk among hippocampal pyramidal neurons, interneurons and astrocytes. Kang and coworkers nicely demonstrated that GABA$_B$Rs on hippocampal astrocytes could be activated upon activation of GABAergic interneurons. The subsequent astrocyte intracellular Ca^{2+} rise was found to trigger the release of glutamate, which then serves as a positive feedback signal to the interneuron to enhance its GABAergic synaptic transmission. This is the first evidence showing the role of astrocyte GABA$_B$Rs involvement in the activity of a neuronal circuit. However, what we have to keep it mind is that the identification of GABA$_B$R on astrocytes, in large part, based on measured Ca^{2+} rises in astrocytes and its sensitivity to GABA$_B$R inhibitors. There are no complementary data from, for example, freshly isolated astrocytes of the same brain region, further supporting the functional expression of GABA$_B$Rs by astrocytes. Furthermore, activation of GABA$_A$Rs in freshly isolated hippocampal astrocytes has been reported to induce an intracellular Ca^{2+} rise attributable to the opening of voltage-gated Ca^{2+} channels on the astrocytes (Fraser et al, 1995). Such a possible secondary effect is a common confounding problem in *in situ* studies. However, studies that do not support Ca^{2+} channel expression in astrocytes also exist. Carmignoto et al (1998) found no evidence of any voltage-gated Ca^{2+} channel expression by hippocampal astrocytes, which supports the view that the [Ca^{2+}]$_i$ rise observed in Kang et al's 1998 study was due to the direct activation of astrocytic GABA$_B$R via a G-protein-mediated IP$_3$

generation of intracellular Ca^{2+} release. Carmignoto et al (1998) only studied astrocytes having Na^+ channel currents, and therefore likely representing the ORA subtype that we have described in freshly isolated preparations from rat hippocampus (Zhou and Kimelberg 2000). It seems that the question of the presence or absence of $GABA_BRs$ on astrocytes in the hippocampus can be best resolved by their molecular expression in freshly isolated GFAP(+) astrocytes which allows a high resolution for immunocytochemical identification (Schools and Kimelberg, 2001). This can be combined with functional studies of Ca^{2+} responses resulting from $GABA_BR$ activation, which can be applied to single, freshly isolated astrocytes (Kimelberg et al, 1997; Cai and Kimelberg, 2000). Data from such studies should then better help to interpret the phenomena observed *in situ*.

6.5.7. The role of astrocytic glutamate receptors in blood flow regulation

The mass of the brain only amounts to 2% of the total body mass, but receives around 20% of the resting cardiac output (Guyton, 2000). It is well-known that cerebral blood flow undergoes wide dynamic changes under physiological and pathological conditions (Guyton 2000). It has also been known since the times Golgi (1885) and Lugaro (1907) that astrocytic processes frequently are in close proximity to both the vasculature and synapses. More recent studies have added the important details that the coverage of blood vessels by the astrocytic foot processes is close to 100% (Peters et al, 1991) and that ensheathment of synapses can vary from 100% to considerably less than that depending on the brain region (Ventura and Harris, 1999). Roy and Sherrington (1890) proposed that the brain has intrinsic mechanisms to control cerebral blood flow (CBF) to correspond with varying metabolic demands but the nature of these mechanisms still remains unclear (Faraci and Heistad, 1998). However, recent studies have provided evidence about how astrocytes may play a role in coupling neuronal activity to CBF, and astrocytic glutamate receptors have been implicated in these processes.

As discussed earlier in this chapter, Porter and McCarthy (1996) provided the first evidence showing that, *in situ*, astrocyte glutamate receptors (mGluR and AMPAR) respond to synaptically released glutamate by a $[Ca^{2+}]_i$ rise. Later studies in cultures (Bezzi et al, 1998) and on astrocytes *in situ* (Pasti et al, 1998; Parri et al, 2001; Aguado et al, 2002) suggested that this intracellular calcium response represents a potential signaling system for reciprocal communication between neurons and astrocytes, including Ca^{2+} oscillations that may mediate the release of glutamate from astrocytes to signal to neurons. Bezzi et al (1998) showed that astrocytes also release prostaglandin E_2 (PGE_2) via a Ca^{2+} -dependent mechanism and, of course, PGE_2 is a potent vasodilating agent (Sagher et al, 1993; Faraci and Heistad, 1998). Alkayed et al (1996, 1997) showed that stimulating astrocytes by adding exogenous glutamate enhanced the release of arachidonic acid (AA) from the astrocyte membrane phospholipid pool, while an astrocyte-specific epoxygenase, P450 2C11 metabolizes the AA to epoxyeicosatrienoic acid (EETs). This compound has been shown to be a potent activator of vascular smooth muscle outward potassium channels (I_{K+OUT}), which in turn leads to the hyperpolarization of smooth muscle, inhibiting the normal activation of voltage-gated Ca^{2+} channels and thereby reducing the influx of Ca^{2+} into smooth muscle to cause smooth muscle relaxation.

Zonta et al (2003) directly measured the luminal diameter of cortical arterioles upon neuronal afferent stimulation in hippocampal slices to provide the first direct evidence that astrocytes can play role in coupling enhanced neuronal activity to arteriole relaxation. This study showed that astrocytic mGluRs serves as the astrocytic sensor for neuronal activation, and one of the vasoactive agents released from astrocytes upon mGluR activation is PGE_2. Experiments on blood flow *in vivo* showed that blockade of mGluR1 and 5 reduced the blood flow increase in the somatosensory cortex during contralateral forepaw stimulation (Zonta et al., 2003). To build on this initial observation we need more information on the properties of the possible astrocyte subtypes surrounding the arterioles for a fuller understanding of the mechanisms underlying this important role of blood flow regulation since Zonta et al (2003) showed that stimulation of astrocytes close to arterioles, which increased $[Ca^{2+}]_i$, did not always induce arteriole dilation. Other than mGluRs, other G-protein coupled astrocytic receptors could also induce astrocytic Ca^{2+} rises. Additionally, Ca^{2+} responses were found in 74% of astrocytes examined by Zonta et al (2003), implying a heterogeneous expression of mGluR5 by hippocampal astrocytes, which is consistent with observations from freshly isolated astrocytes (Cai and Kimelberg, 2000).

6. 6. Conclusions

Contemplation of the data and the suggestions for function of astrocytic glutamate and GABARs in the hippocampus reveals that we know too little about astrocytic properties and functions related to these receptors. Indeed control of blood flow might simply be inferred from the localization of astrocytic processes (end feet) around all the vessels of the brain as the *glial limitans* is carried inward with the vessels as they penetrate from the pia into the brain tissue. The perennial questions to be resolved are do astrocytes control blood flow and if so by what mechanism(s). In spite of the excellent experiments of Zonta et al (2003) mainly in slices just discussed, and before them experiments showing that astrocyte metabolic activation affects blood flow done by the late Marcos Tsacopoulos and colleagues (see review by Tsacopoulos, 2002), we are still unclear as to what extent these observations relate to normal physiological processes. Much the same questions can be addressed to the observations of the influence of neuronal activity on astrocyte activity and visa versa done in slices, as described in other chapters in this book. The more and so-called reductionist approach of using cultures are compromised both by the problem of whether co-cultures reproduce the actual relationships *in situ*, and the demonstrated and widespread problem of culturing altering mRNA expression and the resultant protein synthesis in unpredictable ways. Culture systems are excellent for studying basic cell biological mechanisms but do have severe problems for physiology. Our approach of using acutely isolated cells is, of course, not immune from problems. The isolated cells cannot be used to determine interactions but only the properties of the cells without the confounding variables encountered in slices and the gene expression changes seen in culture, and we can only confidently exclude problems due to isolation damage when results from the isolated cells are in agreement with data from other more intact systems such as slices.

We could only say here that the predictability of the isolated cells will likely be higher than for cultures. As experimentalists we are all subject to a macroscopic version of the Uncertainty Principle applied to the very small, where the detection of electrons by light affects the observations made because, being of similar size and energies, each affects the other (Feynman, 1965). In our experiments the methods determine what will be found and can only approach the unperturbed *in vivo* state (also see introduction, especially Eddington's parable of the fishing net).

Yet in spite of all these well-known problems, advances have and will continue to be made, hopefully at a more rapid pace in the future than in the past, and the chapters in this book and other recent review volumes (Kettenmann and Ransom, 1995; Volterra et al, 2002), do attest to that. We should, perhaps, be comforted with an observation of the founder of the modern scientific method, Sir Isaac Newton, that "the safest method of philosophizing is first to inquire diligently into the nature of things and only then to proceed to hypotheses to explain them." (Christianson, 1984) Two comments here are that science is a school of philosophy (love of wisdom) and now by far the most successful and powerful. And second the quote clearly begs the question of when do we have enough knowledge of "the nature of things" to safely proceed to hypotheses. This is so much a personal choice (again Newton; "it is not for one man to prescribe rules for the studies of another", Christianson, 1984), and for this only the judgment of time tells us when any of us were right.

Acknowledgements. Work presented in this chapter from the authors' laboratory was supported by NIH grant NS 19492 and NSF grant IBN-0136960.

6.7. References

Aguado F, Espinosa-Parrilla JF, Carmona MA, Soriano E (2002) Neuronal activity regulates correlated network properties of spontaneous calcium transients in astrocytes in situ. J Neurosci 22:9430-9444.

Alkayed NJ, Birks EK (1997) Narayanan J, Petrie KA, Kohler-Cabot AE, Harder DR.Role of P-450 arachidonic acid epoxygenase in the response of cerebral blood flow to glutamate in rats. Stroke 28:1066-1072.

Alkayed NJ, Narayanan J, Gebremedhin D, Medhora M, Roman RJ, Harder DR (1996) Molecular characterization of an arachidonic acid epoxygenase in rat brain astrocytes. Stroke 27:971-979.

Bekar LK, Walz W (2002) Intracellular chloride modulates A-type potassium currents in astrocytes. Glia 39:207-216.

Bergles DE, Roberts JD, Somogyi P, Jahr CE (2000) Glutamatergic synapses on oligodendrocyte precursor cells in the hippocampus. Nature 405:187-191.

Bergles DE, Jahr CE (1997) Synaptic activation of glutamate transporters in hippocampal astrocytes. Neuron 19:1297-1308.

Bezzi P, Carmignoto G, Pasti L, Vesce S, Rossi D, Rizzini BL, Pozzan T, Volterra A (1998) Prostaglandins stimulate calcium-dependent glutamate release in astrocytes. Nature 391:281-285.

Bordey A, Sontheimer H (1997) Postnatal development of ionic currents in rat hippocampal astrocytes in situ. J Neurophysiol 78:461-477.

Borges K, Kettenmann H (1995) Blockade of K^+ channels induced by AMPA/kainate receptor activation in mouse oligodendrocyte precursor cells is mediated by Na^+ entry. J Neurosci Res 42:579-593.

Bormann J (1988) Patch-clamp analysis of GABA- and glycine-gated chloride channels. Adv Biochem Psychopharmacol 45:47-60.

Bowman CL, Kimelberg HK (1984) Excitatory amino acids directly depolarize rat brain astrocytes in primary culture. Nature 311:656-659.

Barakat L, Bordey A (2002) GAT-1 and reversible GABA transport in Bergmann glia in slices. J Neurophysiol 88:1407-1419.

Brickley SG, Revilla V, Cull-Candy SG, Wisden W, Farrant M (2001) Adaptive regulation of neuronal excitability by a voltage-independent potassium conductance. Nature 409:88-92.

Burnashev N, Khodorova A, Jonas P, Helm PJ, Wisden W, Monyer H, Seeburg PH, Sakmann B (1992) Calcium-permeable AMPA-kainate receptors in fusiform cerebellar glial cells. Science 256:1566-1570.

Bushong EA, Martone ME, Jones YZ, Ellisman MH (2002) Protoplasmic astrocytes in CA1 stratum radiatum occupy separate anatomical domains. J Neurosci 22:183-192.

Cai Z, Schools GP, Kimelberg HK (2000) Metabotropic glutamate receptors in acutely isolated hippocampal astrocytes: developmental changes of mGluR5 mRNA and functional expression. Glia 29:70-80.

Cai Z, Kimelberg HK (1997) Glutamate receptor-mediated calcium responses in acutely isolated hippocampal astrocytes. Glia 21:380-389.

Carmignoto G, Pasti L, Pozzan T (1998) On the role of voltage-dependent calcium channels in calcium signaling of astrocytes in situ. J Neurosci 18:4637-4645.

Chen N, Ren J, Raymond LA, Murphy TH (2001) Changes in agonist concentration dependence that are a function of duration of exposure suggests N-methyl-D-aspartate receptor nonsaturation during synaptic stimulation. Mol Pharmacol 59:212-219.

Christianson, G. E. In the presence of the creator: Isaac Newton and his Times):p165, 169, 1984. The Free Press.

Cornell-Bell AH, Finkbeiner SM, Cooper MS, Smith SJ (1990) Glutamate induces calcium waves in cultured astrocytes: long-range glial signaling. Science 247:470-473.

Dawson MRL, Levine JM, Reynolds R (2000) NG2-expressing cells in the central nervous system: are they oligodendroglial progenitors? J Neurosci Res 61:471-479.

Dzubay JA, Jahr CE (1999) The concentration of synaptically released glutamate outside of the climbing fiber-Purkinje cell synaptic cleft. J Neurosci 19:5265-5274.

Derouiche A, Frotscher M. (2001) Peripheral astrocyte processes: monitoring by selective immunostaining for the actin-binding ERM proteins. Glia 36:330-341.

Eddington, A (1939) The philosophy of physical science. Cambridge UK, pp16-17, 62.

Faraci FM, Heistad DD (1998) Regulation of the cerebral circulation: role of endothelium and potassium channels. Physiol Rev 78:53-97.

Feynman, R. The Character of Physical Law. 7-173, 1965. The MIT Press. Cambridge, MA and London UK.

ffrench-Constant C, Raff MC (1986) The oligodendrocyte-type-2 astrocyte cell lineage is specialized for myelination. Nature 323:335-338.

Fraser DD, Mudrick-Donnon LA, MacVicar BA (1994) Astrocytic GABA receptors. Glia 11:83-93.

Fraser DD, Duffy S, Angelides KJ, Perez-Velazquez JL, Kettenmann H, MacVicar BA (1995) GABA$_A$/benzodiazepine receptors in acutely isolated hippocampal astrocytes. J Neurosci 15:2720-2732.

Gallo V, Zhou JM, McBain CJ, Wright P, Knutson PL, Armstrong RC (1996) Oligodendrocyte progenitor cell proliferation and lineage progression are regulated by glutamate receptor-mediated K$^+$ channel block. J Neurosci 16:2659-2670.

Golgi, C (1885) Sulla fina anatomia degli organi centrali del sistema nervoso. Riv Sper Fremiat Med Leg Alienazioni Ment 11, 72-123.

Guyton AC and Hall JE (2001), Textbook of Medical physiology, 10th edition, W.S. Saunders Company, Philadelphia.

Haydon PG (2001) GLIA: listening and talking to the synapse. Nat Rev Neurosci 2:185-193.

Hosli E, Hosli L (1990) Evidence for GABAB-receptors on cultured astrocytes of rat CNS: autoradiographic binding studies. Exp Brain Res 80:621-625.

Iino M, Goto K, Kakegawa W, Okado H, Sudo M, Ishiuchi S, Miwa A, Takayasu Y, Saito I, Tsuzuki K, Ozawa S (2001) Glia-synapse interaction through Ca^{2+}-permeable AMPA receptors in Bergmann glia. Science 292:926-929.

Jabs R, Kirchhoff F, Kettenmann H, Steinhäuser C (1994) Kainate activates Ca^{2+}-permeable glutamate receptors and blocks voltage-gated K^+ currents in glial cells of mouse hippocampal slices. Pflugers Arch 426:310-319.

Jonas P, Sakmann B (1992) Glutamate receptor channels in isolated patches from CA1 and CA3 pyramidal cells of rat hippocampal slices. J Physiol 455:143-171.

Kang J, Jiang L, Goldman SA, Nedergaard M (1998) Astrocyte-mediated potentiation of inhibitory synaptic transmission. Nat Neurosci 1:683-692.

Kettenmann H and Ransom B (1995), Neuroglia, New York: Oxford University Press.

Kettenmann H, Schachner M (1985) Pharmacological properties of gamma-aminobutyric acid-, glutamate-, and aspartate-induced depolarizations in cultured astrocytes. J Neurosci 5:3295-3301.

Kimelberg HK (1983) Primary astrocyte cultures--a key to astrocyte function. Cell Mol Neurobiol 3:1-16.

Kimelberg, H. K. (1988) Glial cell receptors. Raven Press, New York.

Kimelberg HK, Cai Z, Rastogi P, Charniga CJ, Goderie S, Dave V, Jalonen TO (1997) Transmitter-induced calcium responses differ in astrocytes acutely isolated from rat brain and in culture. J Neurochem 68:1088-1098.

Kimelberg, H.K. (1995b) Receptors on astrocytes-what possible functions? Neurochem. Intl. 26:27-40.

Kimelberg, H.K., Jalonen, T. and Walz, W. (1993) Regulation of the brain microenvironment: transmitters and ions. In: Astrocytes: Pharmacology and Function. S. Murphy (ed.) Academic Press. pp.193-228.

Kimelberg, H.K. (1990). Cl⁻ transport across glial membranes. In: Chloride Channels and Carriers in Nerve, Muscle and Glial Cells (eds. F.J. Alvarez-Leefmans and J. Russell) Plenum Press, pp 159-191.

Kimelberg HK (1981) Active accumulation and exchange transport of chloride in astroglial cells in culture. Biochim Biophys Acta 646:179-184.

Kindler CH, Pietruck C, Yost CS, Sampson ER, Gray AT (2000) Localization of the tandem pore domain K^+ channel TASK-1 in the rat central nervous system. Brain Res Mol Brain Res 80:99-108.

Kinney GA, Spain WJ (2002) Synaptically Evoked GABA Transporter Currents in Neocortical Glia. J Neurophysiol 88:2899-2908.

Kosaka T, Hama K (1986).Three-dimensional structure of astrocytes in the rat dentate gyrus. J Comp Neurol 249:242-260.

Kressin, K, Kuprijanova, E, Jabs, R, Seifert, G, and Steinhäuser C (1995) Developmental regulation of Na^+ and K^+ conductances in glial cells of mouse hippocampal brain slices. Glia 15:173-87.

Levine JM, Card JP (1987) Light and electron microscopic localization of a cell surface antigen (NG2) in the rat cerebellum: association with smooth protoplasmic astrocytes. J Neurosci 7:2711-2720.

Liu HN, Almazan G (1995) Glutamate induces c-fos proto-oncogene expression and inhibits proliferation in oligodendrocyte progenitors: receptor characterization. Eur J Neurosci 7:2355-2363.

Liu S and Bergles DE (2001) Synaptic activation of $GABA_A$ receptors in hippocampal oligodendrocyt precursor cells. Soc Neurosci Abst 503.10.

LoTurco JJ, Owens DF, Heath MJ, Davis MB, Kriegstein AR (1995) GABA and glutamate depolarize cortical progenitor cells and inhibit DNA synthesis. Neuron 15:1287-1298.

Lugaro E (1907) Sulle Funzioni Della Nevroglia. Riv D Pat Nerv Ment 12:225-233.

Matthias K, Kirchhoff F, Seifert G, Huttmann K, Matyash M, Kettenmann H, Steinhäuser C. (2003) Segregated expression of AMPA-type glutamate receptors and glutamate transporters defines distinct astrocyte populations in the mouse hippocampus. J Neurosci 23:1750-8.

Mothet JP, Parent AT, Wolosker H, Brady RO Jr, Linden DJ, Ferris CD, Rogawski MA, Snyder SH (2000) D-serine is an endogenous ligand for the glycine site of the N-methyl-D-aspartate receptor. Proc Natl Acad Sci U S A 97:4926-4931.

Muller T, Moller T, Berger T, Schnitzer J, Kettenmann H (1992) Calcium entry through kainate receptors and resulting potassium-channel blockade in Bergmann glial cells. Science 256:1563-1566.

Ogata K, Kosaka T (2002). Structural and quantitative analysis of astrocytes in the mouse hippocampus. Neuroscience 113:221-233.

Parri HR, Gould TM, Crunelli V (2001). Spontaneous astrocytic Ca²⁺ oscillations in situ drive NMDAR-mediated neuronal excitation. Nat Neurosci 4:803-812.

Pasti L, Volterra A, Pozzan T, Carmignoto G (1997) Intracellular calcium oscillations in astrocytes: a highly plastic, bidirectional form of communication between neurons and astrocytes in situ. J Neurosci 17:7817-7830.

Pastor A, Chvatal A, Sykova E, Kettenmann H (1995) Glycine- and GABA-activated currents in identified glial cells of the developing rat spinal cord slice. Eur J Neurosci 7:1188-1198.

Peters A, Palay SL and Webster, H.d.F.(1991) The Fine Structure of the Nervous system, Neurons and their supporting cells. Oxford University Press, New York.

Porter JT, McCarthy KD (1997) Astrocytic neurotransmitter receptors in situ and in vivo. Prog Neurobiol 51:439-55.

Porter JT, McCarthy KD (1996) Hippocampal astrocytes in situ respond to glutamate released from synaptic terminals. J Neurosci 16:5073-5081.

Porter JT, McCarthy KD (1995) Adenosine receptors modulate [Ca²⁺]ᵢ in hippocampal astrocytes in situ. J Neurochem 65:1515-1523.

Riquelme R, Miralles CP, De Blas AL (2002) Bergmann Glia GABAₐ Receptors Concentrate on the Glial Processes that Wrap Inhibitory Synapses. J Neurosci 22:10720-10730.

Roy CS, Sherrington C (1890) On the regulation of the blood supply of the brain. J Physiol. 11, 85-108.

Schipke CG, Ohlemeyer C, Matyash M, Nolte C, Kettenmann H, Kirchhoff F (2001) Astrocytes of the mouse neocortex express functional N-methyl-D-aspartate receptors. FASEB J 15:1270-1272.

Sagher O, Zhang XQ, Szeto W, Thai QA, Jin Y, Kassell NF, Lee KS (1993) Live computerized videomicroscopy of cerebral microvessels in brain slices. J Cereb Blood Flow Metab 13:676-682.

Schell MJ, Molliver ME, Snyder SH (1995) D-serine, an endogenous synaptic modulator: localization to astrocytes and glutamate-stimulated release. Proc Natl Acad Sci U S A 92:3948-3952.

Schools GP, Zhou M, Kimelberg HK (2003) NG2 (+) cells freshly isolated from rat hippocampus are GFAP negative and electrophysiologically complex J Neurosci Res (in press)

Schools GP and Kimelberg HK (2001) Metabotropic glutamate receptors in freshly isolated astrocytes from rat hippocampus. Prog Brain Res 132:301-312.

Schools GP and Kimelberg HK (1999) mGluR3 and mGluR5 are the predominant metabotropic glutamate receptor mRNAs expressed in hippocampal astrocytes acutely isolated from young rats. J Neurosci Res 58:533-543.

Schroder W, Seifert G, Huttmann K, Hinterkeuser S, Steinhäuser C (2002).AMPA receptor-mediated modulation of inward rectifier K⁺ channels in astrocytes of mouse hippocampus. Mol Cell Neurosci 19:447-458.

Seifert, G, Zhou, M, and Steinhäuser C (1997) Analysis of AMPA receptor properties during postnatal development of mouse hippocampal astrocytes. J Neurophysiol 78:2916-2923.

Seifert G, Steinhäuser C (1995) Glial cells in the mouse hippocampus express AMPA receptors with an intermediate Ca^{2+} permeability. Eur J Neurosci 7:1872-1881.

Somjen GG (1988) Nervenkitt: notes on the history of the concept of neuroglia. Glia 1:2-9.

Steinhäuser C, Gallo V (1996) News on glutamate receptors in glial cells. Trends Neurosci 19:339-345.

Steinhäuser C, Kressin K, Kuprijanova E, Weber M, Seifert G (1994a) Properties of voltage-activated Na^+ and K^+ currents in mouse hippocampal glial cells *in situ* and after acute isolation from tissue slices. Pflugers Arch 428:610-620.

Steinhäuser C, Jabs R, Kettenmann H (1994b) Properties of GABA and glutamate responses in identified glial cells of the mouse hippocampal slice. Hippocampus 419-435.

Tsacopoulos M (2002) Metabolic signaling between neurons and glial cells: a short review. J Physiol Paris 96:283-288.

Verkhratsky A, Steinhäuser C (2000) Ion channels in glial cells. Brain Res Brain Res Rev 32:380-412.

Ventura R, Harris KM (1999) Three-dimensional relationships between hippocampal synapses and astrocytes. J Neurosci 19:6897-6906.

Volterra A, Magistretti P, and Haydon P. G. (2003) The tripartite synapse; glia in synaptic transmission. Oxford University Press.

Walz W (2002) Chloride/anion channels in glial cell membranes. Glia 40:1-10.

Wolosker H, Blackshaw S, Snyder SH (1999) Serine racemase: a glial enzyme synthesizing D-serine to regulate glutamate-N-methyl-D-aspartate neurotransmission. Proc Natl Acad Sci U S A 96:13409-13414.

Zhao JW, Du JL, Li JS, Yang XL (2000) Expression of GABA transporters on bullfrog retinal Muller cells. Glia 31:104-117.

Zhou M, Kimelberg HK (2002) Heterogeneity of swelling activated chloride currents by astrocytes freshly isolated from rat hippocampus Soc Neurosci Abst. 649.10.

Zhou M, Kimelberg HK (2001) Freshly isolated hippocampal CA1 astrocytes comprise two populations differing in glutamate transporter and AMPA receptor expression. J Neurosci 21:7901-7908.

Zhou M, Kimelberg HK (2000) Freshly isolated astrocytes from rat hippocampus show two distinct current patterns and different $[K^+]_o$ uptake capabilities. J Neurophysiol 84:2746-2757.

Zhou, M., School, GP, and Kimelberg, HK (2000) GFAP mRNA positive glia acutely isolated from rat hippocampus predominantly show complex pattern. Brain res Mol Brain Res 76:121- 131.

Ziak D, Chvatal A, Sykova E (1998) Glutamate-, kainate- and NMDA-evoked membrane currents in identified glial cells in rat spinal cord slice. Physiol Res 47:365-375.

Zonta M, Angulo MC, Gobbo S, Rosengarten B, Hossmann KA, Pozzan T, Carmignoto G (2003) Neuron-to-astrocyte signaling is central to the dynamic control of brain microcirculation. Nat. Neurosci. 6:43-50.

6.8. Abbreviations

AA	Arachidonic acid
AMPARs	α-amino-3 hydroxy-5-methyl-4-isoxazole propionate receptors
CBF	Cerebral blood flow
EETs	Epoxyeicosatrienoic acid
EPSPs	Excitatory postsynaptic potentials
GABA	γ-aminobutyric acid
GABARs	GABA receptors
$GABA_ARs$	$GABA_A$ receptors
$GABA_BRs$	$GABA_B$ receptors
GAT	GABA transporter

GFAP	Glial fibrillary acidic protein
GLAST	L-glutamate/L-aspartate transporter
GLT-1	Glutamate transporter 1
I_{K+OUT}	Outward potassium channel current
I_{Na}^{+}	Sodium channel current
IPSPs	Inhibitory postsynaptic potentials
mEPSPs	Spontaneous miniature excitatory postsynaptic potentials
mGluR	Metabotropic glutamate receptor
NMDA	N-methyl-D-aspartate
OPCs	Oligodendrocyte progenitor cells
ORAs	Outwardly rectifying astrocytes
SC-RT-PCR	Single-cell reverse transcriptase-polymerase chain reaction
I_{Swell, Cl^-}	Swelling activated chloride currents
VRAs	Variably rectifying astrocytes

Chapter 7

Ion channels in astrocytes

Gerald Seifert and Christian Steinhäuser*

Experimental Neurobiology, Neurosurgery
University of Bonn, Sigmund-Freud-Str. 25
53105 Bonn, Germany

*Corresponding author: Christian.Steinhaeuser@ukb.uni-bonn.de

Contents

7.1. Introduction

Work over the past ten years has significantly added to our understanding of astrocyte physiology. A huge number of original reports on astrocyte ion channel properties now are available, and it is beyond the scope of this report to provide a complete survey of this work. Rather, while referring to reviews for detailed information, we tried to focus the reader's attention on acute preparations (brain slices, freshly isolated cells). It should be noted in this context that astrocytes in culture can display a considerable 'plasticity' in functioning and do not always reflect the cells' properties *in vivo*. This report sums up information regarding potential functions that the various ion channels might have in astroglial development and cell-cell signaling, and discusses respective hypotheses. Knowledge is now gradually emerging indicating a role of astrocyte ion channels in central nervous system (CNS) disease. This aspect is also covered, by examining the impact of altered astroglial ion channel expression on injury, such as brain lesions, epilepsy and ischemia.

7.2. Voltage-gated Ca^{2+} channels

7.2.1. Classification of voltage-gated Ca^{2+} channels and their expression by
       astrocytes

Voltage-gated Ca^{2+} channels (Ca_v channels) are ubiquitously expressed by various electrically excitable and non-excitable cell types. By mediating Ca^{2+} influx upon membrane depolarization they constitute an important route for Ca^{2+} delivery necessary to regulate a multitude of intracellular processes, e.g. to ensure cellular metabolism, secretion and gene expression. According to their functional properties, high-voltage activated (L-, N-, P-, Q-, R-type) and low-voltage activated (T-type) channels are distinguished. The voltage-gated transmembrane channel is formed by a principal α_1 subunit that is encoded by several different genes, leading to the functional diversity of Ca_v channels. Based on gene sequence similarity, the current nomenclature subdivides Ca_v channel α_1 subunits into three families: Ca_v1.1-1.4, Ca_v2.1-2.3, and Ca_v3.1-3.3 (Ertel et al., 2000). In addition, auxiliary subunits have been identified that assemble with the α_1 subunit and may modulate its functional properties.

Almost 20 years ago, MacVicar provided the first evidence of the functional expression of Ca_v channels by astrocytes in culture (MacVicar, 1984). Since that time astrocytes of various CNS preparations have been demonstrated to possess these currents. Functional and pharmacological analysis indicated the capability of astrocytes to express L- and T-type Ca^{2+} channels (reviewed by Verkhratsky and Steinhäuser, 2000). Culture data suggested that the expression of Ca_v channels in astrocytes is controlled by neurons (Corvalan et al., 1990) and dependent on the presence of agents in the culture medium which increase the intracellular 3',5'-cyclic adenosine monophosphate (cAMP) level (MacVicar and Tse, 1988; Barres et al., 1989). Under these conditions, membrane depolarization induced both inward currents and a substantial increase in astroglial $[Ca^{2+}]_i$ (up to the μM range) as revealed when combining electrophysiology with Ca^{2+} imaging techniques (reviewed by Verkhratsky et al., 1998).

The molecular identity of the α_1 subunits underlying Ca^{2+} currents in astrocytes remained unclear for a long time. Using the reverse transcription-polymerase chain reaction (RT-PCR) technique, and primers directed to the α_1 gene family and to auxiliary subunits, transcripts encoding Ca_v1.3 (L-type) and two regulatory subunits (α_2, β_3) have been found in Müller cells of the retina. Patch clamp recording confirmed functional expression of L-type Ca_v channels in retinal glial cells (Puro et al., 1996). In primary cultures of cortical astrocytes, MacVicar's group recently identified mRNAs for the α subunits $Ca_v1.2$ and $Ca_v1.3$ (L-types), $Ca_v2.2$ (N-type), $Ca_v2.3$ (R-type) and $Ca_v3.1$ (T-type), but not for $Ca_v2.1$ (P/Q-type). Western blot and immunocytochemistry with subunit-specific antibodies confirmed their presence on a protein level (Latour et al., 2003).

The culture findings raised the question whether functional Ca_v channels are also expressed by astrocytes *in vivo*. Two types of acute preparations, freshly isolated cells and tissue slices, have been used to address this issue. Newman was first to describe Ca_v channels (L-type) in acute glial cells of the retina, both *in situ* and after fresh isolation (Newman, 1985). In another approach, a 'tissue print' method was used to search for Ca_v channels in freshly isolated optic nerve astrocytes. Patch clamp analysis identified two components, L-type and T-type currents, which were downregulated during postnatal development (Barres et al., 1990). A similar expression pattern was found in Müller cells acutely isolated from rabbit retina, where Ca^{2+} current densities reached a maximum at early postnatal days (Bringmann et al., 2000b). Additional evidence for the presence of astroglial Ca_v channels *in vivo* came from a study using microfluorometry to monitor depolarization-induced Ca^{2+} influx in astrocytes acutely isolated from rat hippocampus. The authors reported a reversible, $[Ca^{2+}]_o$-dependent increase in $[Ca^{2+}]_i$ although no transmembrane Ca^{2+} currents could be detected with the patch clamp technique. The increase in $[Ca^{2+}]_i$ was sensitive to the Ca_v channel antagonists verapamil, Cd^{2+} and Co^{2+} but not to dihydropyridines, indicating that the responses were not mediated by 'classical' L-type channels (Duffy and MacVicar, 1994). A verapamil-sensitive increase in $[Ca^{2+}]_i$ upon $[K^+]_o$-induced depolarization was also observed in hippocampal astrocytes *in situ* (Porter and McCarthy, 1995; Duffy and MacVicar, 1996), but electrophysiological properties were not investigated in these studies. Combining Ca^{2+} imaging with patch clamp analysis, different Ca^{2+} current components were identified in a subpopulation of 'complex' glial cells in the juvenile mouse hippocampus (Akopian et al., 1996). These cells were identified as astrocytes by their expression of glutamine synthetase and, later on, of the astrocyte-specific marker, S100β (Seifert et al., 1997). The kinetic and pharmacological properties of the currents indicated expression of T- and L-type channels by these astrocytes (Fig. 7.1). In addition, the authors found a ω-conotoxin GVIA-sensitive current component resembling neuronal N-type Ca^{2+} currents. Using the same preparation from rat, a subsequent study found no indication of functional Ca_v channels in astrocytes (Carmignoto et al., 1998). In light of recent work revealing a co-existence of distinct astroglial cell types with contrasting morphological, functional and antigen profiles (Matthias et al., 2003), it is likely that the two groups analyzed different cell types, which led to different conclusions of astroglial Ca_v channel expression. The aforementioned cell culture studies and findings in spinal cord white matter *in situ* (Agrawal et al., 2000; Brown et al., 2001) confirmed the capacity of astrocytes to express a variety of different Ca_v channel $α_1$ subunits.

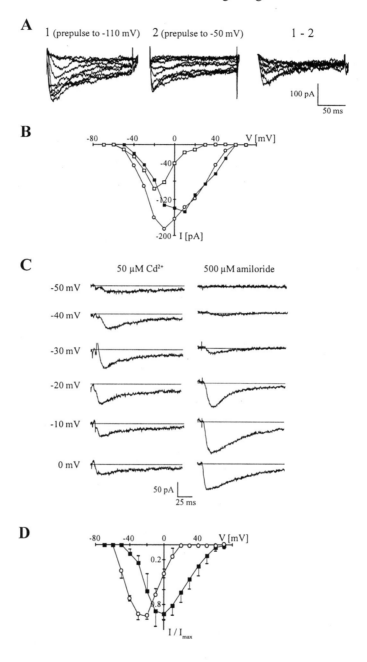

Figure 7.1. Astrocytes in the hippocampus express Ca$_v$ currents. Low voltage activated (LVA) and high voltage activated (HVA) currents were separated due to their distinct inactivation characteristics and modulation by Cd^{2+} and amiloride. (A) Ca$_v$ currents were evoked after hyper- or depolarizing the membrane to –110 mV and –50 mV (duration 1.5 s), respectively, and stepping to increasing depolarizing potentials (–70 to 0 mV). Depolarizing pre-pulses to -

50 mV prior to the recordings isolated a HVA component because LVA currents were almost completely inactivated at this voltage (middle panel). Subtracting the current families isolates LVA currents (right panel). (B) I/V curves of the currents shown in 1 (circles), 2 (filled squares), and 1 -2 (open squares). (C) After pre-pulses to -110 mV, currents were obtained in bath solutions supplemented with either Cd^{2+} (50 µM) or amiloride (500 µM). (D) I/V relations of the peak currents obtained in the presence of Cd^{2+} (open circles) and amiloride (filled squares). Note the positive voltage shift of threshold potential and peak currents mediated by amiloride. Currents (I) are normalized to the maximal current response (I $_{max}$). Recordings were performed in Na^+- and K^+-free, TTX-containing solution. Modified from Akopian et al. (1996), with permission.

7.2.2. Physiological implications

Culture work suggested that Ca^{2+} influx through voltage-gated channels significantly influences astrocyte physiology, e.g. by enhancing gap junctional communication (De Pina-Benabou et al., 2001) or by mediating peripheral benzodiazepine receptor-dependent regulation of astrocyte proliferation (Gandolfo et al., 2001). Although the contribution of Ca_v channels to an elevation of $[Ca^{2+}]_i$ in astrocytes under normal conditions in situ appears to be relatively small, it was recently reported that these channels are necessary for the spontaneous astrocyte Ca^{2+} transients observed in acute slices from various brain regions (Aguado et al., 2002). It remains to be clarified whether 'hot spots' of functional Ca_v channels are crucial for astrocyte physiology. They might mediate locally restricted changes in $[Ca^{2+}]_i$ in subcellular microdomains (Grosche et al., 1999) which are difficult to resolve with whole-cell analyses. Such local changes in $[Ca^{2+}]_i$ could be important for the release of transmitters, cytokines and growth factors from astrocytes, or for modulating the activity of other, Ca^{2+}-sensitive astroglial channels and receptors located in the immediate vicinity of these potential 'hot spots'.

7.2.3. Changes of astroglial Ca_v channel expression in the diseased nervous system

Data are available suggesting a role for astroglial Ca_v channels in epilepsy (reviewed by Steinhäuser and Seifert, 2002). During seizures, $[Ca^{2+}]_o$ decreases at the focus site (Heinemann et al., 1977), leading to epileptiform activity (Haas and Jefferys, 1984). The decrease in $[Ca^{2+}]_o$ was attributed to neuronal Ca^{2+} influx, but astrocytes might well contribute to this phenomenon. Indeed, anticonvulsant compounds (e.g. phenytoin, valproate, flunarizine) at therapeutically relevant concentrations, reduced depolarization-induced increase in $[Ca^{2+}]_i$ in cultured astrocytes (White et al., 1992). The authors speculated that in addition to neurons, Ca_v channels in astrocytes might contribute to $[Ca^{2+}]_o$ depletion and represent targets for antiepileptic drugs. This hypothesis is in line with a study reporting enhanced expression of L-type Ca_v channels ($Ca_v1.2$) in astrocytes in the kainate model of epilepsy (Westenbroek et al., 1998). Interestingly, a similar up-regulation of $Ca_v1.2$ immunoreactivity has now been demonstrated in astrocytes of the hippocampus obtained from epilepsy patients with Ammon's horn sclerosis (AHS) (Djamshidian et al., 2002).

Ca_v channels might also be involved in traumatic spinal cord white matter injury. Immunohistochemistry detected L- and N-type channels in periaxonal astrocytes, and inhibition of those channels during the lesion resulted in an improvement of axonal excitability (Agrawal et al., 2000). The authors speculated that this functional recovery was due to the protection of the astroglial ability to regulate the K^+ homeostasis. Similarly, influx of Ca^{2+} through astroglial L- and T-type channels during white matter ischemia was associated with significant cell death while removal of cytoplasmic Ca^{2+}, via the Na^+/Ca^{2+} exchanger, was protective (Fern, 1998). In hippocampal astrocytes, hypoxia led to enhanced voltage-dependent Ca^{2+} influx (Duffy and MacVicar, 1996). The upregulation of Ca_V channels (particularly $Ca_V1.2$) subsequent to injury, as observed in reactive astrocytes of various brain regions, might represent a compensatory effect promoting astroglial signaling and neuronal survival (Westenbroek et al., 1998).

Changes in Ca^{2+} currents also seem to accompany other diseases. Culture work suggested a role of Ca_V channels in prion protein-induced astrocyte proliferation (Thellung et al., 2000), and downregulation of L- and T-type currents has been reported in acute isolated Müller cells of diseased human retina (Bringmann et al., 2000a).

7.3. Voltage-gated Na^+ channels

7.3.1. Classification and astroglial expression of voltage-gated Na^+ channels

Voltage-gated Na^+ channels (Na_V channels) represent an indispensable prerequisite for initiation and propagation of action potentials. Similar to Ca_V channels, a principal pore-forming α subunit, associated with auxiliary β subunits, forms functional channels. The Na_V channel family comprises 9 different α subunit isoforms, $Na_V1.1$ to $Na_V1.9$. In addition, closely related Na_V channel-like proteins (Na_x) were cloned that have not yet been functionally expressed (Goldin et al., 2000). Atypical Na_x proteins are also expressed by astrocytes, but probably these proteins have a different physiological role and do not function as Na_V channels (Goldin, 2002).

Compelling evidence is now available demonstrating the expression of functional Na_V channels by astrocytes in culture and in situ (reviewed by Verkhratsky and Steinhäuser, 2000). Although the molecular identity of the glial channels has not been systematically assessed it appears that they express the same α subunits as neurons. So far, transcript analysis or immunocytochemistry detected $Na_V1.1$-$Na_V1.3$, $Na_V1.5$ and $Na_V1.6$ in cultured spinal cord astrocytes (Oh et al., 1994; Schaller et al., 1995; Black et al., 1998; Reese and Caldwell, 1999), and it has been proposed that $Na_V1.5$ accounted for the tetrodotoxin (TTX)-resistant Na_V currents observed in a subpopulation of cultured cells (pancake astrocytes) (Black et al., 1998). These cells also contain transcripts for the auxiliary subunits $\beta1$ and $\beta2$ as revealed with RT-PCR (Oh et al., 1997).

In addition, mRNAs encoding $Na_V1.1$-$Na_V1.3$ and $Na_V1.6$ were identified in optic nerve and spinal cord white matter astrocytes in situ (Oh et al., 1994; Schaller et al., 1995). Nevertheless, although Na_V currents have been recorded from astrocytes of various CNS regions (Akopian et al., 1997; Bordey and Sontheimer, 2000), the subunits underlying astroglial Na_V currents in gray matter still remain unclear. In most cases, Na_V currents recorded in situ proved to be TTX-sensitive (but see below). Patch clamp analyses in the developing hippocampus of mouse and rat yielded controversial findings as to the developmental regulation of Na_v currents (Kressin et al., 1995; Bordey and Sontheimer, 1997). In view of the proven heterogeneity of astroglial cell types *in vivo* (Matthias et al., 2003), these differences probably resulted from different criteria applied to select cells for recording in the slice preparation. Glial fibrillary acidic protein (GFAP)-positive astrocytes derived from human embryonic CNS stem cells expressed exceptionally high Na_v current amplitudes, generated action potentials upon current injections, and even displayed spontaneous firing (Gritti et al., 2000). The authors proposed that excitable, immature astrocytes might contribute to neuronal migration and to the modulation of glutamate release during gliogenesis.

Due to limited space clamp, reliable analysis of currents with rapid gating characteristics is difficult to accomplish *in situ*. Hence, acute cell isolation was used to quantify biophysical parameters of astrocyte Na_v currents (Fig. 7.2). In the hippocampus, pharmacological, stationary and kinetic characteristics of the glial currents matched corresponding parameters of neurons in the same brain region (Steinhäuser et al., 1994b). Astrocytes isolated from the rabbit retina, however, possessed Na_v channels with a lower TTX-sensitivity and slower activation kinetics compared with the neuronal counterparts (Clark and Mobbs, 1994). This distinct pharmacology was not found in retinae of other species including human (Chao et al., 1994).

7.3.2. Potential physiological role of astroglial Na_v channels

The physiological role of Na_v channels in astrocytes is still unknown. It has been proposed that they might serve the regulation of $[Na^+]_i$ and thereby control Na^+-dependent transporters such as Na^+/glutamate transporters or the Na^+/K^+ ATPase (Sontheimer et al., 1994), but other data did not support this idea (Rose et al., 1997). Although the contribution of Na_v channel-mediated influx of $[Na^+]_i$ to the whole-cell baseline $[Na^+]_i$ is relatively small, it is conceivable that local increases in $[Na^+]_i$ might be sensed by nearby K^+ inward rectifier (Kir) channels, leading to a reduced K^+ influx and modulation of astrocyte K^+ buffering capacity (Schröder et al., 2002). A Na^+-dependent modulation of Kir channels would be expected to be particularly effective under conditions of enhanced Na_v channel expression as has been observed at specific stages of the cell cycle (proliferating, S-phase arrested astrocytes; MacFarlane and Sontheimer, 2000a) and in astrocytes of the diseased CNS where Kir blockage might add to the neuronal hyperactivity associated with various pathological conditions (see below).

7.3.3. Modified expression of Na_v channels in the diseased nervous system

Evidence is accumulating that the expression of Na_v channels changes in CNS diseases. A dramatic up-regulation of Na_v current density was noticed in cultured astrocytes isolated from a seizure focus of human epileptic tissue. The cells possessed depolarized resting membrane potentials and were even capable of generating action potential-like responses upon current injection (O'Connor et al., 1998). This led the authors suggest that astrocytes overexpressing Na_v channels might support the spread of seizure activity through CNS regions in which synaptic transmission was interrupted due to neuronal cell loss. In the acute human epileptic hippocampus, however, the increase in Na^+ current density was less pronounced (Bordey and Sontheimer, 1998b). No differences in Na_v currents were noticed in a comparative patch-clamp analysis of astrocytes in the CA1 region of the hippocampus removed from patients either with AHS or lesion-associated epilepsy, two forms of temporal lobe epilepsy (TLE) (Hinterkeuser et al., 2000). AHS was characterized by selective neuronal cell loss and reactive gliosis, while the hippocampus of patients with lesion-associated TLE lacked significant histopathological alterations and was used as control-like tissue. Similarly, no increase in astroglial Na_v current amplitudes was observed in the sclerotic hippocampus of kainate-treated rats, an animal model of TLE (Jabs et al., 1997). Thus, the results of the latter two studies did not favor a role for astroglial Na_v channels in epilepsy. The molecular identity of glial Na_v channels in epileptic tissue is still unknown. It remains to be established whether astrocytes associated with epileptic seizure foci express the α isoform $rNa_v1.5a$ as recently suggested (Gersdorff Korsgaard et al., 2001). Enhanced expression of the Na_v channel β1 subunit was reported in a rat model of TLE (Gorter et al., 2002). Since the β subunits can function as cell adhesion molecules (Isom, 2001), the authors speculated that the increase in reactive astrocytes might subserve the cellular or synaptic reorganization characteristic of epileptic tissue.

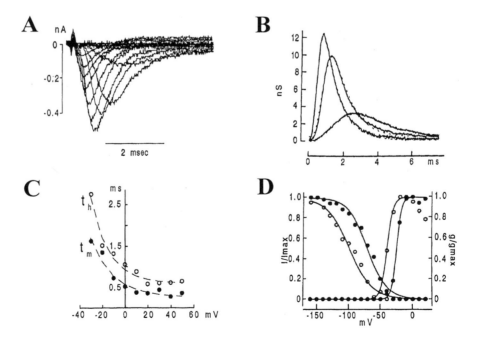

Figure 7.2. Na_v current analysis in acutely isolated Müller cells. (A) Na_v currents were activated in a feline Müller cell (voltage steps from –160 mV to +60 mV, holding potential –80 mV). To remove channel inactivation, conditioning voltage steps to –120 mV preceded test pulses. (B) Currents obtained from a murine Müller cell at –30, 0 and +30 mV were converted to conductances. (C) Time constants for Na_v current activation (t_m, full circles) and

inactivation (t_h, open circles) were determined using the Hodgkin-Huxley model. Data were plotted against step potential and fit to exponential functions (dotted lines). (D) Steady-state activation curves were constructed by plotting normalized conductances (g/g_{max}) as a function of membrane potential. Steady-state inactivation was determined by applying a series of pre-pulses (–160 to –10 mV) prior to the test potential (0 mV), normalizing test currents to maximum response (I/I_{max}), and plotting against pre-pulse potential. Activation and inactivation curves were fit to Boltzmann equations. Reduction of extracellular Ca^{2+} (open circles) produced a negative shift of control activation and inactivation curves (full circles). Modified from Chao et al. (1994), with permission.

Astrocytes of other *in vitro* and *in vivo* lesion models were also characterized by an up-regulated expression of Na_v channels, suggesting that the cells de-differentiated and underwent injury-induced proliferation (MacFarlane and Sontheimer, 1997; Bordey et al., 2001). In cell culture, this process was accompanied by a switch from TTX-sensitive to TTX-resistant Na_v channels (MacFarlane and Sontheimer, 1998).

Na_v channel expression is seriously affected in tumor cells that possess astroglial properties. In human astrocytoma cells, the enhanced Na_v current densities even led to the generation of action potentials upon depolarization (Labrakakis et al., 1997; Bordey and Sontheimer, 1998a). However, it appears unlikely that the glial cells develop such regenerative activity *in vivo*.

7.4. K^+ Channels

K^+ channels constitute the largest and most diverse family of ion channels, and are ubiquitously expressed in many cell types (for review see Coetzee et al., 1999). In contrast to Na_v and Ca_v channels, K^+ channels are formed by more than a single principal (α) subunit that assembles in a homomeric or heteromeric manner within the different gene families. Additional diversity is produced by interaction of α subunits with auxiliary β subunits, and with α subunits that do not form functional channels by themselves. K^+ channels are abundantly expressed by astrocytes where their conductance dominates the overall membrane current pattern (reviewed by Verkhratsky and Steinhäuser, 2000). Although more than 100 K^+ channel genes have been cloned, little is known about the subunits forming K^+ channels in astrocytes.

7.4.1. Voltage-gated and Ca^{2+}-activated K^+ channels possessing six transmembrane domains

Voltage-gated K^+ channels (Kv channels), Ca^{2+}-regulated K^+ channels (SK and BK channels), eag channels and KCNQ channels all belong to the superfamily of K^+ channels possessing six transmembrane domains. Except SK channels, these subfamilies are made up of subunits carrying an intrinsic voltage sensor.

7.4.1.1. Kv channels

So far, eight subfamilies of Kv α subunits have been identified, Kv1 to Kv6, Kv8 and Kv9, which include genes encoding delayed rectifier (K_D) and A-type (K_A) channels. Some of the α subunits (e.g. Kv 5.1, Kv6.1, Kv2.3) and the β subunits

(Kvβ1 - Kvβ3, KCHAP and KCHIP1-3) constitute auxiliary subunits, and their association with α subunits confers new functional properties to the channels.

Astrocytes both in culture and *in situ* are endowed with K_D and K_A currents. Usually, the Kv current densities exceed several fold those of Na_v and Ca_v, which explains the lack of spike generation of astrocytes under physiological conditions (Verkhratsky and Steinhäuser, 2000). K_D and K_A currents in astrocytes of the hippocampus have received particular attention. These currents are particularly abundant in the so-called 'complex cells' (Steinhäuser et al., 1994a) or 'GluR cells' (Matthias et al., 2003) that express the astroglial marker S100β rather than GFAP. The threshold for activation of K_D and K_A was positive to –40 mV, and the currents possessed common pharmacological properties, e.g. sensitivity to tetraethylammonium chloride (TEA) and 4-aminopyridine (4-AP). Freshly isolated cells were used to determine stationary and kinetic properties of K_A (Tse et al., 1992; Steinhäuser et al., 1994b; Zhou and Kimelberg, 2000). During postnatal development, significant changes have been reported with respect to pharmacological and kinetic properties of the currents as well as the relative expression levels of K_D and K_A currents (Kressin et al., 1995; Bordey and Sontheimer, 1997).

K_D and K_A currents are also expressed by astrocytes of other CNS regions, including brain stem (Akopian et al., 1997), spinal cord (Chvátal et al., 1995), cortex (Bordey and Sontheimer, 2000) and retina (Clark and Mobbs, 1994). Müller cells of rabbit retina displayed a similar developmental regulation of Kv currents as hippocampal astrocytes: K_A currents dominated in immature cells and declined during maturation while K_D currents reached maximum in adult animals (Bringmann et al., 2000b). In contrast, mouse Müller cells apparently lack a K_A component (Pannicke et al., 2002). Similarly, Bergmann glial cells of the cerebellum are devoid of K_A, and K_D currents were only observed at early developmental stages (Müller et al., 1994).

Little is known about the subunits coding for glial K_D and K_A currents. Kv1.5 has been detected with immunocytochemistry in hippocampal astrocytes and in Bergmann glia (Roy et al., 1996). By using antisense oligonucleotides specific to Kv1.5 in cultured spinal cord astrocytes, the authors isolated a current component with low TEA-sensitivity and supposed that homomeric Kv1.5 channels contributed to K_D currents in this preparation. RT-PCR, ribonuclease protection assays and immunocytochemistry detected Kv1.6 in cultured cortical astrocytes. Although the cells also contained low levels of Kv1.1 and Kv1.2, the high sensitivity to dendrotoxin suggested that a portion of the K_D currents was mediated by Kv1.6 channels (Smart et al., 1997).

7.4.1.2. Presumed functional role of Kv channels: regulation of astroglial
       proliferation

Although the physiological role of Kv channels in astrocytes yet has to be established, recent evidence suggests the involvement of K_D currents in cell cycle regulation, presumably via modulation of the intracellular pH (Pappas et al., 1994; see Chapter 10). Spinal cord astrocytes in culture displayed a continuous increase in K_D conductance during progression from G1 to S phase. Current blockade arrested the cells in G1, confirming a pivotal role of K_D augmentation for entry into the S phase (MacFarlane and Sontheimer, 2000a). Antisense oligonucleotides and antibody staining identified the subunit Kv1.5 as a crucial regulatory target. Phosphorylation of channel protein by Src family tyrosine kinases, rather than a change in Kv1.5 expression, caused proliferation, and downregulation of Src activity led to reduced K_D current amplitudes and promoted cellular differentiation (MacFarlane and Sontheimer, 2000b).

7.4.1.3. Altered expression of Kv channels in astrocytes under pathological conditions

Upregulation of Kv currents has been observed under pathological conditions accompanied by reactive astrogliosis *in vitro* (K_D and K_A; MacFarlane and Sontheimer, 1997), and in proliferative areas of the cortex *in vivo* (K_D; Bordey et al., 2001). Slightly enhanced K_A current densities were also observed in Müller cells of the diseased human retina, while K_D remained unchanged (Bringmann et al., 2000b). Human hippocampal astrocytes displayed only minor differences in Kv currents when comparing cells from AHS patients with cells analysed in control-like tissue of patients with lesion-associated epilepsy (Hinterkeuser et al., 2000; but see Bordey and Sontheimer, 1998b). Similarly, unchanged Kv current densities were observed upon entorhinal cortex lesion, a deafferentiation model known to initiate reactive gliosis and synaptic reorganisation in the dentate gyrus (Schröder et al., 1999).

Spinal cord white matter astrocytes contain the subunit Kv1.4, which encodes transient K_A channels, both under control conditions and after spinal cord injury. Besides its localization in GFAP-positive astrocytes, a dramatic upregulation of Kv1.4 immunoreactivity after injury was observed in NG2-positive cells (Edwards et al., 2002; see also Chapter 6). A recent study demonstrated that NG2-positive cells cannot be considered a homogeneous cell population and obviously include cells with astroglial properties (Matthias et al., 2003). Reactive astrocytes in the lesioned rat cerebellum expressed the subunits Kv1.1 to Kv1.4, Kv1.6, Kvβ1.1, and a rare splice variant of Kvβ2, Kvβ2.1A, that was not found in normal brain. The latter co-assembles with Kv1.1, Kv1.2 and Kv1.4, conferring modified functional properties to the channel complex and influencing surface expression of α subunits (Akhtar et al., 1999).

The link between K_D currents and regulation of proliferation as demonstrated in cell culture raises the question of the physiological relevance of the mechanism. Activation of α-amino-3-hydroxy-5-methyl-4-isoxazole propionate (AMPA) receptors in astrocytes *in situ* caused a fast, reversible blockage of K_D and K_A currents that was mediated by Na^+ (Jabs et al., 1994; Schröder et al., 2002) (Fig. 7.3) or Ca^{2+} influx through the receptor pore (Müller et al., 1992). Hence, since AMPA receptors of NG2- and GFAP-positive cells are probably activated *in vivo* (Porter and McCarthy, 1996; Bergles et al., 2000; Aguado et al., 2002), K_D blockage might be operative and affect proliferation and differentiation under physiological conditions. In line with this hypothesis is the observation that in cerebellar slice cultures, AMPA receptor activation inhibited the proliferation of NG2-positive cells (Yuan et al., 1998).

7.4.1.4. EAG channels

Members of the three subfamilies of the eag K^+ channels, ether-a-go-go (eag), eag-related (erg) and eag-like (elk), encode voltage-gated K^+ channels with a structure similar to other Kv channels. However, they contain a cyclic nucleotide-binding domain in the C-terminus of the channel protein. Erg-type K^+ currents were reported in hippocampal astrocytes *in situ*, and RT-PCR identified the expression of transcripts encoding erg1. Interestingly, erg immunoreactivity was mostly confined to astrocytes in the hippocampus, and blockade of erg-mediated currents impaired the clearance of extracellular K^+ (Emmi et al., 2000).

7.4.1.5. Ca^{2+} activated K^+ channels

The activity of large conductance Ca^{2+} activated K^+ channels (BK channels; also termed slo or MaxiK channels) depends on both membrane potential and $[Ca^{2+}]_i$. They consist of a α subunit (slo1, slo3) that can co-assemble with β-subunits (KCNMB1-4), which changes pharmacological properties (charybdotoxin-sensitivity) and the Ca^{2+}-sensitivity of the channels in a tissue specific manner (for review see Vergara et al., 1998). Small conductance Ca^{2+} activated K^+ channels (SK channels) are voltage-independent and possess a smaller single channel conductance than BK channels. The α subunits SK1-SK3 are apamin-sensitive and have a single channel conductance of 4-20 pS while SK4 (also termed IK channel) forms apamin-insensitive channels and exhibits a higher unit conductance (20-80 pS). In neurons, BK and SK channels are selectively coupled with N- and L-type Ca_v channels (Marrion and Tavalin, 1998).

Ca^{2+} activated K^+ currents are expressed by cultured astrocytes. Presumed SK (Quandt and MacVicar, 1986) or SK and BK channels (Supattapone and Ashley, 1991; Bychkov et al., 2001) were observed in cortical and striatal astrocytes, respectively. In the latter, a transient increase of both channel types was reported upon activation of endothelin receptors. Cerebellar astrocytes possess Ca^{2+} activated K^+ channels that are triggered by $[Ca^{2+}]_i$ oscillations due to stimulation of group I metabotropic glutamate receptors (Chen et al., 1997). In cultured cortical astrocytes, stimulation of β-adrenoreceptors and serotonin led to the opening of BK (Muyderman et al., 2001) and apamin-sensitive SK channels (Jalonen et al., 1997). Two novel types of Ca^{2+} activated K^+ channels were found in cultured astrocytes, which also expressed transcripts of the β_4 subunit, KCNMB4. These channels displayed a unitary conductance of 71 and 161 pS, were linked to phospholipase C and G-proteins of the G_i/G_o subtype, and were insensitive to apamin, iberiotoxin and charybdotoxin (Gebremedhin et al., 2003).

Less evidence is available for the presence of BK and SK channels in gray matter astrocytes *in situ*. In brain slices of rat hippocampus and cerebellum, immunohistochemistry and ultrastructural analysis revealed co-localisation of astroglial BK channels with aquaporin water channels in perivascular endfeet suggesting the involvement of BK channels in K^+ redistribution and regulation of cerebral blood flow (Price et al., 2002). Müller cells in the rabbit retina express BK channels, and channel activity declined during the first two weeks of postnatal development (Bringmann et al., 2000b). In human and porcine Müller cells, a single-channel conductance of 175 pS was determined, with a half maximal current activation occurring at a $[Ca^{2+}]_i$ of 8.1 μM. The open probability of BK channels was enhanced by cAMP-dependent phosphorylation while activation of protein kinase C (PKC) had the opposite effect (Schopf et al., 1999). Application of glutamate led to a current increase, by shifting channel activation towards more negative potentials (Bringmann and Reichenbach, 1997).

7.4.1.6. Presumed role of Ca^{2+} activated K^+ channels in proliferation and disease

Evidence is available suggesting a role for BK channels in the regulation of proliferation in Müller cells (Puro et al., 1989), presumably by influencing transmembrane Ca^{2+} influx (Kodal et al., 2000). Accordingly, enhanced activity of BK channels appears to underlie the enhanced proliferation typical of retinal diseases such as retinal detachment and proliferative vitreoretinopathy (Bringmann et al., 2000b) (Fig. 7.4). Neuronal Ca^{2+} activated K^+ channels open upon influx of Ca^{2+} through Ca_v channels whereas in retinal Müller cells, BK channel activity followed Ca^{2+} release from intracellular stores via activation of G-protein coupled P2Y receptors (Bringmann et al., 2002). Indeed, enhanced P2Y receptor-mediated increase in $[Ca^{2+}]_i$ and BK channel activation might be relevant to reactive responses of Müller cells, e.g. in proliferative vitreoretinopathy (Francke et al., 2002). Overexpression and increased Ca^{2+} sensitivity of BK channels was also observed in human glioma cells (Liu et al., 2002; Ransom et al., 2002), further supporting a role of BK channels in cellular proliferation and migration.

7.4.2. Inward rectifier K^+ channels

Inwardly rectifying K^+ (Kir) channels belong to the superfamily of two membrane domain channels and lack an intrinsic voltage sensor. Seven subfamilies are distinguished, Kir1 to Kir7. Kir channels are formed by 4 subunits that assemble as homomers or heteromers, and co-assembly of subunits of different Kir families considerably changes channel properties. The channels have a high open probability at negative membrane potentials. Inward rectification results from positively charged polyamines and Mg^{2+}, which plug the channel from the intracellular site in a voltage-dependent manner. Kir channels can be identified by their high sensitivity to extracellular Ba^{2+} that blocks the channels in the sub-mM concentration range. Phospholipids, G-proteins, the intracellular pH and adenosine triphosphate (ATP) modulate channel activity. Members of the ATP-sensitive Kir6 family co-assemble with sulphonylurea receptors to form octameric (4:4) channels which couple electrical activity to the metabolic state of the cell (reviewed by Reimann and Ashcroft, 1999).

7.4.2.1. Regulation of Kir channels during development und physiological implications

Kir channels are abundantly expressed by astrocytes of various CNS regions, including spinal cord, retina, brain stem, cerebellum and hippocampus (Verkhratsky and Steinhäuser, 2000). These channels are predominantly responsible for the maintenance of the astrocyte resting potential that usually stays close to the K^+ equilibrium potential. Kir channels in astrocytes are thought to represent

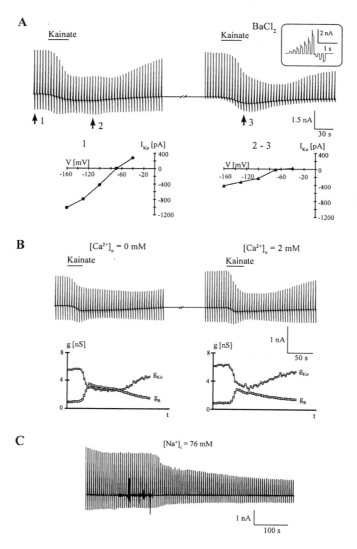

Figure 7.3. Inhibition of Kv and Kir channels by AMPA receptor-mediated increase in $[Na^+]_i$. (A) Whole cell currents were evoked in a hippocampal astrocyte by stepping the membrane to -40, -20, 0, 20, 40, 60, 100, -100, -130 and -160 mV for 100 ms, separated by 100 ms intervals (inset gives responses at higher resolution). This protocol was repetitively applied every 3 s. Note the prominent initial inward currents (left panel, arrow 1). Application of kainate (0.5 mM) blocked Kv currents while there was no consistent increase in overall inward current (arrow 2). After suppressing Kir currents with Ba^{2+} (50 μM), the kainate-induced AMPA receptor current could be isolated at negative voltages in the same cell (right panel). The I/V curves of Kir currents prior to (left) and during (right) application of kainate were given in the lower panels. In the presence of kainate, Kir currents were reduced to 55 % (-100 mV). (B) Kainate (0.5 mM) was applied in nominally Ca^{2+}-free solution (left panel). Then, the same cell was exposed to the agonist in the presence of 2 mM $[Ca^{2+}]_o$. In these two solutions containing different external $[Ca^{2+}]_o$, the Kir conductance was blocked to 45.1 and 48.6 % when

challenged with kainate (lower panels). (C) Increasing $[Na^+]_i$ from 6 to 76 mM via intracellular perfusion blocked both Kv and Kir currents. In this cell, Kir currents were reduced to 55.1 % (-100 mV). Modified from Schröder et al. (2002), with permission.

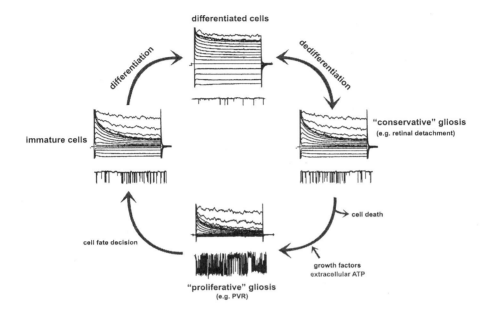

Figure 7.4. K^+ channel activity in Müller cells during ontogeny and gliosis. During differentiation, Müller cells upregulate Kir currents, mediating spatial buffering of K^+ and stabilizing a negative membrane potential. In contrast, BK channel activity is downregulated (middle, left and upper panels). Single BK channel activity was recorded at resting membrane potential (cell-attached mode, pipette potential 0 mV). During 'conservative' gliosis' (e.g. after experimental retinal detachment), Müller cells downregulate Kir currents (middle, right). During 'proliferative' gliosis (e.g. in retinae of patients with proliferative vitreoretinopathy, PVR), the strong (and sustained) downregulation of the Kir conductance and the high activity of BK channels are prerequisites for re-entering the cell cycle (lower panel). Modified from Bringmann et al. (2000b), with permission.

a prerequisite for the regulation of the K^+ homeostasis (Orkand et al., 1966). In the retina, the unequal distribution of K^+ conductances along the Müller cell surface supports the redistribution of locally elevated K^+, a process termed K^+ siphoning (Brew et al., 1986; Newman, 1986). During ontogenesis, an increase in Kir currents accompanies maturation of astrocytes as demonstrated in several gray matter areas and in the retina (Figs. 7.4, 7.5A) (Kressin et al., 1995; Bringmann et al., 2000b; Bordey and Sontheimer, 2000). Neuronal activity is accompanied by a temporary elevation of $[K^+]_o$ causing depolarization of nearby membranes which if uncorrected would produce hyperexcitability. Hence, enhanced Kir channel expression probably is necessary to maintain K^+ homeostasis in the smaller extracellular space of the mature brain (Lehmenkühler et al., 1993). Processes that interfere with Kir channel functioning thus might affect the capacity of astrocytes to buffer $[K^+]_o$. In this context, it should be noted that in hippocampal astrocytes activation of AMPA receptors led to a simultaneous, reversible block of Kir currents. Current inhibition was Ca^{2+}-independent but sensitive to AMPA receptor-mediated influx of Na^+ (Fig. 7.3) (Schröder et al., 2002).

Among the Kir subunits identified in the CNS, Kir4.1 is special because its expression appears to be confined to glial cells. Kir4.1 transcripts and protein have been found in Bergmann glial cells of the cerebellum, astrocytes in the hippocampus, and retinal Müller cells (Takumi et al., 1995; Ishii et al., 1997; Poopalasundaram et al., 2000). In the hippocampus, Kir4.1 transcripts were detected only in a subpopulation of astrocytes possessing Kir currents (Schröder et al., 2002), and high resolution immunocytochemistry localized Kir4.1 channels on astroglial processes wrapping synapses and blood vessels (Higashi et al., 2001). Interestingly, neuronal Kv channels that release K^+ into the extracellular space, are clustered adjacent to astrocytic processes further supporting a role of astroglial Kir channels in K^+ buffering and tuning of the excitability of neuronal membranes (Du et al., 1998). In addition to Kir4.1, hippocampal astrocytes abundantly express subunits of the Kir2 family (Kir2.1-Kir2.3), and among them Kir2.1 and/or Kir2.2 are probably targets of the aforementioned blockade by $[Na^+]_i$ upon AMPA receptor activation (Stonehouse et al., 1999; Schröder et al., 2002).

Müller cells express transcripts encoding Kir4.1 and members of the Kir2, Kir3 and Kir6 families (Raap et al., 2002) but not all of the subunits seem to be expressed on a protein level. Knock-out of Kir4.1 suggested its involvement in the regulation of $[K^+]_o$ (Kofuji et al., 2000). Interestingly, immunocytochemistry found Kir2.1 protein predominantly in direct apposition to neuronal membranes, while Kir4.1 was identified in Müller cell endfeet surrounding retinal blood vessels. This segregated expression of strongly (Kir2.1) and weakly rectifying (Kir4.1) subunits suggests a model of retinal K^+ siphoning in which K^+ influx is mediated by Kir2.1 while K^+ leaves the Müller cell endfeet via Kir4.1 channels (Kofuji et al., 2002). Thereby Kir4.1 channels might cooperate with water channels (aquaporin-4), which are co-localized around the vitreous body and retinal capillaries, to combine K^+ siphoning with water transport in the retina (Nagelhus et al., 1999).

Kir6 subunits co-assemble with sulphonylurea receptors (SUR1, SUR2) to form functional channels (also termed K_{ATP} channels). In cultured astrocytes, K_{ATP} channels regulate gap junctional coupling. Sulfonylureas blocking K_{ATP} channels increased, while K_{ATP} channel openers decreased gap junction permeability. The data suggested that K_{ATP} channel blockade by enhanced intracellular ATP might support the propagation of metabolic substrates within glial networks (Velasco et al., 2000). Electrophysiological and pharmacological analysis confirmed expression of K_{ATP} channels by astrocytes of hippocampus, cerebellum and brain stem in situ (Zawar et al., 1999; Brockhaus and Deitmer, 2000). K_{ATP} currents were primarily observed in astrocytes possessing prominent Kv currents (previously termed 'complex cells' or 'GluR cells'; cf. Matthias et al., 2003) rather than in 'passive cells', and the percentage of cells in which K_{ATP} currents could be activated declined with increasing age. The currents were enhanced by external stimulation with diazoxide and by intracellular cAMP application, indicating a sensitivity of channel activity to protein kinase A-dependent phosphorylation. The molecular identity of astroglial K_{ATP} channels still is a matter of debate. Antibody staining identified Kir6.1 in astrocytes of several brain regions (cerebellum, hypothalamus, hippocampus), preferentially in perisynaptic and peridendritic processes (Thomzig et al., 2001). The authors stated that astrocytes are devoid of Kir6.2 although this conclusion conflicts with other work (Karschin et al., 1998; Zhou et al., 2002). Transcripts for both pore-forming Kir6 subunits were found in Müller cells of the retina (Raap et al., 2002), and co-expression of Kir6.1 and SUR1 was demonstrated on the protein level (Eaton et al., 2002). Kir6.1 seems to co-localize with Kir4.1 in the endfeet which might serve the maintenance of a high K^+ conductance both at high and low ATP levels (Skatchkov et al., 2001). Taken together, functional and immunocytochemical data yet available indicate a heterogeneous expression of K_{ATP} channels, differing in astroglial cell types and CNS regions.

7.4.2.2. Regulation of Kir channels under pathological conditions

Several lines of evidence suggest a down-regulation of astroglial Kir currents in response to injury or in the diseased CNS, which might reflect some kind of de-differentiation, leading to an impaired K^+ buffer capacity of the cells and neuronal hyperexcitability. Reduced Kir currents accompanied reactive gliosis *in vitro* (MacFarlane and Sontheimer, 1997) and were observed under pathological conditions *in situ*, e.g. in Müller cells (Bringmann et al., 2000b) and in gray matter astrocytes in response to entorhinal cortex lesion (Schröder et al., 1999), cortical dysplasia (Bordey et al., 2001), traumatic and ischemic brain injury (D'Ambrosio et al., 1999; Köller et al., 2000), and in epileptic tissue (Bordey and Sontheimer, 1998b; Hinterkeuser et al., 2000) (Figs. 7.4, 7.5B,C). The mechanism(s) underlying this phenomenon are unknown but *in vitro* data suggested that tumor necrosis factor α (TNFα)– or transforming growth factor β1 (TGF-β1)-dependent PKC activation might contribute to current reduction (Köller et al., 1998; Perillan et al., 2002).

The modulation of astroglial Kir expression in human epilepsy attracted particular attention (reviewed by Steinhäuser and Seifert, 2002). TLE is often accompanied by reactive gliosis, and there is compelling evidence that disturbances of ionic concentrations lead to seizure activity. Hence, malfunction of glial inward rectification was speculated to be involved in the development of seizure activity (Bordey and Sontheimer, 1998b). By comparing the effect of Ba^{2+} on stimulus-induced rise in $[K^+]_o$, recent studies provided indirect evidence for a reduction of Kir currents in glial cells of the sclerotic human and rodent hippocampus (Gabriel et al., 1998; Kivi et al., 2000). The authors' hypothesis that diminished astroglial Kir conductances, rather than alterations in passive KCl uptake or Na^+ / K^+ ATPase activity, underlies the reduced $[K^+]_o$ buffering in AHS, was confirmed by patch clamp studies allowing assessment of intrinsic membrane properties of human astrocytes (Hinterkeuser et al., 2000). Subsequent analysis identified the subunit Kir4.1 in these cells (Schröder et al., 2000), but a co-expression of other subunits appears very likely (e.g. Kir6/SUR, Steinhäuser et al., 2000). The question which of the Kir subunits are affected in sclerosis to produce reduced inward rectification still has to be answered although preliminary data identified Kir4.1 as a potential candidate (Seifert et al., 2002). It is yet unclear whether increased astroglial proliferation or rather de-differentiation of formerly mature cells constitutes the basis of the observed loss of astroglial inward rectification in sclerotic epileptic tissue. In any case, this alteration, in conjunction with the proven seizure-induced shrinkage of the extracellular space, would impair spatial K^+ buffering, resulting in stronger and prolonged depolarisation of glial cells and neurons in response to activity-dependent

K$^+$ release. Thus, modified properties of astrocytes might directly contribute to, or even initiate seizure generation and spreading.

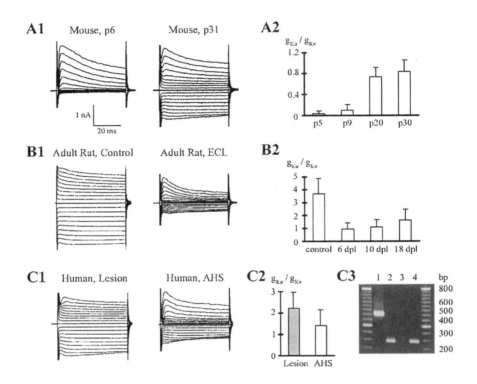

Figure 7.5. Regulation of astroglial Kir currents during ontogenesis, after lesion, and in human temporal lobe epilepsy. (A1) Comparative recordings from hippocampal astrocytes at different postnatal ages. Currents were activated by stepping the membrane between -160 and +20 mV, revealing an increase in Kir currents during development. (A2) After subtraction of background currents, Kir and Kv conductances were calculated at −130 and +20 mV. Comparing the ratio of g_{Kir} / g_{Kv} revealed a significant increase in the relative contribution of g_{Kir} beyond p9. (B1) shows the current pattern of astrocytes in the dentate gyrus of adult control rats and after entorhinal cortex lesion (ECL). Currents were evoked as described in (A1). Prominent background currents and Kir currents were activated in the control astrocyte while reduced inward rectification was evident after ECL. (B2) g_{Kir} and g_{Kv} were determined as described in (A2). Between 6 and 18 days post lesion (dpl), the ratio g_{Kir} / g_{Kv} was significantly lower than in control astrocytes. (C1) Current pattern of hippocampal astrocytes from patients with lesion-associated epilepsy and AHS (same protocol as described in (A1)). (C2) g_{Kir} and g_{Kv} were calculated as described in (A2). A significantly reduced ratio g_{Kir} / g_{Kv} was observed in AHS. (C3) Subsequent to the recording the cytoplasm of human cells was harvested and probed for Kir4.1 and β-actin transcripts. An astrocyte contained mRNAs for Kir4.1 (lane 1) and β-actin (lane 2). In contrast, transcripts for the housekeeping gene, β-actin (lane 4), but not for Kir4.1 (lane 3) were detected in a neuron. Modified from Steinhäuser and Seifert (2002), with permission.

7.4.3. Leak K$^+$ conductance

In many preparations, astrocytes display prominent passive or background currents lacking time- and voltage-dependency. Predominant 'passive' current patterns were also observed in acutely isolated astrocytes (Seifert and Steinhäuser, 1995; Matthias et al., 2003), proving the intrinsic nature of such currents and excluding that they reflected insufficient voltage-clamp control or were generated by gap junction coupling when recording *in situ*. However, isolated cells often display reduced 'passive' currents, which might indicate that the respective channels are primarily located on distal processes that are cut off during preparation. The reversal potential of astroglial 'passive' currents is usually close to the equilibrium potential of K$^+$.

Although the identity of this conductance is still largely unknown, recent work identified members of the two-pore-domain K$^+$ (KCNK) channel family in cultured astrocytes. These channels are open at resting potential and drive it near the K$^+$ equilibrium potential. Channel activity is sensitive to pH, fatty acids, and volatile anaesthetics. Currently, 14 members of this channel family have been cloned. KCNK subunits carry four transmembrane domains, are active as dimers, and are expressed by both excitable and nonexcitable cells in many tissues (for review see Goldstein et al., 2001). Most of the known KCNK subunits have been found in the brain, primarily in neurons (Talley et al., 2001). However, antibodies staining localized KCNK3 (TASK-1) protein in astrocytes of spinal cord white matter, cerebellum and hippocampus (Kindler et al., 2000). Moreover, cultured astrocytes possess transcripts encoding KCNK2 (TASK-1), KCNK9 (TASK-3), and KCNK10 (TREK-2). The principal ability of astrocytes to express KCNK channels was confirmed with electrophysiology. The cells possessed functional background K$^+$ channels with properties resembling cloned KCNK10 channels, including sensitivity to pH, membrane stretch and fatty acids (Gnatenco et al., 2002). Interestingly, a complete loss of astrocytes with predominating background currents has been reported in human AHS (Hinterkeuser et al., 2000). It remains to be demonstrated whether the regulation of KCNK channel expression in astrocytes, by modulating the membrane potential, influences ion homeostasis, uptake mechanisms, and neuron-glia signalling.

7.5. Concluding remarks

Astrocytes express various types of ionic channels, and recent advances in single-cell molecular biological techniques now allow identifying the subunits underlying the respective transmembrane currents, e.g. by correlating transcript expression patterns with functional properties in individual cells. Although a predominating K$^+$ conductance hinders generation of regenerative activity in astrocytes, these cells are not 'passive' but capable of sensing and responding to the activity of neighboring cells. While the functional significance of voltage-gated Na$^+$ and Ca^{2+} channels is still speculative, recent data support the hypothesis that Kv and BK channels in astrocytes are critically involved in cell cycle regulation and differentiation. Kir channels, by regulating [K$^+$]$_o$, are thought to adjust the level of neuronal excitability. However, recent findings also suggest that astrocytes *in vivo* can not be regarded as a homogeneous cell population and based on their different functional properties, certainly serve diverse roles in cell-cell signaling (see Chapters 3 and 4). In addition, ion channel expression in astrocytes varies considerably during development, between different CNS regions and under pathophysiological conditions. This tremendous degree of variability has to be kept in mind in future work devoted to unraveling the role of astroglial ion channels in tuning the neuron-glial circuitry.

Acknowledgement. The authors' work was supported by Bundesministerium für Bildung und Forschung (0311469B) and Deutsche Forschungsgemeinschaft (SFB Tr3). The authors thank Claudia Krebs for comments on the manuscript.

7.6. References

Agrawal SK, Nashmi R, Fehlings MG (2000) Role of L- and N-type calcium channels in the pathophysiology of traumatic spinal cord white matter injury. Neuroscience 99:179-188.

Aguado F, Espinosa-Parrilla JF, Carmona MA, Soriano E (2002) Neuronal activity regulates correlated network properties of spontaneous calcium transients in astrocytes in situ. J Neurosci 22:9430-9444.

Akhtar S, McIntosh P, Bryan-Sisneros A, Barratt L, Robertson B, Dolly JO (1999) A functional spliced-variant of β2 subunit of Kv1 channels in C6 glioma cells and reactive astrocytes from rat lesioned cerebellum. Biochemistry 38:16984-16992.

Akopian G, Kressin K, Derouiche A, Steinhäuser C (1996) Identified glial cells in the early postnatal mouse hippocampus display different types of Ca^{2+} currents. Glia 17:181-194.

Akopian G, Kuprijanova E, Kressin K, Steinhäuser C (1997) Analysis of ion channel expression by astrocytes in red nucleus brain stem slices of the rat. Glia 19:234-246.

Barres BA, Chun LLY, Corey DP (1989) Calcium current in cortical astrocytes: induction by cAMP and neurotransmitters and permissive effect of serum factors. J Neurosci 9:3169-3175.

Barres BA, Koroshetz WJ, Chun LLY, Corey DP (1990) Ion channel expression by white matter glia: the type-1 astroyte. Neuron 5:527-544.

Bergles DE, Roberts JD, Somogyi P, Jahr CE (2000) Glutamatergic synapses on oligodendrocyte precursor cells in the hippocampus. Nature 405:187-191.

Black JA, Dib-Hajj S, Cohen S, Hinson AW, Waxman SG (1998) Glial cells have heart: rH1 Na^+ channel mRNA and protein in spinal cord astrocytes. Glia 23:200-208.

Bordey A, Lyons SA, Hablitz JJ, Sontheimer H (2001) Electrophysiological characteristics of reactive astrocytes in experimental cortical dysplasia. J Neurophysiol 85:1719-1731.

Bordey A, Sontheimer H (1997) Postnatal development of ionic currents in rat hippocampal astrocytes in situ. J Neurophysiol 78:461-477.

Bordey A, Sontheimer H (1998a) Electrophysiological properties of human astrocytic tumor cells in situ: Enigma of spiking glial cells. J Neurophysiol 79:2782-2793.

Bordey A, Sontheimer H (1998b) Properties of human glial cells associated with epileptic seizure foci. Epilepsy Res 32:286-303.

Bordey A, Sontheimer H (2000) Ion channel expression by astrocytes in situ: Comparison of different CNS regions. Glia 30:27-38.

Brew H, Gray PTA, Mobbs P, Attwell D (1986) Endfeet of retinal glial cells have higher densities of ion channels that mediate K^+ buffering. Nature 324:466-468.

Bringmann A, Biedermann B, Schnurbusch U, Enzmann V, Faude F, Reichenbach A (2000a) Age- and disease-related changes of calcium channel-mediated currents in human Muller glial cells. Invest Ophthalmol Vis Sci 41:2791-2796.

Bringmann A, Francke M, Pannicke T, Biedermann B, Kodal H, Faude F, Reichelt W, Reichenbach A (2000b) Role of glial K^+ channels in ontogeny and gliosis: A hypothesis based upon studies on Muller cells. Glia 29:35-44.

Bringmann A, Pannicke T, Weick M, Biedermann B, Uhlmann S, Kohen L, Wiedemann P, Reichenbach A (2002) Activation of P2Y receptors stimulates potassium and cation currents in acutely isolated human Muller (glial) cells. Glia 37:139-152.

Bringmann A, Reichenbach A (1997) Heterogeneous expression of Ca^{2+}-dependent K^+ currents by Muller glial cells. NeuroReport 8:3841-3845.

Brockhaus J, Deitmer JW (2000) Developmental downregulation of ATP-sensitive potassium conductance in astrocytes in situ. Glia 32:205-213.

Brown AM, Westenbroek RE, Catterall WA, Ransom BR (2001) Axonal L-type Ca^{2+} channels and anoxic injury in rat CNS white matter. J Neurophysiol 85:900-911.

Bychkov R, Glowinski J, Giaume C (2001) Sequential and opposite regulation of two outward K^+ currents by ET-1 in cultured striatal astrocytes. Am J Physiol Cell Physiol 281:C1373-C1384.

Carmignoto G, Pasti L, Pozzan T (1998) On the role of voltage-dependent calcium channels in calcium signaling of astrocytes in situ. J Neurosci 18:4637-4645.

Chao TI, Skachkov SN, Eberhardt W, Reichenbach A (1994) Na^+ channels of Müller (glial) cells isolated from retinae of various mammalian species including man. Glia 10:173-185.

Chen JG, Backus KH, Deitmer JW (1997) Intracellular calcium transients and potassium current oscillations evoked by glutamate in cultured rat astrocytes. J Neurosci 17:7278-7287.

Chvátal A, Pastor A, Mauch M, Syková E, Kettenmann H (1995) Distinct populations of identified glial cells in the developing rat spinal cord slice: Ion channel properties and cell morphology. Eur J Neurosci 7:129-142.

Clark BA, Mobbs P (1994) Voltage-gated currents in rabbit retinal astrocytes. Eur J Neurosci 6:1406-1414.

Coetzee WA, Amarillo Y, Chiu J, Chow A, Lau D, McCormack T, Moreno H, Nadal MS, Ozaita A, Pountney D, Saganich M, Vega-Saenz dM, Rudy B (1999) Molecular diversity of K^+ channels. Ann N Y Acad Sci 868:233-285.

Corvalan V, Cole R, de Vellis J, Hagiwara S (1990) Neuronal modulation of calcium channel activity in cultured rat astrocytes. Proc Natl Acad Sci USA 87:4345-4348.

D'Ambrosio R, Maris DO, Grady MS, Winn HR, Janigro D (1999) Impaired K^+ homeostasis and altered electrophysiological properties of post-traumatic hippocampal glia. J Neurosci 19:8152-8162.

De Pina-Benabou MH, Srinivas M, Spray DC, Scemes E (2001) Calmodulin kinase pathway mediates the K^+-induced increase in gap junctional communication between mouse spinal cord astrocytes. J Neurosci 21:6635-6643.

Djamshidian A, Grassl R, Seltenhammer M, Czech T, Baumgartner C, Schmidbauer M, Ulrich W, Zimprich F (2002) Altered expression of voltage-dependent calcium channel α_1 subunits in temporal lobe epilepsy with Ammon's horn sclerosis. Neuroscience 111:57-69.

Du J, Tao-Cheng JH, Zerfas P, McBain CJ (1998) The K^+ channel, Kv2.1, is apposed to astrocytic processes and is associated with inhibitory postsynaptic membranes in hippocampal and cortical principal neurons and inhibitory interneurons. Neuroscience 84:37-48.

Duffy S, MacVicar BA (1994) Potassium-dependent calcium influx in acutely isolated hippocampal astrocytes. Neuroscience 61:51-61.

Duffy S, MacVicar BA (1996) In vitro ischemia promotes calcium influx and intracellular calcium release in hippocampal astrocytes. J Neurosci 16:71-81.

Eaton MJ, Skatchkov SN, Brune A, Biedermann B, Veh RW, Reichenbach A (2002) SUR1 and Kir6.1 subunits of K_{ATP}-channels are co-localized in retinal glial (Muller) cells. NeuroReport 13:57-60.

Edwards L, Nashmi R, Jones O, Backx P, Ackerley C, Becker L, Fehlings MG (2002) Upregulation of Kv 1.4 protein and gene expression after chronic spinal cord injury. J Comp Neurol 443:154-167.

Emmi A, Wenzel HJ, Schwartzkroin PA, Taglialatela M, Castaldo P, Bianchi L, Nerbonne J, Robertson GA, Janigro D (2000) Do glia have heart? Expression and functional role for ether-a-go-go currents in hippocampal astrocytes. J Neurosci 20:3915-3925.

Ertel EA, Campbell KP, Harpold MM, Hofmann F, Mori Y, Perez-Reyes E, Schwartz A, Snutch TP, Tanabe T, Birnbaumer L, Tsien RW, Catterall WA (2000) Nomenclature of voltage-gated calcium channels. Neuron 25:533-535.

Fern R (1998) Intracellular calcium and cell death during ischemia in neonatal rat white matter astrocytes *in situ* . J Neurosci 18:7232-7243.

Francke M, Weick M, Pannicke T, Uckermann O, Grosche J, Goczalik I, Milenkovic I, Uhlmann S, Faude F, Wiedemann P, Reichenbach A, Bringmann A (2002) Upregulation of extracellular ATP-induced Muller cell responses in a dispase model of proliferative vitreoretinopathy. Invest Ophthalmol Vis Sci 43:870-881.

Gabriel S, Eilers A, Kivi A, Kovacs R, Schulze K, Lehmann TN, Heinemann U (1998) Effects of barium on stimulus induced changes in extracellular potassium concentration in area CA1 of hippocampal slices from normal and pilocarpine-treated epileptic rats. Neurosci Lett 242:9-12.

Gandolfo P, Louiset E, Patte C, Leprince J, Masmoudi O, Malagon M, Gracia-Navarro F, Vaudry H, Tonon MC (2001) The triakontatetraneuropeptide TTN increases $[Ca^{2+}]_i$ in rat astrocytes through activation of peripheral-type benzodiazepine receptors. Glia 35:90-100.

Gebremedhin D, Yamaura K, Zhang C, Bylund J, Koehler RC, Harder DR (2003) Metabotropic glutamate receptor activation enhances the activities of two types of Ca^{2+}-activated K^+ channels in rat hippocampal astrocytes. J Neurosci 23:1678-1687.

Gersdorff Korsgaard MP, Christophersen P, Ahring PK, Olesen SP (2001) Identification of a novel voltage-gated Na^+ channel $rNa_v1.5a$ in the rat hippocampal progenitor stem cell line HiB5. Pflugers Arch 443:18-30.

Gnatenco C, Han J, Snyder AK, Kim D (2002) Functional expression of TREK-2 K^+ channel in cultured rat brain astrocytes. Brain Res 931:56-67.

Goldin AL (2002) Evolution of voltage-gated Na^+ channels. J Exp Biol 205:575-584.

Goldin AL, Barchi RL, Caldwell JH, Hofmann F, Howe JR, Hunter JC, Kallen RG, Mandel G, Meisler MH, Netter YB, Noda M, Tamkun MM, Waxman SG, Wood JN, Catterall WA (2000) Nomenclature of voltage-gated sodium channels. Neuron 28:365-368.

Goldstein SA, Bockenhauer D, O'Kelly I, Zilberberg N (2001) Potassium leak channels and the KCNK family of two-P-domain subunits. Nat Rev Neurosci 2:175-184.

Gorter JA, Van Vliet EA, Lopes da Silva FH, Isom LL, Aronica E (2002) Sodium channel beta1-subunit expression is increased in reactive astrocytes in a rat model for mesial temporal lobe epilepsy. Eur J Neurosci 16:360-364.

Gritti A, Rosati B, Lecchi M, Vescovi AL, Wanke E (2000) Excitable properties in astrocytes derived from human embryonic CNS stem cells. Eur J Neurosci 12:3549-3559.

Grosche J, Matyash V, Moller T, Verkhratsky A, Reichenbach A, Kettenmann H (1999) Microdomains for neuron-glia interaction: parallel fiber signaling to Bergmann glial cells. Nat Neurosci 2:139-143.

Haas HL, Jefferys JGR (1984) Low-calcium field burst discharges of CA1 pyramidal neurones in rat hippocampal slices. J Physiol (London) 354:185-201.

Heinemann U, Lux HD, Gutnick MJ (1977) Extracellular free calcium and potassium during paroxsmal activity in the cerebral cortex of the cat. Exp Brain Res 27:237-243.

Higashi K, Fujita A, Inanobe A, Tanemoto M, Doi K, Kubo T, Kurachi Y (2001) An inwardly rectifying K^+ channel, Kir4.1, expressed in astrocytes surrounds synapses and blood vessels in brain. Am J Physiol 281:C922-C931.

Hinterkeuser S, Schröder W, Hager G, Seifert G, Blümcke I, Elger CE, Schramm J, Steinhäuser C (2000) Astrocytes in the hippocampus of patients with temporal lobe epilepsy display changes in potassium conductances. Eur J Neurosci 12:2087-2096.

Ishii M, Horio Y, Tada Y, Hibino H, Inanobe A, Ito M, Yamada M, Gotow T, Uchiyama Y, Kurachi Y (1997) Expression and clustered distribution of an inwardly rectifying potassium channel, K_{AB}-2/Kir4.1, on mammalian retinal Muller cell membrane: Their regulation by insulin and laminin signals. J Neurosci 17:7725-7735.

Isom LL (2001) Sodium channel beta subunits: anything but auxiliary. Neuroscientist 7:42-54.

Jabs R, Kirchhoff F, Kettenmann H, Steinhäuser C (1994) Kainate activates Ca^{2+}-permeable glutamate receptors and blocks voltage-gated K^+ currents in glial cells of mouse hippocampal slices. Pflugers Arch 426:310-319.

Jabs R, Paterson IA, Walz W (1997) Qualitative analysis of membrane currents in glial cells from normal and gliotic tissue in situ: Down-regulation of Na^+ current and lack of P_2 purinergic responses. Neuroscience 81:847-860.

Jalonen TO, Margraf RR, Wielt DB, Charniga CJ, Linne ML, Kimelberg HK (1997) Serotonin induces inward potassium and calcium currents in rat cortical astrocytes. Brain Res 758:69-82.

Karschin A, Brockhaus J, Ballanyi K (1998) KATP channel formation by the sulphonylurea receptors SUR1 with Kir6.2 subunits in rat dorsal vagal neurons in situ. J Physiol (Lond) 509:339-346.

Kindler CH, Pietruck C, Yost CS, Sampson ER, Gray AT (2000) Localization of the tandem pore domain K^+ channel TASK-1 in the rat central nervous system. Mol Brain Res 80:99-108.

Kivi A, Lehmann T, Kovacs R, Eilers A, Jauch R, Meencke HJ, Von Deimling A, Heinemann U, Gabriel S (2000) Effects of barium on stimulus-induced rises of $[K^+]_o$ in human epileptic non-sclerotic and sclerotic hippocampal area CA1. Eur J Neurosci 12:2039-2048.

Kodal H, Weick M, Moll V, Biedermann B, Reichenbach A, Bringmann A (2000) Involvement of calcium-activated potassium channels in the regulation of DNA synthesis in cultured Muller glial cells. Invest Ophthalmol Vis Sci 41:4262-4267.

Kofuji P, Biedermann B, Siddharthan V, Raap M, Iandiev I, Milenkovic I, Thomzig A, Veh RW, Bringmann A, Reichenbach A (2002) Kir potassium channel subunit expression in retinal glial cells: implications for spatial potassium buffering. Glia 39:292-303.

Kofuji P, Ceelen P, Zahs KR, Surbeck LW, Lester HA, Newman EA (2000) Genetic inactivation of an inwardly rectifying potassium channel (Kir4.1 subunit) in mice: Phenotypic impact in retina. J Neurosci 20:5733-5740.

Köller H, Allert N, Oel D, Stoll G, Siebler M (1998) TNFα induces a protein kinase C-dependent reduction in astroglial K^+ conductance. NeuroReport 9:1375-1378.

Köller H, Schroeter M, Jander S, Stoll G, Siebler M (2000) Time course of inwardly rectifying K^+ current reduction in glial cells surrounding ischemic brain lesions. Brain Res 872:194-198.

Kressin K, Kuprijanova E, Jabs R, Seifert G, Steinhäuser C (1995) Developmental regulation of Na^+ and K^+ conductances in glial cells of mouse hippocampal brain slices. Glia 15:173-187.

Labrakakis C, Patt S, Weydt P, Cervos NJ, Meyer R, Kettenmann H (1997) Action potential-generating cells in human glioblastomas. J Neuropathol Exp Neurol 56:243-254.

Latour I, Hamid J, Beedle AM, Zamponi GW, MacVicar BA (2003) Expression of voltage-gated Ca^{2+} channel subtypes in cultured astrocytes. Glia 41:347-353.

Lehmenkühler A, Syková E, Svoboda J, Zilles K, Nicholson C (1993) Extracellular space parameters in the rat neocortex and subcortical white matter during postnatal development determined by diffusion analysis. Neuroscience 55:339-351.

Liu X, Chang Y, Reinhart PH, Sontheimer H, Chang Y (2002) Cloning and characterization of glioma BK, a novel BK channel isoform highly expressed in human glioma cells. J Neurosci 22:1840-1849.

MacFarlane SN, Sontheimer H (1997) Electrophysiological changes that accompany reactive gliosis in vitro. J Neurosci 17:7316-7329.

MacFarlane SN, Sontheimer H (1998) Spinal cord astrocytes display a switch from TTX-sensitive to TTX-resistant sodium currents after injury-induced gliosis in vitro. J Neurophysiol 79:2222-2226.

MacFarlane SN, Sontheimer H (2000a) Changes in ion channel expression accompany cell cycle progression of spinal cord astrocytes. Glia 30:39-48.

MacFarlane SN, Sontheimer H (2000b) Modulation of Kv1.5 currents by Src tyrosine phosphorylation: Potential role in the differentiation of astrocytes. J Neurosci 20:5245-5253.

MacVicar BA (1984) Voltage-dependent calcium channels in glial cells. Science 226:1345-1347.

MacVicar BA, Tse FW (1988) Norepinephrine and cyclic adenosine 3':5'-cyclic monophosphate enhance a nifedipine-sensitive calcium current in cultured rat astrocytes. Glia 1:359-365.

Marrion NV, Tavalin SJ (1998) Selective activation of Ca^{2+}-activated K^+ channels by co-localized Ca^{2+} channels in hippocampal neurons. Nature 395:900-905.

Matthias K, Kirchhoff F, Seifert G, Hüttmann K, Matyash M, Kettenmann H, Steinhäuser C (2003) Segregated expression of AMPA-type glutamate receptors and glutamate transporters defines distinct astrocyte populations in the mouse hippocampus. J Neurosci 23:1750-1758.

Muyderman H, Sinclair J, Jardemark K, Hansson E, Nilsson M (2001) Activation of beta-adrenoceptors opens calcium-activated potassium channels in astroglial cells. Neurochem Int 38:269-276.

Müller T, Fritschy JM, Grosche J, Pratt GD, Möhler H, Kettenmann H (1994) Developmental regulation of voltage-gated K^+ channel and $GABA_A$ receptor expression in Bergmann glial cells. J Neurosci 14:2503-2514.

Müller T, Möller T, Berger T, Schnitzer J, Kettenmann H (1992) Calcium entry through kainate receptors and resulting potassium- channel blockade in Bergmann glial cells. Science 256:1563-1566.

Nagelhus EA, Horio Y, Inanobe A, Fujita A, Haug FM, Nielsen S, Kurachi Y, Ottersen OP (1999) Immunogold evidence suggests that coupling of K^+ siphoning and water transport in rat retinal Muller cells is mediated by a coenrichment of Kir4.1 and AQP4 in specific membrane domains. Glia 26:47-54.

Newman EA (1985) Voltage-dependent calcium and potassium channels in retinal glial cells. Nature 317:809-811.

Newman EA (1986) High potassium conductance in astrocyte endfeet. Science 233:453-454.

O'Connor ER, Sontheimer H, Spencer DD, De Lanerolle NC (1998) Astrocytes from human hippocampal epileptogenic foci exhibit action potential-like responses. Epilepsia 39:347-354.

Oh Y, Black JA, Waxman SG (1994) The expression of rat brain voltage-sensitive Na^+ channel mRNAs in astrocytes. Mol Brain Res 23:57-65.

Oh Y, Lee YJ, Waxman SG (1997) Regulation of Na^+ channel β1 and β2 subunit mRNA levels in cultured rat astrocytes. Neurosci Lett 234:107-110.

Orkand RK, Nicholls JG, Kuffler SW (1966) Effect of nerve impulses on the membrane potential of glial cells in the central nervous system of amphibia. J Neurophysiol 29:788-806.

Pannicke T, Bringmann A, Reichenbach A (2002) Electrophysiological characterization of retinal Müller glial cells from mouse during postnatal development: Comparison with rabbit cells. Glia 38:268-272.

Pappas CA, Ullrich N, Sontheimer H (1994) Reduction of glial proliferation by K^+ channel blockers is mediated by changes in pH_i. NeuroReport 6:193-196.

Perillan PR, Chen M, Potts EA, Simard JM (2002) Transforming growth factor-beta 1 regulates Kir2.3 inward rectifier K^+ channels via phospholipase C and protein kinase C-delta in reactive astrocytes from adult rat brain. J Biol Chem 277:1974-1980.

Poopalasundaram S, Knott C, Shamotienko OG, Foran PG, Dolly JO, Ghiani CA, Gallo V, Wilkin GP (2000) Glial heterogeneity in expression of the inwardly rectifying K^+ channel, Kir4.1, in adult rat CNS. Glia 30:362-372.

Porter JT, McCarthy KD (1995) GFAP-positive hippocampal astrocytes in situ respond to glutamatergic neuroligands with increases in $[Ca^{2+}]_i$. Glia 13:101-112.

Porter JT, McCarthy KD (1996) Hippocampal astrocytes in situ respond to glutamate released from synaptic terminals. J Neurosci 16:5073-5081.

Price DL, Ludwig JW, Mi H, Schwarz TL, Ellisman MH (2002) Distribution of rSlo Ca^{2+}-activated K^+ channels in rat astrocyte perivascular endfeet. Brain Res 956:183-193.

Puro DG, Hwang JJ, Kwon OJ, Chin HM (1996) Characterization of an L-type calcium channel expressed by human retinal Muller (glial) cells. Mol Brain Res 37:41-48.

Puro DG, Roberge F, Chan CC (1989) Retinal glial cell proliferation and ion channels: a possible link. Invest Ophthalmol Vis Sci 30:521-529.

Quandt FN, MacVicar BA (1986) Calcium activated potassium channels in cultured astrocytes. Neuroscience 19:29-41.

Raap M, Biedermann B, Braun P, Milenkovic I, Skatchkov SN, Bringmann A, Reichenbach A (2002) Diversity of Kir channel subunit mRNA expressed by retinal glial cells of the guinea-pig. NeuroReport 13:1037-1040.

Ransom CB, Liu X, Sontheimer H (2002) BK channels in human glioma cells have enhanced calcium sensitivity. Glia 38:281-291.

Reese KA, Caldwell JH (1999) Immunocytochemical localization of NaCh6 in cultured spinal cord astrocytes. Glia 26:92-96.

Reimann F, Ashcroft FM (1999) Inwardly rectifying potassium channels. Curr Opin Cell Biol 11:503-508.

Rose CR, Ransom BR, Waxman SG (1997) Pharmacological characterization of Na^+ influx via voltage- gated Na^+ channels in spinal cord astrocytes. J Neurophysiol 78:3249-3258.

Roy ML, Saal D, Perney T, Sontheimer H, Waxman SG, Kaczmarek LK (1996) Manipulation of the delayed rectifier Kv1.5 potassium channel in glial cells by antisense oligodeoxynucleotides. Glia 18:177-184.

Schaller KL, Krzemien DM, Yarowsky PJ, Krueger BK, Caldwell JH (1995) A novel, abundant sodium channel expressed in neurons and glia. J Neurosci 15:3231-3242.

Schopf S, Bringmann A, Reichenbach A (1999) Protein kinases A and C are opponents in modulating glial Ca^{2+} -activated K^+ channels. NeuroReport 10:1323-1327.

Schröder W, Hager G, Kouprijanova E, Weber M, Schmitt AB, Seifert G, Steinhäuser C (1999) Lesion-induced changes of electrophysiological properties in astrocytes of the rat dentate gyrus. Glia 28:166-174.

Schröder W, Hinterkeuser S, Seifert G, Schramm J, Jabs R, Wilkin GP, Steinhäuser C (2000) Functional and molecular properties of human astrocytes in acute hippocampal slices obtained from patients with temporal lobe epilepsy. Epilepsia 41:S181-S184.

Schröder W, Seifert G, Hüttmann K, Hinterkeuser S, Steinhäuser C (2002) AMPA receptor-mediated modulation of inward rectifier K^+ channels in astrocytes of mouse hippocampus. Mol Cell Neurosci 19:447-458.

Seifert G, Steinhäuser C (1995) Glial cells in the mouse hippocampus express AMPA receptors with an intermediate Ca^{2+} permeability. Eur J Neurosci 7:1872-1881.

Seifert G, Zhou M, Steinhäuser C (1997) Analysis of AMPA receptor properties during postnatal development of mouse hippocampal astrocytes. J Neurophysiol 78:2916-2923.

Seifert G, Becker A, Steinhäuser C (2002) Combining patch-clamp techniques with RT-PCR. In: Neuromethods, Vol. 35: Patch-clamp analysis: Advanced techniques, Walz W, Boulton AA, Baker GB (Eds.), Humana Press, Totowa, NJ, 301-330.

Skatchkov SN, Thomzig A, Eaton MJ, Biedermann B, Eulitz D, Bringmann A, Pannicke T, Veh RW, Reichenbach A (2001) Kir subfamily in frog retina: specific spatial distribution of Kir 6.1 in glial (Muller) cells. NeuroReport 12:1437-1441.

Smart SL, Bosma MM, Tempel BL (1997) Identification of the delayed rectifier potassium channel, Kv1.6, in cultured astrocytes. Glia 20:127-134.

Sontheimer H, Fernandez-Marques E, Ullrich N, Pappas CA, Waxman SG (1994) Astrocyte Na^+ channels are required for maintenance of Na^+/K^+-ATPase activity. J Neurosci 14:2464-2475.

Steinhäuser C, Jabs R, Kettenmann H (1994a) Properties of GABA and glutamate responses in identified glial cells of the mouse hippocampal slice. Hippocampus 4:19-36.

Steinhäuser C, Kressin K, Kuprijanova E, Weber M, Seifert G (1994b) Properties of voltage-activated sodium and potassium currents in mouse hippocampal glial cells in situ and after acute isolation from tissue slices. Pflugers Arch 428:610-620.

Steinhäuser C, Schröder W, Hinterkeuser S, Knott C, Wilkin GP, Thomzig A, Veh R, Seifert G (2000) Inward rectifier K^+ currents in hippocampal astrocytes of patients with temporal lobe epilepsy are mediated by Kir4.1 and Kir6/SUR channels. Soc Neurosci Abstr 26:1837.

Steinhäuser C, Seifert G (2002) Glial membrane channels and receptors in epilepsy: impact for generation and spread of seizure activity. Eur J Pharmacol 447:227-237.

Stonehouse AH, Pringle JH, Norman RI, Stanfield PR, Conley EC, Brammar WJ (1999) Characterisation of Kir2.0 proteins in the rat cerebellum and hippocampus by polyclonal antibodies. Histochem Cell Biol 112:457-465.

Supattapone S, Ashley CC (1991) Endothelin Opens Potassium Channels in Glial Cells. Eur J Neurosci 3:349-355.

Takumi T, Ishii T, Hori Y, Morishige K-I, Takahashi N, Yamada M, Yamashita T, Kiyama H, Sohmiya K, Nakanishi S, Kurachi Y (1995) A novel ATP-dependent inward rectifier potassium channel expressed predominantly in glial cells. J Biol Chem 270:16339-16346.

Talley EM, Solorzano G, Lei Q, Kim D, Bayliss DA (2001) CNS distribution of members of the two-pore-domain (KCNK) potassium channel family. J Neurosci 21:7491-7505.

Thellung S, Florio T, Corsaro A, Arena S, Merlino M, Salmona M, Tagliavini F, Bugiani O, Forloni G, Schettini G (2000) Intracellular mechanisms mediating the neuronal death and astrogliosis induced by the prion protein fragment 106-126. Int J Dev Neurosci 18:481-492.

Thomzig A, Wenzel M, Karschin C, Eaton MJ, Skatchkov SN, Karschin A, Veh RW (2001) Kir6.1 is the principal pore-forming subunit of astrocyte but not neuronal plasma membrane K-ATP channels. Mol Cell Neurosci 18:671-690.

Tse FW, Fraser DD, Duffy S, MacVicar BA (1992) Voltage-activated K^+ currents in acutely isolated hippocampal astrocytes. J Neurosci 12:1781-1788.

Velasco A, Tabernero A, Granda B, Medina JM (2000) ATP-sensitive potassium channel regulates astrocytic gap junction permeability by a Ca^{2+}-independent mechanism. J Neurochem 74:1249 -56 74.

Vergara C, Latorre R, Marrion NV, Adelman JP (1998) Calcium-activated potassium channels. Curr Opin Neurobiol 8:321-329.

Verkhratsky A, Orkand RK, Kettenmann H (1998) Glial calcium: homeostasis and signaling function. Physiol Rev 78:99-141.

Verkhratsky A, Steinhäuser C (2000) Ion channels in glial cells. Brain Res Rev 32:380-412.

Westenbroek RE, Bausch SB, Lin RCS, Franck JE, Noebels JL, Catterall WA (1998) Upregulation of L-type Ca^{2+} channels in reactive astrocytes after brain injury, hypomyelination, and ischemia. J Neurosci 18:2321-2334.

White HS, Skeen GA, Edwards JA (1992) Pharmacological regulation of astrocytic calcium channels: implications for the treatment of seizure disorders. Prog Brain Res 94:77-87.

Yuan X, Eisen AM, McBain CJ, Gallo V (1998) A role for glutamate and its receptors in the regulation of oligodendrocyte development in cerebellar tissue slices. Development 125:2901-2914.

Zawar C, Plant TD, Schirra C, Konnerth A, Neumcke B (1999) Cell-type specific expression of ATP-sensitive potassium channels in the rat hippocampus. J Physiol (London) 514.2:327-341.

Zhou M, Kimelberg HK (2000) Freshly isolated astrocytes from rat hippocampus show two distinct current patterns and different $[K^+]_o$ uptake capabilities. J Neurophysiol 84:2746-2757.

Zhou M, Tanaka O, Suzuki M, Sekiguchi M, Takata K, Kawahara K, Abe H (2002) Localization of pore-forming subunit of the ATP-sensitive K^+-channel, Kir6.2, in rat brain neurons and glial cells. Mol Brain Res 101:23-32.

7.7. Abbreviations

AHS	Ammon's horn sclerosis
AMPA	α-Amino-3-hydroxy-5-methyl-4-isoxazole propionate
4-AP	4-Aminopyridine
ATP	Adenosine triphosphate
BK channels	Large conductance Ca^{2+}-regulated K^+ channels
cAMP	3',5'-cyclic adenosine monophosphate
CNS	Central nervous system
Ca_v channels	Voltage-gated Ca^{2+} channels
eag	Ether-a-go-go
ECL	Entorhinal cortex lesion
elk	eag-like
erg	eag-related
GFAP	Glial fibrillary acidic protein
HVA	High voltage activated Ca^{2+} channel
K_A	A-type Kv channels
K_D	Delayed rectifier Kv channels
Kv	Voltage-gated K^+ channels
LVA	Low voltage activated Ca^{2+} channels
Na_v channels	Voltage-gated Na^+ channels
PKC	Protein kinase C
RT-PCR	Reverse transcription-polymerase chain reaction
SK channels	Small conductance Ca^{2+}-regulated K^+ channels
SUR	Sulphonylurea receptors
TEA	Tetraethylammonium chloride
TGF-β1	Transforming growth factor-β1
TLE	Temporal lobe epilepsy
TNFα	Tumor necrosis factor α
TTX	Tetrodotoxin
$[X^{\pm}]_i$	Intracellular concentration
$[X^{\pm}]_o$	Extracellular concentration

Chapter 8

Specialized channels in astrocytes

Kimberly A. Parkerson and Harald Sontheimer*

Department of Neurobiology and Civitan International Research Center
The University of Alabama at Birmingham, Birmingham, AL 35294 USA

*Corresponding author: hws@nrc.uab.edu

Contents

8.1. Introduction

As discussed in Chapter 7, astrocytes express a large repertoire of ion channels that are reminiscent of those used by excitable cells to generate or propagate electrical signals. In addition, astrocytes also contain more specialized channels that appear to engage in ion and water homeostasis in brain. Most notably, these include anion channels and water-permeable aquaporins. These channels are much less well understood than their voltage-gated cousins. This chapter attempts to provide a concise summary of our current knowledge regarding the molecular, pharmacological and biophysical characteristics of these specialized channels as well as to discuss some of the potential roles for these channels in the biology of astrocytes. The reader is also referred to recent reviews on anion channels in astrocytes (Walz, 2002) and aquaporins in the central nervous system (Badaut et al., 2002;Venero et al., 2001).

8.2 Anion channels

8.2.1. An overview

Like all ion channels, anion channels are integral membrane proteins that allow for the rapid movement of ions across a cellular membrane. Specifically, anion channels mediate the flow of small negatively charged ions, of which chloride is most abundant physiologically. Therefore, anion channels are often referred to as chloride channels (Hille, 2001). Other species that may be permeable include halides such as bromide and iodide as well as non-halides such as bicarbonate and thiocyanate (Hille, 2001). Additionally, it has been suggested that organic osmolytes such as taurine and inositol may permeate certain anion channels (Jackson and Strange, 1993).

Usually, the biophysical characterization of anion channels combines the relative permeabilities of these anions or osmolytes with the mode of activation of the channel, with the sensitivity of the currents to a variety of channel blockers, and with the ability of the channel to undergo functional modulation by different substrates. When considered together, these characteristics provide a good basis by which to compare anion channels, as unfortunately there is currently an absence of single unique characteristics to easily distinguish one channel type from another.

In addition to the large number of biophysically characterized channels, there have also been four major molecular families of anion channels identified. These are the voltage-gated chloride channels (ClCs), the ATP-binding cassette channels, the voltage-dependent anion channels (VDACs), and the Ca^{2+}-activated chloride channels. However, to date, these molecularly identified channels are unable to account for all of those that have been biophysically identified. Therefore, whole gene families of anion channels may as yet be undiscovered (Jentsch et al., 2002).

8.2.2. Biophysical characterization of anion channels in astrocytes

Whole-cell anion currents in cultured rat cortical astrocytes were first described by Bevan and colleagues (1985) and then further characterized by Gray and Ritchie (1986). These studies showed that astrocytes exhibited outward anion currents (corresponding to an inward movement of anions) that activated at membrane potentials positive to −40 mV and showed slight time-dependent inactivation with steps to membrane potentials more positive than +60 mV (Figure 8.1A). The currents increased in amplitude within the few minutes after formation of the whole-cell patch and were supported when bromide replaced chloride in the external bath solution but were reduced when glutamate, ascorbate, methylsulfate, sulfate, isethionate or acetate replaced chloride and completely eliminated when gluconate replaced chloride (Figure 8.1B). Additionally, the currents were inhibited by external application of the stilbene derivatives, 4,4'-diisothiocyanostilbene-2,2'-disulfonic acid (DIDS) and 4-acetamido-4'-isocyanatostilbene-2,2'-disulfonic acid (SITS).

For almost a decade, these two studies remained the only characterization of whole-cell anion currents in astrocytes. However, during this time there were several reports of single-channel anion conductances in astrocytes, and it was shown that astrocytes possessed at least three different types of anion channels (See Table 8.1 for a summary of biophysically identified anion channels in astrocytes). First, Sonnhof (1987) found the presence of large conductance anion channels in approximately 20% of inside-out patches from cultured rat astrocytes, but in less than 1% of cell-attached patches. The channels were characterized by a mean conductance level of 400 pS and exhibited a slight permeability to cations as well as permeability to divalent anions and large anions such as isethionate. However, the channels were impermeant to glutamate and aspartate. In addition, the channels could be divided into two groups: approximately 85% showed the highest probability of opening at the zero-current potential and approximately 15% showed voltage-independent behavior.

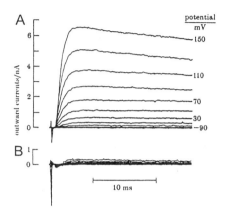

Figure 8.1. Records of the outward currents (whole-cell recording) from a rat cultured astrocyte (with N-methyl-(+)-glucamine gluconate in the pipette). The cell was held at −70 mV, pulsed to −100 mV for 100 ms, and then brought to the potentials indicated. Panel (*b*) shows the same family of records obtained shortly after the sodium chloride of the bathing medium had been replaced by sodium gluconate. [From Gray and Ritchie (1986), with permission.]

Around the same time, Nowak and colleagues (1987) described two types of anion channels in mouse cortical astrocytes. The first type appeared identical to the more prevalent class of channels described by Sonnhof (1987), as the channels exhibited a high probability of opening between −15 mV and +30 mV in symmetrical chloride concentrations, a mean conductance of 385 pS, and a finite cation and substantial isethionate permeability. Interestingly, both Sonnhof (1987) and Nowak and colleagues (1987) referred to the possibility that these large conductance single-channel currents could represent the correlate of the whole-cell anion currents observed by Bevan and colleagues (1985) and Gray and Ritchie (1986); however, they did not reconcile why the activity of these channels required an excised patch in their studies but were readily observable in whole-cell patch recordings in the earlier reports.

The second type of channels in the study by Nowak and colleagues (1987) showed quite different behavior and were unlike any previous anion channels described in astrocytes. These channels exhibited an increased probability of opening upon hyperpolarization and showed a mean conductance of 5 pS. Unfortunately, further characterization of this second anion channel type has not been performed to date.

Table 8.1. Biophysically identified anion channels in astrocytes

Preparation	Configuration	Activation	Conductance	Ion Selectivity	Inhibitors	Modifiers	Special	Reference
Rat	Whole-cell	$V_m > -40$ mV		Cl^- > glut⁻, ascorb⁻				Bevan et al., 1985
Rat	Whole-cell	$V_m > -40$ mV		$Br^- > Cl^-$ > methylSO_4^- > SO_4^{2-} ise⁻ > ace⁻ > gluc⁻	DIDS, SITS	Not internal Ca^{2+}, or addition of cAMP, ATP or Mg^{2+}		Gray and Ritchie, 1986
Rat	Inside-out	~85% at zero-current potential; ~15% voltage-independent	400 pS	Perm to divalent and large anions like ise⁻; not perm to glut⁻ or asp⁻; slight perm to cations			Found in ~20% of inside-out patches; <1% cell-attached patches	Sonnhof, 1987
Mouse	Outside-out	V_m −15 to 30 mV	385 pS	Perm to ise⁻; finite cation perm				Nowak et al., 1987
Mouse	Outside-out	V_m to −100 mV	5 pS					Nowak et al., 1987
Rat	Cell-attached, inside-out	Voltage near zero-current potential	200-300 pS		Zn^{2+}, Cd^{2+}, L-644,711	Increased activity in hypotonicity or after trypsin	More frequent inside-out than cell-attached	Jalonen et al., 1989, 1991; Jalonen, 1993
Rat	Whole-cell	Morphological change and variable voltage-dependency			DIDS, Zn^{2+}	Actin polymerization		Lascola and Kraig, 1996

Table 8.1. Continued

Preparation	Configuration	Activation	Conductance	Ion Selectivity	Inhibitors	Modifiers	Special	Reference
Rat	Inside-out	Spontaneous or following depolarization; active at all potentials	36 pS from −60 to −80 mV; 75 pS from 60 to 80 mV		ATP, DIDS, Zn^{2+}	Actin polymerization	More frequent in stellate than flat cells	Lascola et al., 1998
Rat	Whole-cell	Hypoosmotic stimulation			NPPB, SITS, genistein, typhostin A23, PD98059	Not intracellular Ca^{2+}, but rundown with omission of ATP	Requirement of tyrosine kinases and MAPK for activation	Crepel et al., 1998
Rat	Whole-cell	Hyperpol. from 0 mV holding		$Cl^-=Br^-=I^->F^-$ >cyclamate≥$gluc^-$	9-AC, Cd^{2+}, Zn^{2+}, but not DIDS or SITS	Changes in pH and osmolarity	Long-term dBcAMP incubation before recording	Ferroni et al., 1995, 1997; Fava et al., 2001
Rat	Cell-attached, outside-out	Hyperpol.	Two equidistant levels of 3 and 6 pS				Long-term dBcAMP incubation before recording	Nobile et al., 2000

Jalonen and colleagues (1989, 1991, 1993) characterized a third chloride conductance at the single-channel level in astrocytes. Similar to the channel observed by Sonnhof (1987), this channel described by Jalonen and colleagues (1989, 1991, 1993) was detected more frequently in excised patches than in cell-attached recordings; however it exhibited a smaller single-channel conductance of approximately 200-300 pS. The channel possessed at least five open sublevels, was maximally open at the zero-current potential, and was inhibited by the anion transport blocker L-644,711. Also, millimolar concentrations of zinc or cadmium ions applied to the intracellular side of the membrane blocked the channel at positive potentials. Additionally, unlike other channels described to this point in astrocytes, the frequency of occurrence of channel activity increased in the presence of low osmolarity solution or upon preparation of secondary cell cultures by trypsinization. Therefore, this series of studies by Jalonen and colleagues (1989, 1991, 1993) appeared as the first reports of hypotonic-activated anion channels in astrocytes.

Finally, in the mid-1990's, several independent groups revisited the characterization of whole-cell anion currents in astrocytes. From these studies emerged a more thorough understanding of the regulation of and properties of anion currents that are present in astrocytes. Lascola and Kraig (1996) even provided an explanation of why Gray and Ritchie (1986) may have been successful in observing anion currents in intact astrocytes while others required formation of excised patches.

In their study, Lascola and Kraig (1996) suggested that the presence of anion currents in astrocytes was dependent upon changes in cell morphology and disassembly of the actin cytoskeleton. First, they recorded from flat, control astrocytes and compared these recordings to those of astrocytes rounded up by brief trypsinization, astrocytes converted to a stellate morphology by exposure to serum-free conditions and astrocytes swollen by exposure to hypoosmotic solution. Under control conditions, astrocytes did not express anion currents, whereas outwardly-rectifying anion currents were observed in each of the other three conditions. Lascola and Kraig (1996) pointed out that Gray and Ritchie (1986) also briefly exposed astrocytes to a trypsin-containing solution in order to facilitate whole-cell patching.

Next, Lascola and Kraig (1996) proceeded to show a link between actin cytoskeleton modulation and anion currents in astrocytes. Using agents that either disrupted or stabilized actin polymerization, they showed a dynamic induction or inhibition of whole-cell anion currents, respectively. For example, cytochalasins, which disrupt actin polymerization by shifting the equilibrium between actin polymers and monomers towards monomers, induced anion currents in flat, control astrocytes, whereas phallodin, which stabilizes actin polymers, prevented hypoosmotic activation of anion currents. In a later study, Lascola and colleagues (1998) showed similar modulation of single-channel anion currents upon disruption or stabilization of the actin cytoskeleton (Figure 8.2).

Interesting, however, was that the single-channel currents they recorded appeared to represent a fourth distinct anion channel type in astrocytes. Unlike the anion channels described in single-channel studies above, these channels were clearly outwardly-rectifying, as they exhibited a single-channel conductance of 36 pS between −60 and −80 mV and 75 pS between 60 and 80 mV in symmetrical chloride solutions. Further, ATP, DIDS, and zinc ions blocked the channels.

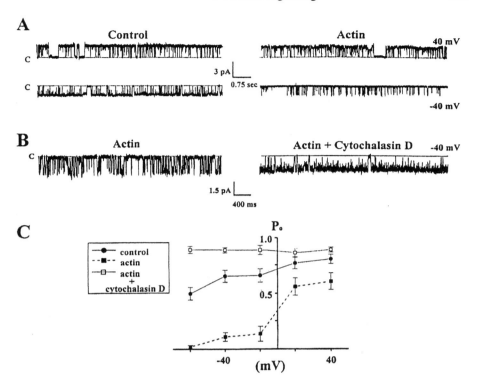

Figure 8.2. Actin and cytochalasin D modulate the open-state probability (P_0) of an outwardly rectifying current at negative potentials. A. The *left* current traces are taken from an inside-out patch initially in control solutions. P_0 at 40 mV was 0.74; P_0 at –40 mV was 0.71. The *right* current traces demonstrate records of the same channel ~5 min after the addition of a mixed solution of actin polymers, short filaments, and monomers (final concentration, 1 mg/ml). Actin applied to the bath caused a dramatic decrease in P_0 at negative potentials. P_0 at –40 mV was 0.05 over 30 sec, whereas at 40 mV P_0 was 0.69 after the addition of actin. B. The current trace on the *left* represents an outwardly rectifying channel at –40 mV after it had been exposed to 1 mg/ml actin. P_0 at –40 mV was 0.23. The current trace on the *right* shows the same channel 17 min after the addition of 10 mM cytochalasin D while the amount of actin in the bath remained unchanged. Channel P_0 increased to 0.95. Note also the marked increase in open channel noise accompanying the increase in P_0. The C adjacent to the *dotted line* indicates the closed state of the channel. C. P_0 is plotted versus membrane potential (mV). Note that the increase in P_0 after the addition of cytochalasin D (unfilled squares) surpasses the P_0 of control patches. Mean P_0 at –40 mV after the addition of cytochalasin D was 0.89 ± 0.02 (n=5), significantly higher (p < 0.05) than the P_0 (0.70 ± 0.04) in control cells. [From Lascola et al. (1998), with permission]

In addition to modulation of anion currents by the cytoskeleton, Crepel and colleagues (1998) showed that other intracellular signaling cascades also contribute to and are critically involved in anion channel activation. In this study, they recorded hypoosmotic-activated anion currents that were similar to those of Lascola and Kraig (1996), and they demonstrated the requirement for tyrosine protein kinases and mitogen-activated protein kinases (MAPK) in activation of the currents.

Hypoosmotic-activated anion currents were blocked by the tyrosine kinase inhibitors, genistein and tyrphostin A23, as well as by the mitogen-activated protein kinase kinase (MEK) inhibitor, PD98059.

Around the same time as these studies were performed on outwardly-rectifying whole-cell anion currents, Ferroni and colleagues (Ferroni et al., 1995, 1997, 2000; Nobile et al., 2000; Fava et al., 2001) studied whole-cell inwardly-rectifying anion currents in astrocytes. Similar to Lascola and Kraig (1996), Ferroni and colleagues (Ferroni et al. 1995, 1997, 2000; Nobile et al., 2000; Fava et al., 2001) had to induce morphological changes in astrocytes in order to observe inwardly-rectifying anion currents. Specifically, they used long-term treatment with dibutyryl-cyclic-AMP (dBcAMP). Under these conditions, hyperpolarizing steps elicited slowly activating inward anion currents. The currents showed no time-dependent inactivation, were not blocked by DIDS, SITS, barium or cesium ions, but were reversibly inhibited by 9-anthracene carboxylic acid (9-AC), cadmium or zinc ions. Additionally, exposure to changes of pH within the physiological range (Ferroni et al., 2000) or to changes in osmolarity (Fava et al., 2001) modulated current amplitudes. Single-channel analysis of these currents revealed two equidistant conductances of 3 and 6 pS (Fava et al., 2001) that possibly represented the same small conductance hyperpolarizing activated currents as earlier recorded by Nowak and colleagues (1987).

In addition to the studies described above on normal astrocytes, there have also been several reports on anion channels in malignantly transformed astrocytes, or gliomas. Jackson and colleagues (1993, 1994) identified and characterized a channel that they termed volume-sensitive organic osmolyte-anion channel (VSOAC) in rat C6 glioma cells. Based on their studies, this channel was permeable to both inorganic and organic anions such as taurine and inositol and represented the major swelling-activated current in these cells. It was blocked by ketoconazole, arachidonic acid, 5-Nitro-2-(3-phenylpropylamino)benzoic acid (NPPB), and 1,9-dideoxyforskolin. Similarly, Roy (1995) showed volume-sensitive anion channels in U-138 glioma cells that were permeable to anionic amino acids, and Jackson and Madsen (1997) found channels with properties identical to VSOAC in human glioma cells following neurosurgical resection.

Anion currents were also reported in STTG1 and D54MG glioma cells by Sontheimer and colleagues (Ullrich and Sontheimer 1996, 1997; Ransom et al, 2001). Unique to these currents is that they were not only reported to activate in response to hypotonic challenge but were also responsible for the resting chloride conductance in these cells under isotonic conditions. These currents were blocked by tamoxifen and NPPB and exhibited an $I-> Cl-$ permeability.

8.2.3. Molecular identification of anion channels in astrocytes

The molecular identification of anion channels in astrocytes is still in its infancy. Of the four major molecular anion channel families, select members of three of these have been examined for expression in astrocytes, namely ClC-2 and ClC-3 of the ClCs (Sik et al., 2000; Stegen et al., 2000), cystic fibrosis transmembrane regulator (CFTR) of the ATP-binding cassette channels (Ballerini et al, 2002) and BR1-VDAC of the VDACs (Dermietzel et al., 1994). However, it should also be mentioned that ClC-4, ClC-5, ClC-6 and ClC-7, other members of the ClCs, have been found in brain (Adler et al., 1997; Brandt and Jentsch 1995; Steinmeyer et al., 1995; Stobrawa et al., 2001).

The ClC family of evolutionarily conserved channels currently consists of nine members (ClC 1-7, ClC-Ka, ClC-Kb) in mammals (Waldegger and Jentsch, 2000). A major boost to the understanding of ClC channels was the recent crystallization of two prokaryotic forms (Dutzler et al., 2002). The study showed that a single CLC channel subunit contained 18 α-helices. Further, a functional channel consisted of a dimeric double-barreled structure of two independent pores, as was first postulated for ClC-0 in *Torpedo marmorata* many years ago (Miller, 1982; Miller and White, 1984).

One member of the ClC family that has been found in astrocytes is ClC-2. ClC-2 was originally isolated and cloned by Thiemann and colleagues (1992) from rat heart and brain and the sequence showed an approximately 50% homology with that of both the *Torpedo* channel ClC-0 and the rat muscle channel ClC-1. When ClC-2 was expressed in *Xenopus* oocytes, electrophysiological analysis revealed a current that activated slowly upon hyperpolarization and showed a $Cl^- \geq Br^- > I^-$ permeability sequence. The current was partially inhibited by the anion channel blockers, 9-AC and diphenylaminecarboxylate, but not affected by DIDS. Additionally, the channel was alternatively activated by extracellular hypotonicity (Grunder et al., 1992).

ClC-2 was detected at the mRNA level by RT-PCR in cultured astrocytes (Stegen et al., 2000) and at the protein level by immmunostaining in the end feet of astrocytes in hippocampal slices (Sik et al., 2000). Also, the inwardly-rectifying anion conductance described above that was characterized by Ferroni and colleagues (Ferroni et al., 1995, 1997, 2000; Nobile et al., 2000, Fava et al., 2001) exhibited features similar to heterologously expressed ClC-2, and the currents were considered to be 'ClC-2 like.' So far, studies such as antisense knockdown to more definitively show that the currents were indeed ClC-2 have not performed in normal astrocytes. However, ClC-2 antisense knockdown experiments were recently performed in D54 glioma cells, and ClC-2 was found to represent an inwardly-rectifying current in these cells (Olsen et al., 2003).

Another member of the ClC family that has been detected in astrocytes is ClC-3. ClC-3 was originally isolated and cloned from rat kidney by Kawasaki and colleagues (1994) and abundant expression of ClC-3 mRNA was found in rat brain. When ClC-3 was expressed in *Xenopus* oocytes, electrophysiological analysis revealed a time-independent current that did not appear to be voltage-dependent and showed an $I^- > Cl^- \approx Br^-$ permeability sequence. Opposite to ClC-2, the current was inhibited by DIDS, but not affected by 9-AC or diphenylamine-2-carboxylate (DPC). ClC-3 currents were also inhibited by the phobol esters that are activators of protein kinase C (PKC). Additionally, Duan and colleagues (1997) showed strong modulation by osmolarity changes of a cardiac clone of ClC-3 when expressed in a fibroblast cell line NIH/3T3, and they suggested a striking similarity of ClC-3 to the swelling-activated anion currents present in native cells. However, since then, efforts to molecularly identify the swelling-activated anion channel have been surrounded by much controversy (for review, Jentsch et al., 2002).

Similar to ClC-2, ClC-3 was detected at the mRNA level in cultured astrocytes (Stegen et al., 2000). However, ClC-3 currents have not been positively identified in normal astrocytes. ClC-3 antisense knockdown experiments were recently performed in D54 glioma cells, and ClC-3 was found to represent a weakly outwardly-rectifying current in these cells (Olsen et al., 2003).

Another chloride channel transcript that has been identified in astrocytes is CFTR, currently the sole member of the ATP-binding cassette channels. Riordan and colleagues (Riordan et al. 1989) originally identified CFTR as the product of the cystic fibrosis gene in 1989. CFTR is a cyclic nucleotide-regulated chloride channel that contains two homologous halves, each consisting of six membrane-spanning and one nucleotide-binding domain (Akabas 2000). Further, a cytoplasmic regulatory domain that contains both protein kinase A (PKA) and PKC phosphorylation sites links the two halves, and the gating of CFTR is controlled by both phosphorylation and ATP binding and hydrolysis (Akabas 2000). Studies have shown that CFTR is blocked by DPC (McCarty et al. 1993) and glybenclamide (Sheppard and Welsh 1992) as well as by certain anions such as I⁻, which is attributed to relatively tight binding of these species within the pore (Linsdell 2001;Tabcharani et al. 1992).

Ballerini and colleagues first detected CFTR in astrocytes using RT-PCR amplification of rat fetal astrocyte RNA (Ballerini et al. 2002). In addition, they observed an efflux of radiolabeled chloride in response to simultaneous activation of PKC and PKA that could be inhibited by preincubation with glybenclamide.

The last anion channel that has been identified in astrocytes is BR-VDAC1, a member of the VDACs, also called porins. It was originally thought that the VDACs were exclusively localized to the outer mitochondrial membrane of eukaryotic cells where they participated in movement of small molecules such as nucleotides as well as ions (Dermietzel et al., 1994). However, recent evidence suggests that some VDACs may also be found in the plasma membrane of eukaryotic cells. Proteins that are highly homologous to mitochondrial VDACs were both isolated from the plasma membrane of a lymphocyte cell line (Thinnes et al., 1989) and found to associate with the γ-aminobutyric acid type A receptor (GABA$_A$) (Bureau et al., 1992).

More recently, Dermietzel and colleagues (1994) isolated and cloned a protein from bovine brain named BR-VDAC1 that was identical to the VDAC identified in lymphocytes. Interestingly, they suggested that the biophysical properties of other VDACs are similar to those of the large-conductance anion channel described by Sonnhof (1987) and Nowak (1987) in astrocytes. Using *in situ* immunohistochemisty, the channel localized to astrocytes, and an antibody against the channel blocked the large-conductance anion channel activity in inside-out patches of astrocytes (Dermietzel et al., 1994). This implied that BR-VDAC1 encoded a functional channel in astrocytic membranes.

8.3. Aquaporins

8.3.1. An overview

The aquaporins are a family of integral membrane proteins that form water-selective channels and serve to increase water permeability of cellular membranes above that conferred by simple lipid-phase water partitioning (Knepper, 1994). The concept of water channels was first postulated in the 1950's (Knepper, 1994); however, it was not until 1988 that the first water channel was identified (Denker et al., 1988). Since then, there have been a total of eleven isoforms of aquaporins

(AQP 0-10) identified in mammals (Matsuzaki et al., 2002). These can be divided into three groups based on permeabilities: AQP0, AQP1, AQP2, AQP4, AQP5, and AQP6 are permeable to water; AQP3, AQP7, AQP8 are permeable to water, glycerol and urea; and AQP9 and AQP10 are permeable to water, purines, pyrimidines, and monocarboxylates (Badaut et al., 2002). Additionally, AQP9 is permeable to glycerol and urea (Badaut et al., 2002).

Based on amino acid sequence, it has been proposed that each aquaporin monomer consists of a single polypeptide chain which transverses the membrane six times (Matsuzaki et al., 2002). The six membrane crossings are formed by two tandem repeats of three α-helices, and the water selectivity of the channels is thought to result from loops containing Asn-Pro-Ala motifs that connect the tandem repeats as shown in Figure 8.3 (Badaut et al., 2002). Further, studies on AQP1 suggest that each monomer forms a water pore and that four pores associate within the plasma membrane to form a functional channel (Agre et al., 1993).

Pharmacologically, many of the aquaporin isoforms show sensitivity to mercury-based reagents. In fact, a cysteine residue, C-189, was identified in AQP1 as the site of binding and inhibition for mercury ions (Preston et al., 1993), and as expected, this residue was absent in the mercurial-insensitive water channel, or AQP4 (Knepper, 1994). Recently, potent inhibition of water permeability was also noted in the presence of silver nitrate or silver sulfadiazine in AQP1-containing red blood cells (Niemietz and Tyerman, 2002) and in the presence of tetraethylammonium ions (TEA^+) in AQP1-expressing *Xenopus* oocytes (Brooks et al., 2000).

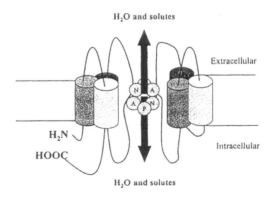

Figure 8.3. Schematic representation of the common aquaporin structure. The aquaporins are formed by two tandem repeats of three membrane-spanning α helices. Two connecting loops, each containing an Asn-Pro-Ala (NPA) motif, are supposed to form the pore in the plasma membrane. [From Badaut et al. (2002), with permission]

8.3.2. Identification of aquaporins in astrocytes

Several different aquaporin isoforms have been identified in brain and/or astrocytes. Probably the best studied of these aquaporins is AQP4 which was cloned independently from both lung and rat brain in 1994 (Hasegawa et al., 1994; Jung et al., 1994). In fact, with the exception of the choroid plexus, where AQP1 is abundantly expressed (Nielsen et al., 1993), mechanisms of water transport within the brain were largely unidentified until the discovery of AQP4 (Jung et al., 1994).

Following the cloning of AQP4, several studies examined its cellular and subcellular localization within brain *in situ*. Jung and colleagues (1994) performed Northern blots and *in situ* hybridization on rat brain slices. They found that AQP4 mRNA probes hybridized to total RNA from the cerebral cortex, cerebellum and brainstem of mature, but not fetal rat brain. Further, *in situ* hybridization showed high expression of AQP4 mRNA at the pial surface of the brain, in the ependymal lining system, in the paraventricular and supraoptic nuclei, and in several neuronal cell layers. Badaut and colleagues (2002) confirmed a similar distribution of AQP4 protein within the brain and further showed a colocalization of AQP4 with glial fibrillary acidic protein (GFAP). In two other studies, AQP4 protein expression was also largely restricted to glial cells in brain, optic nerve and retina (Nagelhus et al., 1998; Nielsen et al., 1997). Interestingly, within the glial cells, AQP4 protein expression was highly polarized with strongest expression noted in astrocytic membranes directly contacting capillaries and the pia mater (Nielsen et al., 1997).

Expression of AQP4 protein was also demonstrated in cultured astrocytes; however, a polarized expression pattern within the cells was not maintained (Nicchia et al., 2000). Importantly, cultured astrocytes exhibited a temperature- and mercury-insensitive swelling in response to osmotic changes (Nicchia et al., 2000), suggesting a potential functional contribution of AQP4 to water homeostasis within astrocytes and the brain. Supportive of such a role, deletion of AQP4 in mice increased survival and decreased swelling of astrocytic end feet following water intoxication as shown in Figure 8.4 (Manley et al., 2000). Deletion of AQP4 in mice also improved neurological outcome following middle cerebral artery occlusion (Manley et al., 2000).

In addition to AQP4, several other aquaporin isoforms have been detected in astrocytes *in situ* and in culture. AQP9 mRNA was first discovered in astrocytes in 1998 (Tsukaguchi et al., 1998), and AQP9 protein was found in brain in 2001 (Elkjaer et al., 2000). However, in the latter study, AQP9 protein was not detected in either astrocytes or neurons. This was reexamined by Badaut and colleagues (2001) who found AQP9 immunolabeling of astrocytic processes bordering the subarachnoid space and ventricles. Recently, Yamamoto and colleagues (2001b) additionally showed the presence of AQP3, AQP5, and AQP8 mRNA in cultured astrocytes by RT-PCR, but *in situ* localization or immunolabeling has not yet been performed.

Complementing the identification and localization of aquaporins, other studies have also examined some of the mechanisms for regulation of aquaporin expression in astrocytes and the brain. Both AQP1 and AQP4 were upregulated in the neoplastic cells within brain tumors (Saadoun et al., 2002a, 2002b), and the degree of upregulation correlated with the grade of the tumor. AQP9 immunolabeling was upregulated in astrocytes within periinfarct areas following transient ischemia (Badaut et al., 2001). AQP4 mRNA was upregulated in reactive astrocytes following brain injury that disrupted the blood-brain barrier (Vizuete et al., 1999), whereas hypoxia induced a decrease in AQP 4, 5, and 9 mRNA expression in the brain (Yamamoto et al., 2001b). Also, activation of PKC by 12-O-tetradecanoylphorbol-13-acetate (TPA) caused a decrease in AQP4 and AQP9 mRNA and protein expression (Nakahama et al., 1999; Yamamoto et al., 2001a), and activation of PKA by dBcAMP caused a decrease in AQP5 mRNA and protein expression, an increase in AQP9 mRNA and protein expression and no change in AQP4 mRNA and protein expression (Yamamoto et al., 2002).

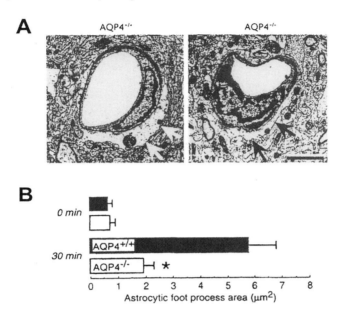

Figure 8.4. Localization and quantitation of cerebral edema following water intoxication. A, Transmission electron micrograph showing edematous cerebral cortex at 30 min. Note the swollen astrocytic foot process in brain from AQP $4^{+/+}$ (white arrows) and AQP $4^{-/-}$ mice. Scale bar represents 3 μm. B. Quantitation of pericapillary astrocyte foot process area. There was significantly less (*, p < 0.005) swelling of the astrocyte foot processes in the AQP $4^{-/-}$ mice following 30 min of water intoxication. [From Manley et al. (2000), with permission]

8.4. Functional roles of anion channels and aquaporins in astrocytes

8.4.1 Cell volume control

Most cells possess mechanisms to control or regulate their volume (Lang et al., 1998), and volume regulation has been clearly demonstrated for cultured astrocytes in response to hypotonic challenge (Kimelberg and Frangakis, 1985; Olson et al., 1986). One of the mechanisms proposed in volume regulation is activation of separate cation and anion channels. Anion channels seem particularly suited to this role in astrocytes. As discussed above, activation of astrocytic anion channels requires shape and/or volume changes (Lascola and Kraig, 1996). Importantly, evidence points to active accumulation of Cl$^-$ and a Cl$^-$ equilibrium potential positive to that of the K$^+$-dominated resting potential of cultured astrocytes (Kimelberg, 1981; Kettenmann, 1987; Walz and Mukerji, 1988; Bevensee et al., 1997; Bekar and Walz, 2002). Therefore, an outward driving force exists for Cl$^-$.

Indeed, cultured astrocytes exhibit a depolarization (Kimelberg and O'Connor, 1988; Kimelberg and Kettenmann, 1990) during volume regulation that is consistent with activation of anion channels. Further, Pasantes-Morales and colleagues (1993, 1994) showed that volume regulation of astrocytes was inhibited by the K^+ channel blocker, quinidine, and the anion channel blocker, DIDS, and Parkerson and Sontheimer (2003) showed a dependence of volume regulation on anion flux and an inhibition of volume regulation by anion channel blockers (Figure 8.5).

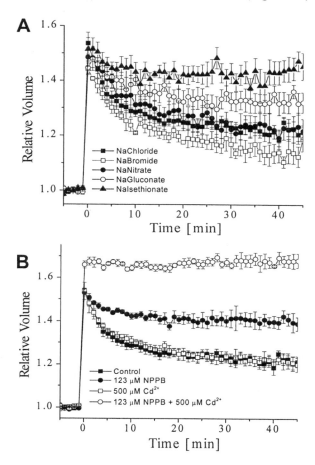

Figure 8.5. Anion channels contribute to volume regulation of astrocytes. A. Comparison of volume regulation under control conditions and after overnight anion substitutions (filled squares, control; open squares, bromide⁻; filled circles, nitrate⁻, open circles, gluconate⁻; filled triangles, isethionate⁻). B. Inhibition of volume regulation by anion channel blockers (filled squares, control; open squares, Cd^{2+}; filled circles, NPPB; open circles, NPPB + Cd^{2+}). [Modified from Parkerson and Sontheimer (2003), with permission]

Undoubtedly, water movements are also associated with the flux of ions during volume regulation in order to dissipate osmotic gradients, although experiments have not been performed to directly implicate aquaporins in astrocytes. However, the Ca^{2+}-activated K^+ channel, rSlo, which is postulated to play a role in cell volume changes has been shown to localize with AQP4 in rat astrocyte perivascular endfeet

(Price et al., 2002). Also, as described above, evidence does suggest an involvement of AQP4 in astrocytic swelling as deletion of AQP4 in mice reduced brain edema following water intoxication and middle cerebral artery occlusion (Manley et al., 2000).

8.4.2. Ion Homeostasis

Proper functioning of the nervous system is highly dependent upon the maintenance of relatively constant ion concentrations, and many studies have examined the processes involved in regulation of the brain microenvironment. In particular, astrocytes have been implicated in the uptake or buffering of extracellular K^+ (Orkand et al., 1966). Walz (1987) suggested that within the physiological range of 1.5 to 12 mM extracellular K^+, uptake of K^+ into astrocytes occurs through activation of the Na-K-2Cl transporter. However, within the pathological range of 25 to 100 mM extracellular K^+, uptake of K^+ into astrocytes occurs through a passive channel-mediated KCl accumulation. Walz and Mukerji (1988) suggested that the channel-mediated Cl^- component might occur through previously described voltage-dependent anion channels. In another study, Walz and Wuttke (1999) found that astrocytes in the gliotic stratum radiatum of the hippocampal slice cooperatively use both transporter and channel-mediated mechanisms within even the physiological range of K^+ concentrations. Therefore, anion channels might play a role in K^+ uptake at all concentrations within reactive astrocytes.

As in volume regulation, water fluxes must necessarily accompany the ion fluxes during K^+ buffering. The role of aquaporins in K^+ buffering has not been investigated within astrocytes of the brain. However, in Müller cells of the retina, AQP4 was shown to localize with the K^+ channel, Kir4.1 (Figure 8.6), which is thought to mediate for K^+ siphoning in the retina (Nagelhus et al., 1999).

A more recent role postulated for anion channels in ion homeostasis is in transmembrane chloride movements associated with GABAergic synaptic transmission (Sik et al., 2000). Sik and colleagues (2000) examined the distribution of ClC-2 within the hippocampus and found a laminar distribution of positively labeled astrocytic processes that associated with neuronal GABAergic terminals. They suggested that such a distribution might allow astrocytes to siphon and deliver Cl^- to specific areas within the brain. Specifically, release of Cl^- near GABAergic synapses would enhance the inward driving force for Cl^- into those neurons and hence the efficacy of GABAergic transmission.

8.4.3. Cell migration

Gliomas exhibit an intense ability to migrate into and invade surrounding brain tissue. This process involves shape and/or volume changes, and it has been proposed that these changes are mediated through fluxes of ions. In fact, the K^+ and Cl^- channel blockers, TEA^+ and tamoxifen, effectively inhibited glioma cell migration when assayed in transwell migration assays, brain aggregate invasion assays, and slice invasion assays (Soroceanu et al., 1999). Interestingly, activation of volume-activated anion currents was also detected during spontaneous movement of cultured glioma cells, and the anion channel blocker, NPPB, inhibited both these currents and transwell migration. Therefore, a model of glioma cell invasion was developed by

Sontheimer and colleagues (Soroceanu et al., 1999; Ransom et al., 2001) in which salt and water efflux via cation, anion, and likely aquaporin channels at the leading edge of the glioma cell allow the cell to initially shrink and invade constrained spaces within the brain (Figure 8.7). Such a requirement of coupled cation, anion and water fluxes in the context of cell migration might more generally apply to other migratory cells. These include embryonic neurons and glia as well as stem cells, all of which migrate in a similarly constricted and tortuous extracellular space.

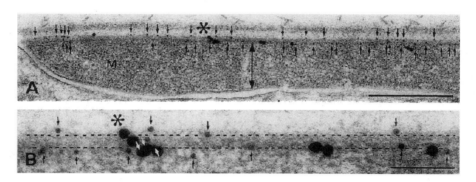

Figure 8.6. Double-immunogold labeling of Kir4.1 (small particles) and AQP4 (large particles) in vitreal Müller cell membranes. A,B. Note, in A, that the Müller cell endfoot (M) is selectively labeled at its inner (vitreal) aspect (both aspects indicated by double arrow). The vitreal plasma membrane (between dashed lines in B) is obliquely cut, allowing labeling at the two sides to be distinguished. Small black arrows indicate Kir4.1 labeling, while small white arrows indicate AQP4 labeling. Asterisks indicate corresponding points at the vitreal surface (part of A is enlarged in B). [From Nagelhus et al. (1999), with permission]

8.5. Future Directions

As conveyed in this chapter, only now are we beginning to gain an understanding of how anions and water transverse the astrocytic membrane. In part, this new understanding is the result of cloning of the genes that encode for anion and water channels and of identifying specific molecular tools that allow us to probe for and to perturb channel expression in a selective manner. These new tools are essential, as currently available pharmacological inhibitors are insufficient.

To date, we still do not understand whether or how anion and water flux across astrocytric membranes are coupled. Electron microscopic studies demonstrate colocalization of these channels and support the generally held view that water movement across membranes is tightly coupled to anion flux. However, future studies are needed to delineate the molecular and physiological interaction of anion and water fluxes. Similarly, the preliminary evidence for a gating of anion channels by changes in the cell cytoskeleton and/or cell shape is intriguing. Yet, we have little knowledge as to the molecular linkage between these processes. In light of the fundamental importance of cytoskeletal interactions with anion and water channels, these studies might be of general importance and reveal novel mechanisms of channel gating that also apply to other related ion channels.

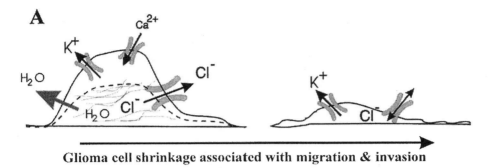

Glioma cell shrinkage associated with migration & invasion

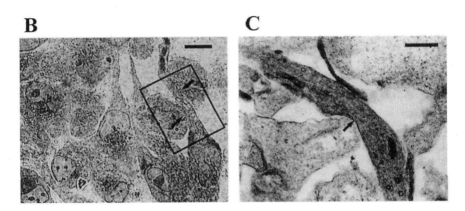

Figure 8.7. A, Model representing glioma cell shape and volume-adaptive changes that occur during invasion in spatially restricted conditions. These changes, accompanied by water loss and cytoskeletal rearrangements, are mediated by ion fluxes through Cl⁻ and K⁺ ion channels and other ion transport mechanisms. B, Semithin section through a coculture of tumor spheroids and fetal brain aggregates, stained with toluidine blue. Glioma cells are seen advancing through two normal rat brain cells (arrows). Scale bar, 20 μm. C, Area of detail of the same preparation as in B, analyzed by transmission electron microscopy. Glioma cells are easily recognized because of the abundance of ribosomes and other organelles that incorporate lead citrate and give a darker appearance. Arrows indicate area of contact between an elongated tumor cell and two other membranes, presumably of the fetal rat brain. Scale bar, 1 μm. [From Soroceanu et al. (1999), with permission.]

Ultimately, one of the main goals in astrocytic biology remains to elucidate the roles that astrocytes play in brain function and disease. Unlike any other organ in the body, the brain exists in a confined space defined by the bony cavity of the skull. This cavity limits any significant changes in overall cell volume. This constraint is immediately apparent in injury and disease conditions such as the prominent brain swelling (edema) following acute head injury or the peritumoral edema associated with brain neoplasia. Studying the role of anion and water channels in this context presents a major challenge, as the underlying conditions cannot readily be reconstructed *in vitro* or *in situ*. Physiological methods do not permit the study of astrocytic function without compromising the integrity of the skull, and even in brain slice preparations, the extracellular space is greatly perturbed. Therefore, much effort is needed to build a body of knowledge from which we can at least infer the role of these channels in the disease process, and, importantly, in the physiological process that normally prevents disease. As a starting point, we must undertake a detailed analysis of anion channels expressed by astrocytes *in vivo* rather than *in vitro* both at the physiological and molecular level. We must use antisense and transgenic strategies to delineate the relative importance of subsets of these channels to anion and water homeostasis. Also, we must study the activation properties of anion channels under conditions that mimic the disease process. Ideally, all these studies will utilize genetic tools to selectively eliminate subsets of channels in order to examine their relative contribution to anion, volume and water homeostasis. Finally, these data may allow us to design specific transgenic animals in which to test the hypothesis that defined anion and water channels confer a brain specific function on astrocytes that is concerned with anion, volume, and water homeostasis.

8.6. References

Adler DA, Rugarli EI, Lingenfelter PA, Tsuchiya K, Poslinski D, Liggitt HD, Chapman VM, Elliott RW, Ballabio A, Disteche CM (1997) Evidence of evolutionary up-regulation of the single active X chromosome in mammals based on Clc4 expression levels in Mus spretus and Mus musculus. Proc Natl Acad Sci USA 94: 9244-9248.

Agre P, Preston GM, Smith BL, Jung JS, Raina S, Moon C, Guggino WB, Nielsen S (1993) Aquaporin CHIP: the archetypal molecular water channel. Am J Physiol 265: F463-F476.

Akabas, MH (2000) Cystic fibrosis transmembrane conductance regulator. Structure and function of an epithelial chloride channel. J Biol Chem. 275: 3729-3732.

Badaut J, Hirt L, Granziera C, Bogousslavsky J, Magistretti PJ, Regli L (2001) Astrocyte-specific expression of aquaporin-9 in mouse brain is increased after transient focal cerebral ischemia. J Cereb Blood Flow Metab 21: 477-482.

Badaut J, Lasbennes F, Magistretti PJ, Regli L (2002) Aquaporins in brain: distribution, physiology, and pathophysiology. J Cereb Blood Flow Metab 22: 367-378.

Ballerini P, Di Iorio P, Ciccarelli R, Nargi E, D'Alimonte I, Traversa U, Rathbone MP, Caciagli F (2002) Glial cells express multiple ATP binding cassette proteins which are involved in ATP release. Neuroreport 13: 1789-1792.

Bekar LK, Walz W (2002) Intracellular chloride modulates A-type potassium currents in astrocytes. Glia 39: 207-216.

Bevan S, Chiu SY, Gray PTA, Ritchie JM (1985) The presence of voltage-gated sodium, potassium and chloride channels in rat cultured astrocytes. Proc Roy Soc Lond B: Biol Sci B225: 299-313.

Bevensee MO, Apkon M, Boron WF (1997) Intracellular pH regulation in cultured astrocytes from rat hippocampus. I. Role of HCO3-. J Gen Physiol 110: 453-465.

Brandt S, Jentsch TJ (1995) ClC-6 and ClC-7 are two novel broadly expressed members of the ClC chloride channel family. FEBS Letters 377: 15-20.

Brooks HL, Regan JW, Yool AJ (2000) Inhibition of aquaporin-1 water permeability by tetraethylammonium: involvement of the loop E pore region. Mol Pharmacol 57: 1021-1026.

Bureau MH, Khrestchatisky M, Heeren MA, Zambrowicz EB, Kim H, Grisar TM, Colombini M, Tobin AJ, Olsen RW (1992) Isolation and cloning of a voltage-dependent anion channel-like Mr 36,000 polypeptide from mammalian brain. J Biol Chem 267: 8679-8684.

Crepel V, Panenka W, Kelly ME, MacVicar BA (1998) Mitogen-activated protein and tyrosine kinases in the activation of astrocyte volume-activated chloride current. J Neurosci 18: 1196-1206.

Denker BM, Smith BL, Kuhajda FP, Agre P (1988) Identification, purification, and partial characterization of a novel Mr 28,000 integral membrane protein from erythrocytes and renal tubules. J Biol Chem 263: 15634-15642.

Dermietzel R, Hwang T-K, Buettner R, Hofer A, Dotzler E, Kremer M, Deutzmann R, Thinnes FP, Fishman GI, Spray DC, Siemen D (1994) Cloning and in situ localization of a brain-derived porin that constitutes a large-conductance anion channel in astrocytic plasma membranes. PNAS 91: 499-503.

Duan D, Winter C, Cowley S, Hume JR, Horowitz B (1997) Molecular identification of a volume-regulated chloride channel. Nature 390: 417-421.

Dutzler R, Campbell EB, Cadene M, Chait BT, MacKinnon R (2002) X-ray structure of a ClC chloride channel at 3.0 A reveals the molecular basis of anion selectivity. Nature 415: 287-294.

Elkjaer M, Vajda Z, Nejsum LN, Kwon T, Jensen UB, Amiry-Moghaddam M, Frokiaer J, Nielsen S (2000) Immunolocalization of AQP9 in liver, epididymis, testis, spleen, and brain. Biochem Biophys Res Commun 276: 1118-1128.

Fava M, Ferroni S, Nobile M (2001) Osmosensitivity of an inwardly rectifying chloride current revealed by whole-cell and perforated-patch recordings in cultured rat cortical astrocytes. FEBS Lett 492: 78-83.

Ferroni S, Marchini C, Nobile M, Rapisarda C (1997) Characterization of an inwardly rectifying chloride conductance expressed by cultured rat cortical astrocytes. Glia 21: 217-227.

Ferroni S, Marchini C, Schubert P, Rapisarda C (1995) Two distinct inwardly rectifying conductances are expressed in long term dibutyryl-cyclic-AMP treated rat cultured cortical astrocytes. FEBS Lett 367: 319-325.

Ferroni S, Nobile M, Caprini M, Rapisarda C (2000) pH modulation of an inward rectifier chloride current in cultured rat cortical astrocytes. Neurosci 100: 431-438.

Gray PT, Ritchie JM (1986) A voltage-gated chloride conductance in rat cultured astrocytes. Proc Roy Soc Lond B: Biol Sci 228: 267-288.

Grunder S, Thiemann A, Pusch M, Jentsch TJ (1992) Regions involved in the opening of cic-2 chloride channel by voltage and cell volume. Nature 360: 759-62.

Hasegawa H, Ma T, Skach W, Matthay MA, Verkman AS (1994) Molecular cloning of a mercurial-insensitive water channel expressed in selected water-transporting tissues. J Biol Chem 269: 5497-5500.

Hille B (2001) Ion Channels of Excitable Membranes. Sunderland: Sinauer.

Jackson PS, Madsen JR (1997) Identification of the volume-sensitive organic osmolyte anion channel in human glial cells. Pediatr Neurosurg 27: 286-291.

Jackson PS, Morrison R, Strange K (1994) The volume-sensitive organic osmolyte-anion channel VSOAC is regulated by nonhydrolytic ATP binding. Am J Physiol 267: C1203-C1209.

Jackson PS, Strange K (1993) Volume-sensitive anion channels mediate swelling-activated inositol and taurine efflux. Am J Physiol 265: t-500.

Jalonen T (1993) Single-channel characteristics of the large-conductance anion channel in rat cortical astrocytes in primary culture. Glia 9: 227-237.

Jalonen T, Johansson S, Holopainen I, Oja SS, Arhem P (1989) A high-conductance multi-state anion channel in cultured rat astrocytes. Acta Physiol 136: 611-612.

Jalonen T, Varga V, Hartikainen K, Janaky R, Oja SS (1991) Anion conductance blocked by divalent cations in cultured rat astrocytes. Ann N Y Acad Sci 633: 583-585.

Jentsch TJ, Stein V, Weinreich F, Zdebik AA (2002) Molecular structure and physiological function of chloride channels. Physiol Rev 82: 503-568.

Jung JS, Bhat RV, Preston GM, Guggino WB, Baraban JM, Agre P (1994) Molecular characterization of an aquaporin cDNA from brain: candidate osmoreceptor and regulator of water balance. Proc Natl Acad Sci U S A 91: 13052-13056.

Kawasaki M, Uchida S, Monkawa T, Miyawaki A, Mikoshiba K, Marumo F, Sasaki S (1994) Cloning and expression of a protein kinase c-regulated chloride channel abundantly expressed in rat brain neuronal cells. Neuron 12: 597-604.

Kettenmann H (1987) K+ and Cl- uptake by cultured oligodendrocytes. Can J Physiol & Pharmacol 65: 1033-1037.

Kimelberg HK (1981) Active accumulation and exchange transport of chloride in astroglial cells in culture. Biochim Biophys Acta 646: 179-184.

Kimelberg HK, Frangakis MV (1985) Furosemide- and bumetanide-sensitive ion transport and volume control in primary astrocyte cultures from rat brain. Brain Res 361: 125-134.

Kimelberg HK, Kettenmann H (1990) Swelling-induced changes in electrophysiological properties of cultured astrocytes and oligodendrocytes. I. Effects on membrane potentials, input impedance and cell-cell coupling. Brain Res 529: 255-261.

Kimelberg HK, O'Connor E (1988) Swelling of astrocytes causes membrane potential depolarization. Glia 1: 219-224.

Knepper MA (1994) The aquaporin family of molecular water channels. Proc Natl Acad Sci U S A 91: 6255-6258.

Lang F, Busch GL, Ritter M, Volkl H, Waldegger S, Gulbins E, Haussinger D (1998) Functional significance of cell volume regulatory mechanisms. Physiol Rev 78: 247-306.

Lascola CD, Kraig RP (1996) Whole-cell chloride currents in rat astrocytes accompany changes in cell morphology. J Neurosci 16: 2532-2545.

Lascola CD, Nelson DJ, Kraig RP (1998) Cytoskeletal actin gates a Cl- channel in neocortical astrocytes. J Neurosci 18: 1679-1692.

Linsdell P (2001) Relationship between anion binding and anion permeability revealed by mutagenesis within the cystic fibrosis transmembrane conductance regulator chloride channel pore. J Physiol 531: 51-66.

Manley GT, Fujimura M, Ma T, Noshita N, Filiz F, Bollen AW, Chan P, Verkman AS (2000) Aquaporin-4 deletion in mice reduces brain edema after acute water intoxication and ischemic stroke. Nat Med 6: 159-163.

Matsuzaki T, Tajika Y, Tserentsoodol N, Suzuki T, Aoki T, Hagiwara H, Takata K (2002) Aquaporins: a water channel family. Anat Sci Int 77: 85-93.

McCarty NA, McDonough S, Cohen BN, Riordan JR, Davidson N, Lester HA (1993) Voltage-dependent block of the cystic fibrosis transmembrane conductance regulator Cl- channel by two closely related arylaminobenzoates. J Gen Physiol 102: 1-23.

Miller C (1982) Open-state substructure of single chloride channels from Torpedo electroplax. Philos Trans R Soc Lond B Biol Sci 299: 401-411.

Miller C, White MM (1984) Dimeric structure of single chloride channels from Torpedo electroplax. Proc Natl Acad Sci U S A 81: 2772-2775.

Nagelhus EA, Horio Y, Inanobe A, Fujita A, Haug FM, Nielsen S, Kurachi Y, Ottersen OP (1999) Immunogold evidence suggests that coupling of K+ siphoning and water transport in rat retinal Muller cells is mediated by a coenrichment of Kir4.1 and AQP4 in specific membrane domains. Glia 26: 47-54.

Nagelhus EA, Veruki ML, Torp R, Haug FM, Laake JH, Nielsen S, Agre P, Ottersen OP (1998) Aquaporin-4 water channel protein in the rat retina and optic nerve: polarized expression in Muller cells and fibrous astrocytes. J Neurosci 18: 2506-2519.

Nakahama K, Nagano M, Fujioka A, Shinoda K, Sasaki H (1999) Effect of TPA on aquaporin 4 mRNA expression in cultured rat astrocytes. Glia 25: 240-246.

Nicchia GP, Frigeri A, Liuzzi GM, Santacroce MP, Nico B, Procino G, Quondamatteo F, Herken R, Roncali L, Svelto M (2000) Aquaporin-4-containing astrocytes sustain a temperature- and mercury-insensitive swelling in vitro. Glia 31: 29-38.

Nielsen S, Nagelhus EA, Amiry-Moghaddam M, Bourque C, Agre P, Ottersen OP (1997) Specialized membrane domains for water transport in glial cells: high-resolution immunogold cytochemistry of aquaporin-4 in rat brain. J Neurosci 17: 171-180.

Nielsen S, Smith BL, Christensen EI, Agre P (1993) Distribution of the aquaporin CHIP in secretory and resorptive epithelia and capillary endothelia. Proc Natl Acad Sci U S A 90: 7275-7279.

Niemietz CM, Tyerman SD (2002) New potent inhibitors of aquaporins: silver and gold compounds inhibit aquaporins of plant ʳⁿᵈ human origin. FEBS Lett 531: 443-447.

Nobile M, Pusch M, Rapisarda C, Ferroni , 000) Single-channel analysis of a ClC-2-like chloride conductance in cultured rat cortical astrocytes. Febs Letters 479: 10-14.

Nowak L, Ascher P, Berwald-Netter Y (1987) Ionic channels in mouse astrocytes in culture. J Neurosci 7: 101-109.

Olsen ML, Schade S, Lyons SA, Sontheimer H (2003) Expression of voltage-gated chloride channels in human glioma cells. J Neurosci submitted.

Olson JE, Sankar R, Holtzman D, James A, Fleischhacker D (1986) Energy-dependent volume regulation in primary cultured cerebral astrocytes. J Cell Physiol 128: 209-215.

Orkand RK, Nicholls JG, Kuffler SW (1966) Effect of nerve impulses on the membrane potential of glial cells in the central nervous system of amphibia. J Neurophysiol 29: 788-806.

Parkerson KA, Sontheimer H (2003) Contribution of Chloride Channels to Volume Regulation of Cortical Astrocytes. Am J Physiol (Cell Physiol), in press.

Pasantes-Morales H, Murray RA, Lilja L, Moran J (1994) Regulatory volume decrease in cultured astrocytes. i. potassium- and chloride-activated permeability. Am J Physiol 266: Pt 1):C165-71.

Preston GM, Jung JS, Guggino WB, Agre P (1993) The mercury-sensitive residue at cysteine 189 in the CHIP28 water channel. J Biol Chem 268: 17-20.

Price DL, Ludwig JW, Mi H, Schwarz TL, Ellisman MH (2002) Distribution of rSlo Ca(2+)-activated K(+) channels in rat astrocyte perivascular endfeet. Brain Res 956: 183-193.

Ransom CB, O'Neal JT, Sontheimer H (2001) Volume-activated chloride currents contribute to the resting conductance and invasive migration of human glioma cells. J Neurosci 21: 7674-7683.

Riordan JR, Rommens JM, Kerem B, Alon N, Rozmahel R, Grzelczak Z, Zielenski J, Lok S, Plavsic N, Chou JL, et al (1989) Identification of the cystic fibrosis gene: cloning and characterization of complementary DNA. Science 245: 1066-1073.

Roy G (1995) Amino acid current through anion channels in cultured human glial cells. J Membr Biol 147: 35-44.

Saadoun S, Papadopoulos MC, Davies DC, Bell BA, Krishna S (2002a) Increased aquaporin 1 water channel expression in human brain tumours. Br J Cancer 87: 621-623.

Saadoun S, Papadopoulos MC, Davies DC, Krishna S, Bell BA (2002b) Aquaporin-4 expression is increased in oedematous human brain tumours. J Neurol Neurosurg Psych 72: 262-265.

Sanchez-Olea R, Moran J, Martinez A, Pasantes-Morales H (1993) Volume-activated Rb+ transport in astrocytes in culture. Am J Physiol 264: C836-C842.

Sheppard DN, Welsh MJ (1992) Effect of ATP-sensitive K+ channel regulators on cystic fibrosis transmembrane conductance regulator chloride currents. J Gen Physiol 100: 573-591.

Sik A, Smith RL, Freund TF (2000) Distribution of chloride channel-2-immunoreactive neuronal and astrocytic processes in the hippocampus. Neurosci 101: 51-65.

Sonnhof U (1987) Single voltage-dependent K+ and Cl- channels in cultured rat astrocytes. Can J Physiol Pharmacol 65: 1043-1050.

Soroceanu L, Manning TJ, Jr., Sontheimer H (1999) Modulation of glioma cell migration and invasion using Cl- and K+ ion channel blockers. J Neurosci 19: 5942-5954.

Stegen C, Matskevich I, Wagner CA, Paulmichl M, Lang F, Broer S (2000) Swelling-induced taurine release without chloride channel activity in Xenopus laevis oocytes expressing anion channels and transporters. Biochim Biophys Acta 1467: 91-100.

Steinmeyer K, Schwappach B, Bens M, Vandewalle A, Jentsch TJ (1995) Cloning and functional expression of rat clc-5, a chloride channel related to kidney disease. J Biol Chem 270: 31172-31177.

Stobrawa SM, Breiderhoff T, Takamori S, Engel D, Schweizer M, Zdebik AA, Bosl MR, Ruether K, Jahn H, Draguhn A, Jahn R, Jentsch TJ (2001) Disruption of ClC-3, a chloride channel expressed on synaptic vesicles, leads to a loss of the hippocampus. Neuron 29: 185-196.

Tabcharani JA, Chang XB, Riordan JR, Hanrahan JW (1992) The cystic fibrosis transmembrane conductance regulator chloride channel. Iodide block and permeation. Biophys.J 62: 1-4.

Thiemann A, Grunder S, Pusch M, Jentsch TJ (1992) A chloride channel widely expressed in epithelial and non- epithelial cells. Nature 356: 57-60.

Thinnes FP, Gotz H, Kayser H, Benz R, Schmidt WE, Kratzin HD, Hilschmann N (1989) [Identification of human porins. I. Purification of a porin from human B-lymphocytes (Porin 31HL) and the topochemical proof of its expression on the plasmalemma of the progenitor cell.]. Biol Chem Hoppe Seyler 370: 1253-1264.

Tsukaguchi H, Shayakul C, Berger UV, Mackenzie B, Devidas S, Guggino WB, van Hoek AN, Hediger MA (1998) Molecular characterization of a broad selectivity neutral solute channel. J Biol Chem 273: 24737-24743.

Ullrich N, Sontheimer H (1996) Biophysical and pharmacological characterization of chloride currents in human astrocytoma cells. Am J Physiol (Cell Physiol) 270: C1511-C1521.

Ullrich N, Sontheimer H (1997) Cell cycle-dependent expression of a glioma-specific chloride current: proposed link to cytoskeletal changes. Am J Physiol 273 (Pt 1): C1290-1297.

Venero JL, Vizuete ML, Machado A, Cano J (2001) Aquaporins in the central nervous system. Prog Neurobiol 63: 321-336.

Vizuete ML, Venero JL, Vargas C, Ilundain AA, Echevarria M, Machado A, Cano J (1999) Differential upregulation of aquaporin-4 mRNA expression in reactive astrocytes after brain injury: potential role in brain edema. Neurobiol Dis 6: 245-258.

Waldegger S, Jentsch TJ (2000) From tonus to tonicity: Physiology of CLC chloride channels. J Am Soc Nephrol 11: 1331-1339.

Walz W (1987) Swelling and potassium uptake in cultured astrocytes. Can J Physiol Pharmacol 65: 1051-1057.

Walz W (2002) Chloride/anion channels in glial cell membranes. Glia 40: 1-10.

Walz W, Mukerji S (1988) KCl movements during potassium-induced cytotoxic swelling of cultured astrocytes. Exp Neurol 99: 17-29.

Walz W, Wuttke WA (1999) Independent mechanisms of potassium clearance by astrocytes in gliotic tissue. J Neurosci Res 56: 595-603.

Yamamoto N, Sobue K, Fujita M, Katsuya H, Asai K (2002) Differential regulation of aquaporin-5 and -9 expression in astrocytes by protein kinase A. Brain Res Mol Brain Res 104: 96-102.

Yamamoto N, Sobue K, Miyachi T, Inagaki M, Miura Y, Katsuya H, Asai K (2001a) Differential regulation of aquaporin expression in astrocytes by protein kinase C. Brain Res Mol Brain Res 95: 110-116.

Yamamoto N, Yoneda K, Asai K, Sobue K, Tada T, Fujita Y, Katsuya H, Fujita M, Aihara N, Mase M, Yamada K, Miura Y, Kato T (2001b) Alterations in the expression of the AQP family in cultured rat astrocytes during hypoxia and reoxygenation. Brain Res Mol Brain Res 90: 26-38.

8.7. Abbreviations

ClC	Voltage-gated chloride channel
CFTR	Cystic fibrosis transmembrane regulator
dBcAMP	Dibutyryl-cyclic-AMP

DIDS	4,4'-diisothiocyanatostilbene-2-2'-disulfonic acid
DPC	Diphenylamine-2-carboxylate
$GABA_A$	γ-aminobutyric acid type A receptor
GFAP	Glial fibrillary acidic protein
MAPK	Mitogen-activated protein kinase
MEK	Mitogen-activated protein kinase kinase
9-AC	9-anthracene carboxylic acid
NPPB	5-Nitro-2-(3-phenylpropylamino)benzoic acid
PKA	Protein kinase A
PKC	Protein kinase C
SITS	4-acetamido-4'-isocyanatostilbene-2-2'-disulfonic acid
TEA^+	Tetraethylammonium ion
VDAC	Voltage-dependent anion channel
VSOAC	Volume-sensitive organic osmolyte-anion channel

Chapter 9

Glutamate uptake by astroglia

Dwight E. Bergles[1]* and Jeffrey D. Rothstein[2]

Departments of Neuroscience [1] and Neurology [2]
Johns Hopkins University School of Medicine
725 N. Wolfe St., WBSB 813, Baltimore, MD 21205 USA

Corresponding author: dbergles@jhmi.edu

Contents

9.1. Introduction

Glutamate is the predominant excitatory neurotransmitter in the central nervous system (CNS), and as a result is continually secreted from cells. It is essential that vesicular release result in fluctuations in the concentration of glutamate that are spatially and temporally constrained, to restrict signaling to defined contacts and to allow signaling to be sustained at high frequencies. Although dilution of glutamate in the extracellular space and diffusion away from receptors work to rapidly dissipate the local spikes in glutamate concentration generated following release, the small volume of the extracellular space and the short distance between neighboring synapses creates difficulties for restricting glutamate transients to individual synaptic sites. Unlike the neuromuscular junction, where acetylcholine is inactivated through the action of an extracellular enzyme, there is no evidence that glutamate is similarly degraded following release. Instead, the actions of glutamate are ultimately terminated by uptake back into cells, a task accomplished primarily by a family of high affinity, Na^+-dependent transporters (see review by Danbolt, 2001). Five different glutamate transporter genes have been identified, encoding at least six different transporters, which exhibit distinct patterns of expression in the CNS. Although we have learned a great deal about these transporters, significant questions remain about the properties of each transporter type, the mechanisms by which they are regulated and their individual roles in the CNS. In this review, we outline the properties of the glutamate transporters expressed in astroglial cells, the significance of these transporters for signaling at synapses, and their potential involvement in human disease.

9.2. Association of astroglial cells with synapses

Astroglial cells (astrocytes and Bergmann glial cells) extend highly ramified processes into the surrounding neuropil (see Chapter 3). Lamellar sheets that project from these fine processes often come in close proximity to and in some cases completely wrap or ensheath synaptic terminals (Spacek, 1971; Palay and Chan-Palay, 1974; Spacek, 1985; Kosaka and Hama, 1986; Ventura and Harris, 1999). The branching of these processes is so extensive that it has been estimated that a single hippocampal astrocyte occupies a volume of ~ 66,000 μm^3 and may come in contact with as many as 140,000 synapses (Bushong et al., 2002). Because astrocytes occupy restricted domains, with little or no overlap occurring between the processes of adjacent cells, it is likely that a single astrocyte is responsible for clearing glutamate from within this entire region. This is a striking proposition, when one considers that each synaptic vesicle contains about 4,000 molecules of glutamate (Riveros et al., 1986), that many synapses appear to release multiple vesicles in response to a single action potential (Wadiche and Jahr, 2001; Oertner et al., 2002), and that neurons can sustain firing rates of thousands of impulses per second.

Although it is commonly stated that astrocytes ensheath synapses, the fraction of the perimeter of the synapse that is bordered by an astrocyte process varies dramatically between brain regions, and between synapses within a particular region (Spacek, 1985; Ventura and Harris, 1999). In the molecular layer of the cerebellum both parallel fiber and climbing fiber synapses formed with Purkinje neurons are essentially completely ensheathed by Bergmann glial cells (Palay and Chan-Palay, 1974; Spacek, 1985). In contrast, in the stratum radiatum region of the hippocampus, where Schaffer collateral-commissural fibers of CA3 pyramidal neurons form synapses with CA1 pyramidal neurons, only about 57 % of synapses are in contact with an astrocyte process, and this contact extends over less than half of the perimeter of the synapse (Ventura and Harris, 1999). It is not yet known if these structures represent snapshots of dynamic interactions or long-lasting associations between astrocytes and synapses. It is an intriguing possibility that the amount of ensheathment may be correlated with the level of activity that a particular input experiences, but this has not been conclusively demonstrated. Nevertheless, the importance of synaptic ensheathment for glutamate clearance has been shown in several brain regions, including the hypothalamus and cerebellum. The magnocellular nuclei of the hypothalamus undergo dramatic structural re-arrangements during lactation, a period characterized by intense neuronal activity (Theodosis and Poulain, 1993). During lactation, the processes of astroglial cells retract from synapses, a change that presumably acts to place transporters further from sites of release. Consistent with this hypothesis, transporter inhibition causes greater activation of presynaptic metabotropic glutamate receptors in virgin or post-lactating animals when astrocytes are more closely associated with synapses (Oliet et al., 2001). These results indicate that there is a greater dependence on transporters for clearance when astrocytes are associated with synapses. Surprisingly, the opposite phenomenon has been observed in the cerebellum. In normal brain, the tight ensheathment of Purkinje cell synapses by Bergmann glial processes appears to ensure that glutamate is removed rapidly and that tightly packed synapses are effectively isolated from one another (Palay and Chan-Palay, 1974). When the processes of Bergmann glial cells are forced to retract from synapses, clearance is compromised and glutamate remains elevated near receptors for much longer (Iino et al., 2001). It is possible that the higher density of synapses in the cerebellum accounts for the differential effect of ensheathment in this region; when ensheathment is prevented and astroglial transporters are removed, glutamate may be able to diffuse to neighboring synapses and prolong synaptic currents.

These studies indicate that the close association of astroglial cells with excitatory synapses creates a barrier to diffusion and brings glutamate transporters closer to sites of release. Although many questions remain to be answered about how such associations are initiated and maintained, recent results suggest that glutamate itself may be involved in these processes by signaling through ionotropic glutamate receptors in astroglial membranes (Iino et al., 2001); however, the low expression of these receptors by astrocytes (Bergles and Jahr, 1998; Zhou and Kimelberg, 2001), suggests that other mechanisms also must be involved. The study of interactions between astrocytes and synapses pose significant challenges because the fine processes of astroglia often consist of two opposed membranes with little cytoplasm (Spacek, 1985). Although such structures can be observed in fixed tissue using electron microscopy, it has not yet been possible to resolve the finest astroglial ramifications with light microscopy, a necessity for studying dynamic changes in size and location of these structures relative to synapses in real time.

Table 9.1. Astroglial glutamate transporter subtypes

Glutamate transporter subtype	Human homologue	Cell type	Anatomic localization	References
GLAST	EAAT1	Bergman glia, Astrocytes	Cerebellum> cortex, spinal cord	(Storck et al., 1992; Shashidharan and Plaitakis, 1993)
GLT1	EAAT2	Astroglia	Throughout brain and spinal cord	(Danbolt et al., 1992; Shashidharan et al., 1994; Tanaka et al., 1997b)
GLT1b	EAAT2b	Astrocytes and Neurons	Throughout brain, spinal cord	(Utsunomiya-Tate et al., 1997a; Chen et al., 2002a; Schmitt et al., 2002)

9.3. Glutamate transporter expression by astroglia

The family of glutamate transporters first cloned in rodents and later in humans constitutes a unique group of proteins distinct from other neurotransmitter transporter families. To date, there are five principal Na^+-dependent glutamate transporters that have been cloned in human and rodent tissue. This family, known as the excitatory amino acid transporters (EAATs), is comprised of 5 molecular subtypes: EAAT1 (GLAST) EAAT2 (GLT-1), EAAT3 (EAAC1), EAAT4 and EAAT5 (Danbolt et al., 1998b). The rodent forms (parentheses) of the proteins are highly homologous to human subtypes. As a family, these transporters all exhibit localization within the CNS, although their cellular distribution varies widely depending on the particular region of the CNS examined and the cell type identified. Only EAAT1 and EAAT2 are astroglial in localization (Rothstein et al., 1994; Furuta et al., 1997b; Danbolt et al., 1998b) (Table 8.1). EAAT1, although present throughout the brain, is prominently expressed by Bergmann glia and is the only glutamate transporter expressed in the region of the cochlea near inner hair cells (Ottersen et al., 1998). EAAT2 (GLT-1) is the most prevalent glutamate transporter, and immunohistochemical analyses clearly demonstrate that EAAT2 protein is widely distributed within astrocytes throughout the gray mater of the brain and spinal cord (Figure 9.1). In fact, it is estimated that up to 1% of all brain protein is EAAT2. Unlike EAAT1, EAAT2 mRNA can be found in some neurons, but multiple immunohistochemical studies using antibodies directed at many different EAAT2 epitopes have not been able to identify expression of the EAAT2 protein in neurons under normal conditions (but see (Chen et al., 2002b). However, under conditions of neural injury, rare neurons appear to express EAAT2 protein (Martin et al., 1997), although the functional significance of this expression is not known.

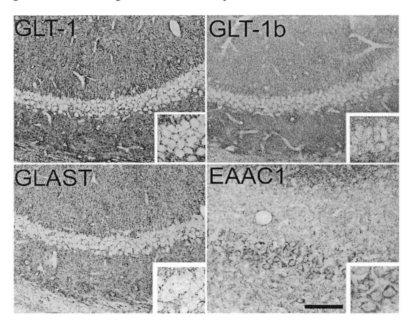

Figure 9.1. Immunolocalization of glutamate transporters in the hippocampus. Astroglial glutamate transporters GLAST and GLT-1 are exclusively localized to neuropil, and neurons appear immunonegative (inset). The GLT-1 splice variant, GLT-1b, has a distribution almost identical to GLT-1, although very low level immunoreactivity may be apparent in neurons (inset). Conversely, the neuronal glutamate transporter EAAC1 is present in various hippocampal neurons, with an obvious enrichment in the cytoplasm (inset). Scale bar = 50 μm.

During development, the pattern of astroglial expression is distinct - EAAT1/GLAST is the dominant protein expressed by astroglia throughout the brain (Furuta et al., 1997a). Only late in development does the expression of GLT-1 in astroglia increase. The peak of EAAT expression occurs approximately 7 - 14 days postnatal, with maximal expression of GLT-1 observed in astrocytes, a period that corresponds with the time of synapse maturation. Notably, rare axons exhibit GLT-1 immunoreactivity during development (Furuta et al., 1997a), and there is evidence that some neurons express GLT-1 *in vitro* (Mennerick et al., 1998).

At the subcellular level, both EAAT1 and EAAT2 are highly localized to astroglial plasma membranes with a much smaller pool of cytoplasmic protein. Ultrastructural studies, using pre- and post-embedding gold methods, suggest that these transporters tend to be localized near synaptic complexes, with a distinct membrane compartmentalization and polarization (Rothstein et al., 1994; Chaudhry et al., 1995; Lehre et al., 1995; Danbolt et al., 1998b; Danbolt et al., 1998a). Subsequent to the cloning of GLT-1/EAAT2, various mRNA-spliced isoforms were identified in tissues throughout the body. These splice variants included altered sequences for either the amino- or carboxy-terminal coding domains. To date, only one of the truncated EAAT2/GLT-1 species has been identified at the protein level in astrocytes; EAAT2b/GLT-1b is a truncated EAAT2 with a novel 11 amino acid carboxy-terminal domain (Utsunomiya-Tate et al., 1997b; Chen et al., 2002c). *In vitro* studies suggest that the GLT1b variant has pharmacological/physiological properties identical to the full-length astroglial EAAT2/GLT-1; however, unlike EAAT2, the spliced variant has an obvious postsynaptic density-95/discs large/zona occludens (PDZ) binding domain in the unique sequence. This region may provide a potential site for regulation through interaction with other proteins, though the functional significance of this splicing is not yet known.

9.4. Biophysical properties of astroglial glutamate transporters

Transporters must move glutamate across the plasma membrane against an electrochemical gradient. This opposing force is a consequence of the negative charge carried by glutamate, which must move against the negative resting membrane potential of astrocytes, and the higher concentration of glutamate in the astrocyte cytosol relative to that in the extracellular fluid (at equilibrium). In order to overcome these opposing forces, glutamate transporters harness the energy stored in the electrochemical gradients for various ions (Na^+, K^+, and H^+), dissipating ion gradients set up by the Na^+/K^+- ATPase, rather than consuming ATP directly. The movement of each glutamate molecule into the cell is accompanied by the movement of three Na^+ and one H^+, and one K^+ is counter transported from inside the cell to the outside to complete the cycle (Klockner et al., 1993; Zerangue and Kavanaugh, 1996; Levy et al., 1998). Although there is general agreement about the involvement of Na^+ and K^+ and the number of these ions that move per cycle, there remains disagreement about whether a H^+ moves into the cell or a OH^- is transported out (Zerangue and Kavanaugh, 1996; Auger and Attwell, 2000), as both can account for the net acidification of the cytoplasm that occurs during glutamate uptake (Bouvier et al., 1992).   Nevertheless, this stoichiometry has the power to achieve a transmembrane concentration gradient of a million fold or greater at equilibrium (Zerangue and Kavanaugh, 1996).   In addition, as a result of this unbalanced coupling to ions, glutamate uptake is an electrogenic process in which a net two positive charges are deposited into the cell during each transport cycle. As might be expected given the dependence on the movement of charged species, the process of glutamate transport is highly voltage-dependent, with the rate of uptake changing e-fold per 56 mV (Wadiche et al., 1995b) (Figure 9.2a).

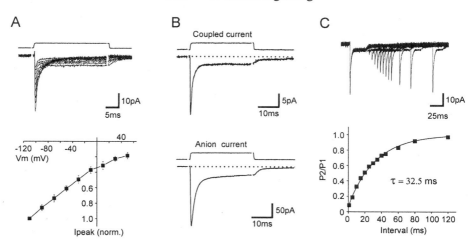

Figure 9.2. Biophysical properties of GLT-1 transporters. A, Coupled (stoichiometric) transporter currents recorded from an outside-out patch removed from a HEK cell expressing GLT-1. The upper trace shows the duration that L-glutamate (10 mM) was applied. The patch was held at voltages from –110 mV to 50 mV. The graph below shows the peak amplitude of the transporter current at these voltages. B, Comparison of the kinetics of L-glutamate-evoked GLT-1 transporter currents recorded in the absence (Coupled current, K-gluconate internal solution) or presence of permeant anions (Anion current, K-thiocyanate internal solution). C, Time course of recovery of the peak amplitude of GLT-1 transporter currents from the steady-state level. Below is a plot of the fractional recovery of the peak amplitude of the transporter current over time. All experiments were performed at room temperature. Adapted from (Bergles et al., 2002).

In addition to the charge movement that drives glutamate translocation and transporter cycling, glutamate transporters also allow certain anions (primarily Cl⁻ under physiological conditions) to flow across the membrane in a manner that is uncoupled from the movement of glutamate (Wadiche et al., 1995a; Eliasof and Jahr, 1996); reversing the Cl⁻ gradient alters the direction of Cl⁻ movement but does not affect the net accumulation of glutamate. This behavior is quite unlike that of the other family of plasma membrane neurotransmitter transporters, those responsible for the uptake of γ-aminobutyric acid (GABA), glycine, and monoamines, for which substrate movement is directly coupled to Cl⁻ (Lu and Hilgemann, 1999). The flux of anions through glutamate transporters is enhanced when glutamate is bound, but also occurs as a constitutive leak though transporters in the absence of glutamate. Among the astroglial transporters, GLAST has a higher permeability to anions than GLT-1 (Wadiche et al., 1995a). It is important to note that the flux of Cl⁻, the Cl⁻ conductance, under physiological conditions is extremely small for all glutamate transporters except EAAT5, a transporter expressed exclusively in the retina (Arriza et al., 1997). It has been estimated based on fluctuation analysis that the unitary conductance of GLAST is less than one femtosiemen (1×10^{-15} Siemens) (Wadiche and Kavanaugh, 1998), more than 1000 times smaller than the conductance of a typical GABA$_A$ receptor chloride channel. Thus, the flux of Cl⁻ through GLT-1 and GLAST does not contribute significantly to the voltage change produced by transporter cycling. The significance of the anion conductance is not yet known, but this Cl⁻ flux could be involved in regulating biochemical processes within the cell (Higashijima et al., 1987). The selectivity of the transporter anion channel follows the chaotropic sequence, with anions such as SCN⁻ (thiocyanate), NO₃⁻ (nitrate), and ClO₄⁻ (perchlorate) (Wadiche et al., 1995a) exhibiting a much higher permeability than Cl⁻. Because many more of these anions flow across the membrane than coupled charges, the currents produced during transporter cycling are amplified when these anions are included in the internal solution (Figure 9.2b). Such manipulations have made it possible to monitor transporter activity in outside-out patches where it is difficult to resolve the movement of coupled charges (Bergles and Jahr, 1997; Otis et al., 1997; Wadiche and Kavanaugh, 1998; Otis and Kavanaugh, 2000).

Studies of GLT-1 and GLAST transporters expressed in heterologous systems have shown that their affinity for glutamate is between 20 and 100 μM (the range reflects the fact that transporters exhibit different affinities in different expression systems) (Arriza et al., 1994), and require more than 50 ms on average to complete one cycle (Wadiche et al., 1995b). Although cycling is relatively slow, the peak transporter current produced by rapid application of glutamate to outside-out patches reaches a peak in < 100 μs (Figure 9.2a), indicating that they bind glutamate extremely rapidly. Similar studies of transporter currents in patches suggest that cycling of native transporters may be more rapid, as the peak response to glutamate recovered with a time constant of ~ 10 ms at near physiological temperatures (Bergles and Jahr, 1997)(Figure 9.2c). However, these measurements are highly dependent on the recording conditions (the concentration of internal and external ions, glutamate, etc.), and there have been no direct measurements of transporter cycling rates in intact tissue. It should also be noted that this rapid recovery could also occur if transporters are inefficient and allow glutamate to unbind to the outside. Indeed, chemical-kinetic models of both GLAST (Wadiche and Kavanaugh, 1998) and GLT-1 (Bergles et al., 2002) based on these and other data suggest that that the efficiency, defined as the probability that glutamate once bound to the transporter is translocated and released to the inside (and the cycle completed), is only about 0.5. Thus, for these two transporters glutamate is as likely to eventually unbind back to the outside as it is to be transported in. The slow turnover rate and low efficiency of transporters has led to the hypothesis that over the time course of a single synaptic event they may function primarily as buffers, rapidly lowering the concentration by merely binding glutamate (Tong and Jahr, 1994; Diamond and Jahr, 1997)(but see (Mennerick et al., 1999). Because transporters are more abundant than receptors, particularly in extrasynaptic regions, they will be more likely to encounter stray glutamate. Surprisingly, comparisons of the biophysical properties of GLAST and GLT-1 have provided few clues to explain why GLAST is the predominant transporter in the developing nervous system, why both transporters are expressed in most astroglial cells, or why GLT-1 predominates in the hippocampus and forebrain and GLAST predominates in the cerebellum and cochlea.

9.5. Physiological properties of astroglia

The net uptake of glutamate by transporters is influenced by ion gradients, transmembrane voltage, and the concentration of glutamate in the cytosol. Given the high density of transporters in astroglial membranes, it is perhaps not surprising that the physiological properties of these cells are uniquely suited for glutamate uptake. Astroglia throughout the CNS exhibit a low membrane resistance (typically less than 50 mΩ), due to extensive coupling with other cells through gap junctions, and the presence of K^+ channels that are open at rest. Because of this high resting conductance to K^+, the membrane potential of astroglial cells is -90 to -100 mV, essentially the same as the equilibrium potential for K^+ (Kuffler et al., 1966). What impact do these properties have on the uptake of glutamate? As discussed above, glutamate translocation is dependent on extracellular Na^+; one or two of these Na^+ bind before glutamate and this binding is voltage-dependent (Wadiche et al., 1995b). Thus, the highly negative resting potential of astroglia will force more transporters to be loaded with Na^+, ensuring they are competent to bind and translocate glutamate. Additional steps within the transport cycle are also likely to be voltage-dependent, including the glutamate translocation steps themselves, and the binding and counter-transport of K^+ (Wadiche and Kavanaugh, 1998; Otis and Kavanaugh, 2000; Bergles et al., 2002). As a result, both transport efficiency and speed of transporter cycling also will increase at more negative voltages (Figure 9.2a). Furthermore, because of their low membrane resistance, the membrane potential of astroglial cells deviates little from rest under physiological conditions (Orkand et al., 1966; Amzica et al., 2002); enormous currents are necessary to produce even small voltage changes (Figure 9.3a). Thus, astroglial cells maintain a transmembrane voltage that is highly favorable for the net uptake of glutamate, and they restrict deviations away from this potential.

The concentration of glutamate in the cytosol also influences the efficiency of transport. When the intracellular level of glutamate is high, it is more likely to rebind the transporter at the intracellular face before Na^+ unbinds, and force reverse transport. The level of free glutamate in the astroglial cytosol is thought to be between 100 μM and 5 mM (Attwell et al., 1993), significantly lower than the 10 – 15 mM glutamate found in neurons. The glutamate concentration is kept low in astroglia by the activity of glutamine synthetase, an enzyme that converts glutamate to glutamine. Thus, the action of this enzyme allows transporters in astroglia to function with higher efficiency. For reverse transport to occur, both glutamate and Na^+ must be available at the intracellular face of the membrane. Because the thin perisynaptic processes of astroglia have such a small volume, the movement of relatively few ions could lead to large changes in concentration and voltage. The extensive gap junctional coupling between adjacent astroglial (Figure 9.3c-d) will help dissipate local accumulations of Na^+ that might occur during intense neuronal activity, reducing the likelihood that transport will be inhibited. However, it should be noted that little is known about the conditions in perisynaptic astrocyte processes, precisely where maximal transporter activity occurs.

9.6. Astroglial glutamate transporters in synaptic signaling

The release of glutamate into the small volume of the synaptic cleft produces a nearly instant rise in concentration (to > 1 mM), ensuring that a sufficient quantity of glutamate is available to reliably activate receptors. Following release, the glutamate transient dissipates rapidly by diffusion and dilution, such that after 100 μs the concentration decreases to a few hundred micromolar (Clements et al., 1992; Clements, 1996; Diamond and Jahr, 1997); the remaining concentration may take tens of milliseconds to return to baseline (Bergles et al., 1997). These estimates of the time course of glutamate in the synaptic cleft are based on studies of glutamate receptor kinetics, inhibition of receptors by low affinity antagonists, and the time course of glutamate transporter currents. However, they are dependent on a number of variables (the concentration of glutamate in a vesicle, the rate of glutamate release, the rate of glutamate diffusion, the properties of receptors at synapses, etc.), for which there are few direct measurements. In addition, the diversity of synaptic morphology, and the wide variation in release probability, glial ensheathment, and transporter expression between synapses, indicate that there is likely to be great variation in the time course of extracellular glutamate between different synapses. Recent studies indicating that the rate of glutamate release from vesicles can vary over time, raising the possibility that glutamate transients may vary over time at a single synapse (Liu et al., 1999; Renger et al., 2001). Nevertheless, there is considerable evidence from many different brain regions that glutamate transporters dictate the rate of clearance of glutamate from the extracellular space, and thus the length of time that glutamate is capable of binding to receptors. Animals that have had the expression of GLT-1 (Rothstein et al., 1996a; Tanaka et al., 1997b) or GLAST (Rothstein et al., 1996a; Watase et al., 1998a) reduced or eliminated, show elevated levels of glutamate in the cerebrospinal fluid, indicating that astroglial transporters are critical for maintaining a low ambient level of glutamate. In the absence of these transporters, glutamate accumulates in the extracellular space and causes severe pathological sequels (see section 9.8 below).

In addition to setting the glutamate "tone", the level of ambient glutamate, transporters also can influence the size and duration of responses at individual synapses. By virtue of their high density and strategic location, transporters influence how much glutamate is available to bind to receptors (Tong and Jahr, 1994; Diamond and Jahr, 1997). This is particularly true for receptors found outside the cleft, where transporters and receptors are juxtaposed (Brasnjo and Otis, 2001; Chen and Diamond, 2002; Clark and Cull-Candy, 2002). Undoubtedly, the level of interaction between transporters and receptors will depend on the densities of receptors and transporters near release sites, their relative affinities (binding and unbinding rates) for glutamate, and the frequency of glutamate release at these and neighboring sites. Studies of the involvement of transporters in synaptic signaling have primarily examined the effect of selective transporter antagonists on the amplitude and time course of synaptic currents. Unfortunately, non-transportable, subtype-selective antagonists for each transporter are not yet available. The compounds that are most suitable for studies in brain slices are dihydrokainate (DHK), which is 100 times more selective for GLT-1 (Arriza et al., 1994), and DL-*threo*-*b*-Benzyloxyaspartic acid (TBOA) which inhibits all transporters with an affinity of between 4 - 15 μM (Shimamoto et al., 1998; Shigeri et al., 2001). Because of this paucity of transporter inhibitors, studies of transporter knockout animals, and animals in which the expression of a particular transporter has been reduced through treatment with antisense oligonucleotides, have been invaluable in understanding the roles played by different transporters. Nevertheless, such animals may exhibit compensation (for example, in the expression and distribution of other transporters or receptors), which have in most cases not yet been examined thoroughly. For these reasons, the results obtained from the study of these animals should be interpreted with caution.

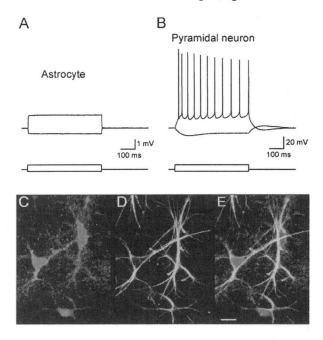

Figure 9.3. Physiological properties of astrocytes. A, Membrane potential response of an astrocyte to injection of – 60 pA and 140 pA through the whole-cell electrode. Note the small change in membrane potential induced by this current. Vm = – 92 mV. B, Injection of the same amount of current in a CA1 pyramidal neuron elicits large fluctuations in voltage. Vm = – 65 mV. C, Immunodetection of biocytin in a hippocampal slice following loading of one astrocyte with biocytin through the recording electrode. Multiple cells are labeled because biocytin diffused through gap junctions. D, GFAP immunoreactivity of the same region of the slice. E, Overlay of panels C and D illustrating that the cells containing biocytin were GFAP immunopositive. Scale bar = 10 μm.

The involvement of transporters in synaptic signaling has been evaluated most extensively in the hippocampus and cerebellum. These two regions exhibit differences in transporter expression, receptor expression, astroglial ensheathment and glutamate clearance. The results obtained from the study of these two regions are described here in order to provide an indication of the complexity of transporter actions at different synapses. The Schaffer collateral-commissural projection from regions CA3 to CA1 in the hippocampus form *en passant* axo-dendritic synapses characterized by a single release site. As described above, these synapses vary greatly in their degree of ensheathment by astrocytes. Three transporters contribute to glutamate uptake in this region: GLAST (EAAT1), GLT-1 (EAAT2), and EAAC1 (EAAT3), with GLT-1 the most abundant. Stimulation of these fibers triggers glutamate transporter currents in astrocytes that are mediated by GLT-1 and GLAST transporters (Figure 9.4). These currents begin rapidly following stimulation, indicating that glutamate diffuses from the cleft within a fraction of a millisecond after release. Inhibition of GLT-1 through the application of DHK slows transmitter clearance (Figure 9.4a), but does not alter miniature or evoked *a*-Amino-3-hydroxy-

5-methyl-4-isoxazolepropionic acid receptor (AMPAR)-mediated currents in CA1 pyramidal neurons, and produces variable effects on evoked N-methyl-D-aspartate receptor (NMDAR) currents (Hestrin et al., 1990). These results suggest that diffusion, dilution, and desensitization are the primary determinants of the decay of these currents. However, other studies indicate that clearance of glutamate from the cleft is delayed in GLT-1 knockout mice (Tanaka et al., 1997b; Katagiri et al., 2001), and studies using DHK suggest that GLT-1 restricts spillover of glutamate between synapses (Asztely et al., 1997). Although it is likely that the vast majority of GLT-1 transporters responsible for this uptake are present in astrocyte membranes, the potential involvement of GLT-1 transporters located in nerve terminals cannot be ruled out (Berger and Hediger, 1998). Block of all glutamate transporters by the application of TBOA produces both a standing inward current in CA1 pyramidal neurons through tonic activation of NMDA receptors, and a slowing of the decay kinetics of evoked NMDA responses (Arnth-Jensen et al., 2002). These results suggest that the duration of NMDA receptor activation is determined, in part, by transporter-mediated clearance. It is not yet known if the receptors involved in this prolongation are located within the cleft or in extrasynaptic membranes; however, this effect was also observed in paired recordings from pyramidal neurons in cultured slices, suggesting that synchronous activation of many axons is not necessary to observe this phenomenon (Arnth-Jensen et al., 2002). Because the binding of two glutamate molecules is necessary to gate the NMDA receptor, it is possible that the prolongation observed is due to the presence of receptors that already have one glutamate molecule bound, and thus require less glutamate for activation. That is, the effects observed could be explained by the increase in ambient glutamate rather than a decrease in clearance near receptors. There is evidence that neuronal transporters (EAAC1) also may be involved in clearance away from these receptors, as evoked NMDA receptor currents in pyramidal neurons decay more slowly at depolarized potentials, a manipulation that inhibits uptake (Diamond, 2001). This difference in NMDA receptor kinetics at hyperpolarized and depolarized potentials is not seen when postsynaptic transport is inhibited with removal of internal K^+, suggesting that this effect cannot be explained by the intrinsic voltage-dependence of the NMDA receptor. These studies point to an involvement of astroglial (primarily GLT-1) transporters in the hippocampus controlling the length of time that NMDA receptors are exposed to glutamate, and the distance that glutamate diffuses following release.

Parallel fiber synapses in the cerebellum also are formed *en-passant*, but unlike those in the hippocampus are tightly ensheathed by astroglial processes. Synaptic excitation of Purkinje neurons is achieved through the activity of AMPA and metabotropic glutamate receptors (mGluRs), as NMDA receptors are not present at these sites, and GLT-1, GLAST, EAAC1, and a fourth transporter, EAAT4, accomplish uptake in this region. EAAT4 is a unique transporter, in that it is expressed only by Purkinje neurons in this region and it has a 10-fold higher affinity for glutamate than the other glutamate transporters (Fairman et al., 1995). Unlike the hippocampus, DHK has little effect on AMPA excitatory postsynaptic currents (EPSCs) in this region, consistent with the higher level of GLAST expression. In addition, few differences in the kinetics of AMPA EPSCs were observed between wild type and GLAST knockout mice, indicating that GLAST does not shape clearance near these receptors, or that other transporters are able to compensate for the absence of GLAST. However, global inhibition of glutamate uptake in this region has profound effects on AMPA receptor currents (Barbour et al., 1994; Takahashi et al., 1995); transporter inhibition induces a decrease in amplitude and a slowing of the decay kinetics of AMPA EPSCs, effects that are even more apparent when desensitization is removed. These results suggest that the tight ensheathment of these synapses slows diffusion allowing glutamate to repeatedly bind to these low affinity receptors. The effects of transporter inhibition are even more profound for responses mediated by mGluRs located perisynaptically. When glutamate transporters are blocked with TBOA, mGluR-mediated currents can be evoked with fewer stimuli and are enhanced in both amplitude and duration (Brasnjo and Otis, 2001). These effects can be mimicked, at least qualitatively, when only uptake into Purkinje cells is reduced, suggesting that EAAT4 and perhaps also EAAC1 are important for clearing glutamate away from these receptors. The lack of selective antagonists against GLAST has hampered attempts to define the role of astroglial transport in this region.

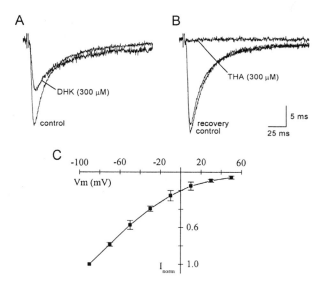

Figure 9.4. Synaptic activation of astrocyte glutamate transporters. A, Evoked glutamate transporter currents recorded from an astrocyte in the stratum radiatum region of area CA1 in an acute hippocampal slice. Application of DHK (300 μM) decreased the amplitude and slowed the kinetics of this response, indicating that GLT-1 transporters contribute to this current and that clearance of glutamate is slowed when this transporter is inhibited. B, Subsequent application of THA (300 μM), a non-selective transporter antagonist completely blocked this response, indicating that the evoked response is mediated by glutamate transporters. C, Current-to-voltage relationship of evoked transporter currents recorded from an astrocyte at potentials between –100 and 50 mV. All responses were recorded with a KNO_3-based internal solution. Adapted from (Bergles and Jahr, 1997).

Together these results indicate that transporters and receptors compete for the glutamate that is released during excitatory synaptic transmission, and that at some synapses transporters determine how much glutamate is available to bind to receptors.

The slow cycling of transporters and rapid rate of glutamate diffusion suggest that the effects of transporters on EPSCs are likely to be mediated largely by binding of glutamate to transporters rather than repeated cycling. Although transporters are unlikely to be saturated by the glutamate released in a single vesicle (Lehre and Danbolt, 1998; Diamond and Jahr, 2000), it is not yet known what proportion of each class of transporter is activated, and what fraction of transporters undergo multiple cycles (and/or multiple binding events) during the release of glutamate at these different synapses.

9.7. Glutamate transporter regulation

Numerous investigations have begun to dissect molecular mechanisms responsible for the regulation of astroglial glutamate transporters. This regulation can occur at several levels - protein expression through gene activation or transcript stabilization, increased translation of protein, trafficking of cytosolic from subcellular compartments to plasma membrane, and direct biochemical modification of the proteins, leading to altered kinetic activity. The first evidence that transporters were subject to acute regulation came from studies of lesions of neuronal pathways. Disruption of axonal inputs to striatum and hippocampus leads to a marked down regulation of GLT-1 and GLAST expression and function (Ginsberg et al., 1995; Levy et al., 1995; Ginsberg et al., 1996). Recovery of synaptic connectivity reverses this effect, suggesting a role for neuronal proteins or cell-cell contacts in regulating astroglial transporter expression. Subsequent *in vitro* studies have confirmed that neuronal secreted factors appear to potently regulate the expression of EAAT1 and EAAT2 (Gegelashvili et al., 1997; Swanson et al., 1997b; Zelenaia et al., 2000). Factors known to alter GLT-1/GLAST expression include: epidermal growth factors, glial derived neurotrophic factor, transforming growth factor beta, as well as dibutyryl cyclic AMP and the pituitary adenylate cyclase-activating polypeptide (PACAP) (Ganel et al., 1998; Figiel and Engele, 2000) (Fig. 9.5). In some cases, protein expression may be increased cytosolically, without concomitant expression of functional protein on the plasma membrane. The exact cellular events responsible for altering transporter expression are not known, but some studies suggest that phosphatidylinositol 3-kinase and/or nuclear transcription factor kappa B are involved. The EAAT2 promoter was recently cloned, and studies using reporter constructs confirmed that several molecular events, including interaction with nuclear transcription factor kappa B, can act to alter EAAT2 gene expression (Su et al., 2003). Overall, these studies demonstrate that soluble factors acting on astrocytes can lead to enhanced transporter expression.

A number of studies have defined a role for protein kinase C (PKC) in the regulation of both GLAST and GLT-1. PKC delta inhibition appears to produce dramatic loss of GLAST, presumably due to increased degradation (Susarla and Robinson, 2003). Similarly, drug induced PKC activation can also lead to loss of GLT-1 cell surface trafficking in selected *in vitro* preparations (Robinson, 2002; Gonzalez et al., 2003). In addition to biochemical regulation, it is likely that protein-protein interactions could also serve to modulate astroglial EAATs. Several glutamate transporter interacting proteins (GTRAPs) have been identified for the neuronal glutamate transporters EAAT3 and EAAT4, (Jackson et al., 2001; Lin et al., 2001), and it is likely that similar proteins may exist to regulate astroglial glutamate transporters (Marie et al., 2002). How these biochemical events interact to regulate transporters *in vivo* is, however, not yet fully understood.

9.8. Transporters and disease

The studies described above clearly establish an important role for astroglial glutamate transporters in normal synaptic activity, and have begun to highlight a complex, highly regulated process responsible for controlling their expression and activity. But what about dysfunction? Is there evidence to suggest that dysfunction of these proteins occurs and contributes to disease? Initial antisense knockdown studies established a prominent role for the astroglial glutamate transporters GLAST and GLT-1, but not neuronal glutamate transport in the normal maintenance of extracellular glutamate levels (Rothstein et al., 1996b). Furthermore, these studies and later gene inactivation studies determined that the majority of biochemical inactivation of extracellular glutamate - as much as 95% of all glutamate transporter - is due to GLT-1 activity (Rothstein et al., 1996b; Tanaka et al., 1997a; Watase et al., 1998b). Furthermore, these studies defined a central role for GLT-1 in excitotoxic neurodegeneration. Loss of GLT-1 expression in adult animals leads to subacute neuronal degeneration and paralysis, while loss of GLT-1 at birth is associated with epilepsy and death. In addition, susceptibility to cerebellar and cortical ischemic injury is increased with loss of GLT-1 or GLAST protein expression (Tanaka et al., 1997a; Watase et al., 1998b).

A more defined role for astroglial transporters comes from study of some neurodegenerative diseases. Amyotrophic lateral sclerosis (ALS) is an adult onset fatal neuromuscular disease characterized by progressive weakness of muscles and respiratory failures. At the cellular level, the cortical, brain stem and spinal cord motor neurons degenerate in people suffering from this disease. The disease is largely sporadic, but some familial forms are associated with mutations of the enzyme copper zinc superoxide dismutase (SOD1) (Cleveland and Rothstein, 2001). Transgenic over expression of the mutant protein in mice accurately recapitulates the disease. Initial biochemical studies established a profound deficit of glutamate transport in affected human and mouse tissue (Rothstein et al., 1992; Howland et al., 2002). Subsequently, a specific loss of GLT-1/EAAT2 protein – but not other glutamate transporters was found in ALS with almost complete loss of protein expression in motor cortex and spinal cord (Rothstein et al., 1995; Howland et al., 2002) (Figure 9.6). The mechanisms for loss of astroglial EAAT2 is not yet known. Several molecular and biochemical process may contribute including the abnormal splicing of the gene product and oxidative damage to the protein (Trotti et al., 1997; Lin et al., 1998; Trotti et al., 1999). Loss of EAAT2 expression may reflect an astroglial response to neuronal injury, although at least some studies document the loss of EAAT2 quite early in the course of the disease. Based on the animal studies described above, it is presumed that the loss of EAAT2/GLT-1 contributes to neurodegeneration that occurs in the human and rodent forms of the disease. Therefore, replacement of the lost protein or enhancement of other glutamate transporters might be expected to alter the disease course. Consistent with this hypothesis, recent studies suggest that over expression of the wild-type protein in transgenic mouse models of ALS significantly delays onset of disease and delays death (Sutherland et al., 2001; Guo et al., 2003). Interestingly, studies of other mouse models of human disease, and analysis of human tissue directly, also have documented a selective loss of astroglial transporters in diseases such as Huntington's chorea (Lievens et al., 2001).

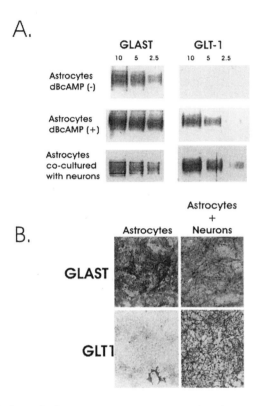

Figure 9.5. Regulation of glutamate transporter expression in astrocytes. A, Purified astrocytes *in vitro* selectively express GLAST, but not GLT-1. Western blots confirm that astrocyte GLT-1 expression is induced and GLAST expression is increased by incubation with Dibutyryl-cAMP (dbcAMP, 0.15 mM) and by co-culture with neurons. Numbers above the lanes denote mg protein loaded onto the lanes. B, Mixed cultures of astrocytes and neurons demonstrating the dramatic increase in expression of GLT-1 in the somas and processes of astrocytes. Adapted from: (Swanson et al., 1997a).

The astroglial glutamate transporters are essential for the maintenance of low extracellular levels of glutamate, and thus loss of that principal function is associated with excitotoxic neurodegeneration. But glutamate transporters may also function in a more metabolic capacity to regulate the levels of intracellular glutamate. The neuronal glutamate transporter EAAT3/EAAC1 is localized on pre-synaptic GABAergic terminals (He et al., 2000), and this unusual location appears to be linked it to its role as a metabolic transport. By transporting the glutamate into presynaptic terminals, EAAT3 provides glutamate as a precursor for the synthesis of the neurotransmitter GABA. Newly synthesized, synaptically releasable pools of GABA appear to rely on EAAC1/EAAT3 transport (Sepkuty et al., 2002; Mathews and Diamond, 2003), and loss of this activity is associated with epileptiform activity and seizures (Sepkuty et al., 2002). Whether this particular pathway contributes to human epilepsies, and whether astroglial transporters are similarly linked to neurotransmitter pools, awaits further study.

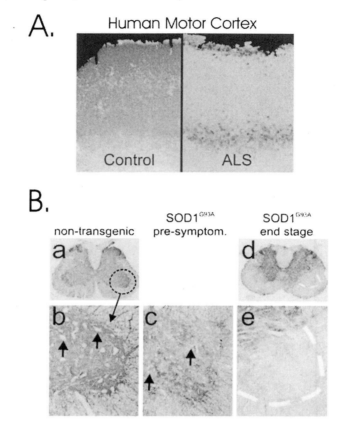

Figure 9.6. Decreased expression of EAAT2/GLT-1 in ALS. A, Dramatic loss of cortical EAAT2 protein expression in a patient with ALS. Only rare astrocytes in layers 1 and 6 continue to express the transporter protein. B, In a transgenic rat ALS model that over expresses the G93A mutant of SOD1, GLT-1 immunoreactive protein is present in spinal cord neuropil (a,b). However, prior to clinical disease, the expression of GLT-1 appears to decrease around motor neurons (arrows) and by late disease (c) there is a complete, focal loss of GLT-1 immunoreactivity in the ventral gray neuropil (d,e). Adapted from (Rothstein et al., 1995; Howland et al., 2002).

9.9. Conclusions

Although we are only beginning to understand the dynamic interactions between receptors and transporters, it is clear that binding of glutamate by transporters and eventual uptake influences both the level of ambient glutamate in the extracellular space, and the duration that receptors are exposed to glutamate following release at synapses. Because transporters are present at a much higher density in astroglial membranes, and these cells exhibit properties that are more favorable for net uptake of glutamate, it is likely that astroglia are largely responsible for these effects. Nevertheless, uncertainties about the level of expression of GLT-1 by neurons, and the possibility that a few strategically located transporters could similarly influence receptor activation, raise the possibility that transporters in neuronal membranes may also contribute significantly to glutamate clearance at synapses. The lack of subtype-selective antagonists suitable for blocking each transporter has limited our ability to address the specific roles served by each transporter, and their similar biophysical properties have not revealed why synapses have evolved to use multiple transporters for clearance. Understanding the role of individual transporters is essential for understanding how changes in activity and expression of different transporters alters glutamate-dependent signaling between both neurons and glial cells, and how such alterations impact human disease. Although studies have shown that transporter activity can be altered through direct modification by phosphorylation and through interaction with other proteins, little is known about the extent and manner in which their activity is regulated under physiological conditions. Given their potential involvement in physiological processes as diverse as synapse formation, transmitter recycling, energy metabolism, and synaptic plasticity, future studies of glutamate transporters will undoubtedly reveal further details of how astroglia and neurons interact to support signaling at synapses, and how disruption of transport impacts central nervous system physiology.

9.10. References

Amzica F, Massimini M, Manfridi A (2002) Spatial buffering during slow and paroxysmal sleep oscillations in cortical networks of glial cells in vivo. J Neurosci 22:1042-1053.

Arnth-Jensen N, Jabaudon D, Scanziani M (2002) Cooperation between independent hippocampal synapses is controlled by glutamate uptake. Nat Neurosci 5:325-331.

Arriza JL, Eliasof S, Kavanaugh MP, Amara SG (1997) Excitatory amino acid transporter 5, a retinal glutamate transporter coupled to a chloride conductance. Proc Natl Acad Sci U S A 94:4155-4160.

Arriza JL, Fairman WA, Wadiche JI, Murdoch GH, Kavanaugh MP, Amara SG (1994) Functional comparisons of three glutamate transporter subtypes cloned from human motor cortex. J Neurosci 14:5559-5569.

Asztely F, Erdemli G, Kullmann DM (1997) Extrasynaptic glutamate spillover in the hippocampus: dependence on temperature and the role of active glutamate uptake. Neuron 18:281-293.

Attwell D, Barbour B, Szatkowski M (1993) Nonvesicular release of neurotransmitter. Neuron 11:401-407.

Auger C, Attwell D (2000) Fast removal of synaptic glutamate by postsynaptic transporters. Neuron 28:547-558.

Barbour B, Keller BU, Llano I, Marty A (1994) Prolonged presence of glutamate during excitatory synaptic transmission to cerebellar Purkinje cells. Neuron 12:1331-1343.

Berger UV, Hediger MA (1998) Comparative analysis of glutamate transporter expression in rat brain using differential double in situ hybridization. Anat Embryol (Berl) 198:13-30.

Bergles DE, Jahr CE (1997) Synaptic activation of glutamate transporters in hippocampal astrocytes. Neuron 19:1297-1308.

Bergles DE, Jahr CE (1998) Glial contribution to glutamate uptake at Schaffer collateral-commissural synapses in the hippocampus. J Neurosci 18:7709-7716.

Bergles DE, Dzubay JA, Jahr CE (1997) Glutamate transporter currents in bergmann glial cells follow the time course of extrasynaptic glutamate. Proc Natl Acad Sci U S A 94:14821-14825.

Bergles DE, Tzingounis AV, Jahr CE (2002) Comparison of coupled and uncoupled currents during glutamate uptake by GLT-1 transporters. J Neurosci 22:10153-10162.

Bouvier M, Szatkowski M, Amato A, Attwell D (1992) The glial cell glutamate uptake carrier countertransports pH-changing anions. Nature 360:471-474.

Brasnjo G, Otis TS (2001) Neuronal glutamate transporters control activation of postsynaptic metabotropic glutamate receptors and influence cerebellar long-term depression. Neuron 31:607-616.

Bushong EA, Martone ME, Jones YZ, Ellisman MH (2002) Protoplasmic astrocytes in CA1 stratum radiatum occupy separate anatomical domains. J Neurosci 22:183-192.

Chaudhry FA, Lehre KP, van Lookeren CM, Ottersen OP, Danbolt NC, Storm-Mathisen J (1995) Glutamate transporters in glial plasma membranes: highly differentiated localizations revealed by quantitative ultrastructural immunocytochemistry. In, pp 711-720.

Chen S, Diamond JS (2002) Synaptically released glutamate activates extrasynaptic NMDA receptors on cells in the ganglion cell layer of rat retina. J Neurosci 22:2165-2173.

Chen W, Aoki C, Mahadomrongkul V, Gruber CE, Wang GJ, Blitzblau R, Irwin N, Rosenberg PA (2002a) Expression of a variant form of the glutamate transporter GLT1 in neuronal cultures and in neurons and astrocytes in the rat brain. 22:2142-2152.

Chen W, Aoki C, Mahadomrongkul V, Gruber CE, Wang GJ, Blitzblau R, Irwin N, Rosenberg PA (2002b) Expression of a variant form of the glutamate transporter GLT1 in neuronal cultures and in neurons and astrocytes in the rat brain. J Neurosci 22:2142-2152.

Chen W, Aoki C, Mahadomrongkul V, Gruber CE, Wang GJ, Blitzblau R, Irwin N, Rosenberg PA (2002c) Expression of a variant form of the glutamate transporter GLT1 in neuronal cultures and in neurons and astrocytes in the rat brain. In, pp 2142-2152.

Clark BA, Cull-Candy SG (2002) Activity-dependent recruitment of extrasynaptic NMDA receptor activation at an AMPA receptor-only synapse. J Neurosci 22:4428-4436.

Clements JD (1996) Transmitter timecourse in the synaptic cleft: its role in central synaptic function. Trends Neurosci 19:163-171.

Clements JD, Lester RA, Tong G, Jahr CE, Westbrook GL (1992) The time course of glutamate in the synaptic cleft. Science 258:1498-1501.

Cleveland DW, Rothstein JD (2001) From charcot to lou gehrig: deciphering selective motor neuron death in als. In, pp 806-819.

Danbolt NC, Storm-Mathisen J, Kanner BI (1992) An [Na+ + K+]coupled L-glutamate transporter purified from rat brain is located in glial cell processes. Neuroscience 51:295-310.

Danbolt NC, Lehre KP, Dehnes Y, Chaudhry FA, Levy LM (1998a) Localization of transporters using transporter-specific antibodies. In, pp 388-407.

Danbolt NC, Chaudhry FA, Dehnes Y, Lehre KP, Levy LM, Ullensvang K, Storm-Mathisen J (1998b) Properties and localization of glutamate transporters. In, pp 23-43.

Diamond JS (2001) Neuronal glutamate transporters limit activation of NMDA receptors by neurotransmitter spillover on CA1 pyramidal cells. J Neurosci 21:8328-8338.

Diamond JS, Jahr CE (1997) Transporters buffer synaptically released glutamate on a submillisecond time scale. J Neurosci 17:4672-4687.

Diamond JS, Jahr CE (2000) Synaptically released glutamate does not overwhelm transporters on hippocampal astrocytes during high-frequency stimulation. J Neurophysiol 83:2835-2843.

Eliasof S, Jahr CE (1996) Retinal glial cell glutamate transporter is coupled to an anionic conductance. Proc Natl Acad Sci U S A 93:4153-4158.

Fairman WA, Vandenberg RJ, Arriza JL, Kavanaugh MP, Amara SG (1995) An excitatory amino-acid transporter with properties of a ligand-gated chloride channel. Nature 375:599-603.

Figiel M, Engele J (2000) Pituitary adenylate cyclase-activating polypeptide (PACAP), a neuron- derived peptide regulating glial glutamate transport and metabolism. In, pp 3596-3605.

Furuta A, Rothstein JD, Martin LJ (1997a) Glutamate transporter protein subtypes are expressed differentially during rat CNS development. In, pp 8363-8375.

Furuta A, Martin LJ, Lin CL, Dykes-Hoberg M, Rothstein JD (1997b) Cellular and synaptic localization of the neuronal glutamate transporters excitatory amino acid transporter 3 and 4. In, pp 1031-1042.

Ganel R, Ho T, Sakal C, Steiner J, Dykes-Hoberg M, Robinson MB, Rothstein JD (1998) Excitotoxicity and neurodegeneration - a novel therapeutic approach. In: Society for Neuroscience, p 2069 (2825.2019).

Gegelashvili G, Danbolt NC, Schousboe A (1997) Neuronal soluble factors differentially regulate the expression of the GLT1 and GLAST glutamate transporters in cultured astroglia. In, pp 2612-2615.

Ginsberg SD, Martin LJ, Rothstein JD (1995) Regional deafferentation down-regulates subtypes of glutamate transporter proteins. In, pp 2800-2803.

Ginsberg SD, Rothstein JD, Price DL, Martin LJ (1996) Fimbria-fornix transections selectively down-regulate subtypes of glutamate transporter and glutamate receptor proteins in septum and hippocampus. In, pp 1208-1216.

Gonzalez MI, Bannerman PG, Robinson MB (2003) Phorbol myristate acetate-dependent interaction of protein kinase Calpha and the neuronal glutamate transporter EAAC1. In, pp 5589-5593.

Guo H, Lai L, Butchbach ME, Stockinger MP, Shan X, Bishop GA, Lin CL (2003) Increased expression of the glial glutamate transporter EAAT2 modulates excitotoxicity and delays the onset but not the outcome of ALS in mice. In: Hum Mol Genet.

He Y, Janssen WG, Rothstein JD, Morrison JH (2000) Differential synaptic localization of the glutamate transporter EAAC1 and glutamate receptor subunit GluR2 in the rat hippocampus. In, pp 255-269.

Hestrin S, Sah P, Nicoll RA (1990) Mechanisms generating the time course of dual component excitatory synaptic currents recorded in hippocampal slices. Neuron 5:247-253.

Higashijima T, Ferguson KM, Sternweis PC (1987) Regulation of hormone-sensitive GTP-dependent regulatory proteins by chloride. J Biol Chem 262:3597-3602.

Howland DS, Liu J, She Y, Goad B, Maragakis NJ, Kim B, Erickson J, Kulik J, DeVito L, Psaltis G, DeGennaro LJ, Cleveland DW, Rothstein JD (2002) Focal loss of the glutamate transporter EAAT2 in a transgenic rat model of SOD1 mutant-mediated amyotrophic lateral sclerosis (ALS). In, pp 1604-1609.

Iino M, Goto K, Kakegawa W, Okado H, Sudo M, Ishiuchi S, Miwa A, Takayasu Y, Saito I, Tsuzuki K, Ozawa S (2001) Glia-synapse interaction through Ca2+-permeable AMPA receptors in Bergmann glia. Science 292:926-929.

Jackson M, Song W, Liu MY, Jin L, Dykes-Hoberg M, Lin CI, Bowers WJ, Federoff HJ, Sternweis PC, Rothstein JD (2001) Modulation of the neuronal glutamate transporter EAAT4 by two interacting proteins. In, pp 89-93.

Katagiri H, Tanaka K, Manabe T (2001) Requirement of appropriate glutamate concentrations in the synaptic cleft for hippocampal LTP induction. Eur J Neurosci 14:547-553.

Klockner U, Storck T, Conradt M, Stoffel W (1993) Electrogenic L-glutamate uptake in Xenopus laevis oocytes expressing a cloned rat brain L-glutamate/L-aspartate transporter (GLAST-1). J Biol Chem 268:14594-14596.

Kosaka T, Hama K (1986) Three-dimensional structure of astrocytes in the rat dentate gyrus. J Comp Neurol 249:242-260.

Kuffler SW, Nicholls JG, Orkand RK (1966) Physiological properties of glial cells in the central nervous system of amphibia. J Neurophysiol 29:768-787.

Lehre KP, Danbolt NC (1998) The number of glutamate transporter subtype molecules at glutamatergic synapses: chemical and stereological quantification in young adult rat brain. J Neurosci 18:8751-8757.

Lehre KP, Levy LM, Ottersen OP, Storm-Mathisen J, Danbolt NC (1995) Differential expression of two glial glutamate transporters in the rat brain: quantitative and immunocytochemical observations. In, pp 1835-1853.

Levy LM, Warr O, Attwell D (1998) Stoichiometry of the glial glutamate transporter GLT-1 expressed inducibly in a Chinese hamster ovary cell line selected for low endogenous Na+-dependent glutamate uptake. J Neurosci 18:9620-9628.

Levy LM, Lehre KP, Walaas SI, Storm-Mathisen J, Danbolt NC (1995) Down-regulation of glial glutamate transporters after glutamatergic denervation in the rat brain. In, pp 2036-2041.

Lievens JC, Woodman B, Mahal A, Spasic-Boscovic O, Samuel D, Kerkerian-Le Goff L, Bates GP (2001) Impaired glutamate uptake in the R6 Huntington's disease transgenic mice. In, pp 807-821.

Lin CI, Orlov I, Ruggiero AM, Dykes-Hoberg M, Lee A, Jackson M, Rothstein JD (2001) Modulation of the neuronal glutamate transporter EAAC1 by the interacting protein GTRAP3-18. In, pp 84-88.

Lin CL, Bristol LA, Jin L, Dykes-Hoberg M, Crawford T, Clawson L, Rothstein JD (1998) Aberrant RNA processing in a neurodegenerative disease: the cause for absent EAAT2, a glutamate transporter, in amyotrophic lateral sclerosis. In, pp 589-602.

Liu G, Choi S, Tsien RW (1999) Variability of neurotransmitter concentration and nonsaturation of postsynaptic AMPA receptors at synapses in hippocampal cultures and slices. Neuron 22:395-409.

Lu CC, Hilgemann DW (1999) GAT1 (GABA:Na+:Cl-) cotransport function. Steady state studies in giant Xenopus oocyte membrane patches. J Gen Physiol 114:429-444.

Marie H, Billups D, Bedford FK, Dumoulin A, Goyal RK, Longmore GD, Moss SJ, Attwell D (2002) The amino terminus of the glial glutamate transporter GLT-1 interacts with the LIM protein Ajuba. In: Mol Cell Neurosci, pp 152-164.

Martin LJ, Brambrink AM, Lehmann C, Portera-Cailliau C, Koehler R, Rothstein J, Traystman RJ (1997) Hypoxia-ischemia causes abnormalities in glutamate transporters and death of astroglia and neurons in newborn striatum. 42:335-348.

Mathews GC, Diamond JS (2003) Neuronal glutamate uptake Contributes to GABA synthesis and inhibitory synaptic strength. In, pp 2040-2048.

Mennerick S, Dhond RP, Benz A, Xu W, Rothstein JD, Danbolt NC, Isenberg KE, Zorumski CF (1998) Neuronal expression of the glutamate transporter GLT-1 in hippocampal microcultures. In, pp 4490-4499.

Mennerick S, Shen W, Xu W, Benz A, Tanaka K, Shimamoto K, Isenberg KE, Krause JE, Zorumski CF (1999) Substrate turnover by transporters curtails synaptic glutamate transients. J Neurosci 19:9242-9251.

Oertner TG, Sabatini BL, Nimchinsky EA, Svoboda K (2002) Facilitation at single synapses probed with optical quantal analysis. Nat Neurosci 5:657-664.

Oliet SH, Piet R, Poulain DA (2001) Control of glutamate clearance and synaptic efficacy by glial coverage of neurons. Science 292:923-926.

Orkand RK, Nicholls JG, Kuffler SW (1966) Effect of nerve impulses on the membrane potential of glial cells in the central nervous system of amphibia. J Neurophysiol 29:788-806.

Otis TS, Kavanaugh MP (2000) Isolation of current components and partial reaction cycles in the glial glutamate transporter EAAT2. J Neurosci 20:2749-2757.

Otis TS, Kavanaugh MP, Jahr CE (1997) Postsynaptic glutamate transport at the climbing fiber-Purkinje cell synapse. Science 277:1515-1518.

Ottersen OP, Takumi Y, Matsubara A, Landsend AS, Laake JH, Usami S (1998) Molecular organization of a type of peripheral glutamate synapse: the afferent synapses of hair cells in the inner ear. Prog Neurobiol 54:127-148.

Palay SL, Chan-Palay V (1974) In: Cerebellar Cortex - Cytology and Organization. Berlin: Springer.

Renger JJ, Egles C, Liu G (2001) A developmental switch in neurotransmitter flux enhances synaptic efficacy by affecting AMPA receptor activation. Neuron 29:469-484.

Riveros N, Fiedler J, Lagos N, Munoz C, Orrego F (1986) Glutamate in rat brain cortex synaptic vesicles: influence of the vesicle isolation procedure. Brain Res 386:405-408.

Robinson MB (2002) Regulated trafficking of neurotransmitter transporters: common notes but different melodies. In, pp 1-11.

Rothstein JD, Martin LJ, Kuncl RW (1992) Decreased glutamate transport by the brain and spinal cord in amyotrophic lateral sclerosis. In, pp 1464-1468.

Rothstein JD, Van Kammen M, Levey AI, Martin LJ, Kuncl RW (1995) Selective loss of glial glutamate transporter GLT-1 in amyotrophic lateral sclerosis. In, pp 73-84.

Rothstein JD, Martin L, Levey AI, Dykes-Hoberg M, Jin L, Wu D, Nash N, Kuncl RW (1994) Localization of neuronal and glial glutamate transporters. In, pp 713-725.

Rothstein JD, Dykes-Hoberg M, Pardo CA, Bristol LA, Jin L, Kuncl RW, Kanai Y, Hediger MA, Wang Y, Schielke JP, Welty DF (1996a) Knockout of glutamate transporters reveals a major role for astroglial transport in excitotoxicity and clearance of glutamate. Neuron 16:675-686.

Rothstein JD, Dykes-Hoberg M, Pardo CA, Bristol LA, Jin L, Kuncl RW, Kanai Y, Hediger MA, Wang Y, Schielke JP, Welty DF (1996b) Knockout of glutamate transporters reveals a major role for astroglial transport in excitotoxicity and clearance of glutamate. In, pp 675-686.

Schmitt A, Asan E, Lesch KP, Kugler P (2002) A splice variant of glutamate transporter GLT1/EAAT2 expressed in neurons: cloning and localization in rat nervous system. Neuroscience 109:45-61.

Sepkuty JP, Cohen AS, Eccles C, Rafiq A, Behar K, Ganel R, Coulter DA, Rothstein JD (2002) A neuronal glutamate transporter contributes to neurotransmitter GABA synthesis and epilepsy. In, pp 6372-6379.

Shashidharan P, Plaitakis A (1993) Cloning and characterization of a glutamate transporter cDNA from human cerebellum. Biochim Biophys Acta 1216:161-164.

Shashidharan P, Huntley GW, Meyer T, Morrison JH, Plaitakis A (1994) Neuron-specific human glutamate transporter: molecular cloning, characterization and expression in human brain. Brain Res 662:245-250.

Shigeri Y, Shimamoto K, Yasuda-Kamatani Y, Seal RP, Yumoto N, Nakajima T, Amara SG (2001) Effects of threo-beta-hydroxyaspartate derivatives on excitatory amino acid transporters (EAAT4 and EAAT5). J Neurochem 79:297-302.

Shimamoto K, Lebrun B, Yasuda-Kamatani Y, Sakaitani M, Shigeri Y, Yumoto N, Nakajima T (1998) DL-threo-beta-benzyloxyaspartate, a potent blocker of excitatory amino acid transporters. Mol Pharmacol 53:195-201.

Spacek J (1971) Three-dimensional reconstructions of astroglia and oligodendroglia cells. Z Zellforsch Mikrosk Anat 112:430-442.

Spacek J (1985) Three-dimensional analysis of dendritic spines. III. Glial sheath. Anat Embryol (Berl) 171:245-252.

Storck T, Schulte S, Hofmann K, Stoffel W (1992) Structure, expression, and functional analysis of a Na(+)-dependent glutamate/aspartate transporter from rat brain. Proc Natl Acad Sci U S A 89:10955-10959.

Su ZZ, Leszczyniecka M, Kang DC, Sarkar D, Chao W, Volsky DJ, Fisher PB (2003) Insights into glutamate transport regulation in human astrocytes: cloning of the promoter for excitatory amino acid transporter 2 (EAAT2). In, pp 1955-1960.

Susarla BT, Robinson MB (2003) Rottlerin, an inhibitor of protein kinase Cdelta (PKCdelta), inhibits astrocytic glutamate transport activity and reduces GLAST immunoreactivity by a mechanism that appears to be PKCdelta-independent. In, pp 635-645.

Sutherland ML, Martinowich K, Rothstein JD (2001) EAAT2 overexpression plays a neuroprotective role in the SOD1 G93A model of amyotrophic lateral sclerosis. In: Society for Neuroscience Abstracts.

Swanson RA, Liu J, Miller JW, Rothstein JD, Farrell K, Stein BA, Longuemare MC (1997a) Neuronal regulation of glutamate transporter subtype expression in astrocytes. J Neurosci 17:932-940.

Swanson RA, Liu J, Miller JW, Rothstein JD, Farrell K, Stein BA, Longuemare MC (1997b) Neuronal regulation of glutamate transporter subtype expression in astrocytes. In, pp 932-940.

Takahashi M, Kovalchuk Y, Attwell D (1995) Pre- and postsynaptic determinants of EPSC waveform at cerebellar climbing fiber and parallel fiber to Purkinje cell synapses. J Neurosci 15:5693-5702.

Tanaka K, Watase K, Manabe T, Yamada K, Watanabe M, Takahashi K, Iwama H, Nishikawa T, Ichihara N, Hori S, Takimoto M, Wada K (1997a) Epilepsy and exacerbation of brain injury in mice lacking the glutamate transporter GLT-1. In, pp 1699-1702.

Tanaka K, Watase K, Manabe T, Yamada K, Watanabe M, Takahashi K, Iwama H, Nishikawa T, Ichihara N, Kikuchi T, Okuyama S, Kawashima N, Hori S, Takimoto M, Wada K (1997b) Epilepsy and exacerbation of brain injury in mice lacking the glutamate transporter GLT-1. Science 276:1699-1702.

Theodosis DT, Poulain DA (1993) Activity-dependent neuronal-glial and synaptic plasticity in the adult mammalian hypothalamus. Neuroscience 57:501-535.

Tong G, Jahr CE (1994) Block of glutamate transporters potentiates postsynaptic excitation. Neuron 13:1195-1203.

Trotti D, Rolfs A, Danbolt NC, Brown RH, Jr., Hediger MA (1999) SOD1 mutants linked to amyotrophic lateral sclerosis selectively inactivate a glial glutamate transporter. In, p 848.

Trotti D, Rizzini BL, Rossi D, Haugeto O, Racagni G, Danbolt NC, Volterra A (1997) Neuronal and glial glutamate transporters possess an SH-based redox regulatory mechanism. In, pp 1236-1243.

Utsunomiya-Tate N, Endou H, Kanai Y (1997a) Tissue specific variants of glutamate transporter GLT-1. FEBS Lett 416:312-316.

Ventura R, Harris KM (1999) Three-dimensional relationships between hippocampal synapses and astrocytes. J Neurosci 19:6897-6906.

Wadiche JI, Kavanaugh MP (1998) Macroscopic and microscopic properties of a cloned glutamate transporter/chloride channel. J Neurosci 18:7650-7661.

Wadiche JI, Jahr CE (2001) Multivesicular release at climbing fiber-Purkinje cell synapses. Neuron 32:301-313.

Wadiche JI, Amara SG, Kavanaugh MP (1995a) Ion fluxes associated with excitatory amino acid transport. Neuron 15:721-728.

Wadiche JI, Arriza JL, Amara SG, Kavanaugh MP (1995b) Kinetics of a human glutamate transporter. Neuron 14:1019-1027.

Watase K, Hashimoto K, Kano M, Yamada K, Watanabe M, Inoue Y, Okuyama S, Sakagawa T, Ogawa S, Kawashima N, Hori S, Takimoto M, Wada K, Tanaka K (1998a) Motor discoordination and increased susceptibility to cerebellar injury in GLAST mutant mice. Eur J Neurosci 10:976-988.

Watase K, Hashimoto K, Kano M, Yamada K, Watanabe M, Inoue Y, Okuyama S, Sakagawa T, Ogawa S, Kawashima N, Hori S, Takimoto M, Wada K, Tanaka K (1998b) Motor discoordination and increased susceptibility to cerebellar injury in GLAST mutant mice. In, pp 976-988.

Zelenaia O, Schlag BD, Gochenauer GE, Ganel R, Song W, Beesley JS, Grinspan JB, Rothstein JD, Robinson MB (2000) Epidermal growth factor receptor agonists increase expression of glutamate transporter GLT-1 in astrocytes through pathways dependent on phosphatidylinositol 3-kinase and transcription factor NF-kappaB. In, pp 667-678.

Zerangue N, Kavanaugh MP (1996) Flux coupling in a neuronal glutamate transporter. Nature 383:634-637.

Zhou M, Kimelberg HK (2001) Freshly isolated hippocampal CA1 astrocytes comprise two populations differing in glutamate transporter and AMPA receptor expression. J Neurosci 21:7901-7908.

9.11. Abbreviations

AMPA	a-Amino-3-hydroxy-5-methyl-4-isoxazolepropionic acid
ATP	Adenosine 5'-triphosphate
EAATs	Excitatory amino acid transporters
EPSC	Excitatory postsynaptic current
CNS	Central nervous system (CNS)
DHK	Dihydrokainate
GABA	γ-aminobutyric acid
GTRAP	Glutamate transporter interacting proteins
mGluR	Metabotropic glutamate receptor
NMDA	N-methyl-D-aspartate
PKC	Protein kinase C
TBOA	DL-*threo-b*-Benzyloxyaspartic acid
THA	DL-*threo*-b-Hydroxyaspartic acid

Chapter 10

pH regulation and acid/base-mediated transport in glial cells

Joachim W. Deitmer

Abteilung für Allgemeine Zoologie, FB Biologie
Universität Kaiserslautern, P.B. 3049
D-67653 Kaiserslautern, Germany

Corresponding author: deitmer@rhrk.uni-kl.de

Contents

10.1. Introduction

In nerve and glial cells and in the extracellular spaces of nervous systems pH changes can be evoked by neuronal activity, by neurotransmitters, by active cellular pH regulation, by secondary transporters carrying acid/base equivalents, and by metabolic processes. In particular, neurotransmission mediated by glutamate, γ-aminobutyric acid (GABA) or glycine as the transmitters, is associated with intra- and extracellular pH changes, which can be large and rapid, not unlike some intracellular calcium transients. However, *unlike* those intracellular calcium changes that rise and then recover, pH shifts can occur in two directions, namely in acid and alkaline directions. Indeed, because several acid/base fluxes with different time courses may be elicited by a stimulus, e.g., by a brief train of action potentials, the pH changes, particularly in the extracellular spaces, may be multiphasic. These changes in extracellular pH (pH_o) may in turn affect the electrical and synaptic activity of neurons.

Rapid pH transients may actually be signals rather than only a result of inadequate homeostatic acid-base regulation. Analogous to the signaling pattern of other ions, such as calcium and potassium, transient shifts of protons and bicarbonate, together with the gas carbon dioxide, may influence or initiate functional processes in the nervous system, including pH-induced changes of neuronal excitability, the modulation of gap junctions and thus of electrical synapses and the glial syncytium, transport processes in which acid or base is involved, and the control of enzyme activities. Proton signaling in cells and in local extracellular domains, particularly in the vicinity of synapses, could well contribute to information processing in nervous systems (Chesler and Kaila, 1992; Deitmer and Rose 1996), and to slowing of potential shifts associated with neuronal activity.

Functionally, pH_o changes will modify processes at the extracellular surface of cells, resulting in the modulation of neuronal excitability and synaptic transmission, as well as of a variety of membrane carriers. For instance, ionotropic glutamate receptors of the N-methyl-D-aspartate (NMDA) type are highly sensitive to pH_o, and synaptic transmission via these receptors is suppressed if pH_o falls below 7.0 (Traynelis and Cull-Candy, 1990). Furthermore, since synaptic vesicles are acidic (pH 5.6, Miesenbock et al., 1998), a transient, local, fall of extracellular pH is associated with their exocytosis during synaptic transmission, suggesting that pH changes at the synapse occur, and may influence, synaptic transmission. Indeed, a transient inhibition of presynaptic Ca^{2+} current in mammalian photoreceptors, presumably due to an acidification in the synaptic cleft, has been reported (DeVries, 2001).

Extracellular acidification itself may gate acid-sensing ion channels (ASICs), a family of amiloride-sensitive Na^+ channels which contribute to synaptic plasticity in the central nervous system (Wemmie et al., 2002). ASIC null mice had reduced excitatory postsynaptic potentials and NMDA receptor activation during high-frequency stimulation of hippocampal neurons. Moreover, loss of ASICs impaired hippocampal long-term potentiation, and ASIC null mice displayed defective spatial learning and eye blink conditioning. ASICs also affect a range of sensory functions that includes perception of gentle touch, harsh touch, heat, sour taste, and pain (Bianchi and Driscoll, 2002).

10.2. The acid-base gradient

The cytosolic pH of animal cells is actively maintained at a value usually between 7.0 and 7.2, which is similar to, or a little lower than, the pH value of the extracellular body fluids (7.2-7.4). The proton equilibrium potential hence ranges between −10 and −20 mV in most animal cells. At a negative cell membrane potential of brain cells between −40 and −90 mV, the total H^+ gradient therefore amounts to 20-80 mV. Acid must be actively extruded by the cells against this electrochemical gradient, which requires energy. In most cells the energy is provided by the Na^+ gradient, which drives the Na^+/H^+ exchanger (NHE) and other acid/base transport systems. The NHE is the most prominent and ubiquitous transport protein for acid extrusion in animal cells (Harris and Fliegel, 1999; Putney et al., 2002) and maintains the cytoplasm at a more alkaline pH than the acid/base electrochemical equilibrium across the plasma membrane, which can be calculated to be around 6.5 or less in most animal cells. When cells become alkaline, base equivalents are extruded mainly by the anion exchanger (AE) Cl^-/HCO_3^- counter-transport.

The need for active maintenance of the cytosolic pH is usually explained by the steep pH dependence of many enzymatic processes in cells, which have their optimum at a pH of around 7.0 or higher. Although the proton gradient across animal plasma membranes is not very large, and amounts to only about half the size of the Na^+ gradient, it is also a significant source of energy, which can be used to fuel secondary transport (see below).

10.3. Intraglial pH regulation

Like many other cell types, glial cells use a variety of acid/base transport systems for their intracellular pH (pH_i) regulation (Fig. 10.1). As with most cells, glial cells use NHE and a Cl^-/HCO_3^- exchanger, and like most *epithelial* cells they use a Na^+/HCO_3^- cotransporter, which is apparently not active in neurons and most non-epithelial cells. In most studies, the Na^+/HCO_3^- cotransporter was detected during addition or removal of CO_2/HCO_3^-. Addition of CO_2/HCO_3^- resulted in an intracellular alkaline shift and a rise in intracellular Na^+ (Na^+_i), while removal of CO_2/HCO_3^- reversed these pH_i and Na^+_i changes (Fig. 10.2A). Simultaneously, the glial membrane hyperpolarized and depolarized, respectively, during these buffer changes due to reversibility of this electrogenic cotransporter (Deitmer 1991). When voltage-clamped, outward and inward currents, respectively, were recorded under these conditions (Munsch and Deitmer 1994).

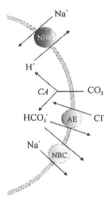

Figure 10.1. The main acid/base-regulating transport systems across the glial cell membrane: Na^+/H^+ exchanger (NHE), Cl^-/HCO_3^- exchanger (or anion exchanger, AE), and $Na^+-HCO_3^-$ cotransporter (NBC). Carbonic anhydrase (CA) catalyses CO_2, diffusing into the cell, to H^+ and HCO_3^-.

As in epithelial cells, the $Na^+-HCO_3^-$ cotransporter in glial cells could be inhibited by stilbene derivatives, such as DIDS, SITS or DNDS (4,4'-diisothiocyanatostilbene-2,2'-disulfonic acid; 4-acetamino-4'-isothiocyanato-stilbene-2,2'-disulfonic acid; dinitrostilbene-disulfonic acid), but was unaffected by amiloride. In cultured rat astrocytes, DIDS partly blocked pH_i recovery and the CO_2/HCO_3^--dependent outward current (Brune et al 1994) as had been shown in leech glial cells (Deitmer and Schlue 1989; Deitmer 1991). These CO_2/HCO_3^--dependent pH_i shifts and membrane potential changes were dependent upon the presence of Na^+_o, but not on $[Cl^-]_o$ or $[Cl^-]_i$. There was a reversible rise in Na^+_i during the exposure to CO_2/HCO_3^- in leech glial cells (Fig. 10.2; Deitmer 1992) and in cultured rat hippocampal astrocytes (Rose and Ransom 1996).

Reduction of the pH_o by reducing the HCO_3^- concentration evoked an inward current in leech glial cells (Deitmer 1991; Munsch and Deitmer 1994) and rat astrocytes (Brune et al 1994). The NBC (sodium-bicarbonate cotransporter) is electrogenic and cotransports one Na^+ with two HCO_3^- (Deitmer and Schlue, 1989; Deitmer and Schneider, 1995). This is consistent with activation of an outward-going electrogenic Na^+-HCO_3^- cotransport. When CO_2/HCO_3^- is introduced, e.g. when changing from a non-bicarbonate, HEPES-buffered saline to a CO_2/HCO_3^--buffered saline, NBC is activated in the inward direction, leading to a membrane hyperpolarization, an intracellular alkalinization and a rise in Na^+_i (Fig. 10.2 A).

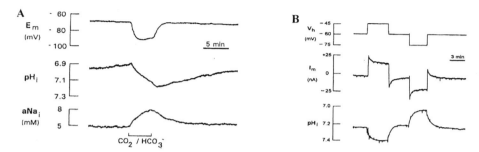

Figure 10.2. *A.* Intracellular recording of membrane potential (E_m), of pH (pH_i) and intracellular Na activity (aNa_i) in the leech giant glial cell *in situ*, when exposed to a saline buffered with 5% CO_2, 25 mM HCO_3^-, maintaining the pH of the saline constant at 7.4, using pH- and Na^+-selective microelectrodes (from Deitmer and Schneider, 1995). *B.* Voltage steps ± 15 mV from a holding potential, V_h, of –60 mV) applied to a voltage-clamped leech giant glial cell in CO_2/ HCO_3^--buffered saline causes changes in membrane current (I_m) and pH_i, as expected from activation of the electrogenic sodium-bicarbonate cotransporter (NBC).

The transport of Na^+ and HCO_3^- can operate in both directions, depending on the pH_i and pH_o (and HCO_3^-), the $[Na^+]_i$ and the membrane potential (Fig. 10.2; Deitmer, 1991; Deitmer and Schneider, 1995). The cotransporter could also be reversed in retinal Müller glial cells (Newman 1991), i.e. operating inwardly *and* outwardly, depending on the thermodynamic conditions. This is also reflected by the pH_i changes induced by slow voltage steps in voltage-clamped leech giant neuropil glial cells (Fig. 10.2 B). De- and hyper- polarizing voltage steps resulted in an intraglial alkalinization and acidification, respectively, providing an extrapolated change of one pH unit/110 mV membrane potential change, supporting a stoichiometry of 2 HCO_3^-: 1 Na^+ (Deitmer and Schneider 1995). The cotransporter appears to have a remarkably high affinity for HCO_3^-, since it was found to be active even in the nominal absence of CO_2/HCO_3^-, when the extracellular bicarbonate concentration is usually less than 0.3 mM due to air-CO_2 (Deitmer and Schneider, 1998). Expressed in frog oocytes, the NBC is so effective that it significantly contributes to the apparent cytosolic buffer capacity (Becker et al., 2004), and may thus enhance the efficacy of other acid/base transport systems.

The NBC has been described in nearly all types of macroglial cells, including astrocytes, oligodendrocytes, Schwann cells and retinal Müller glial cells (*cf.* Deitmer and Rose, 1996). A stoichiometry of 1 Na^+: 2 HCO_3^- has also been reported for the mammalian renal NBC expressed in frog oocytes (Heyer et al., 1999). The NBCs from human kidney and rat brain have recently been cloned, and expressed in frog oocytes (Romero et al., 1997; Giffard et al., 2000). *In situ* hybridization revealed NBC mRNA expression throughout the rat central nervous system, with particularly high levels in the olfactory bulb, the hippocampus dentate gyrus, and the cerebellum (Schmitt et al., 2000).

10.4. pH shifts during neuronal activity

Studies on central nervous systems of both vertebrates and invertebrates have shown that neuronal activity leads to defined pH_o and pH_i changes (Deitmer and Rose, 1996). These consist of mono- or multiphasic pH shifts indicating that they might originate from multiple sources and/or via multiple processes. Due to the increase in $[K^+]_o$ and to excitatory neurotransmitters, glial cells may respond to the activity of neighboring neurons with a substantial depolarization of their cell membrane, accompanied by an intracellular alkalinization. In the rat cortex, the stimulus-evoked glial depolarization is accompanied by an intracellular alkalinization of astrocytes, the amplitude of which is dependent on the amplitude of the glial depolarization (Chesler and Kraig, 1989). In the extracellular space (ECS), the same nerve stimulation, which elicits an intraglial alkalinization, evokes an acid transient in the ECS. Interestingly, while the intraglial pH shift was unaffected by the carbonic anhydrase (CA) inhibitor ethoxyzolamide, the extracellular acid transient was converted to a large alkaline transient following inhibition of CA activity (Rose and Deitmer, 1995b). This suggests that these pH_o changes are greatly affected by the activity of extracellular and/or intracellular CA.

Several lines of evidence suggest that the depolarization-induced alkalinization of glial cells in both vertebrate and invertebrate preparations is due to inward transport of bicarbonate via the electrogenic Na^+-HCO_3^- cotransport (NBC) activated by the K^+-induced membrane depolarization (Deitmer and Szatkowski, 1990; Grichtchenko and Chesler, 1994; Pappas and Ransom, 1994; Bevensee et al., 1997). In the cortex, the glial alkaline shift was partly inhibited in Na^+-free saline and turned into a small acidification when the K^+-induced depolarization was reduced by the application of Ba^{2+}, (Chesler and Kraig, 1989; Grichtchenko and Chesler, 1994). The stimulus-induced alkalinization of the leech giant glial cell was turned into an acidification by all experimental protocols suppressing the activation of the NBC: (1) by voltage-clamping the glial cell (Fig. 10.3A; Rose and Deitmer, 1994), (2) in the presence of the stilbene, DIDS and (3) in CO_2, HCO_3^--free saline (Rose and Deitmer, 1995a; Rose and Deitmer, 1995b). Suppressing the glial depolarization during nerve root stimulation not only reversed the intraglial pH change, but also introduced an alkaline pH_o transient, which preceded the extracellular acidification (Fig. 10.3B; Rose and Deitmer, 1994).

Glial cells have a variety of transmitter receptors coupled to ion channels (see Chapter 7). The activation of these transmitter receptors can induce pH transients in nervous systems, which either emerge directly in response to the action of neurotransmitters themselves by both HCO_3^--dependent and -independent mechanisms, or are secondary to membrane potential changes (Chesler and Kaila, 1992; Munsch and Deitmer, 1994). The majority of available data relates to pH changes induced by GABA and glutamate, while the effects of other transmitters on pH_o or pH_i in the nervous system have been investigated in only a few systems. It has become clear, however, that there may be complex interactions between transmitter effects on both glial cells and neurons and pH_o or pH_i changes, including not only the activation of ionotropic receptor-operated channels, but also transmitter carriers, which may contribute to acid/base fluxes (see below).

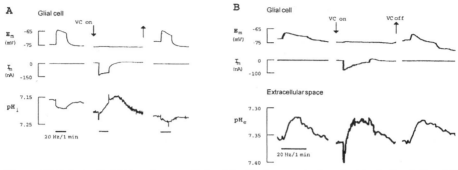

Figure 10.3. Intraglial (*A*) and extracellular (*B*) pH changes during electrical stimulation (20 Hz for 1 min) of a side nerve of an isolated leech ganglion, when the glial cell is held in current-clamp, or in voltage-clamp to suppress the membrane potential change. Note that the intracellular alkalinization is converted to an acidification (*A*), while an extracellular alkaline transient becomes apparent when voltage-clamping the glial cell (*B*). (From Rose and Deitmer, 1994).

Perturbations of pH can induce a variety of changes in cellular functions in nervous systems, from the activation or inhibition of ionic currents, to alterations in overall neuronal excitability, and to modulation of enzyme activities (Chesler 1990; Deitmer and Rose 1996). In glial cells in particular, pH shifts may be associated with acid/base secretion, lactate transport, cell volume changes, glutamate uptake and glutamine efflux, alteration in gap junctional communication and metabolic processes. Some of these pH-dependent processes are linked to, or might induce, a cascade of H^+-induced signals in nervous systems. For example, pH modulation of gap junctions might result in a pH-dependence of transmitter release through hemi-channels in the glial cell membrane, as suggested for ATP and glutamate (Cotrina et al., 2000; Yeh et al., 2003). pH-dependent Cl^- regulation in neurons and glial cells, and HCO_3^--permeable channels activated by GABA or glycine, may affect synaptic inhibition in nervous systems (Kaila, 1994).

10.5. Acid/base changes during metabolic shuttling

The products of the enzymatic processing of CO_2, protons and bicarbonate, might be employed to drive two cotransporters, which use bicarbonate and protons as co-substrates, the NBC and the monocarboxylate transporter (MCT), respectively (see Fig. 10.4). The MCT proteins belong to a family of transporters including multiple isoforms, which carry monocarboxylate anions, such as lactate, pyruvate, acetoacetate etc., in cotransport with a proton in an electroneutral manner across the cell membrane (Halestrap and Price, 1999). Their activity can result in the release of lactate or other monocarboxylates from astroglial cells into the extracellular spaces. The monocarboxylic acids are then taken up by neurons via the neuronal MCT isoforms and are consumed to generate ATP (Magistretti et al., 1999).

The lactate in astroglial cells is produced from glycolysis, whereby pyruvate, instead of being channeled into the tricarboxylic acid (TCA) cycle, is converted into lactate by lactate dehydrogenase (LDH) isoform 5 (Dringen et al., 1993; Bittar et al., 1996; Magistretti et al., 1999). From the 36 ATP derived from one glucose, two are retained by the glial cells during glycolysis, while 34 ATP can be transferred to neurons in the form of lactate. The release of lactate from glial cells and the uptake of lactate into neurons, a process which is suggested by a number of studies (Walz and Mukieri, 1988; Dringen et al., 1993; Poitry-Yamate et al., 1995; Hu and Wilson, 1997; Schurr et al., 1997; Bouzier et al., 2000; Vega et al., 2003), but also be disputed (Chih et al., 2001), would enable a major transfer of energy from glial cells to neurons. The direction of this transfer is also favored by the different substrate affinities of the glial MCT-1 and the neuronal MCT-2, which are almost one order of magnitude apart (Bröer et al., 1997; Bröer et al., 1998; Halestrap and Price, 1999); glial MCT-1 has a K_m value for lactate of 3-5 mM, and neuronal MCT-2 has a K_m value for lactate of 0.5 mM.

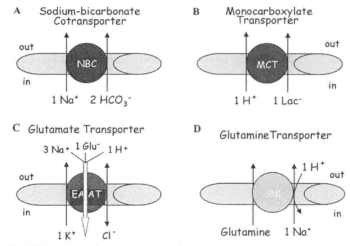

Figure 10.4. Stoichiometry of transport proteins reported to be functional in the cell membrane of glial cells, transporting acid/base equivalents. A. The sodium-bicarbonate cotransporter (NBC), which transports one sodium ion with two bicarbonate ions. This transporter is hence electrogenic and dependent on the membrane potential. It may function as an extruder of bicarbonate, which enhances the buffering capacity of the extracellular spaces. B. The monocarboxylate transporter (MCT), which mediates the cotransport of one monocarboxylate anion, such as lactate or pyruvate, with one proton. Different isoforms appear to exist in glial cells and neurons MCT1 and MCT2, respectively. C. The excitatory amino acid transporter (EAAT), which mediates high-affinity uptake of glutamate. In glial cells, primarily EAAT1 (GLAST) and EAAT2 (GLT-1) have been identified, while EAAT3-5 are found in neurons. According to its role to take up the excitatory neurotransmitter glutamate, these transporters are found in synaptic domains. Some EAATs can be associated with a chloride conductance, the significance of which is yet unclear. D. Amino acid transporter SN1 ("N system"), one of several transporter families mediating glutamine transport. Glutamine is released by glial cells and taken up by neurons as part of the glutamate/glutamine cycle.

The lactate taken up by neurons is converted to pyruvate, catalyzed by LDH-1. Pyruvate is then channeled into the TCA cycle and ultimately generates ATP and CO_2 by oxidative metabolism. Neurons need a sufficient level of ATP (Attwell and Laughlin, 2001), which they can derive from glucose as well as from lactate, to maintain their electrical and synaptic activity (Schurr et al., 1988, 1999; Izumi et al., 1997). During energy deprivation, added monocarboxylates have been shown to be neuroprotective in acute brain slices, isolated optic nerve and neuronal cultures (Izumi et al., 1997; Schurr et al., 1997; 2001; Maus et al., 1999; Wender et al., 2000; Cater et al., 2001).

In a hypothetical scenario (Fig. 10.5; see also Deitmer, 2002), when neurons are active, CO_2 leaves the neurons by diffusing through the cell membrane into the extracellular spaces, and from there into glial cells. Due to the high CA activity in astroglial cells, CO_2 is converted to protons and bicarbonate, and hence creates a persisting gradient of CO_2 into the glial cells. Subsequently, protons and bicarbonate are extruded from the glial cytoplasm, or are otherwise consumed. A high glial CA activity works toward establishing an equilibrium between CO_2, H^+ and HCO_3^-, thus enabling continuous diffusion of CO_2 into the glial cells. Intracellular HCO_3^- would activate the NBC in the glial membrane in the outward direction, sustained by the production of HCO_3^-. Together with HCO_3^-, Na^+ is extruded by the NBC against a steep gradient. This could subsequently activate NHE, which would then short-circuit the extrusion of Na^+ and HCO_3^- by the NBC. However, glial cell pH, due to the presence of NBC, is less dominated by NHE (Brune et al., 1994; Bevensee et al., 1997; Deitmer and Schneider, 1998). In addition, in most cell types activation of NHE requires an pH_i value lower than 7 and is significantly reduced at lower pH_o, as induced e.g. by neuronal activity (Deitmer and Rose, 1996; Putney et al., 2002).

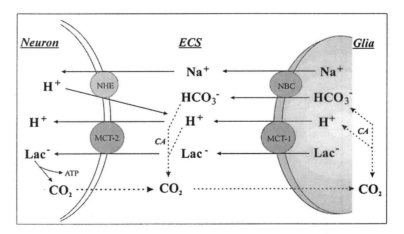

Figure 10.5. Cartoon illustrating some possibly related and functionally linked acid-base transporters across the cell membrane of a neuron (left) and a glial cell (right) in the brain. CO_2 diffusing into glial cells is converted into H^+ and HCO_3^- catalyzed by carbonic anhydrase (CA). Intraglial protons are used to drive lactate out of the glial cell via the monocarboxylate transporter (MCT-1), and intraglial bicarbonate activates the sodium-bicarbonate cotransport (NBC). Lactate is taken up by the neuron via MCT-2 in a cotransport with a proton, which is extruded from the neuron via Na^+/H^+ exchange (NHE). In the neuron, lactate is metabolized

resulting in the generation of ATP and CO_2; the latter diffuses across the cell membrane out of the neuron into the neighboring glial cell. The possibility of CO_2 recycling is indicated by the formation of CO_2, catalyzed by CA in the extracellular space (ECS), and the subsequent diffusion of CO_2 back into the glial cell. High activity of CA would ensure rapid equilibration of CO_2, H^+ and HCO_3^-, and hence the continuous flow of CO_2 into glial cells. This would result in net secretion of sodium and lactate from glial cells (after Deitmer, 2002).

The extrusion of HCO_3^- may counteract extracellular acidosis (as e.g. induced by lactate secretion or NHE activity), and enhances the extracellular buffering capacity (Thomas et al., 1991). The HCO_3^- may also be converted during the consumption of protons to CO_2 by *extracellular* CA activity, thus recycling CO_2, which would then again diffuse into the glial cells (Fig. 10.5, dotted lines). This process is not expected to promote significant CO_2 re-diffusion back into the glial cells, however, since a major part of the CA activity in the brain has been located in the glial compartment (Cammer, 1984; Sapirstein et al., 1984). There is also evidence for extracellular (interstitial) location of CA activity (Deitmer, 1992; Tong et al., 2000), which enhances lactate transport across cell membranes of glial cells and neurons (Svichar and Chesler, 2003).

The Na^+ extrusion via the NBC, which can be stimulated by lowering pH_o (Deitmer, 1991), would relieve some of the load resting on the glial Na/K-ATPase, which has to cope with a potentially large Na^+ influx associated with various sodium-driven processes in glial cells, particularly the high-affinity glutamate uptake. However, a direct link between the NBC and the Na/K-ATPase in the manner suggested here has not yet been shown. The bicarbonate-driven sodium efflux might save energy, which glial cells can either deliver to neurons, or use themselves to prevent the dissipation of the sodium gradient, which in turn may lead to a calcium overload (Attwell and McLaughlin, 2001), and, possibly, to apoptosis (Choi, 1992).

10.6. Protons are also associated with glutamate and glutamine transport

Glutamate uptake via the excitatory amino acid transporters (EAATs), which is mainly fuelled by the inwardly directed Na^+ gradient, also transport H^+ into the cell (Anderson and Swanson, 2000; Danbolt, 2001; see Chapter 9). Thus, during increased activity of excitatory neurons releasing glutamate, glial EAAT1 and EAAT2, corresponding to GLAST and GLT-1, respectively, are activated and acidify the cytosol during the uptake of this neurotransmitter (Amato et al., 1994; Deitmer and Schneider, 1998). The glutamate is either metabolized, or, more commonly, converted to glutamine by the ATP-consuming glutamine synthetase, and as such recycled via the glutamate-glutamine shuttle (Hertz et al., 1999).

Glutamine, which is not a neurotransmitter, can be transported out of the glial cells and taken up by neurons, where it is converted back to glutamate by aminase activity (Fig. 10.4). Both astrocytes and neurons exhibit a variety of neutral amino acid transporters that transport glutamine and other amino acids (Bröer and Brookes, 2001). One of the systems related to glutamine transport in astrocytes is the system N transport (SN1), which cotransports one glutamine with one Na^+ in exchange for one H^+ in an electroneutral transfer (Chaudhry et al., 1999). In addition, a H^+ conductance has been suggested for the SN1-mediated glutamine transport, which is not stoichiometrically coupled to the amino acid transport (Chaudhry et al., 2001). Due to the steep gradient of glutamine, this transport system can mediate both influx and efflux of glutamine. We could recently identify the SN1 system as one of the major pathways for glutamine efflux from cultured rat astrocytes (Deitmer et al., 2003). The other glutamine transporters used by glial cells and neurons, such as L (a Na^+-independent pathway preferring bulky and branched-chain substrates typified by leucine, hence 'L') and A (a Na^+-dependent pathway preferring short-chain substrates typified by alanine, hence 'A') transport systems, however, are not associated with the transport of acid or base, although they may exhibit some pH sensitivity (Bröer and Brookes, 2001).

10.7. Functional interactions

Neuronal firing of action potentials induces the release of neurotransmitter(s) and K^+ into the extracellular spaces. There is evidence that neuronal activity can also lead to a considerable rise in the brain lactic acid level (Fox et al., 1988; Fray et al., 1996). Due to the consumption of metabolic energy, which neurons primarily employ to maintain their own ionic gradients, neurons take up lactate via the neuronal MCT-2 and release CO_2. This, in turn, might lead, directly or indirectly, to the activation of the following processes in glial cells (Fig. 10.6; Deitmer 2000): The neurotransmitter glutamate activates metabotropic receptors in the glial membrane, leading to an intraglial calcium transient induced by inositol-1,4,5-trisphosphate-mediated calcium release from intracellular organelles, which can increase the membrane K^+ permeability. Glutamate is also taken up by the glial cell, leading to an increased glucose uptake and glycolysis (presumably stimulated by enhanced ATP consumption). Glutamate is converted to glutamine, which is exported via neutral amino acid transporters, such as SN1. Lactate, as the product of glycolysis, is secreted via the MCT-1 and taken up by neurons via MCT-2. CO_2 is rapidly processed with the aid of carbonic anhydrases (CA), stimulating HCO_3^- secretion via the NBC (Fig 10.4).

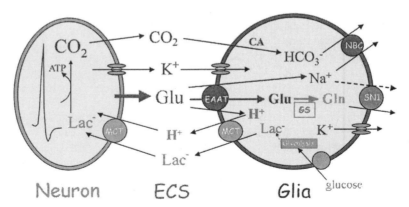

Figure 10.6. Summary of neuron-glia interactions. An active neuron (left), which fires action potentials and releases glutamate and potassium, has an increased energy consumption, which leads to lactate uptake via neuronal MCT, and eventually CO_2 release. The glial cell (right) is activated and responds in a multiple fashion: Glutamate activates metabotropic receptors (1),

which leads to calcium signalling (2), and, in turn, increases the potassium permeability (3). Glutamate is also taken up by the glial cell via the EAAT (4). Uptake of glucose (5), which is fed into glycolysis, leads to the formation of lactate, which is secreted in a co-transport with protons via the glial MCT (6), and subsequently taken up into neurons via the neuronal MCT (6). CO_2 is processed (7), catalyzed by carbonic anhydrases (CA), and the bicarbonate is secreted in cotransport with sodium via the NBC (8) (modified from Deitmer, 2000).

This list of coupled glial functions with direct or indirect involvement of acid/base-coupled transports is likely to be incomplete, as the glutamate uptake and the Na^+-HCO_3^- cotransport could be extended by a number of additional neurotransmitter and ion transporters, respectively, but it demonstrates that linking these processes may effectively enhance the transport of metabolites under energy-saving conditions. The essential features of this scenario are that net glutamate uptake into, and net lactate secretion from, glial cells, occur *co-operatively* under conditions of CO_2 processing and are supported by a high NBC activity. The Na/K-ATPase could afford to operate at moderate background rates, and most of the metabolic energy derived from the glucose that is taken up, could be transferred in the form of lactate to energy-demanding neurons (Tsacopoulos and Magistretti, 1996; Magistretti et al., 1999; Deitmer, 2000).

10.8. Conclusions

For nearly all events related to pH changes in nervous tissue, the presence of CO_2 and HCO_3^- has a great impact on neuronal functions. HCO_3^- determines the buffering capacity to a large extent; the presence of the CO_2/ HCO_3^- enables HCO_3^- flux through $GABA_A$ receptor channels and thereby modifies the inhibitory synaptic potentials, and stimulates the powerful glial electrogenic Na^+- HCO_3^- cotransporter and other carriers such as Na^+-dependent and Na^+-independent Cl^-/ HCO_3^- exchange. CO_2, as a gas that easily permeates membranes, rapidly dissipates from any location where it is formed through cells and tissues, and together with a high enzyme activity of carbonic anhydrase provides an effective and high buffer capacity even at relatively low concentrations. Considering H^+ transients as signals, CO_2, HCO_3^- and carbonic anhydrase are essential elements in this signaling, determining the shape of the pH shifts in time and space within nervous systems. Glial cells appear to play a particularly significant role in most of these processes.

Acknowledgements. Some of the own studies discussed in this article have been supported by grants from the Deutsche Forschungsgemeinschaft.

10.9. References

Amato A, Ballerini L, Attwell D (1994) Intracellular pH changes produce by glutamate uptake in rat hippocampal slices. J Neurophysiol 72:1686-1696.

Anderson CM, Swanson RA (2000) Astrocyte glutamate transport: Review of properties, regulation, and physiological functions. Glia 32:1-14.

Attwell D, Laughlin SB (2001) An energy budget for signaling in the grey matter of the brain. J Cereb Blood Flow Metab 21:11-33.

Becker, H., Bröer, S. & Deitmer, J.W. (2004) Facilitated lactate transport by MCT1 when co-expressed with the sodium-bicarbonate cotransporter (NBC) in Xenopus oocytes. Biophys. J. 86, 235-247.

Bevensee MO, Apkon M, Boron WF (1997) Intracellular pH regulation in cultured astrocytes from rat hippocampus. II. Electrogenic Na/HCO3 cotransport. J Gen Physiol 110:467-483.

Bianchi L, Driscoll M (2002) Protons at the gate: DEG/EnaC ion channels help us feel and remember. Neuron 34:337-340.

Bittar PG, Charnay Y, Pellerin L, Bouras C, Magistretti PJ (1996) Selective distribution of lactate dehydrogenase isoenzymes in neurons and astrocytes of human brain. J Cereb Blood Flow Metab 16:1079-1089.

Bröer S, Brookes N (2001) Transfer of glutamine between astrocytes and neurons. J Neurochem 77:705-19.

Bröer S, Rahman B, Pellegri G, Pellerin L, Martin JL, Verleysdonk S, Hamprecht B, Magistretti PJ (1997) Comparison of lactate transport in astroglial cells and monocarboxylate transporter 1 (MCT 1) expressing Xenopus laevis oocytes. Expression of two different monocarboxylate transporters in astroglia cell and neurons. J Biol Chem 272:30096–30102.

Bröer S, Schneider HP, Bröer A, Rahman B, Hamprecht B, Deitmer JW (1998) Characterization of the monocarboxylate transporter 1 expressed in Xenopus laevis oocytes by changes in cytosolic pH. Biochem J 333:167-174.

Brune T, Fetzer S, Backus K., Deitmer JW (1994) Evidence for electrogenic sodium-bicarbonate cotransport in cultured rat cerebellar astrocytes. Pflügers Arch 429:64-71.

Bouzier A., Thiaudiere E, Biran M, Rouland R, Canioni P, Merle M (2000) The metabolism of [3-(13)C]lactate in the rat brain is specific of a pyruvate carboxylase-deprived compartment. J Neurochem 75:480-486.

Cammer W (1984) Carbonic anhydrase in oligodendrocytes and myelin in the central nervous system. Ann NY Acad Sci 429:494-497.

Cater HL, Benham CD, Sundstrom LE (2001) Neuroprotective role of monocarboxylate transport during glucose deprivation in slice cultures of rat hippocampus. J Physiol 531.2:459-66.

Chaudhry FA, Reimer RJ, Krizaj D, Barber D, Storm-Mathiesen J, Copenhagen DR, Edwards RH (1999) Molecular analysis of System N suggests novel physiological roles in nitrogen metabolism and synaptic transmission. Cell 99:769-780.

Chaudhry FA, Krizaj D, Larsson P, Reimer RJ, Wreden C, Storm-Mathisen J, Copenhagen D, Kavanaugh M, Edwards R (2001) Coupled and uncoupled proton movement by amino acid transport system N. EMBO J 20:7041-7051.

Chesler M, Kraig RP (1989) Intracellular pH transients of mammalian astrocytes. J Neurosci 9:2011-2019.

Chesler M (1990) The regulation and modulation of pH in the nervous system. Progr Ncurobiol 34:401-427.

Chesler M, Kaila K (1992) Modulation of pH neunronal activity. Trends Neurosci 15:396-402.

Chih CP, Lipton P, Roberts EL Jr (2001) Do active cerebral neurons really use lactate rather than glucose? Trends Neurosci 24:573-578.

Choi DW (1992) Excitotoxin cell death. J Neurobiol 23:1261-1276.

Cotrina ML, Lin JH, Lopez-Garcia JC, Naus CC, Nedergaard M (2000). ATP-mediated glia signaling. J Neurosci 20:2835-44.

Deitmer JW (1991) Electrogenic sodium-dependent bicarbonate secretion by glial cells of the leech central nervous system. J Gen Physiol 98:637-655.

Deitmer JW (1992a) Bicarbonate-dependent changes of intracellular sodium and pH in identified leech glial cells. Plügers Arch 420:584-589.

Deitmer JW (1992b) Evidence for glial control of extracellular pH in the leech central nervous system. Glia 5:43-47.

Deitmer JW (2000) Glial strategy for metabolic shuttling and neuronal function. BioEssays 22:747-752.

Deitmer JW, Szatkowski M (1990) Membrane potential dependence of intracellular pH regulation by identified glial cells in the leech central nervous system. J Physiol 421:617-631.

Deitmer JW, Schlue WR (1989) An inwardly directed electrogenic sodium-bicarbonate cotransport in leech glial cells. J Physiol (Lond) 411:179-194.

Deitmer JW, Schneider HP (1995) Voltage-dependent clamp of intracellular pH of identified leech glial cells. J Physiol (Lond) 485:157-166.

Deitmer JW, Schneider H-P (1998) Acid-base transport across the leech giant glial cell membrane at low external bicarbonate concentrations. J Physiol 512.2:459-469.

Deitmer JW, Rose CR (1996) pH regulation and proton signalling by glial cells. Progr Neurobiol 48:73-103.

Deitmer JW, Schneider HP (2000) Enhancement of glutamate uptake transport by CO2/bicarbonate in the leech giant glial cell. Glia 30:392-400.

Deitmer, J.W., Bröer, A. & Bröer, S. (2003) Glutamine efflux from astrocytes is mediated by multiple pathways. J. Neurochem. 87, 127-135.

DeVries SH (2001) Exocytosed protons feedback to suppress the Ca2+ current in mammalina cone photoreceptors. Neuron 32:1107-1117.

Dringen R, Gebhardt R, Hamprecht B (1993) Glycogen in astrocytes: possible function as lactate supply for neighboring cells. Brain Res 623:208-214.

Fox PT, Raichle ME, Mintun MA, Dence C (1988) Nonoxidative glucose consumption during focal physiologic neural activity. Science 241:462-464.

Fray AE, Boutelle M, Fillenz M (1996) The mechanisms controlling physiologically stimulated changes in rat brain glucose and lactate: a microdialysis study. J Physiol (Lond) 496:49-57.

Giffard RG, Papadopoulous MC, van Hooft AC, Xu L, Giuffrida R, Monyer H (2000) The electrogenic sodium bicarbonate cotransporter: developmental expression in rat brain and possible role in acid vulnerability. J Neurosci 20:1001-1008.

Grichtenko JJ, Chesler M (1994) Depolarization-induced alkalinization of astrocytes in gliotic hippocampal slices. Neuroscience 62:1071-1078.

Halestrap AP, Price NT (1999) The proton-linked monocarboxylate transporter (MCT) family: structure, function and regulation. Biochem J 343:281-299.

Harris C, Fliegel L (1999) Amiloride and the Na^+/H^+ exchanger protein: mechanism and significance of inhibition of the Na^+/H^+ exchanger. Int J Mol Med 3:315-321.

Hertz L, Dringen R, Schousboe A, Robinson SR (1999) Astrocytes: Glutamate producers for neurons. J Neurosci Res 57:417-428.

Heyer M, Müller-Berger S, Romero MF, Boron WF, Frömter E (1999) Stoichiometry of the rat kidney Na+-HCO3-cotransporter expressed in Xenopus laevis oocytes. Eur J Physiol 438:322-329.

Hu Y, Wilson GS (1997) A temporary local energy pool coupled to neuronal activity: fluctuations of extracellular lactate levels in rat brain monitored with rapid-response enzyme-based sensor. J Neurochem 69:1484-1490.

Izumi Y, Benz AM, Katsuki H, Zorumski CF (1997) Endogenous monocarboxylates sustain hippocampal synaptic function and morphological integritiy during energy deprivation. J Neurosci 17:9448-9457.

Magistretti PJ, Pellerin L, Rothman DL, Shulman RG (1999) Energy on demand. Science 283:496-497.

Maus M, Marin P, Israel M, Glowinski J, Premont J (1999) Pyruvate and lactate protect striatal neurons against N-methl-D-aspartate-induced neurotoxcity. Eur J Neurosi 11:3215-3224.

Miesenbock G, De Angelis DA, Rothman JE (1998) Visualizing secretion and synaptic transmission with pH-sensitive green fluorescent proteins. Nature 394:192-195.

Munsch T, Deitmer JW (1994) Sodium-bicarbonate cotransport current in dentified leech glial cells. J Physiol 474:43-55.

Newman EA (1991) Sodium-bicarbonate cotransport in retinal Müller (glial) cells of the salamander. J Neurosci 11:3972-3983.

Pappas CA, Ransom,B (1994) Depolarization-induced alkalinization (DIA) in rat hippocampal astrocytes. J Neurophysiol 72:2816-2826.

Poitry-Yamate CL, Poitry S, Tsacopoulos M (1995) Lactate released by Müller glial cells is metabolized by photoreceptors from mammalia retina. J Neurosci 15:5179-5191.

Putney LK, Denker SP, Barber DL (2002) The changing face of the Na^+/H^+ exchanger, NHE1: structure, regulation, and cellular actions. Annu Rev Pharmacol Toxicol 42:527-52. Review.

Romero MF, Hediger MA, Boulpaep EL, Boron WF (1997) Expression cloning and characterization of a renal electrogenic Na^+/HCO_3^- cotransporter. Nature 387:409-413.

Rose CR, Deitmer JW (1994) Evidence that glial cells modulate extracellular pH transients induced by neuronal activity in the leech central nervous system. J Physiol 481.1:1-5.

Rose CR, Deitmer JW (1995a) Stimulus-evoked changes of extra- and intracellular pH in the leech central nervous system. I. Bicarbonate dependence. J Neurophysiol 73:125-131.

Rose CR, Deitmer JW (1995b) Stimulus-evoked changes of extra- and intracellular pH in the leech central nervous system. II. Mechanisms and maintenance of pH homeostasis. J Neurophysiol 73:132-140.

Rose CR, Ransom B (1996) Intracellular sodium homeostasis in rat hippocampal astrocytes. J Physiol (Lond) 491:573-587.

Sapirstein VS, Strocchi P, Gilbert JM (1984) Properties and function of brain carbonic anhydrase. Ann NY Acad Sci 429:481-493.

Schmitt BM, Berger UV, Douglas RM, Bevensee MO, Hediger MA, Haddad GG, Boron WF (2000) Na/HCO3 cotransporters in rat brain: expression in glia, neurons and choroid plexus. J Neurosci 20:6839-6848.

Schurr A, West CA, Rigor BM (1988) Lactate-supported synaptic function in the rat hippocampal slice preparation. Science 240:1326-1328.

Schurr A, Payne RS, Miller JJ, Rigor BM (1997) Brain lactate is an obligatory aerobic energy substrate for functional recovery after hypoxia: further in vitro validation. J Neurochem 69:423-426.

Schurr A , Miller JJ, Payn RS, Rigor BM (1999) An increase in lactate output by brain tissue serves to meet the energy needs of glutamate-activated neurons. J Neurosci 19, 34-39.

Schurr A,. Payne RS, Miller JJ, Tseng MT, Rigor BM (2001). Blockade of lactate transport exacerbated delayed neuronal damage in a rat model of cerebral ischemia. Brain Res 895:268-272.

Svichar N, Chesler M (2003) Surface carbonic anhydrase activity on astrocytes and neurons facilitate lactate transport. Glia 41:415-419.

Tsacopoulos M, Magistretti PJ (1996) Metabolic coupling between glia and neurons. J Neurosci 16: 877-885.

Thomas RC, Coles JA, Deitmer JW (1991) Homeostatic muffling. Nature 350:564.

Tong CK, Brion LP, Suarez C, Chesler M (2000). Interstitial carbonic anhydrase (CA) activity in brain is attributable to membrane-bound CA type IV. J Neurosci 20:8247-8253.

Traynelis SF, Cull-Candy SG (1990) Proton inhibition of N-methyl-D-aspartate receptors in cerebellar neurons. Nature 345:347-50.

Vega C, Martiel JL, Drouhault D, Burckhart MF, Coles JA (2003) Uptake of locally applied deoxyglucose, glucose and lactate by axons and Schwann cells of rat vagus nerve. J. Physiol 546:551-564.

Walz W, Mukerji S (1988) Lactate production and release in cultured astrocytes. Neurosci Lett 86:296.300.

Wemmie JA, Chen J, Askwith CC, Hruska-Hagermann AM, Price MP, Nolan BC, Yoder PG, Lamani E, Hoshi T, Freeman JH, Welsh MJ (2002) The Acid-Activated Ion Channel ASIC Contributes to Synaptic Plasticity, Leaning and Memory. Neuron 34:463-477.

Wender R, Brown AM, Fern R, Swanson RA, Farrell K, Ranson BR (2000) Astrocytic glycogen influences axon function and survival during glucose deprivation in central white matter. J Neurosci 15:6804-6810.

Ye ZC, Wyeth MS, Baltan-Tekkok S, Ransom BR (2003) Functional hemichannels in astrocytes: a novel mechanism of glutamate release. J Neurosci 23:3588-96.

10.10. Abbreviations

AE	Anion exchanger
ASICs	Acid-sensing ion channels
DIDS	4,4'-diisothiocyanatostilbene-2,2'-disulfonic acid
DNDS	Dinitrostilbene-disulfonic acid
EAATs	Excitatory amino acid transporters
CA	Carbonic anhydrase
GABA	γ-aminobutyric acid
LDH	Lactate deydrogenase
MCT	Monocarboxylate transporter
NBC	Sodium-bicarbonate cotransporter
pH_i	Intracellular pH
pH_o	Extracellular pH
SITS	4-acetamino-4'-isothiocyanato-stilbene-2,2'-disulfonic acid
SN1	System N transport
$[X^{\pm}]_i$	Intracellular concentration of ion X
$[X^{\pm}]_o$	Extracellular concentration of ion X

Chapter 11

Glial-neuronal interactions and brain energy metabolism

Angus M. Brown[1], Selva Baltan Tekkök[2] and Bruce R. Ransom[2]*

[1] MRC Applied Neuroscience Group, Biomedical Sciences, University of Nottingham
Queens Medical Center, Nottingham, UK, and
[2] Department of Neurology, University of Washington, 1959 Pacific St. NE
Seattle, WA 98195 USA

*Corresponding author: bransom@u.washington.edu

Contents

11. 1. Introduction

Golgi, more than a century ago, suggested that glial cells provide nutritive support for neurons. He based this on his microscopic observations that glial cells are positioned between blood vessels and neurons, and their endfeet intimately surround blood vessels (Andriezen, 1893; Cajal, 1995). The anatomic arrangement of astrocytes, neurons and capillaries suggested that nutrients might be taken up preferentially by astrocytes. Astrocytes would then 'share' these nutrients with nearby neurons (Figure 11.1A). This old idea gained a degree of modern plausibility as more was learned about brain energy metabolism, and it was discovered that astrocytes are the only cells in the mammalian brain that contain significant glycogen (Cataldo and Broadwell, 1986a), the storage form of glucose. These refinements in the evolution of the nutritive hypothesis are shown in Figure 11.1B. The transfer of energy substrate (e.g. glucose or monocarboxylates) occurs across brain extracellular space (ECS), which is so narrow that molecules released from one cell diffuse almost instantly to adjacent cells (Nicholson, 1995). A crucial permissive feature of this scheme is that nearly every neuron in the brain shares common ECS with adjacent astrocytes.

Several aspects of this hypothesis are appealing. For one thing, it makes sense of a special design feature in the brain, namely the close and nearly universal apposition of glial endfeet to nutritive capillaries (Figure 11.2) (Nedergaard et al., 2003; Simard et al., 2003). It also suggests a mechanism whereby astrocyte glycogen, the sole energy store in brain, could be shared with neurons. Despite the appeal of this scheme, however, early experiments were not supportive (e.g. (Wolfe and Nicholls, 1967)). In their brilliant review of glial cells published 30 years ago, Kuffler and Nichols (Kuffler and Nicholls, 1966) summed up the situation as follows: "...*in our opinion, no convincing demonstration has yet been made to show that substances are, in fact, exchanged between neurons and glia across the narrow intercellular clefts. Such an observation is a prerequisite for the theory that certain glial cells serve either as storage sites for the benefit of neurons or as distributing channels*". Recent studies have resurrected this theory and provided 'proof of principle' that glial cells can provide fuel to neurons. The role of glycogen in this glial-neuronal interaction has also been partially clarified. Here we review the evidence supporting the idea that glial cells provide energy substrate to neurons. We also point out areas of continued uncertainty.

11.2. Brain metabolism

It is widely accepted that the human brain has minimal amounts of endogenous energy reserves (Stryer, 1995; Frier and Fisher, 1999; Garrett and Grisham, 1999) and uses only glucose as an energy substrate (Clarke and Sokoloff, 1999; Chih and Roberts Jr., 2003). It should be noted, however, that under special conditions (such as starvation, diabetes, breast-feeding in neonates, and experimental intervention) other metabolic substrates can successfully substitute for glucose as sources of energy to sustain brain function (Clarke and Sokoloff, 1999). For example, carefully controlled studies have shown that IV infusion of mannose can act as a suitable substitute for glucose (Sloviter and Kamimoto, 1970). This may not be too surprising as mannose is an epimer of glucose (Champe and Harvey, 1994), but galactose, the other epimer of glucose is ineffective as an energy substrate, even in tissue culture conditions (Wiesinger et al., 1997). *In vitro* studies, where vascular supply is irrelevant and nutrition is provided by diffusion from a bath, confirm that both gray and white matter operate normally if lactate (or a number of other select substrates) is substituted for glucose (Schurr et al., 1988; Brown et al., 2001). Interestingly, studies on neurons using radio-labeled lactate have shown that even in the presence of glucose, the majority of the CO_2 produced is radio-labeled implying that the carbon source was lactate (Larrabee, 1983; Poitry-Yamate et al., 1995; Larrabee, 1996; Bouzier-Sore et al., 2003). The ability to use substrates other than glucose for energy metabolism is a feature of all the main cells in the central nervous system (CNS), including oligodendrocytes (Sanchez-Abarca et al., 2001). This is a crucial point. It is the selective admission by the blood-brain-barrier of glucose over other substrates, not the incapacity of the brain to use other substrates, which limits the brain's diet to glucose under normal conditions. These facts, of course, leave unanswered the fate of glucose once it crosses cerebral capillaries. It could, of course, be preferentially taken up by one cell type and metabolized to another form for consumption by another cell type. In the absence of concrete information on this point, it has been generally assumed that glia and neurons dine exclusively on glucose (Chih and Roberts Jr., 2003).

Such is the human brain's requirement for energy substrate (glucose) and oxygen by which to optimally metabolize it, that at rest the brain accounts for about 50% and 20% of whole body glucose and oxygen consumption, respectively (Clarke and Sokoloff, 1999). As the human brain comprises only about 2% of body weight this implies a high basal metabolic rate, and indeed only kidney cortex and heart muscle have higher metabolic rates (Ganong, 1989). To ensure a constant, continuous supply of glucose to the brain, complex hormonal homeostatic mechanisms have evolved to maintain blood glucose at a constant level (~ 4 - 7 mM) (Garrett and Grisham, 1999). In young adult brain, average values for glucose consumption, O_2 consumption and cerebral blood flow are 5.5 mg/100g/min, 3.5ml/100g/min and 57 ml/100g/min, respectively (Clarke and Sokoloff, 1999). The brain extracts about 50% of the oxygen and 10% of the glucose from arterial blood. The fate of any extracted glucose that is surplus to these requirements is unknown. It is probably distributed in part as lactate, pyruvate and various other metabolic intermediates between glucose and its ultimate products, CO_2 and H_2O, none of which are released from brain into the blood in sufficient amounts to be detectable as significant arteriovenous differences (Sokoloff, 1992). This suggests that the brain does not have the capacity to store excess glucose efficiently (see below), further reinforcing the concept that the brain requires a continuous, uninterrupted supply of glucose, and is at the mercy of the systemic circulation to deliver adequate glucose.

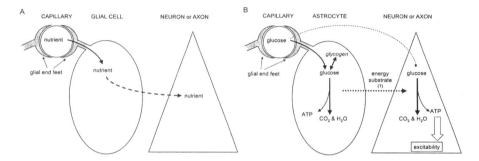

Figure 11.1. Schematic diagrams of how glial cells and neurons might interact with one and other in terms of energy metabolism. A) Golgi proposed that glia feed neurons. For anatomic reasons, nutrient was suspected of entering glia first and then being transported to neurons. B) More contemporary version of this theory of glial-neuronal interaction. Astrocytes enwrap capillaries with their endfeet. In the brain, only astrocytes contain glycogen, the storage form of glucose. Glucose could diffuse between astrocyte endfeet and make its way directly to neurons (dashed line). Alternatively, glucose might preferentially enter astrocytes and be shuttled to neurons as glucose or as some other form of energy substrate after conversion.

Mechanisms have evolved that store excess glucose in the periphery in times of plenty and release the stored glucose into the blood in times of famine to maintain normal blood glucose levels (i.e. euglycemia or normoglycemia) (Stryer, 1995). Even under conditions of prolonged starvation where liver glycogen is depleted, fat and protein are metabolized to glucose and ketone bodies to ensure that the brain receives a constant supply of utilizable energy substrate (Stryer, 1995). The devastating consequences of stroke are surely irrefutable evidence of the unforgiving nature of brain tissue when deprived, however temporarily, of its blood supply.

In tissue culture studies astrocytes have a higher rate of glucose utilization than neurons (22.3 vs. 6.3 nmol/mg protein/min) (Sokoloff et al., 1977). Given that the ratio of neuron:astrocyte volume is probably close to 1:1, these data suggest that the majority of brain glucose utilization occurs in astrocytes, not neurons. Once inside the astrocyte, a substantial portion of the glucose is metabolized to lactate in a series of eleven enzymatically-controlled steps, the Embden Meyerhoff pathway or glycolysis. Some glucose is aerobically metabolized to CO_2 and H_2O but adult astrocytes are capable of prolonged function under entirely anaerobic conditions (Goldberg and Choi, 1993; Ransom and Fern, 1996; Rose et al., 1998). In fact, even under aerobic conditions, astrocytes process a significant amount of glucose in an anaerobic fashion (Ransom and Fern, 1996), which is to say they release large amounts of lactate (Walz and Mukerji, 1988). Astrocytes, but not neurons, release more lactate in the presence of higher extracellular glucose or K^+ concentrations (Walz and Mukerji, 1988).

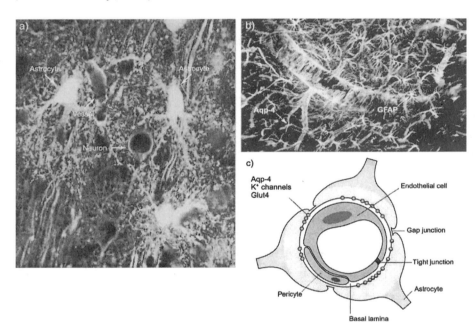

Figure 11.2. Astrocytes, neurons and blood vessels have complex spatial and functional relationships. A) Spatial organization of astrocytes, neurons and vessels in rat cortex. Astrocytes, expressing green fluorescent protein (yellow), extend into the neuropil a dense thicket of fine processes that intimately surround neurons (stained for microtubule-associated protein 2 (blue). A small vessel is outlined by astrocyte endfeet. B) Astrocytes strongly express the water channel protein aquaporin (aqp-4; red). Immunohistochemistry for GFAP (white) does not stain the endfeet as uniformly as does staining for aquaporin. C) Functional anatomy of the gliovascular interface. Many channels and transporters are clustered in the membranes of astrocyte endfeet that abut brain capillaries.

The initial step in glucose metabolism is phosphorylation by the enzyme hexokinase, which has a low K_m (0.1 mM) and V_{max}, making it a high affinity, low capacity enzyme (Champe and Harvey, 1994). Thus, at the concentrations of glucose under normal conditions, phosphorylation of glucose is a rate-limiting step in the formation of lactate (Champe and Harvey, 1994). Astrocytes do not possess glucokinase, the liver enzyme, which has a much higher K_m and V_{max} than hexokinase, allowing glucokinase to deal rapidly with large deliveries of intracellular glucose. Hexokinase phosphorylates glucose to glucose-6-phosphate (G-6-P), which can be metabolized in three separate reactions, namely glycolysis in which pyruvate or lactate is formed, glycogen synthesis in which excess G-6-P is converted to the carbohydrate storage macromolecule glycogen, or the pentose phosphate pathway which creates NADPH essential for glycolysis. In order for glucose to be released from cells, G-6-P must be dephosphorylated by glucose-6-phosphatase. Although this enzyme may be present in astrocytes, it has very low or negligible activity (Magistretti, 1997; Gotoh et al., 2000), and it is widely accepted that astrocytes do not release glucose (Dringen et al., 1993, but see Forsyth et al., 1996). As mentioned above, astrocytes do release other metabolic substrates, especially lactate (Walz and Mukerji, 1988; Dringen et al., 1993; Magistretti et al., 1993a), but also pyruvate, α-ketoglutarate, citrate and malate at lower concentrations. Therefore, although astrocytes and hepatocytes both contain glycogen, astrocytes are not 'brain hepatocytes'; rather than exporting glucose, as is the case with hepatocytes, astrocytes export significant amounts of lactate and are thus more analogous to skeletal muscle cells. While it is well established that astrocytes *in vitro* release large amount of lactate, this cannot be easily confirmed *in vivo*. A second point of contention is the question of what happens to the lactate that astrocytes release.

11.3. Glucose entry into brain

We have described the need by the brain for blood-borne glucose, but how does glucose gain access to brain tissue? Brain capillaries are the starting place for this discussion. Astrocytic endfeet almost totally encircle nutritive capillaries (see Figure 11.2), a unique anatomic arrangement not seen elsewhere in the body. This is not fully appreciated when astrocytes are stained for glial fibrillary acidic protein (GFAP), the standard astrocyte marker. As shown in Figure 11.2A, astrocyte endfeet are more reliably demonstrated using an antibody for the water channel protein, aquaporin4 (Nedergaard et al., 2003; Simard et al., 2003). The endfeet form a cellular barrier encountered by glucose leaving capillaries, but this is not an impermeant barrier; the endfeet are not 'zippered' shut against paracellular diffusion by tight junctions, as are the capillary endothelial cells. While peri-capillary astrocyte endfeet are likely to serve more than one purpose in the brain, including water regulation (del Zoppo and Hallenbeck, 2000), blood flow control (Anderson and Nedergaard, 2003; Zonta et al., 2003), and modulation of the blood-brain-barrier (del Zoppo and Hallenbeck, 2000) (Figure 11.2), they are undeniably well-suited for capturing glucose. Consistent with such a role, astrocyte endfeet express glucose transporter 1 (glut 1), the same transporter expressed by endothelial cells (Vannucci et al., 1997). In contrast to astrocytes, neurons make no direct contact with capillaries. These anatomical arrangements suggest, but certainly do not prove, that uptake into astrocytes is the preferred mode of glucose entry into the brain (i.e. Figure 11.1B). In fact, as it relates to mammalian brains, this idea remains very controversial (Chih and Roberts Jr., 2003; Pellerin and Magistretti, 2003b).

If astrocytes did take up the majority of glucose, how would energy substrate be delivered to neurons (and presumably to other brain cells, as well)? This question is discussed more thoroughly below, but one point is important to re-emphasize; astrocytes probably do not release glucose. When glucose enters astrocytes it is rapidly phosphorylated to G-6-P, trapping the glucose inside the cell. To exit the cell as glucose, phosphate must be cleaved from G-6-P by glucose-6-phosphatase, an enzyme that astrocytes appear to lack (Gotoh et al., 2000, but see Forsyth et al., 1996). Given that astrocytes are unlikely to release glucose themselves, the fact that low concentrations of glucose (~2.5 mM) can be measured in brain ECS implies that some glucose, at least, must diffuse around astrocyte endfeet into brain parenchyma (Silver and Erecinska, 1994; Hu and Wilson, 1997); it should be noted, however, that others have measured much lower levels of ECS glucose in awake animals (~0.5 mM) (Fellows and Boutelle, 1993; Lowry et al., 1998). Neurons express glucose transporter protein 3 (glut 3) and, therefore, can take up glucose directly from the brain ECS. Intense neural activity leads to increased glucose uptake (Hu and Wilson, 1997) and might cause rapid depletion of glucose in brain ECS. Unfortunately, currently available enzyme electrodes for measuring extracellular glucose concentration ($[glucose]_o$) are too large and too slow to provide an adequate level of resolution (Hu and Wilson, 1997). More data regarding the dynamics of brain $[glucose]_o$ are badly needed to help resolve questions about glucose utilization at rest and during hypoglycemia or intense stimulation.

Despite the intriguing spatial and physiological features of astrocyte endfeet, the predominating view at this time is that CNS neurons have access to glucose and take it up directly as their preferred energy substrate. This view is being actively challenged in two specific settings, namely during periods of heightened brain activity and when glucose is in short supply (see below). In the later case, at least, there is now clear evidence that astrocytes transfer energy substrate to neurons in the form of a monocarboxylate, probably lactate.

While it seems unlikely that all the glucose entering the brain is taken up by astrocytes, a modified form of this hypothesis remains plausible and can be stated as follows: astrocytes take up glucose in excess of their metabolic needs and redistribute this in the form of a useable energy substrate to neurons. This perspective is compatible with some glucose bypassing astrocytes to be directly taken up by neurons (and other brain cells). What is the role of astrocyte glycogen in this hypothesis? In general, it would serve as a readily accessible reserve of glucose residues for the astrocyte's own energy needs and/or for export to fuel-deficient neighbors.

11.4. Energy transfer from glial cells to neurons

The first solid evidence of glial transfer of energy substrate to neurons was obtained in studies on the honeybee drone retina. In this structure, the neural elements, the photoreceptors, contain mitochondria and produce energy mainly by oxidative phosphorylation (Tsacopoulos et al., 1994). They are surrounded by glial-like cells that are filled with glycogen, contain few if any mitochondria, and produce energy by glycolysis. Only the glial-like cells take up glucose and, consistent with this, they alone have significant hexokinase activity. Energy metabolism in the photoreceptors increases when they are activated by light and they signal nearby glial-like cells to increase their uptake of glucose; the nature of this signal has not been firmly established, but it may be NH_4^+ released by the photoreceptors (Tsacopoulos et al., 1997). What then do the photoreceptors use for fuel? Elegant biochemical experiments indicate that the photoreceptors take up and oxidize alanine released by the glial-like cells (Tsacopoulos et al., 1994). Alanine is taken up by a Na^+-dependent transporter and converted to pyruvate, which can enter the tricarboxylic acid cycle. Consistent with its role as the main energy supply for the photoreceptors, alanine is present in high concentration in the ECS (Cardinaud et al., 1994).

Experiments analogous to those described above in the honeybee retina have been carried out in the rabbit retina (Poitry-Yamate et al., 1995). The major difference is that mammalian retinal glial cells, Muller cells, produce lactate, not alanine, for export to the adjacent photoreceptors. It is important to recall that lactate is an excellent fuel for oxidative cells. It can be converted back to pyruvate and produces nearly as much ATP as glucose (1 glucose – 36 ATP, 2 lactate – 34 ATP). If given the choice, rabbit photoreceptors prefer lactate to glucose as a fuel. This preference for lactate over glucose as an energy substrate has also been confirmed for cultured rat forebrain neurons (Bouzier-Sore et al., 2003). Consistent with the idea that mammalian astrocytes might shuttle fuel to neurons (and other brain cells) as lactate is the 'odd' metabolic tendency of astrocytes to export large amounts of lactate to the extracellular space even under aerobic conditions (Walz and Mukerji, 1988; Abi-Saab et al., 2002).

The honeybee experiments revealed 'coupling' between neural activity and glial glucose uptake. Magistretti and colleagues pursued this question in rodents and have developed a model for activity-dependent metabolic coupling between astrocytes and neurons (Bouzier-Sore et al., 2002) (Figure 11.3). Astrocytes are the essential third element of glutamate synapses, in addition to the pre- and post-synaptic neurons. They remove about 95% of the glutamate that is released from the presynaptic terminal via glial-specific glutamate transporters (Anderson and Swanson, 2000). The energy drain of glutamate removal and subsequent metabolism, specifically, accumulation of intracellular Na^+ necessitating its active removal by Na^+-K^+ ATPase and conversion of glutamate to glutamine by ATP-requiring glutamine synthetase, lowers ATP and activates glycolysis and glucose uptake (Magistretti and Pellerin, 1999). The greater the neural activity, the greater is the Na^+ load and the downstream need for restorative glycolytic activity in astrocytes. This effectively 'couples' neuronal activity to glucose uptake (albeit in astrocytes), a well-known feature of normal brain metabolism. Experimental support for this hypothesis includes the fact that glutamate stimulates glycolysis in astrocytes and that blocking Na^+-K^+ ATPase with ouabain completely inhibits glutamate-induced glycolysis (Pellerin and Magistretti, 1994; Pellerin and Magistretti, 2003a). It is also supported by recent data in which knockout mice lacking either of the astrocyte-specific glutamate transporters, GLAST or GLT-1, exhibited decreased glucose uptake in response to increased synaptic activation (Voutsinos-Porche et al., 2003).

The Magistretti-Pellerin model also proposes that lactate released by astrocytes during heightened glycolysis is taken up by the neighboring neurons and oxidized. Indeed, this step has given the scheme its name: astrocyte-neuron lactate shuttle hypothesis or ANLSH. Ironically, it may be the weakest link in the hypothesis. The step involving transfer of lactate to nearby active neurons remains unproven and has attracted detailed criticism (Chih et al., 2001). Concerns raised include the following (Chih et al., 2001): 1) Why wouldn't neurons satisfy their energy needs by using more glucose? Neurons, like all brain cells, possess a glycolytic pathway that is tightly coupled to energy demand; low levels of ATP activate hexokinase and accelerate glycolysis. This control mechanism would allow active neurons to rapidly increase glucose uptake to meet their energy needs. 2) The pathway for increasing lactate import is via lactate dehydrogenase (LDH), and increased energy demand does not activate this enzyme. 3) If glucose were available in the ECS, it would essentially compete with lactate for access to the energy metabolism pathways for kinetic and thermodynamic reasons (see (Chih et al., 2001) for details). In a rebuttal statement, the authors of the ANLSH emphasize that this idea remains an hypothesis (Pellerin and Magistretti, 2003b). They point to accumulating experimental work that is consistent with the theory, without conclusively proving it. Moreover, there is now 'proof of principle' in the extreme circumstance of hypoglycemia (Wender et al., 2000; Brown et al., 2003). Likewise, some of the latest data on lactate and glucose concentrations in brain ECS indicate that lactate is consistently higher than glucose (Abi-Saab et al., 2002), favorable circumstances for neurons to use lactate in favor of glucose for energy metabolism, e.g., (Bouzier-Sore et al., 2003). Only more experimental work can settle this question.

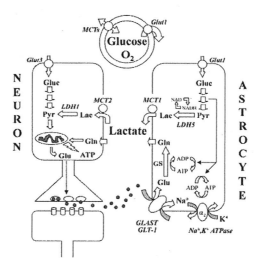

Figure 11.3. Proposed mechanism by which active neurons could signal astrocytes to increase glucose uptake and export lactate for neuronal energy metabolism. Neural activity leads to synaptic release of glutamate (Glu), which is taken up by astrocytes via the Na^+-dependent glutamate transporters GLAST and GLT-1. This results in massive Na^+ flux into the astrocytes, and activates the Na^+, K^+ ATPase. In astrocytes, glutamate is converted to glutamine (Gln) by glutamine synthetase (GS). Because glutamine synthetase and the Na^+, K^+ ATPase consume ATP, glucose uptake (via Glut1) and glycolysis are enhanced. Pyruvate (Pyr) is converted to lactate (Lac) by lactate dehydrogenase (LDH5 isoform in astrocytes). Lactate is released from astrocytes via the monocarboxylate transporter MCT1 into the extracellular space. The energy demand of active neurons can be met by glucose (via Glut3) or lactate uptake (via monocarboxylate transporter MCT2). The hypothesis holds that lactate may be preferentially taken up by the active neurons to serve as fuel for ATP production or a carbon source for glutamate synthesis.

The role that astrocyte glycogen might play in the ANLSH has not been explored. It is clear that glycogen turns over rapidly in the brain (Watanabe and Passonneau, 1974) and that turnover can be activated selectively. For example, glycogen breakdown is increased in "barrel fields" in rat somatosensory cortex when the facial whiskers that project to this area are manually stimulated (Swanson, 1992). This result is compatible with the idea that glycogen breakdown is stimulated by synaptic activity and contributes glycolytic fuel to meet the heightened metabolic demand in astrocytes (Magistretti, 1999). Whether astrocyte glycogen also contributes to net lactate export is not known but this is certainly known to occur under conditions of metabolic stress (Dringen et al., 1993).

This scheme, of course, is primarily relevant for synaptic regions of the brain, i.e. gray matter. The mechanism that 'couples' axonal activity to glucose utilization in white matter is not established. Because axonal activity produces proportional increases in extracellular potassium ion concentration ($[K^+]_o$) (Connors et al., 1982), and increases in $[K^+]_o$ raise astrocyte glucose utilization (Salem et al., 1975; Walz and Mukerji, 1988), it is tempting to speculate that activity-dependent changes in $[K^+]_o$ in white matter play an analogous role to glutamate release in gray matter.

Finally, the coupling model discussed here may represent the explanation for the results in certain types of functional brain imaging (Magistretti and Ransom, 2002). Positron emission tomography with 18F-deoxyglucose (FDG PET) measures regional glucose utilization in relation to neural activity. Given that glutamate release is the signature of cortical activation, glutamate's subsequent effects on astrocyte glucose uptake would plausibly explain FDG PET signals.

11.5. Glycogen

Glycogen is a complex molecule consisting of a protein backbone, glycogenin, and up to 30,000 glucose residues. One of the cellular advantages of condensing many glucose molecules into a single large molecule of glycogen is that it reduces osmotic pressure. It represents a readily mobilized storage form of glucose and is found in most mammalian tissues, including the brain. Glycogen in the brain is found almost exclusively in astrocytes (Cataldo and Broadwell, 1986b) and at concentrations far lower than in liver or skeletal muscle (about 2 to 5% of the level in the liver (Villar-Palasi and Larner, 1960)), although the amounts measured in previous studies may have been significantly underestimated for technical reasons (Cruz and Dienel, 2002). Astrocytes possess the enzymes glycogen synthase (Pellegri et al., 1996) and glycogen phosphorylase (Pfeiffer-Guglielmi et al., 2003), which control synthesis and catabolism of glycogen, respectively. In fasted animals, liver glycogen falls dramatically but brain glycogen does not change significantly (Villar-Palasi and Larner, 1960).

There are about 100 g of glycogen in the liver and 400 g of glycogen in resting muscle. Thus glycogen accounts for 1 - 2 % of the weight of muscle (30 - 100 µmol/g) and 6 - 8% of the weight of liver (100 - 500 µmol/g) (Shulman et al., 1995). Estimates of human brain glycogen are between 2 and 5 µmol/g (Swanson et al., 1989), although this has recently been revised upward to 6 - 8 µmol/g (Cruz and Dienel, 2002), and thus there is about 0.5 - 1.5 g of glycogen in the human brain, or about 0.1% of total brain weight. The relatively low concentration of brain glycogen coupled with the high metabolic rate of the brain cause glycogen to be neglected as a meaningful energy reserve. There was another reason, of course, to ignore glycogen. There was no obvious way that glycogen in astrocytes could have any benefit for neurons or other glial cells. Presuming for the moment that glycogen could assist all cells in the brain, calculations based on cortical metabolic rate and estimations of free glucosyl units released from measured glycogen content, suggested that glycogen could only support cortical function for three minutes in the absence of glucose (Siesjö, 1978). This was a period of redemption hardly worth talking about. The idea that this concept, i.e. benefit of astrocyte glycogen for general brain metabolism, might be worth testing experimentally would not emerge for many years.

The introduction of insulin therapy to treat schizophrenia (i.e. insulin-induced hypoglycemia) prompted some of the earliest studies on brain glycogen. Measurements of glycogen in the adult dog subjected to varying degrees of hypoglycemia indicated that glycogen content fell first in areas of the brain with the highest metabolic rates (Chesler and Himwich, 1944; Rinkel and Himwich, 1959), demonstrating a connection between glycogen and brain function. These initial functional studies were not followed up, as the majority of subsequent studies focused on the effect of a variety of experimental maneuvers on glycogen content (Hof et al., 1988; Magistretti et al., 1993b; Hamai et al., 1999; Bernard-Helary et al., 2000; Cruz and Dienel, 2002). These studies revealed a wide variety of compounds that altered glycogen content including glucose, insulin, K^+, vasoactive intestinal peptide (VIP), norepinephrine and general anesthetics.

In vitro, astrocyte glycogen is rapidly degraded when glucose is withdrawn (Dringen et al., 1993), and glycogen falls rapidly *in vivo* during ischemia, with a time course that is closely related to ATP depletion and accumulation of lactate (Swanson et al., 1989) (see also (Ransom and Fern, 1997)). Neurons grown in astrocyte-rich cultures are less severely injured by glucose withdrawal than are neurons in astrocyte-poor cultures (Swanson and Choi, 1993). This benefit appeared to derive from the presence of greater amounts of glycogen in the astrocyte-rich cultures, because depleting glycogen negated the benefit (Swanson and Choi, 1993). Two possible mechanisms for this outcome, not mutually exclusive, were suggested but not tested: 1) Astrocytes themselves utilize the energy from glycogen breakdown to prevent the accumulation of toxic levels of glutamate (removing it by a Na^+-gradient-dependent transporter as discussed above); or 2) Glycogen provides fuel to neurons to sustain their energy metabolism.

Studies on central nervous system (CNS) white matter (i.e. rodent optic nerve) have clearly established that astrocyte glycogen can provide fuel to brain cells when glucose is in short supply. Optic nerve function, measured as the compound action potential (CAP), persists for about 20-30 minutes at 37° C in the absence of glucose (Ransom and Fern, 1997; Fern et al., 1998; Brown et al., 2003). This observation suggested the hypothesis that during glucose withdrawal astrocyte glycogen is converted to lactate and transported into axons to act as an energy source. Consistent with this idea, glycogen content of the optic nerve falls to a low stable level during glucose withdrawal with a time course that corresponds well to the time course of CAP failure (Figure 11.4). If glycogen content is increased, this extends the duration of optic nerve function in the absence of glucose (Wender et al., 2000), and vice versa when glycogen content is diminished prior to glucose removal (Brown and Ransom, 2002). There is direct and linear relationship between glycogen content and latency to CAP failure during glucose withdrawal (Brown and Ransom, 2002). These results indicate that astrocyte glycogen in white matter is readily available to axons, mainly as lactate (or possibly pyruvate), during glucose withdrawal. If lactate transport by monocarboxylate transporters is blocked pharmacologically, the benefit of glycogen in sustaining function during aglycemia is lost (Wender et al., 2000).

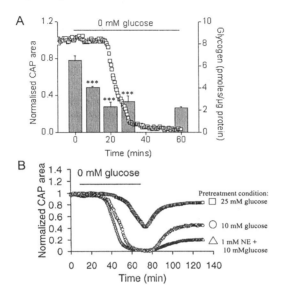

Figure 11.4. Glycogen content and optic nerve excitability during glucose deprivation. A). In the absence of glucose, glycogen content (right axis) declines over time and reaches a low stable level at 30 min. Optic nerve excitability, measured as normalized area under the compound action potential (CAP; left axis) declines in the absence of glucose (each open square is average CAP area). Note that the CAP is maintained for 20 min in the absence of glucose before decline begins, which corresponds to the time when glycogen reaches its nadir. B) Incubation of optic nerves with 25 mM glucose (open squares) increases glycogen content and incubation with norepinephrine (NE, open triangles) reduces glycogen content. Control nerves (incubated in 10 mM glucose, open circles) show ~45% CAP recovery after 60 min of aglycemia. Nerves with increased glycogen content show increased CAP recovery and nerves with decreased glycogen show worse recovery.

During high frequency CNS axon discharge (four minutes of 100 Hz stimulation), glycogen content falls even in the presence of normal bath glucose (Brown et al., 2003) (Figure 11.5). If lactate transport is blocked during high frequency discharge, axon function fails, suggesting that lactate is moving from astrocytes to axons under these conditions. Astrocyte glycogen, therefore, has the ability to 'buffer' the energy substrate content in the immediate vicinity of neural elements whose activity and corresponding energy demands vary widely (Brown et al., 2003). This result suggests the possibility that glycogen might abet the energy transactions associated with such phenomena as learning and memory where intense bursts of synaptic activity induce synaptic plasticity. These findings indicate important roles for glycogen in both pathological and normal circumstances. They also provide the surest evidence available that astrocytes can share fuel with their neural neighbors (Figure 11.6). This lends plausibility to the notion that lactate released from astrocytes might serve as energy substrate for neurons even under normal conditions (see above). The possible advantage of such a system is that, lactate transferred to neurons can be metabolized without the initial expense of the ATP necessary to phosphorylate glucose. Because nearly every neuron has astrocyte neighbors, the delivery of lactate might be more efficient and reliable than depending on diffusion of glucose from more distant capillaries.

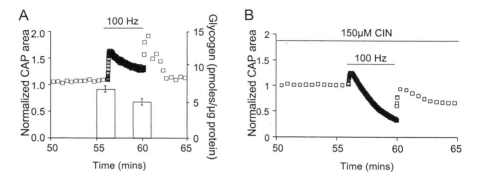

Figure 11.5. Glycogen breaks down to lactate to support axon function during high frequency discharge in optic nerve. (A) High frequency stimulation (100 Hz for 4 min) causes an activity dependent drop in glycogen content (columns, right axis) and a temporary increase in CAP area (open squares, left axis). Optic nerves are incubated in 10 mM glucose. (B) The MCT2 blocker cinnamic acid (CIN) caused the area under CAP to decline during high frequency stimulation in 10 mM glucose (compare to panel A). This suggests that lactate derived from glycogen breakdown must shuttle to axons to maintain excitability (i.e. CAP amplitude) during intense activity, even in the presence of glucose.

Glycogen levels in astrocytes are regulated by various neurotransmitters and peptide modulators. Monoamine neurotransmitters (noradrenaline, serotonin and histamine), peptides such as VIP, and adenosine and ATP are glycogenolytic in the brain (Magistretti et al., 1981; Magistretti et al., 1986). Interestingly, the rapid glycogenolysis mediated by VIP, noradrenaline and adenosine is followed by a slow upregulation of glycogen content (Sorg and Magistretti, 1992). In some instances, astrocyte glycogen content can be increased by insulin (Magistretti et al., 1993c). While the brain mainly expresses non-insulin sensitive glucose transporters, the insulin sensitive glucose transporter 4 (GLUT 4) is expressed in certain areas. It appears that insulin receptors are expressed in exactly those parts of the brain that express GLUT 4, suggesting that insulin's effect on glycogen content may be mediated by enhanced glucose transport (Brown et al., 2002).

11.6 Glycogen and the CNS axons during aglycemia: the model

Based on the data reviewed, a model can be constructed showing how glycogen protects axons during glucose removal (Figure 11.6). This model, of course, is also relevant when intense neural activity causes axon energy demands to exceed the availability of glucose. The enzyme lactate dehydrogenase (LDH) can exist as five different isozymes depending on the tetrameric association of the two subunits, H and M. The kinetic properties of the various isozymes differ in terms of their affinity for various substrates and inhibition by end-products (Garrett and Grisham, 1999). The isozyme designated LDH-5 preferentially converts pyruvate to lactate, a process that does not require oxygen, thus leading to the widely held concept that lactate is the anaerobic product of tissues unable to carry out oxidative metabolism (e.g. exercising muscle). Astrocytes, which have less active oxidative enzymes than neurons (Friede, 1962), express LDH-5 and can readily convert pyruvate to lactate. Conversely, neurons stain exclusively with anti-H (LDH-1) antibodies, the subunit combination that preferentially oxidizes lactate to pyruvate (Bittar et al., 1996).

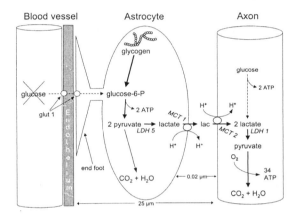

Figure 11.6. Glycogen sustains CNS axons during aglycemia. During aglycemia, astrocyte glycogen is degraded to lactate and transported to neighboring axons. Axons take up lactate and convert it to pyruvate for energy metabolism. See text section 11.6 for details.

The heterogeneous cellular distribution of monocarboxylate transporters (MCTs) also suggests one-way traffic of lactate from astrocytes to neurons. MCTs shuttle lactate and pyruvate across cell membranes using a proton symport (Poole and Halestrap, 1993). There are several isoforms of MCT: MCT-1 is expressed in tissue that exports lactate, and MCT-2 is expressed in tissue that consumes lactate (Jackson and Halestrap, 1996; Broer et al., 1997). Consistent with their presumed role as lactate exporters, astrocytes express MCT-1 (Koehler-Stec et al., 1998; Halestrap and Price, 1999). Neurons, on the other hand, express MCT-2 and are ideally suited for lactate uptake at low substrate concentrations (Halestrap and Price, 1999). The cellular distribution of LDH isozymes and MCT isoforms, therefore, facilitates lactate export from astrocytes and uptake by nearby axons. It should be stated for completeness sake that the exact distribution of these important proteins has not been confirmed in white matter but is assumed based on the distribution pattern seen in gray matter.

In the absence of glucose, lactate would be formed from glycogenolysis in astrocytes and immediately delivered to the ECS where it could be taken up by adjacent axons. As mentioned above, in the presence of O_2, lactate can be readily used to produce abundant ATP. It is not known if the flow of lactate from astrocytes to axons is regulated in any way during aglycemia. This could be important to ensure that the rate of glycogen breakdown 'matches' the energy demands of both the host astrocytes and the at-risk axons.

11.7. References

Abi-Saab WM, Maggs DG, Jones T, Jacob R, Srihari V, Thompson J, Kerr D, Leone P, Krystal JH, Spencer DD, During MJ, Sherwin RS (2002) Striking differences in glucose and lactate levels between brain extracellular fluid and plasma in conscious human subjects: effects of hyperglycemia and hypoglycemia. J Cereb Blood Flow Metab 22:271-279.

Anderson CM, Swanson RA (2000) Astrocyte glutamate transport: review of properties, regulation, and physiological functions [In Process Citation]. Glia 32:1-14.

Anderson CM, Nedergaard M (2003) Astrocyte-mediated control of cerebral microcirculation. Trends Neurosci 26:340-344; author reply 344-345.

Andriezen WL (1893) On a system of fibre-like cells surrounding the blood vessels of the brain of man and mammals, and its physiological significance. Int Monatsschr Anat Physiol 10:532-540.

Bernard-Helary K, Lapouble E, Ardourel M, Hevor T, Cloix JF (2000) Correlation between brain glycogen and convulsive state in mice submitted to methionine sulfoximine. Life Sci 67:1773-1781.

Bittar PG, Charnay Y, Pellerin L, Bouras C, Magistretti PJ (1996) Selective distribution of lactate dehydrogenase isoenzymes in neurons and astrocytes of human brain. J Cereb Blood Flow Metab 16:1079-1089.

Bouzier-Sore AK, Merle M, Magistretti PJ, Pellerin L (2002) Feeding active neurons: (re)emergence of a nursing role for astrocytes. J Physiol Paris 96:273-282.

Bouzier-Sore AK, Voisin P, Canioni P, Magistretti PJ, Pellerin L (2003) Lactate is a preferential oxidative energy substrate over glucose for neurons in culture. J Cereb Blood Flow Metab 23:1298-1306.

Broer S, Rahman B, Pellegri G, Pellerin L, Martin JL, Verleysdonk S, Hamprecht B, Magistretti PJ (1997) Comparison of lactate transport in astroglial cells and monocarboxylate transporter 1 (MCT 1) expressing Xenopus laevis oocytes. Expression of two different monocarboxylate transporters in astroglial cells and neurons. J Biol Chem 272:30096-30102.

Brown AM, Ransom BR (2002) Neuroprotective effects of increased extracellular Ca(2+) during aglycemia in white matter. J Neurophysiol 88:1302-1307.

Brown AM, Wender R, Ransom BR (2001) Ionic mechanisms of aglycemic axon injury in mammalian central white matter. J Cereb Blood Flow Metab 21:385-395.

Brown AM, Tekkok SB, Ransom BR (2003) Glycogen regulation and functional role in mouse white matter. J Physiol 549:501-512.

Brown AM, Westenbroek RE, Baltan Tekkok S, Ransom BR (2002) Functional insulin receptors are selectively expressed on CNS astrocytes. Soc Neurosci Abstr:(#581.512).

Cajal R (1995) Histology of the Nervous System. New York: Oxford University Press.

Cardinaud B, Coles JA, Perrottet P, Spencer AJ, Osborne MP, Tsacopoulos M (1994) The composition of the interstitial fluid in the retina of the honeybee drone: implications for the supply of substrates of energy metabolism from blood to neurons. Proc R Ros Lond [Biol] 257:49-58.

Cataldo AM, Broadwell RD (1986a) Cytochemical identification of cerebral glycogen and glucose-6- phosphatase activity under normal and experimental conditions. II. Choroid plexus and ependymal epithelia, endothelia and pericytes. J Neurocytol 15:511-524.

Cataldo AM, Broadwell RD (1986b) Cytochemical identification of cerebral glycogen and glucose-6- phosphatase activity under normal and experimental conditions. I. Neurons and glia. J Electron Microscopy Technique 3:413-437.

Champe PC, Harvey RA (1994) Lippincott's Illustrated reviews: Biochemistry, 2 Edition. Philadelphia: Lippincott Williams and Wilkins.

Chesler A, Himwich HE (1944) Effect of insulin hypoglycaemia on glycogen content of parts of the central nervous system of the dog. Arch Neurol Psychiat 52:114-116.

Chih CP, Roberts Jr EL (2003) Energy substrates for neurons during neural activity: a critical review of the astrocyte-neuron lactate shuttle hypothesis. J Cereb Blood Flow Metab 23:1263-1281.

Chih CP, Lipton P, Roberts EL, Jr. (2001) Do active cerebral neurons really use lactate rather than glucose? Trends Neurosci 24:573-578.

Clarke DD, Sokoloff L (1999) Circulation and energy metabolism of the brain. In: Basic Neurochemistry: Molecular, Cellular and Medical Aspects, 6th Edition (Siegel GS, Agranoff B, eds), pp 637-669. Philadelphia: Lippincott-Raven Pubs.

Connors BW, Ransom BR, Kunis DM, Gutnick MJ (1982) Activity-dependent K$^+$ accumulation in the developing rat optic nerve. Science 216:1341-1343.

Cruz NF, Dienel GA (2002) High glycogen levels in brains of rats with minimal environmental stimuli: implications for metabolic contributions of working astrocytes. J Cereb Blood Flow Metab 22:1476-1489.

del Zoppo GJ, Hallenbeck JM (2000) Advances in the vascular pathophysiology of ischemic stroke. Thromb Res 98:73-81.

Dringen R, Gebhardt R, Hamprecht B (1993) Glycogen in astrocytes: possible function as lactate supply for neighboring cells. Brain Res 623:208-214.

Fellows LK, Boutelle MG (1993) Rapid changes in extracellular glucose levels and blood flow in the striatum of the freely moving rat. Brain Res 604:225-231.

Fern R, Davis P, Waxman SG, Ransom BR (1998) Axon conduction and survival in CNS white matter during energy deprivation: a developmental study. J Neurophysiol 79:95-105.

Forsyth R, Fray A, Boutelle M, Fillenz M, Middleditch C, Burchell A (1996) A role for astrocytes in glucose delivery to neurons? Dev Neurosci 18:360-370.

Friede RL (1962) Cytochemistry of normal and reactive astrocytes. J Neuropathol Exp Neurol 21:471-478.

Frier BM, Fisher BM (1999) Hypoglycaemia in Clinical Diabetes. New York: John Wiley & Sons, Ltd.

Ganong WF (1989) Review of Medical Physiology. Norwalk, Connecticut: Appleton and Lange.

Garrett RH, Grisham CM (1999) Biochemistry: Second Edition, 2 Edition. Fort Worth: Saunders College Publishing.

Goldberg MP, Choi DW (1993) Combined oxygen and glucose deprivation in cortical cell culture: calcium-dependent and calcium-independent mechanisms of neuronal injury. J Neurosci 13:3510-3524.

Gotoh J, Itoh Y, Kuang TY, Cook M, Law MJ, Sokoloff L (2000) Negligible glucose-6-phosphatase activity in cultured astroglia. J Neurochem 74:1400-1408.

Halestrap AP, Price NT (1999) The proton-linked monocarboxylate transporter (MCT) family: structure, function and regulation. Biochem J 343 Pt 2:281-299.

Hamai M, Minokoshi Y, Shimazu T (1999) L-glutamate and insulin enhance glycogen synthesis in cultured astrocytes from the rat brain through different intracellular mechanisms. J Neurochem 73:400-407.

Hof PR, Pascale E, Magistretti PJ (1988) K+ at concentrations reached in the extracellular space during neuronal activity promotes a Ca2+-dependent glycogen hydrolysis in mouse cerebral cortex. J Neurosci 8:1922-1928.

Hu Y, Wilson GS (1997) Rapid changes in local extracellular rat brain glucose observed with an in vivo glucose sensor. J Neurochem 68:1745-1752.

Jackson VN, Halestrap AP (1996) The kinetics, substrate, and inhibitor specificity of the monocarboxylate (lactate) transporter of rat liver cells determined using the fluorescent intracellular pH indicator, 2',7'-bis(carboxyethyl)-5(6)-carboxyfluorescein. J Biol Chem 271:861-868.

Koehler-Stec EM, Simpson IA, Vannucci SJ, Landschulz KT, Landschulz WH (1998) Monocarboxylate transporter expression in mouse brain. Am J Physiol 275:E516-524.

Kuffler SW, Nicholls JG (1966) The physiology of neuroglial cells. Ergeb Physiol 57:1-90.

Larrabee MG (1983) Lactate uptake and release in the presence of glucose by sympathetic ganglia of chicken embryos and by neuronal and nonneuronal cultures prepared from these ganglia. J Neurochem 40:1237-1250.

Larrabee MG (1996) Partitioning of CO_2 production between glucose and lactate in excised sympathetic ganglia, with implications for brain. J Neurochem 67:1726-1734.

Lowry JP, O'Neill RD, Boutelle MG, Fillenz M (1998) Continuous monitoring of extracellular glucose concentrations in the striatum of freely moving rats with an implanted glucose biosensor. J Neurochem 70:391-396.

Magistretti PJ (1997) Coupling of cerebral blood flow and metabolism. In: Primer of cerebrovascular diseases (Welch KMA, Caplan LR, Reis DJ, Siesjö BK, Weir B, eds), pp 70-75: Academic Press.

Magistretti PJ (1999) Cellular and molecular bases of brain energy metabolism. In: Fundamental Neuroscience (Zigmond M, Bloom FE, Landis S, Roberts J, Squire L, eds), pp 389-413: Academic Press.

Magistretti PJ, Pellerin L (1999) The role of astrocytes in coupling synaptic activity to glucose utilization in the brain. NIPS 14:177-182.

Magistretti PJ, Ransom BR (2002) Astrocytes. In: Neuropsychopharmacology (Davis KL, Charney D, Coyle JT, Nemeroff C, eds), pp 133-146. Philadelphia, PA: Lippincott Williams and Wilkins.

Magistretti PJ, Hof P, Martin JL (1986) Adenosine stimulates glycogenolysis in mouse cerebral cortex : a possible coupling mechanism between neuronal activity and energy metabolism. JN 6:2558-2562.

Magistretti PJ, Sorg O, Martin J-L (1993a) Regulation of glycogen metabolism in astrocytes: physiological, pharmacological, and pathological aspects. In: Astrocytes: Pharmacology and Function, pp 243-265: Academic Press.

Magistretti PJ, Morrison JH, Shoemaker WJ, Sapin V, Bloom FE (1981) Vasoactive intestinal polypeptide induced glycogenolysis in mouse cortical slices : a possible regulatory mechanism for the local control of energy metabolism. PNAS 78:6535-6539.

Magistretti PJ, Sorg O, Yu N, Martin JL, Pellerin L (1993b) Neurotransmitters regulate energy metabolism in astrocytes: implications for the metabolic trafficking between neural cells. Dev Neurosci 15:306-312.

Magistretti RJ, Sorg O, Martin J-L (1993c) Regulation of glycogen metabolism in astrocytes: Physiological, pharmacological and pathological aspects. In: Astrocytes: Pharmacology and Function (Murphy S, ed), pp 243-265. San Diego: Academic.

Nedergaard M, Ransom BR, Goldman S (2003) New roles for astrocytes: Redefining the functional architecture of the brain (review). TINS 26:523-530.

Nicholson C (1995) Extracellular space as the pathway for neuron-glial cell interaction. In: Neuroglia (Kettenmann H, Ransom BR, eds), pp 387-397. New York: Oxford University Press.

Pellegri G, Bittar PG, Martin J-L, Magistretti PJ (1996) Differential distribution of lactate transporters and lactate dehydrogenase (LDH) isozymes: evidence for an astrocyte-neuron lactate cycle. Soc Neurosci Abstr.

Pellerin L, Magistretti PJ (1994) Glutamate uptake into astrocytes stimulates aerobic glycolysis: a mechanism coupling neuronal activity to glucose utilization. PNAS 91:10625-10629.

Pellerin L, Magistretti PJ (2003a) How to balance the brain energy budget while spending glucose differently. J Physiol 546:325.

Pellerin L, Magistretti PJ (2003b) Food for thought: challenging the dogmas. J Cereb Blood Flow Metab 23:1282-1286.

Pfeiffer-Guglielmi B, Fleckenstein B, Jung G, Hamprecht B (2003) Immunocytochemical localization of glycogen phosphorylase isozymes in rat nervous tissues by using isozyme-specific antibodies. J Neurochem 85:73-81.

Poitry-Yamate CL, Poitry S, Tsacopoulos M (1995) Lactate released by Muller glial cells is metabolized by photoreceptors from mammalian retina. J Neurosci 15:5179-5191.

Poole RC, Halestrap AP (1993) Transport of lactate and other monocarboxylates across mammalian plasma membranes. Am J Physiol 264:C761-782.

Ransom BR, Fern R (1996) Anoxic-Ischemic glial cell injury: Mechanisms and Consequences. In: Tissue oxygen deprivation (Haddad G, Lister G, eds), pp 617-652. New York: Marcel Dekker, Inc.

Ransom BR, Fern R (1997) Does astrocytic glycogen benefit axon function and survival in CNS white matter during glucose deprivation? Glia 21:134-141.

Rinkel M, Himwich HE (1959) Insulin Treatment in Psychiatry. New York: Philosophical Library, Inc.

Rose CR, Waxman SG, Ransom BR (1998) Effects of glucose deprivation, chemical hypoxia, and simulated ischemia on Na+ homeostasis in rat spinal cord astrocytes. J Neurosci 18:3554-3562.

Salem RD, Hammerschlag R, Brancho H, Orkand RK (1975) Influence of potassium ions on accumulation and metabolism of (14C)glucose by glial cells. Brain Res 86:499-503.

Sanchez-Abarca LI, Tabernero A, Medina JM (2001) Oligodendrocytes use lactate as a source of energy and as a precursor of lipids. Glia 36:321-329.

Schurr A, West CA, Rigor BM (1988) Lactate-supported synaptic function in the rat hippocampal slice preparation. Science 240:1326-1328.

Shulman RG, Bloch G, Rothman DL (1995) In vivo regulation of muscle glycogen synthase and the control of glycogen synthesis. Proc Natl Acad Sci U S A 92:8535-8542.

Siesjö BK (1978) Brain energy metabolism. New York: John Wiley & Sons.

Silver IA, Erecinska M (1994) Extracellular glucose concentration in mammalian brain: continuous monitoring of changes during increased neuronal activity and upon limitation in oxygen supply in normo-, hypo-, and hyperglycemic animals. J Neurosci 14:5068-5076.

Simard M, Arcuino G, Takano T, Liu QS, Nedergaard M (2003) Signaling at the gliovascular interface. J Neurosci 23:9254-9262.

Sloviter HA, Kamimoto T (1970) The isolated, perfused rat brain preparation metabolizes mannose but not maltose. J Neurochem 17:1109-1111.

Sokoloff L (1992) The brain as a chemical machine. Prog Brain Res 94:19-33.

Sokoloff L, Reivich M, Kennedy C, Des Rosiers MH, Patlak CS, Pettigrew KD, Sakurada O, Shinohara M (1977) The [14C]deoxyglucose method for the measurement of local cerebral glucose utilization: theory, procedure, and normal values in the conscious and anesthetized albino rat. J Neurochem 28:897-916.

Sorg O, Magistretti PJ (1992) Vasoactive intestinal peptide and noradrenaline exert long-term control on glycogen levels in astrocytes: blockade by protein synthesis inhibition. JN 12:4923-4931.

Stryer L (1995) Pentose phosphate pathway and gluconeogenesis. In: Biochemistry, fourth Edition, pp 559-580. New York: W.H. Freeman.

Swanson RA (1992) Physiologic coupling of glial glycogen metabolism to neuronal activity in brain. Can J Physiol Pharmacol 70:S138-144.

Swanson RA, Choi DW (1993) Glial glycogen stores affect neuronal survival during glucose deprivation in vitro. J Cereb Blood Flow Metab 13:162-169.

Swanson RA, Sagar SM, Sharp FR (1989) Regional brain glycogen stores and metabolism during complete global ischaemia. Neurol Res 11:24-28.

Tsacopoulos M, Poitry-Yamate CL, Poitry S (1997) Ammonium and Glutamate Released by Neurons Are Signals Regulating the Nutritive Function of a Glial Cell. J Neurosci 17:2383-2390.

Tsacopoulos M, Veuthey AL, Saravelos SG, Perrottet P, Tsoupras G (1994) Glial cells transform glucose to alanine, which fuels the neurons in the honeybee retina. J Neurosci 14:1339-1351.

Vannucci SJ, Maher F, Simpson IA (1997) Glucose transporter proteins in brain: delivery of glucose to neurons and glia. Glia 21:2-21.

Villar-Palasi C, Larner J (1960) Levels of activity of the enzymes of glycogen cycle in rate tissues. Arch of Biochem and Biophys 86:270-273.

Voutsinos-Porche B, Bonvento G, Tanaka K, Steiner P, Welker E, Chatton JY, Magistretti PJ, Pellerin L (2003) Glial glutamate transporters mediate a functional metabolic crosstalk between neurons and astrocytes in the mouse developing cortex. Neuron 37:275-286.

Walz W, Mukerji S (1988) Lactate release from cultured astrocytes and neurons: a comparison. Glia 1:366-370.

Watanabe H, Passonneau JV (1974) The effect of trauma on cerebral glycogen and related metabolites and enzymes. Brain Research 66:147-159.

Wender R, Brown AM, Fern R, Swanson RA, Farrell K, Ransom BR (2000) Astrocytic glycogen influences axon function and survival during glucose deprivation in central white matter. J Neurosci 20:6804-6810.

Wiesinger H, Hamprecht B, Dringen R (1997) Metabolic pathways for glucose in astrocytes. Glia 21:22-34.

Wolfe DE, Nicholls JG (1967) Uptake of radioactive glucose and its conversion to glycogen by neurons and glial cells in the leech central nervous system. J Neurophysiol 30:1593-1609.

Zonta M, Angulo MC, Gobbo S, Rosengarten B, Hossmann KA, Pozzan T, Carmignoto G (2003) Neuron-to-astrocyte signaling is central to the dynamic control of brain microcirculation. Nat Neurosci 6:43-50.

11.8. Abbreviations

ANLSH	Astrocyte-neuron lactate shuttle hypothesis
ATP	Adenosine triphosphate
CAP	Compound action potential
CIN	Cinnamic acid
CNS	Central nervous system
ECS	Extracellular space
FDG PET	18F-deoxyglucose positron emission tomography
$[glucose]_o$	Extracellular glucose concentration
G-6-P	Glucose-6-phosphate
GFAP	Glial fibrillary acidic protein
Gln	Glutamine
Glu	Glutamate
Glut 1,3,4	Glucose transporter 1,3,4
GS	Glutamine synthetase
$[K^+]_o$	Extracellular potassium ion concentration
Lac	Lactate
LDH	Lactate dehydrogenase
MCT	Monocarboxylate transporters
MON	Mouse optic nerve
NADPH	Nicotinamide adenine dinucleotide phosphate hydrogenase
Pyr	Pyruvate
VIP	Vasoactive intestinal peptide

Chapter 12

Calcium signaling in glia

Helmut Kettenmann* and Carola G. Schipke

Max-Delbrück Center for Molecular Medicine, Cellular Neurosciences,
Robert-Rössle-Str. 10, 13092 Berlin, Germany

*Corresponding author: hketten@mdc-berlin.de

Contents

12.1. Astrocytes

12.1.1. Voltage gated Ca^{2+} channels and capacitative Ca^{2+} entry control Ca^{2+} influx

The expression of voltage-gated Ca^{2+} channels on astrocytes in culture has already been shown 20 years ago (MacVicar, 1984). A detailed investigation has recently identified a large variety of subtypes present in cultured cells, both on the protein and mRNA level, namely α_{1B} (N-type), α_{1C} (L-type), α_{1D} (L-type), α_{1E} (R-type), and α_{1G} (T-type), but not $\alpha 1A$ (P/Q-type) channels (Latour et al., 2003). The expression of Ca^{2+} channels in astrocytes in situ is controversial. There was no evidence found for Ca^{2+} channels in astrocytes in acute slices from the visual cortex or the CA1 hippocampal region of developing rats and the depolarization-induced $[Ca^{2+}]_i$ increases in astrocytes was solely attributed to the activation of metabotropic receptors by neurotransmitters, such as glutamate, released by synaptic terminals upon depolarization (Carmignoto et al., 1998). In contrast, freshly isolated astrocytes from 2-6 week old rat hippocampi showed verapamil-sensitive increases in Ca^{2+} due to depolarization by high K^+ supporting the presence of voltage-gated Ca^{2+} channels (Fraser et al., 1995). For more details on Ca^{2+} channels see also Chapter 7.

Depletion of intracellular cytoplasmic Ca^{2+} stores activates a Ca^{2+} entry channel located on the plasma membrane to refill the stores and this event is also termed capacitative Ca^{2+} entry. The capacitative Ca^{2+} entry can be blocked by La^{3+} or by low extracellular $[Ca^{2+}]_o$ concentrations. Capacitative Ca^{2+} entry is part of the observed Ca^{2+} transient, e.g., elicited by glutamate in cultured astrocytes (Pizzo et al., 2001) or by endothelin (ET) in Bergmann glial cells from cerebellar slices (Tuschick et al., 1997): The ET-triggered Ca^{2+} increase in Ca^{2+}-free solution was shorter in duration since it lacked the capacitative component. Re-addition of extracellular Ca^{2+} to a normal level briefly after the ET application induced an intracellular Ca^{2+} increase in Bergmann glia that is due to the activated capacitative Ca^{2+} entry to refill the stores.

12.1.2. Astrocytes have different intracellular compartments for the accumulation and release of Ca^{2+}

Astrocytes have different compartments for the intracellular accumulation and release of Ca^{2+}. The classical release channel located intracellularly on the endoplasmic reticulum is the inositol trisphosphate receptor (InsP$_3$R). Signaling via most metabotropic receptors in astrocytes is linked to the phospholipase C pathway. Via activation of phospholipase C, InsP$_3$ is formed which gates the InsP$_3$R and Ca^{2+} is released from the endoplasmic stores. Another release channel on the endoplasmic reticulum is the ryanodine receptor (RyR). Astrocytes specifically express the RyR3 subtype and not the suptypes 1 or 2 (Matyash et al., 2002). RyRs also modulate cell motility. In a wound-healing assay cell motility was strongly attenuated in astrocytes cultured from homozygous RyR type 3 knockout mice (Matyash et al., 2002).

There exist two distinct Ca^{2+} storage compartments within the endoplasmic reticulum, one associated with the release via RyR; the other one is linked to a (cyclopiazonic acid-sensitive) Ca^{2+} pump associated with release via InsP$_3$Rs. The latter one has a larger storage capacity and only this compartment is linked to metabotropic purinergic and glutamatergic signaling. The stores are filled, however, by the same type of pump, the Na^+/Ca^{2+} exchanger (Golovina et al., 1996; Golovina and Blaustein, 2000). Another second messenger that has recently been identified to cause Ca^{2+} release from intracellular stores is cyclic ADP ribose. It triggers a Ca^{2+} response in cultured astrocytes and is linked to the control of glutamate and GABA release (Verderio et al., 2001).

A second type of organelle involved in Ca^{2+} homeostasis in astrocytes is the mitochondrion: Ca^{2+} buffering via uptake into mitochondria provides a potent mechanism to regulate the localized spread of astrocytic Ca^{2+} signals. Preventing mitochondrial Ca^{2+} uptake broadens the Ca^{2+} signals by slowing the rate of decay of cytosolic $[Ca^{2+}]_i$ transients. Thus mitochondria act as Ca^{2+} buffers and shorten Ca^{2+} signals (Boitier et al., 1999).

12.1.3. Neurotransmitters lead to an increase in intracellular Ca^{2+} levels

Astrocytes express a variety of ionotropic and metabotropic transmitter receptors linked to Ca^{2+} signaling. In this chapter we have focused on those receptors which are not only identified in cell culture, but also in astrocytes from intact tissue or in freshly isolated cells.

Bergmann glial cells express AMPA-type glutamate receptors with a high Ca^{2+}-permeability as demonstrated by combining patch clamping and imaging in cerebellar slices. This unusual high Ca^{2+}-permeability of the AMPA receptor in these cells is due to a lack of the GluR2 subunit which confers Ca^{2+} impermeability into the receptor complex (Muller et al., 1992; Burnashev et al., 1992). Blocking the Ca^{2+}-permeability of these receptors by introducing the GluR2 subunit into Bergmann glial cells strongly impairs synaptic transmission at the parallel fibre Purkinje-cell synapse (Iino et al., 2001). Calcium influx can also occur through NMDA-type glutamate receptor. Astrocytes of the mouse neocortex express functional NMDA-receptors in situ and activation of these receptors leads to a local increase in cytosolic Ca^{2+} in the processes of astrocytes (Schipke et al., 2001). Metabotropic glutamate receptors were identified in Bergmann glial cells in situ (Kirischuk et al., 1999). The large topic of glutamatergic signaling from and to astrocytes will be discussed in a separate chapter (Chapter 15).

The inhibitory transmitter GABA triggers $[Ca^{2+}]_i$ increase in astrocytes by acting both via ionotropic $GABA_A$ and metabotropic $GABA_B$ receptors. Since astrocytes accumulate Cl⁻, activation of $GABA_A$ receptors leads to membrane depolarization sufficient to activate voltage gated Ca^{2+} channels. This leads to an influx of Ca^{2+} and that has been demonstrated on freshly isolated astrocytes from rat hippocampus (Fraser et al., 1995). Activity of interneurons in the hippocampus activates $GABA_B$ receptors in surrounding astrocytes. In response to $GABA_B$ receptor activation astrocytes potentiate inhibitory transmission (Kang et al., 1998).

In cultured astrocytes the (co-)transmitter ATP can induce Ca^{2+} signaling both via activation of metabotropic P2Y-type and ionotropic P2X-type receptors. The activation triggers an increase in Ca^{2+} and a cationic conductance (Walz et al., 1994). In Bergmann glial cells in cerebellar slices, only P2Y-type receptors linked to Ca^{2+} mobilization from intracellular stores could be detected, but no P2X-receptor mediated responses (Kirischuk et al., 1995b). Purinergic signaling also acts back on glial cells which is discussed in the section on calcium waves and the whole issue of ATP-mediated signaling is also treated in a different chapter (Chapter 14). Adenosine receptors have a modulatory effect on Ca^{2+} signaling in astrocytes. They increase the sensitivity of Ca^{2+} signals triggered by glutamate and ATP (Jimenez et al., 1999; Toms and Roberts, 1999).

In a slice preparation from the hippocampus, nerve-fiber stimulation in the stratum oriens/alveus evoked a long-lasting inward current and increased the $[Ca^{2+}]_i$ level in astrocytes. This form of neuron-glia interaction was mediated by acetylcholine (Araque et al., 2002).

Further transmitter receptors linked to astrocyte Ca^{2+} signaling include adrenergic receptors, muscarinic cholinergic and histaminergic as studied in hippocampal or cerebellar slices (Shelton and McCarthy, 2000; Kirischuk et al., 1996; Duffy and MacVicar, 1995).

12.1.4. Other substances that lead to an increase in astrocyte cytosolic Ca^{2+}

Astrocyte Ca^{2+} responses are not only triggered by transmitters, but also by substances released during inflammation, released from endothelial cells and by mediators related to pathology. Peptides involved in the complement factor cascade can enter the brain during a disturbance of the blood brain barrier, but are also produced by brain cells. These peptides trigger Ca^{2+} signaling in astrocytes. Stimulation of complement factor 3a (C3a)- and C5a-receptors with C3a or C5a, respectively, leads to an increase in intracellular calcium in cultured astrocytes (Sayah et al., 2003).

The envelope glycoprotein gp120 of the human immune deficiency virus has been shown to induce Ca^{2+} signals in astrocytes cultured from the cerebellar cortex (Codazzi et al., 1995) whereas neurons do not show any response to the activation with gp120. This protein plays an important role in modulating the glial pathways leading to neuronal death during HIV-infection (Bezzi et al., 2001). Another neuropeptide that acts on astrocytes is ET. ET has been shown to induce Ca^{2+} transients in Bergmann glial cells in acute slices from mouse brain. Bergmann glial cells are endowed with functional ET-B receptors which induce the generation of intracellular Ca^{2+} signals by activation of Ca^{2+} release from $InsP_3$-sensitive intracellular stores followed by a secondary Ca^{2+} influx (Tuschick et al., 1997). Another substance involved in Ca^{2+} signaling in Bergmann glial cells is nitric oxide (NO). The NO-triggered increase in $[Ca^{2+}]_i$ is due to Ca^{2+} influx from the extracellular space and not to release from cytoplasmic stores. NO also triggers Ca^{2+} transients in cultured astrocytes. Using patch-clamping and imaging techniques, it was shown that NO is released from parallel fibres after electrical stimulation and that NO serves as a signaling substance to the neighboring Bergmann glia cells (Matyash et al., 2001).

Lysophosphatidic acid (LPA) is a phospholipid mediator with a variety of biological activities. LPA is able to stimulate the expression of various genes encoding for cytokines, including nerve growth factor, interleukin-1beta (IL-1β), IL-3 and IL-6 (Tabuchi et al., 2000). In cultured astrocytes, LPA increases $[Ca^{2+}]_i$ and causes morphological changes (Steiner et al., 2002). The variability of astrocytic properties in different brain regions becomes evident as LPA-induced responses vary among astrocytes from different brain regions (Steiner et al., 2002).

12.1.5. $[Ca^{2+}]_i$ can increase in small compartments of astrocytes, the microdomains

Parallel fibre stimulation can trigger locally confined Ca^{2+} signals in small compartments of Bergmann glia processes, the microdomains. These locally confined responses can be elicited with a single stimulation. Moreover, independently occurring spontaneous activity can also be recorded within different microdomains within the same cell. By analyzing three-dimensional reconstructions of processes, morphological correlates to the microdomains could be identified. These cellular compartments do have the same dimensions of several μm as observed for the localized Ca^{2+} signals. The microdomains contain small membrane leaflets that are only tens of nm thick, they ensheathe synapses, contain mitochondria and may serve to synchronize ensembles of synapses (Grosche et al., 1999; Grosche et al., 2002), (Fig. 12.1; see also Chapter 3). Also, NMDA-receptor mediated influx of Ca^{2+} into astrocytes is restricted to fine processes, and did not spread to the cell soma as studied in acute slices from the neocortex preparations (Schipke et al., 2001). Thus, astrocytes can be considered as cells with multiple functional and structural compartments. In contrast to the local signaling may be the wide-range form of signaling in between astrocytes, the so-called calcium waves.

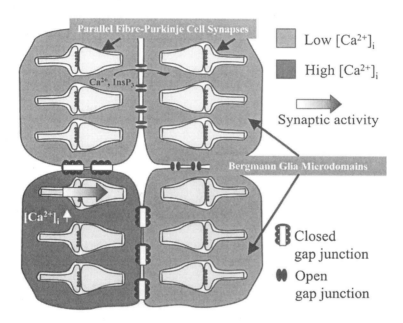

Figure 12.1. Schematic diagram of the proposed interaction between Bergmann glial microdomains and parallel fibre-Purkinje cell synapses. The activity of a subset of synapses within one microdomain triggers a Ca^{2+} response in this microdomain (lower left). If there is a feedback signal (such as glutamate release), it will act back on all synapses in this microdomain. The $[Ca^{2+}]_i$ increase leads to a closure of gap junctions leading to an electrical isolation of this one microdomain while the remaining domains remain coupled and thus can exchange metabolites and electrical signals (Muller et al., 1996).

12.1.6. Ca^{2+} waves in astrocytes are a form of long-distance signaling

Astrocytes exhibit a form of long distance signaling, termed Ca^{2+} waves, that is the propagation of Ca^{2+} transients within an astrocyte population. These Ca^{2+} waves can spread hundreds of μm thereby activating hundreds of cells and have been described to occur in primary cultures (Cornell-Bell et al., 1990), slice cultures (Dani et al., 1992), the isolated retina (Newman and Zahs, 1997; Newman, 2001) and acute slices from brain (Schipke et al., 2002). In parallel with the propagation of calcium waves, ATP (Wang et al., 2000) and glutamate concentrations can increase in the extracellular space (Innocenti et al., 2000). The mechanisms leading to the release of these transmitters are still under debate, but there is a difference in Ca^{2+} dependence: ATP release is Ca^{2+}-independent and the ATP wave can propagate independently from the Ca^{2+} wave (Wang et al., 2000). In contrast, the release of glutamate only occurs in parallel with the increase in Ca^{2+} (Parpura et al., 1994; Bezzi et al., 1998; Pasti et al., 2001). Toxins that interfere with the SNARE-complex block the glutamate release, a finding that suggests a Ca^{2+} dependent vesicular release mechanism comparable with synaptic exocytosis (Jeftinija et al., 1997; Bezzi et al., 1998; Araque et al., 2000). The release of ATP is inhibited by flufenamic acid, a non-specific gap junction and hemichannel blocker, suggesting a release mechanism via connexin hemichannels (Stout et al., 2002). Recently, a connexin hemichannel–dependent release has also been described for glutamate. Removal of extracellular Ca^{2+} caused an influx of Lucifer Yellow and at the same time a release of glutamate from cultured rat hippocampal astrocytes. Both events are blocked by the gap junction blockers octanol, heptanol and carbenoxolone (Ye et al., 2003). Taken together, these results show that Ca^{2+} activity spreads wave-like within the astrocyte population and that these waves are accompanied by release of transmitters (Fig. 12.2).

12.1.7. Ca^{2+} waves in culture, mechanisms of propagation

Ca^{2+} waves spread within the astrocytic population with a speed of $10 - 20$ μm/s and thus orders of magnitude slower than neuronal signal propagation. Two different mechanisms have been described to explain how the Ca^{2+} wave propagates within an astrocytic network in culture: 1. the intra- and intercellular diffusion of second messengers via gap junctions between highly coupled astrocytes with subsequent Ca^{2+} release from intracellular stores (Giaume and Venance, 1998; Venance et al., 1998; also Chapter 13), and 2. the release of ATP from astrocytes into the extracellular space followed by purinergic receptor activation on neighboring cells, which, in turn, leads to elevation of $[Ca^{2+}]_i$ (Guthrie et al., 1999; Wang et al., 2000; Arcuino et al., 2002).

These two mechanisms do not occur independently of each other. As the major gap junction protein, astrocytes express connexin (Cx) 43. Deletion of Cx43 potentiated the response after activation of purinergic receptors by ATP and UTP. The reduction in gap junctional communication in astrocytes cultured from Cx43 knock-out animals thus goes along with a functional switch in the expression of P2Y nucleotide receptor subtypes (Scemes et al., 2000).

Pharmacological studies and Western blot analysis indicate that there is a reciprocal regulation of $P2Y_1$ receptor and $P2Y_4$ receptor expression levels, such that downregulation of Cx43 (using an antisense approach) leads to decreased expression of the adenine-sensitive $P2Y_1$ receptor and increased expression of the uridine-sensitive $P2Y_4$ receptor. This change in P2Y receptor subtypes was paralleled by changes in the mode of calcium wave propagation (Suadicani et al., 2003).

Recent evidence indicates that P2Y receptor subtypes differ in their ability to generate Ca^{2+} signaling in cultured spinal cord astrocytes. While $P2Y_2$ receptor activation triggers a single $[Ca^{2+}]_i$ transient, $P2Y_1$ receptor activation elicits rapid $[Ca^{2+}]_i$ oscillations when the specific ligands were applied once per minute. Less frequent application did not elicit such oscillations. Moreover, Ca^{2+} responses mediated by either receptor exhibit slow depression (Fam et al., 2003).

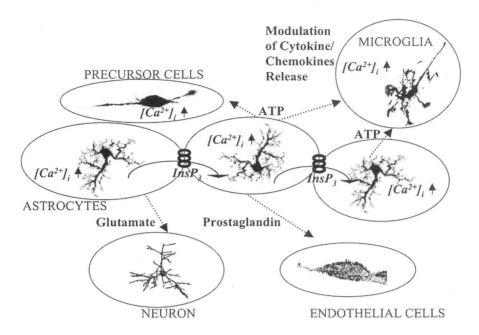

Figure 12.2. Schematic diagram showing the interactions and intercellular communication via Ca^{2+} signals between different glial cells (astrocytes, precursor cells, microglial cells), neurons and endothelial cells. Summarized are data from in situ studies. Astrocytes can communicate intracellular Ca^{2+} signals to neighboring astrocytes. The signal can spread in between astrocytes via diffusion of the second messenger InsP$_3$ through gap junctions of these highly coupled cells or via the release of ATP (middle row). The communication between astrocytes and precursor cells and astrocytes and microglia is achieved by ATP released from astrocytes that activates purinergic receptors on those cell types (upper row). Activation of purinergic receptors on precursor cells and micrcoglia leads to an increase in $[Ca^{2+}]_i$ levels. Astrocytic calcium wave propagation in the intact tissue can thus influence also these cells. E.g. cytokine release from microglia is dependent s on $[Ca^{2+}]i$ levels. As indicated, also astrocytes themselves can release a number of substances after elevation of $[Ca^{2+}]_i$. Glutamate released from astrocytes can trigger responses in neighboring neurons. Signaling from astrocytes to endothelial is achieved via prostaglandin-release from astrocytes that acts on endothelial cells (lower row).

12.1.8. Ca^{2+} waves can be elicited in tissue

So far there are only few reports on astrocytic Ca^{2+} wave propagation in living tissue. First evidence came from a study on hippocampal organotypic slices. Activation of neuronal activity triggered astrocyte Ca^{2+} waves, and these waves travel with a similar speed as described in culture (Dani et al., 1992). Subsequently Newman and Zahs (Newman and Zahs, 1997) established that an astrocytic Ca^{2+} wave can propagate within the isolated retina, and they showed that the wave recruits Müller cells, a radial glial cell with some astrocyte features. The wave spreads via ATP release and concomitant purinergic receptor activation and is not influenced by blockers of gap junctions (Newman, 2001). In acutely isolated brain tissue, a glial

Ca^{2+} wave that comprises astrocytes and glial precursor cells, can be elicited electrically (Schipke et al., 2002). This wave, elicited in white matter, also travels to grey matter and is mediated by release of ATP and subsequent activation of purinergic receptors and involves Ca^{2+} release from cytoplasmic stores (Fig. 12.2).

12.1.9. Mediators of inflammation can affect Ca^{2+} signaling and waves

Tumor necrosis factor alpha (TNFα), a major proinflammatory cytokine, reduces the glutamate induced $[Ca^{2+}]_i$ increase in astrocytes within 1 h of incubation (Koller et al., 2001). In turn, TNFα release from astrocytes can be rapidly triggered by the activation of the chemokine receptor CXCR4 with stromal cell-derived factor 1 (SDF-1). TNFα release is accompanied by a $[Ca^{2+}]_i$ increase and release of glutamate and prostaglandins. The response is augmented in the presence of activated microglia (Bezzi et al., 2001). CXCR4 also binds the human immunodeficiency virus envelope protein gp120 and indeed gp 120 elicits Ca^{2+} signals in astrocytes (Codazzi et al., 1995) and binds to the CXCR4 receptor on astrocytes.

IL-1β is another major proinflammatory cytokine and differentially regulates P2 receptor-mediated and gap junction-mediated pathways. Intercellular Ca^{2+} wave transmission in IL-1β-treated cultures was potentiated compared with control despite a marked reduction in gap-junctional coupling. Conversely, transmission of Ca^{2+} waves via the P2 receptor-mediated pathway was potentiated in IL-1β treated cultures (John et al., 1999).

The cytokine interferon-gamma (IFN-γ) is expressed by T cells and natural killer cells and can modulate astrocyte function during a T cell invasion into the brain. Application of IFN-γ to astrocyte cultures causes an increase in the frequency of spontaneously occurring Ca^{2+} signals. This increased activity is associated with an increase in the amount of ATP released (Verderio and Matteoli, 2001).

12.1.10. Spontaneous Ca^{2+} activity

Astrocytes exhibit changes in the cytosolic Ca^{2+} concentration not only in response to stimuli, but also as spontaneous events. In culture, these spike-like responses ranged from resting levels of 50-250 nM to as high as 1-2 µM. The spikes were found to be irregular in frequency and amplitude and had a duration of tens of seconds. They could occur independently in a population of astrocytes, but were frequently synchronized in confluent cultures (Fatatis and Russell, 1992). This spontaneous activity can also be observed in acute tissue preparations (Nett et al., 2002). Neurons can influence the spontaneous Ca^{2+} activity in astrocytes. A network analysis revealed that neurons and astrocytes exhibit a synchronized, spontaneous Ca^{2+} activity in brain slices. Decreasing spontaneous $[Ca^{2+}]_i$ transients in neurons by tetrodotoxin (TTX) does not alter the number of active astrocytes, but it impairs their synchronous network activity. Thus spontaneous activity in astrocytes and neurons is patterned into correlated neuronal/astrocytic networks in which neuronal activity regulates the network properties of astrocytes (Aguado et al., 2002). There is also a feedback of astrocytes onto neurons: spontaneous astrocytic Ca^{2+} oscillations can trigger slowly decaying NMDA receptor-mediated inward currents in neurons located close to active astrocytes (Parri et al., 2001).

12.1.11. Astrocyte - endothelial cell Ca^{2+} signaling

Astrocytes enwrap blood vessels with their endfeet and are therefore in the strategic position to convey signals from neurons to the blood system. Since blood flow is modulated by neuronal activity, astrocytes could be the mediators between brain activity and local blood supply. Little is known, however, about pathways of communication between astrocytes and endothelial cells. Like astrocytes, endothelial cells respond to a variety of stimuli with an increase of $[Ca^{2+}]_i$ that is propagated to adjacent cells as an intercellular Ca^{2+} wave (Leybaert et al., 1998). In co-culture, intercellular Ca^{2+} waves, induced by mechanical stimulation of a single cell, propagate from astrocytes to endothelial cells and vice versa. Intercellular Ca^{2+} waves could also be induced by flash photolysis of pressure-injected caged $InsP_3$ and also by applying the flash to remote noninjected cells. Interestingly, Ca^{2+} waves induced by flash photolysis propagated from endothelial cells to astrocytes but not from astrocytes to endothelial cells, even though caged $InsP_3$ diffused between the two cell types. Even more remarkably, flash photolysis of caged Ca^{2+} (NP-EGTA) resulted in an increase of $[Ca^{2+}]_i$ but did not initiate an intercellular Ca^{2+} wave (Leybaert et al., 1998). In contrast, mechanical damage of a single astrocyte triggers a large intercellular Ca^{2+} wave that propagates to surrounding astrocytes and also to even remotely (several hundred μm) located endothelial cells. The mechanism is similar to that shown for the astrocyte Ca^{2+} wave propagation in retina or corpus callosum, namely release of ATP and subsequent activation of purinergic receptors on neighboring cells (both, astrocytes and endothelial cells) (Paemeleire and Leybaert, 2000; Fig. 12.2).

Recent work has provided evidence for the functional coupling of neuronal activity, astrocyte Ca^{2+} signaling and vessel diameter (Zonta et al., 2003). In rat cortical slices the dilation of arterioles triggered by neuronal activity is dependent on $[Ca^{2+}]_i$ oscillations in astrocytes. The Ca^{2+} signals elicited by neuronal activity were mediated by the activation of metabotropic glutamate receptors. Inhibition of the astrocyte Ca^{2+} responses resulted in the impairment of activity-dependent vasodilation, whereas activation of single astrocytes that were in contact with arterioles triggered vessel relaxation. A cyclooxygenase product is centrally involved in this astrocyte-mediated control of arterioles: blocking the prostaglandin forming enzyme cyclooxygenase by acetylsalicylic acid (aspirin) led to only small if any dilations of vessels in response to astrocyte stimulation. Blockade of metabotropic glutamate receptors in an in vivo model had an impact on the coupling of neuronal activity and blood flow. Forepaw stimulation did, under normal conditions, increase blood flow in the somatosensory cortex as measured with Laser-Doppler flowmetry. In the presence of mGluR antagonists this coupling was impaired (Zonta et al., 2003). Thus, astrocyte Ca^{2+} signals are key elements to couple neuronal activity to blood flow.

12.2. Oligodendrocytes

12.2.1. Ca^{2+} channel expression in oligodendrocytes is developmentally regulated

The expression of Ca^{2+} channels undergoes marked changes in the development of oligodendrocytes as studied in cell culture. Immature precursor cells express two different types of Ca^{2+} channels, high and low voltage gated channels distinguished by their peak activation. While the majority of precursor cells expressed only one of the two current types, in 30% of all cells both types of current could be identified (Verkhratsky et al., 1990). The expression of the Ca^{2+} channels was strongly correlated with the expression of Na^+ channels. More mature precursor cells lacked Ca^{2+} and Na^+ channels. Large Ca^{2+} currents were recorded at later stages of oligodendrocyte development correlated with the expression of the O10 antigen (Blankenfeld et al., 1992).

The channels are unevenly distributed across the membrane. In glial precursor cells from both retina and cortex, small depolarizations activated $[Ca^{2+}]_i$ transients in processes indicating the presence of low-voltage-activated Ca^{2+} channels. Larger depolarizations (with 50 mM K^+) additionally activated high-voltage-activated Ca^{2+} channels in the soma. An uneven distribution of Ca^{2+} channels was also observed in mature oligodendrocytes; $[Ca^{2+}]_i$ transients in processes were considerably larger than in the soma. Recovery of $[Ca^{2+}]_i$ levels after the voltage-induced influx was achieved by the activity of the plasmalemmal Ca^{2+} pump, while mitochondria played a minor role in restoring $[Ca^{2+}]_i$ levels after an influx through voltage-operated channels (Kirischuk et al., 1995a). While the above mentioned studies were performed in culture, Ca^{2+} channel activity was also reported from glial precursor cells of the developing corpus callosum. In contrast, Ca^{2+} currents could not be recorded from oligodendrocytes in situ. This could be due to a preferential localization of Ca^{2+} channels on distal processes where the voltage clamp control is insufficient to depolarize the membrane to the activation threshold (Berger et al., 1992).

12.2.2. AMPA receptors mediate Ca^{2+} influx through the receptor pore and by activation of voltage-gated channels

Responses to glutamate in cells of the oligodendrocyte lineage have been reported in culture (Gilbert et al., 1984; Kettenmann et al., 1984) and in brain slices (Berger et al., 1992). While NMDA did not trigger a current response, the glutamate response was mimicked by kainate indicating the presence of AMPA/kainate type receptors (Berger et al., 1992). AMPA/kainate-type glutamate receptors activated a cationic conductance which was accompanied by two additional responses: (i) an increase in $[Ca^{2+}]_i$ mediated by depolarization and a subsequent activation of voltage-gated Ca^{2+} channels and (ii) a transient blockade of a delayed rectifying K^+ current. The blockade of the K^+ current was not due to the increase in $[Ca^{2+}]_i$ since it was also observed in Ca^{2+}-free bathing solution when no increase in $[Ca^{2+}]_i$ was detectable after exposure to kainate. In contrast to precursor cells, oligodendrocytes responded weakly or not at all to glutamate or related ligands (Borges et al., 1994). Glutamate acting at AMPA receptors increased mRNA and protein levels of the transcription factor NGFI-A in purified rat cortical O-2A progenitors. The increase in the immediate early gene expression was mediated by an increase in $[Ca^{2+}]_i$. Thus, activation of glutamate receptors could regulate oligodendrocyte development by having rapid effects at the genomic level (Pende et al., 1994).

Besides triggering Ca^{2+} entry via activation of Ca^{2+} channels, AMPA receptors can directly conduct Ca^{2+} ions. AMPA receptors lacking the GluR2 subunit are highly Ca^{2+} permeable (Wisden and Seeburg, 1993). These Ca^{2+} permeable receptors are upregulated in a defined developmental time window: In oligodendroglial progenitors and immature oligodendrocytes the GluR3 and GluR4 subunits are transiently upregulated and this subunit composition is preferentially assembled in these cells. In contrast, oligodendroglial pre-progenitors or mature oligodendrocytes express the GluR2 subunit and thus express a low Ca^{2+} permeability (Itoh et al., 2002; Deng et al., 2003).

Activation of either AMPA or kainate receptors is toxic to oligodendrocytes if combined with a Ca^{2+} influx (Sanchez-Gomez and Matute, 1999). The differential regulation of edited GluR2-free, and hence Ca^{2+}-permeable, AMPA-GluR explains the selective susceptibility to excitotoxicity of cells at these stages of oligodendroglial differentiation.

12.2.3. Depolarization by GABA and glycine trigger Ca^{2+} influx

GABA evokes transient increases in $[Ca^{2+}]_i$ in cultured early precursor cells (Kirchhoff and Kettenmann, 1992). These cells are characterized by a high density of $GABA_A$ receptors (Kettenmann et al., 1991) and Ca^{2+} channels (Blankenfeld et al., 1992). The response is mediated by $GABA_A$ receptors, since muscimol mimicked and bicuculline and picrotoxin blocked the $[Ca^{2+}]_i$ increase. The GABA mediated $[Ca^{2+}]_i$ increase could also be blocked by the Ca^{2+} channel blocker nifedipine or by omitting Ca^{2+} from the bath. In contrast, $[Ca^{2+}]_i$ levels were not affected in oligodendrocytes. This could be due to the low level of $GABA_A$ receptor density (Blankenfeld et al., 1992) which may not sufficiently depolarize oligodendrocytes to the threshold of Ca^{2+} channel activation. Similarly, glycine induces an increase in $[Ca^{2+}]_i$ in cortical oligodendrocyte progenitor cells also due to membrane depolarization and activation of voltage-gated Ca^{2+} channels (Belachew et al., 2000).

12.2.4. Oligodendrocytes express functionally distinct intracellular Ca^{2+} stores

Besides the endoplasmic reticulum, mitochondria also serve as Ca^{2+} stores. In glial precursor cells cultured from rabbit retina, the fluorescence signal of active mitochondria was confined to the tips of processes, while in oligodendrocytes an even distribution was found (Kirischuk et al., 1995a). Mitochondria are found in groups of three or more in oligodendrocyte processes (Simpson and Russell, 1996). In glial precursor cells, the mitochondrial uncoupler CCCP generated an increase in the cytoplasmic calcium concentration $[Ca^{2+}]_i$ in regions corresponding to the concentration of mitochondria. In mature oligodendrocytes CCCP evoked a $[Ca^{2+}]_i$ elevation without significant spatial heterogeneity (Kirischuk et al., 1995a). Mitochondria play an active role in Ca^{2+} signaling: stimulation of muscarinic acetylcholine receptors activates propagating Ca^{2+} wave fronts in oligodendrocytes and the waves are dependent on mitochondrial location and function (Simpson and Russell, 1996). Mitochondria are only found in intimate association with these sites possessing high density endoplasmic reticulum proteins such as the sarcoplasmic-endoplasmic reticulum Ca^{2+}-ATPase which fills the stores (Simpson and Russell, 1997). This indicates that mitochondria and InsP$_3$R Ca^{2+} release channels form structural units (Simpson et al., 1997). These are also functional units: $[Ca^{2+}]_i$ elevations in the cytosol evoked by kainate were translated into long-lasting $[Ca^{2+}]_i$ elevations in subpopulations of mitochondria. Thus, Ca^{2+} uptake into some mitochondria is activated both by Ca^{2+} entry into cells or release from stores (Simpson and Russell, 1998). Ryanodine receptors also participate in Ca^{2+} signaling. Mitochondrial depolarization is accompanied by Ca^{2+} puffs and waves within the oligodendrocytes. Mitochondria even seem to be involved in the initiation sites of waves (Haak et al., 2002). Besides mitochondria and InsP$_3$ receptors, RyR also participate in Ca^{2+} signaling. Oligodendrocytes express the specific Ca^{2+} release channel subtypes RyR3 and InsP$_3$R2 in patches along their processes. RyRs are coexpressed with InsP$_3$Rs in some patches, but InsP$_3$Rs are also found alone. This heterogeneous distribution is likely the cause of the distinct Ca^{2+} response pattern elicited by agonists of ryanodine and InsP$_3$Rs, respectively (Haak et al., 2001).

12.2.5. Metabotropic receptors linked to Ca^{2+} signaling are differentially expressed during development

Some metabotropic receptors linked to Ca^{2+} signaling have been identified on cells of the oligodendrocyte lineage as revealed in tissue culture. Oligodendrocyte precursors express metabotropic glutamate receptors of the mGluR1/5 subtype (Luyt et al., 2003) and nicotinic acetylcholine receptors (Rogers et al., 2001). Ligands for both receptors induced Ca^{2+} oscillations. In a subset of cells nicotine triggered intracellular free Ca^{2+} oscillations that continued in the presence of nicotine over a period of 2 to 3 min. Oligodendrocytes express bradykinin receptors (Stephens et al., 1993), and responded to carbachol, histamine and norepinephrine with a $[Ca^{2+}]_i$ transient (Takeda et al., 1995).

In cultured cells of the oligodendrocyte lineage as well as in oligodendrocytes from mouse corpus callosum slices, ATP induced a transient increase of $[Ca^{2+}]_i$ in late precursors and oligodendrocytes but not in early glial precursor cells from retinal and cortical cultures and from corpus callosum slices. Elevation of $[Ca^{2+}]_i$ is due to a Ca^{2+} liberation from intracellular stores as this is the case for most metabotropic Ca^{2+} signaling (Kirischuk et al., 1995b).

The calcium-sensing receptor (CaSR) is a member of a growing family of heptahelical receptors with an unusually large extracellular domain. In cultured rat oligodendrocytes, Ca^{2+} induced stimulation of phosphatidylinositol hydrolysis with an EC$_{50}$ of 1.4 mM and increased $[Ca^{2+}]_i$ (Ferry et al., 2000). The CaSR is expressed in immature oligodendrocytes and may be functionally linked to cellular proliferation (Chattopadhyay et al., 1998).

12.3. Microglia

Most studies described in this chapter have been performed in cell culture and we should be aware that the cultured microglia represents a cell in a (more or less) defined stage of activation. In the normal brain, microglia are present in their resting form characterized by a ramified morphology. Pathologic events trigger an activation program in these cells which ultimately transforms them into cytotoxic, phagocytosing cells which release a variety of cytokines and can migrate to the sites of injury. This transformation is accompanied by a change in the membrane current pattern. Cells patch-clamped in freshly isolated slices are closest to the resting form and thus to the situation in the normal brain. These ramified cells express almost no voltage- and time-gated currents. In a model of injury, the facial nerve lesion, the microglia expressed inwardly rectifying K^+ currents about 12 h post-lesion. This current pattern also characterizes the unstimulated microglia in culture on which most studies were performed described in this chapter. 24 h post-lesion an additional outwardly rectifying K^+ is expressed and this current pattern matches that of bacterial endotoxin lipopolysaccharide (LPS)-stimulated microglia in culture. With each increasing numbers of K^+ channels, the membrane potential is stabilized at more negative values and thus activation correlates with membrane hyperpolarization (Boucsein et al., 2000). Since the reversal potential for Ca^{2+} is at a positive membrane potential, microglial activation also correlates with an increased driving force for Ca^{2+} across the cell membrane.

12.3.1. A variety of receptors elicit Ca^{2+} signaling

Microglial cells express a large variety of transmembrane receptors which trigger an increase in $[Ca^{2+}]_i$ after activation. These include classical transmitter receptors such as glutamate receptors. Metabotropic glutamate receptor mGlu5a mRNA was found in cultured microglia and the metabotropic glutamate receptor ligand $(1S,3R)$-1-aminocyclopentane-1,3-dicarboxylic acid (trans-ACPD)-induced transient calcium signals (Boddeke et al., 1999). Ionotropic glutamate receptors mainly contain the AMPA-preferring subunits GluR1 and GluR4, but also contain Ca^{2+}-impermeable GluR2 subunits and thus are not essential elements in glutamate mediated Ca^{2+} signaling (Noda et al., 2000). Carbachol and norepinephrine acting via muscarinic acetylcholine and adrenergic receptors trigger increases in $[Ca^{2+}]_i$ via release from intracellular stores (Whittemore et al., 1993; Zhang et al., 1998). Both endothelin (ET)-1 and ET-3 increased $[Ca^{2+}]_i$ concentration via ET-B receptors (Moller et al., 1997a).

A number of cytokines trigger a transient increases in $[Ca^{2+}]_i$. Stimulation with the chemokine CCL21 induced intracellular Ca^{2+} transients and chemotaxis in cultured microglia acting via the CXCR3 receptor (Biber et al., 2001; Rappert et al., 2002). Fractalkine induced $[Ca^{2+}]_i$ transients and, at high concentrations, oscillatory mobilization of intracellular Ca^{2+} from the stores (Boddeke et al., 1999). The presence of voltage gated Ca^{2+} channels on microglia is under debate. In a work on chemokine induced Ca^{2+} signaling macrophage inflammatory protein-1α (MIP-1α) directly evoked $[Ca^{2+}]_i$ responses while the CC chemokine RANTES acting via CCR3, and eotaxin activate L-type Ca^{2+} channels (Hegg et al., 2000).

Sphingosine-1-phosphate or LPA triggered an increase in $[Ca^{2+}]_i$ which caused the activation of Ca^{2+}-dependent K^+ channels (Schilling et al., 2002). Although LPA induced increases in the $[Ca^{2+}]_i$ concentration in both mouse and rat microglia, the responses differed substantially. The Ca^{2+} signal in rat microglia occurred primarily through Ca^{2+} influx via the plasma membrane, whereas the Ca^{2+} signal in mouse microglia was due to release from intracellular stores (Moller et al., 2001). Further receptors linked to rapid $[Ca^{2+}]_i$ increase include the protease activated receptor (PAR)1 activated by thrombin (Moller et al., 2000).

Purinergic receptors linked to Ca^{2+} signaling were first identified in cultured mouse microglial cells (Walz et al., 1993). The ATP-induced Ca^{2+} response involved both, Ca^{2+} influx through ionotropic receptors and Ca^{2+} release from intracellular pools, whereas UTP selectively stimulated intracellular Ca^{2+} release indicating that these microglial cells express the ionotropic P2X-type and the metabotropic P2Y-type receptors (Toescu et al., 1998). Moreover, P2Y receptor stimulation triggered the activation of a K^+ current. The presence of functional purinergic receptors could also be verified in situ. Patch-clamp recordings from identified microglial cells in acute slices of adult mouse brain indicated the expression of $P2Y_1$ and $P2Y_{2/4}$ receptors linked to the activation of the K^+ current and P2X receptors including $P2X_7$ linked to the activation of the non-selective cationic current (Boucsein et al., 2003). A similar diverse expression was found on immature ameboid microglia from slices of early postnatal corpus callosum. These cells were most likely in the phase of CNS invasion during development (Haas et al., 1996). Thus, microglial cells *in situ* and in culture express different purinergic receptors with distinct sensitivity and functional coupling.

12.3.2. Depletion of intracellular Ca^{2+} stores can trigger a chronic Ca^{2+} influx

UTP is a good tool for stimulating Ca^{2+} release from intracellular stores. When this Ca^{2+} release was stimulated in the absence of extracellular Ca^{2+}, the re-addition of extracellular Ca^{2+} caused a large rebound $[Ca^{2+}]_i$ increase in mouse brain microglia. Following this rebound, $[Ca^{2+}]_i$ did not return to the initial resting level, but remained elevated for long periods of time (up to 20 min), at a higher steady-state level. Both the amplitude of the rebound $[Ca^{2+}]_i$ transient and the new plateau level strongly correlated with the degree of intracellular Ca^{2+} depletion, indicating the chronic activation of a store-operated Ca^{2+} entry pathway. The elevated steady-state $[Ca^{2+}]_i$ level was associated with a significant increase in the plasma membrane permeability to Ca^{2+}, as changes in extracellular Ca^{2+} were reflected in rapid changes of $[Ca^{2+}]_i$. Similarly, blocking plasmalemmal Ca^{2+} channels with the non-specific open channel blocker La^{3+} caused a decrease in $[Ca^{2+}]_i$, despite the continuous presence of Ca^{2+} ions in the extracellular medium. After the establishment of the new, elevated steady-state $[Ca^{2+}]_i$ level, stimulation of uridine-sensitive $(P2Y_{2/4})$ metabotropic purinoceptors did not induce a $[Ca^{2+}]_i$ response. In addition, application of thapsigargin, a blocker of the pump responsible for Ca^{2+} uptake into the stores failed to affect $[Ca^{2+}]_i$. All these data indicate that the maximal depletion of intracellular Ca^{2+} stores determines the long-term activation of a plasma membrane Ca^{2+} entry pathway. This activation appears to be associated with a significant decrease in the capability of the intracellular Ca^{2+} stores to take up cytosolic Ca^{2+} once they have been strongly depleted (Toescu et al., 1998).

The activity of the Ca^{2+} release activated Ca^{2+} channel (CRAC) was studied using the patch-clamp technique. It could be activated by dialyzing the cell with the Ca^{2+} chelator BAPTA, and the current appeared within about 10 minutes. Using proper isolation solutions, a unitary Na^+ conductance of 42.5 pS through the Ca^{2+} channel was determined. The CRAC current is enhanced by cAMP and is differentially regulated by protein kinase A and protein kinase C (Hahn et al., 2000).

12.3.3. Microglial activation and some cytokines trigger a chronic increase of $[Ca^{2+}]_i$

Microglial cells are activated by any type of CNS injury and this activation affects many microglial properties including migration, proliferation, release of substances including NO and cytokines, phagocytosis or antigen presentation. LPS is a classical tool to activate microglia. In culture, LPS led to a chronic elevation of basal $[Ca^{2+}]_i$ in microglial cells along with a suppression of evoked calcium signaling, as indicated by reduced $[Ca^{2+}]_i$ transients upon stimulation with UTP and C5a. Experimentally lowering $[Ca^{2+}]_i$ by buffering the cytoplasm with BAPTA restored much of the signaling efficacy. Moreover, BAPTA strongly attenuated the LPS-induced release of NO and the cytokines TNFα, interleukin-6, interleukin-12, macrophage inflammatory protein-1α (MIP-1α) and the CXC chemokine KC. By experimental elevation of basal $[Ca^{2+}]_i$, using the ionophore ionomycin, UTP induced calcium signals were suppressed thus mimicking LPS treatment, but failed to induce cytokine release activity on its own. Thus chronic elevation of basal $[Ca^{2+}]_I$ attenuates receptor-triggered Ca^{2+} signaling. Moreover, increased $[Ca^{2+}]_i$ is required, but by itself not sufficient, for release of NO and cytokines. Elevation of basal $[Ca^{2+}]_i$ could thus prove a central element in the regulation of some executive functions in activated microglia (Hoffmann et al., 2003; Fig. 12.3).

The cytokines TNFα, IL-1ß and IFN-γ also induce a chronic increase in $[Ca^{2+}]_i$, yet by different mechanisms. TNFα elicited an increase in $[Ca^{2+}]_i$ to a plateau level due to release of Ca^{2+} from an as yet unidentified intracellular source distinct from InsP$_3$-sensitive stores (McLarnon et al., 2001). IFN-γ caused a progressive increase in $[Ca^{2+}]_i$ to a plateau level due to chronic activation of a Ca^{2+} entry pathway (Franciosi et al., 2002). Similarly, IL-1β caused a slow, progressive increase in $[Ca^{2+}]_i$ in human microglia, but the IL-1β-induced responses involve both a Ca^{2+} entry pathway and a mechanism of intracellular release (Goghari et al., 2000).

12.3.4. Microglia can sense astrocyte Ca^{2+} waves

Pathologic impacts in the brain lead to a widespread activation of microglial cells far beyond the site of injury. Recently, it has been demonstrated that astrocyte Ca^{2+} waves can trigger responses in microglial cells in culture (Verderio and Matteoli, 2001) and in brain slices (Schipke et al., 2001). In acute slices from corpus callosum, Ca^{2+} signals can be triggered by electrical stimulation or local ATP ejection and propagate as waves within those cells that were loaded with a Ca^{2+}-sensitive dye. These Ca^{2+} waves were not recorded from microglial cells since only macroglial cells, astrocytes and oligodendrocytes and their precursors preferentially take up the dye. The mechanism of propagation is due to ATP release and activation of purinergic receptors. To test whether microglial cells respond to the wave, cells were labeled with a dye-coupled lectin to identify them in the slice and membrane currents were recorded with the patch-clamp technique. When the wave passed by, a current with the characteristics of a purinergic response was activated. Thus, microglial cells sense glial Ca^{2+} waves (Schipke et al., 2001; Fig. 12.2). In culture, repeated stimulations of microglial cells by astrocyte-released ATP activated P2X$_7$ purinergic receptor, eventually leading to microglial apoptosis. IFN-γ increased ATP release and potentiated the P2X$_7$-mediated cytolytic effect (Verderio and Matteoli, 2001).

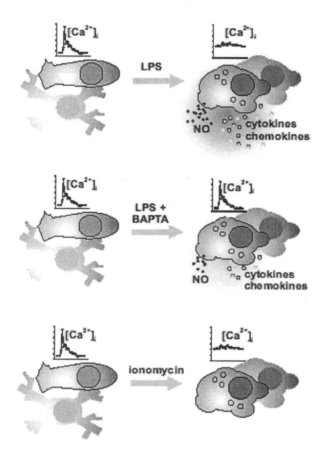

Figure 12.3. Schematic summary of the experimentally induced adaptations of microglia. Unstimulated microglial cells (shown on the left) in vitro typically appearing with a short-processed, non-branched or rod-shaped morphology responded to UTP and C5a receptor stimulation with the generation of a $[Ca^{2+}]_i$ transient, but did not show signs of release activity - similarly to the 'resting' ramified microglia of the normal brain tissue. A challenge of these cells under pathological conditions, as mimicked by a treatment with bacterial LPS, led to a complex morphological and functional transformation known as microglial activation. LPS-activated cells were characterized by an elevated basal $[Ca^{2+}]_i$ level along with a suppressed ability to generate receptor-triggered Ca^{2+} signals. Strong release of NO as well as cyto- and chemo- kines was measured. LPS treatment in the presence of BAPTA nearly restored the receptor signaling efficacy, paralleled by an almost back-to-normal basal $[Ca^{2+}]_i$ and an attenuated release performance. On the other hand, direct enforcement of a rise in basal $[Ca^{2+}]_i$ by microglial incubation with ionomycin also suppressed the signal amplitudes, but failed to trigger an LPS-like release pattern. Together, these observations suggest that an elevated basal $[Ca^{2+}]_i$ participates in the functional adjustment of activated microglia, without being the sole cytosolic control element for executive features, such as NO and cyto/chemokine production (adapted from Hoffmann et al.).

12.3.5. Purinergic receptors control microglial release activity

TNFα is a major inflammatory cytokine and is released from microglial cells upon activation, e.g. by LPS. ATP also can potently stimulate TNFα release in rat cultured brain microglia, concomitant with TNFα mRNA expression. The ATP induced TNFα release is mimicked by a P2X$_7$ receptor-selective agonist suggesting the involvement of P2X$_7$ receptors, which include a large pore. A sustained Ca^{2+} influx correlated with the TNFα release and the release was Ca^{2+}-dependent. ATP-induced TNFα release was also regulated independently of Ca^{2+}, namely by the p38 mitogen-activated protein kinase (Hide et al., 2000).

Another P2X$_7$ receptor mediated mechanism controls plasminogen release. ATP stimulated the release of plasminogen from microglia in a concentration-dependent manner within 10 min. The influx of Ca^{2+} is essential for the onset of the release: Suppression of the Ca^{2+} increase during ATP stimulation prevented the release while an experimental elevation of [Ca^{2+}]$_i$ via a ionophore stimulated release. Thus, ATP, by activating P2X$_7$ receptors triggers an increase in [Ca^{2+}]$_i$ which stimulates the release of plasminogen from microglia (Inoue et al., 1998).

Purinergic receptors also influence the process of microglial activation. When cultured microglial cells are stimulated with LPS, they release a number of cytokines such as TNFα, IL-6, IL-12 and MIP-1α and also NO. This release activity starts after several hours and a substantial release can be measured after 24h. Chronic incubation with purinergic ligands attenuated this release activity indicating that purinergic receptor activation counteracts microglial activation (Boucsein et al., 2003; Fig. 12.2). This seems at first glance a contradiction to the above-mentioned study on TNFα release. However, Hide and Tanaka (Hide et al., 2000) found the most pronounced effect with high concentrations of ATP (3 mM) while LPS-induced TNFα release was most efficiently suppressed at 100 μM. This could indicate that the suppressing effect is mediated via metabotropic receptors while P2X$_7$ receptor activation stimulates release. The suppressing effect of purinergic receptors on microglial activation is supported by the observation that the synthesis of the inflammation-related protein microglial response factor-1 (MRF)-1 is suppressed by ATP in cultured rat microglia. The *mrf-1* gene encodes a 17-kDa protein with a single Ca^{2+}-binding (EF-hand) motif and is expressed specifically in microglia. Selective activation of P2X$_7$ receptors mimicked the response which is Ca^{2+}-dependent and could be mimicked by experimental elevation of [Ca^{2+}]$_i$. These results indicate that ATP selectively suppresses MRF-1 synthesis at the transcription level via Ca^{2+} influx through P2X$_7$ receptors (Kaya et al., 2002).

12.3.6. Ca^{2+} control of microglial migration

Complement fragment C5a is a chemotactic substance for microglial cells. Application of C5a triggers, within few seconds, an intense ruffling of microglial membranes followed by lamellipodia extension accompanied by a rapid rearrangement of the actin cytoskeleton (Nolte et al., 1996). Also, C5a generated biphasic [Ca^{2+}]$_i$ transients in microglial cells from neonatal corpus callosum slices and in cell culture. These Ca^{2+} signals are due to Ca^{2+} release from internal pools and subsequent activation of Ca^{2+} entry controlled by the filling state of the intracellular

Ca^{2+} pools. Pertussis toxin (PTX) inhibited both, the C5a- and C3a-triggered $[Ca^{2+}]_i$ responses, indicating the involvement of PTX-sensitive G-proteins in the signal transduction chain (Moller et al., 1997b). $[Ca^{2+}]_i$ transients were, however, not a prerequisite for triggering the increase in motility; motility could be repeatedly evoked by C5a in nominally Ca^{2+}-free solution, while Ca^{2+} signals occurred only upon the first stimulation. Moreover, conditions mimicking $[Ca^{2+}]_i$ transients were not able to induce any motility reaction, suggesting that $[Ca^{2+}]_i$ transients are not necessary for, but are associated with, microglial motility. Motile activity is, however, restricted to a defined concentration range of $[Ca^{2+}]_i$ since either lowering or increasing $[Ca^{2+}]_i$ impaired motility.

12.3.7. Microglial cells sense pH shifts and NH_4^+

Changes in extracellular pH accompany neuronal activity and pathological conditions are mainly associated with acidosis. An extracellular alkaline shift leads to an increase in $[Ca^{2+}]_i$ concomitant with an intracellular alkaline shift. Application of NH_3/NH_4^+ caused an initial rapid alkalinization followed by a slow recovery towards the resting level, while application of alkaline (pH 8.2) solution triggered a slower rise in the intracellular pH. The $[Ca^{2+}]_i$ elevation triggered by NH_3/NH_4^+ and an extracellular alkaline shift were caused by different mechanisms: extracellular alkalinization induced a transmembrane Ca^{2+} entry, whereas NH_3/NH_4^+ triggered Ca^{2+} release from thapsigargin-sensitive intracellular pools. The mobilization of intracellular Ca^{2+} caused by NH_3/NH_4^+ was dependent on activation of phospholipase C (Minelli et al., 2000).

12.4. References

Aguado F, Espinosa-Parrilla JF, Carmona MA, Soriano E (2002) Neuronal activity regulates correlated network properties of spontaneous calcium transients in astrocytes in situ. J Neurosci 22: 9430-9444.

Araque A, Li N, Doyle RT, Haydon PG (2000) SNARE protein-dependent glutamate release from astrocytes. J Neurosci 20: 666-673.

Araque A, Martin ED, Perea G, Arellano JI, Buno W (2002) Synaptically released acetylcholine evokes Ca2+ elevations in astrocytes in hippocampal slices. J Neurosci 22: 2443-2450.

Arcuino G, Lin JH, Takano T, Liu C, Jiang L, Gao Q, Kang J, Nedergaard M (2002) Intercellular calcium signaling mediated by point-source burst release of ATP. Proc Natl Acad Sci U S A 99: 9840-9845.

Belachew S, Malgrange B, Rigo JM, Rogister B, Leprince P, Hans G, Nguyen L, Moonen G (2000) Glycine triggers an intracellular calcium influx in oligodendrocyte progenitor cells which is mediated by the activation of both the ionotropic glycine receptor and Na+-dependent transporters. Eur J Neurosci 12: 1924-1930.

Berger T, Schnitzer J, Orkand PM, Kettenmann H (1992) Sodium and Calcium Currents in Glial Cells of the Mouse Corpus Callosum Slice. Eur J Neurosci 4: 1271-1284.

Bezzi P, Carmignoto G, Pasti L, Vesce S, Rossi D, Rizzini BL, Pozzan T, Volterra A (1998) Prostaglandins stimulate calcium-dependent glutamate release in astrocytes. Nature 391: 281-285.

Bezzi P, Domercq M, Brambilla L, Galli R, Schols D, De Clercq E, Vescovi A, Bagetta G, Kollias G, Meldolesi J, Volterra A (2001) CXCR4-activated astrocyte glutamate release via TNFalpha: amplification by microglia triggers neurotoxicity. Nat Neurosci 4: 702-710.

Biber K, Sauter A, Brouwer N, Copray SC, Boddeke HW (2001) Ischemia-induced neuronal expression of the microglia attracting chemokine Secondary Lymphoid-tissue Chemokine (SLC). Glia 34: 121-133.

Blankenfeld GG, Verkhratsky AN, Kettenmann H (1992) Ca2+ Channel Expression in the Oligodendrocyte Lineage. Eur J Neurosci 4: 1035-1048.

Boddeke EW, Meigel I, Frentzel S, Biber K, Renn LQ, Gebicke-Harter P (1999) Functional expression of the fractalkine (CX3C) receptor and its regulation by lipopolysaccharide in rat microglia. Eur J Pharmacol 374: 309-313.

Boitier E, Rea R, Duchen MR (1999) Mitochondria exert a negative feedback on the propagation of intracellular Ca2+ waves in rat cortical astrocytes. J Cell Biol 145: 795-808.

Borges K, Ohlemeyer C, Trotter J, Kettenmann H (1994) AMPA/kainate receptor activation in murine oligodendrocyte precursor cells leads to activation of a cation conductance, calcium influx and blockade of delayed rectifying K+ channels. Neuroscience 63: 135-149.

Boucsein C, Kettenmann H, Nolte C (2000) Electrophysiological properties of microglial cells in normal and pathologic rat brain slices. Eur J Neurosci 12: 2049-2058.

Boucsein C, Zacharias R, Farber K, Pavlovic S, Hanisch UK, Kettenmann H (2003) Purinergic receptors on microglial cells: functional expression in acute brain slices and modulation of microglial activation in vitro. Eur J Neurosci 17: 2267-2276.

Burnashev N, Khodorova A, Jonas P, Helm PJ, Wisden W, Monyer H, Seeburg PH, Sakmann B (1992) Calcium-permeable AMPA-kainate receptors in fusiform cerebellar glial cells. Science 256: 1566-1570.

Carmignoto G, Pasti L, Pozzan T (1998) On the role of voltage-dependent calcium channels in calcium signaling of astrocytes in situ. J Neurosci 18: 4637-4645.

Chattopadhyay N, Ye CP, Yamaguchi T, Kifor O, Vassilev PM, Nishimura R, Brown EM (1998) Extracellular calcium-sensing receptor in rat oligodendrocytes: expression and potential role in regulation of cellular proliferation and an outward K+ channel. Glia 24: 449-458.

Codazzi F, Menegon A, Zacchetti D, Ciardo A, Grohovaz F, Meldolesi J (1995) HIV-1 gp120 glycoprotein induces [Ca2+]i responses not only in type-2 but also type-1 astrocytes and oligodendrocytes of the rat cerebellum. Eur J Neurosci 7: 1333-1341.

Cornell-Bell AH, Finkbeiner SM, Cooper MS, Smith SJ (1990) Glutamate induces calcium waves in cultured astrocytes: long-range glial signaling. Science 247: 470-473.

Dani JW, Chernjavsky A, Smith SJ (1992) Neuronal activity triggers calcium waves in hippocampal astrocyte networks. Neuron 8: 429-440.

Deng W, Rosenberg PA, Volpe JJ, Jensen FE (2003) Calcium-permeable AMPA/kainate receptors mediate toxicity and preconditioning by oxygen-glucose deprivation in oligodendrocyte precursors. Proc Natl Acad Sci U S A 100: 6801-6806.

Duffy S, MacVicar BA (1995) Adrenergic calcium signaling in astrocyte networks within the hippocampal slice. J Neurosci 15: 5535-5550.

Fam SR, Gallagher CJ, Kalia LV, Salter MW (2003) Differential frequency dependence of P2Y1- and P2Y2- mediated Ca2+ signaling in astrocytes. J Neurosci 23: 4437-4444.

Fatatis A, Russell JT (1992) Spontaneous changes in intracellular calcium concentration in type I astrocytes from rat cerebral cortex in primary culture. Glia 5: 95-104.

Ferry S, Traiffort E, Stinnakre J, Ruat M (2000) Developmental and adult expression of rat calcium-sensing receptor transcripts in neurons and oligodendrocytes. Eur J Neurosci 12: 872-884.

Franciosi S, Choi HB, Kim SU, McLarnon JG (2002) Interferon-gamma acutely induces calcium influx in human microglia. J Neurosci Res 69: 607-613.

Fraser DD, Duffy S, Angelides KJ, Perez-Velazquez JL, Kettenmann H, MacVicar BA (1995) GABAA/benzodiazepine receptors in acutely isolated hippocampal astrocytes. J Neurosci 15: 2720-2732.

Giaume C, Venance L (1998) Intercellular calcium signaling and gap junctional communication in astrocytes. Glia 24: 50-64.

Gilbert P, Kettenmann H, Schachner M (1984) gamma-Aminobutyric acid directly depolarizes cultured oligodendrocytes. J Neurosci 4: 561-569.

Goghari V, Franciosi S, Kim SU, Lee YB, McLarnon JG (2000) Acute application of interleukin-1beta induces Ca(2+) responses in human microglia. Neurosci Lett 281: 83-86.

Golovina VA, Bambrick LL, Yarowsky PJ, Krueger BK, Blaustein MP (1996) Modulation of two functionally distinct Ca2+ stores in astrocytes: role of the plasmalemmal Na/Ca exchanger. Glia 16: 296-305.

Golovina VA, Blaustein MP (2000) Unloading and refilling of two classes of spatially resolved endoplasmic reticulum Ca(2+) stores in astrocytes. Glia 31: 15-28.

Grosche J, Kettenmann H, Reichenbach A (2002) Bergmann glial cells form distinct morphological structures to interact with cerebellar neurons. J Neurosci Res 68: 138-149.

Grosche J, Matyash V, Moller T, Verkhratsky A, Reichenbach A, Kettenmann H (1999) Microdomains for neuron-glia interaction: parallel fiber signaling to Bergmann glial cells. Nat Neurosci 2: 139-143.

Guthrie PB, Knappenberger J, Segal M, Bennett MVL, Charles AC, Kater SB (1999) ATP released from astrocytes mediates glial calcium waves. J Neurosci 19: 520-528.

Haak LL, Grimaldi M, Smaili SS, Russell JT (2002) Mitochondria regulate Ca2+ wave initiation and inositol trisphosphate signal transduction in oligodendrocyte progenitors. J Neurochem 80: 405-415.

Haak LL, Song LS, Molinski TF, Pessah IN, Cheng H, Russell JT (2001) Sparks and puffs in oligodendrocyte progenitors: cross talk between ryanodine receptors and inositol trisphosphate receptors. 21: 3860-3870.

Haas S, Brockhaus J, Verkhratsky A, Kettenmann H (1996) ATP-induced membrane currents in ameboid microglia acutely isolated from mouse brain slices. Neuroscience 75: 257-261.

Hahn J, Jung W, Kim N, Uhm DY, Chung S (2000) Characterization and regulation of rat microglial Ca(2+) release-activated Ca(2+) (CRAC) channel by protein kinases. Glia 31: 118-124.

Hegg CC, Hu S, Peterson PK, Thayer SA (2000) Beta-chemokines and human immunodeficiency virus type-1 proteins evoke intracellular calcium increases in human microglia. Neuroscience 98: 191-199.

Hide I, Tanaka M, Inoue A, Nakajima K, Kohsaka S, Inoue K, Nakata Y (2000) Extracellular ATP triggers tumor necrosis factor-alpha release from rat microglia. J Neurochem 75: 965-972.

Hoffmann A, Kann O, Ohlemeyer C, Hanisch UK, Kettenmann H (2003) Elevation of basal intracellular calcium as a central element in the activation of brain macrophages (microglia): suppression of receptor-evoked calcium signaling and control of release function. J Neurosci 23: 4410-4419.

Iino M, Goto K, Kakegawa W, Okado H, Sudo M, Ishiuchi S, Miwa A, Takayasu Y, Saito I, Tsuzuki K, Ozawa S (2001) Glia-synapse interaction through Ca2+-permeable AMPA receptors in Bergmann glia. Science 292: 926-929.

Innocenti B, Parpura V, Haydon PG (2000) Imaging extracellular waves of glutamate during calcium signaling in cultured astrocytes. J Neurosci 20: 1800-1808.

Inoue K, Nakajima K, Morimoto T, Kikuchi Y, Koizumi S, Illes P, Kohsaka S (1998) ATP stimulation of Ca2+ -dependent plasminogen release from cultured microglia. Br J Pharmacol 123: 1304-1310.

Itoh T, Beesley J, Itoh A, Cohen AS, Kavanaugh B, Coulter DA, Grinspan JB, Pleasure D (2002) AMPA glutamate receptor-mediated calcium signaling is transiently enhanced during development of oligodendrocytes. J Neurochem 81: 390-402.

Jeftinija S, Jeftinija K, Stefanovic G (1997) Cultured astrocytes express proteins involved in vesicular glutamate release. Brain Res. 750:41-47.

Jimenez AI, Castro E, Mirabet M, Franco R, Delicado EG, Miras-Portugal MT (1999) Potentiation of ATP calcium responses by A2B receptor stimulation and other signals coupled to Gs proteins in type-1 cerebellar astrocytes. Glia 26: 119-128.

John GR, Scemes E, Suadicani SO, Liu JS, Charles PC, Lee SC, Spray DC, Brosnan CF (1999) IL-1beta differentially regulates calcium wave propagation between primary human fetal astrocytes via pathways involving P2 receptors and gap junction channels. Proc Natl Acad Sci U S A 96: 11613-11618.

Kang J, Jiang L, Goldman SA, Nedergaard M (1998) Astrocyte-mediated potentiation of inhibitory synaptic transmission. Nat Neurosci 1: 683-692.

Kaya N, Tanaka S, Koike T (2002) ATP selectively suppresses the synthesis of the inflammatory protein microglial response factor (MRF)-1 through Ca(2+) influx via P2X(7) receptors in cultured microglia. Brain Res 952: 86-97.

Kettenmann H, Blankenfeld GV, Trotter J (1991) Physiological properties of oligodendrocytes during development. Ann N Y Acad Sci 633: 64-77.

Kettenmann H, Orkand RK, Lux HD (1984) Some properties of single potassium channels in cultured oligodendrocytes. Pflugers Arch 400: 215-221.

Kirchhoff F, Kettenmann H (1992) GABA Triggers a [Ca2+]i Increase in Murine Precursor Cells of the Oligodendrocyte Lineage. Eur J Neurosci 4: 1049-1058.

Kirischuk S, Kirchhoff F, Matyash V, Kettenmann H, Verkhratsky A (1999) Glutamate-triggered calcium signaling in mouse bergmann glial cells in situ: role of inositol-1,4,5-trisphosphate-mediated intracellular calcium release. Neuroscience 92: 1051-1059.

Kirischuk S, Neuhaus J, Verkhratsky A, Kettenmann H (1995a) Preferential localization of active mitochondria in process tips of immature retinal oligodendrocytes. Neuroreport 6: 737-741.

Kirischuk S, Scherer J, Kettenmann H, Verkhratsky A (1995b) Activation of P2-purinoreceptors triggered Ca2+ release from InsP3-sensitive internal stores in mammalian oligodendrocytes. J Physiol 483 (Pt 1): 41-57.

Kirischuk S, Tuschick S, Verkhratsky A, Kettenmann H (1996) Calcium signaling in mouse Bergmann glial cells mediated by alpha1-adrenoreceptors and H1 histamine receptors. Eur J Neurosci 8: 1198-1208.

Koller H, Trimborn M, von Giesen H, Schroeter M, Arendt G (2001) TNFalpha reduces glutamate induced intracellular Ca(2+) increase in cultured cortical astrocytes. Brain Res 893: 237-243.

Latour I, Hamid J, Beedle AM, Zamponi GW, MacVicar BA (2003) Expression of voltage-gated Ca2+ channel subtypes in cultured astrocytes. Glia 41: 347-353.

Leybaert L, Paemeleire K, Strahonja A, Sanderson MJ (1998) Inositol-trisphosphate-dependent intercellular calcium signaling in and between astrocytes and endothelial cells. Glia 24: 398-407.

Luyt K, Varadi A, Molnar E (2003) Functional metabotropic glutamate receptors are expressed in oligodendrocyte progenitor cells. J Neurochem 84: 1452-1464.

MacVicar BA (1984) Voltage-dependent calcium channels in glial cells. Science 226: 1345-1347.

Matyash M, Matyash V, Nolte C, Sorrentino V, Kettenmann H (2002) Requirement of functional ryanodine receptor type 3 for astrocyte migration. FASEB J 16: 84-86.

Matyash V, Filippov V, Mohrhagen K, Kettenmann H (2001) Nitric oxide signals parallel fiber activity to Bergmann glial cells in the mouse cerebellar slice. Mol Cell Neurosci 18: 664-670.

McLarnon JG, Franciosi S, Wang X, Bae JH, Choi HB, Kim SU (2001) Acute actions of tumor necrosis factor-alpha on intracellular $Ca(2+)$ and $K(+)$ currents in human microglia. Neuroscience 104: 1175-1184.

Minelli A, Lyons S, Nolte C, Verkhratsky A, Kettenmann H (2000) Ammonium triggers calcium elevation in cultured mouse microglial cells by initiating $Ca(2+)$ release from thapsigargin-sensitive intracellular stores. Pflugers Arch 439: 370-377.

Moller T, Contos JJ, Musante DB, Chun J, Ransom BR (2001) Expression and function of lysophosphatidic acid receptors in cultured rodent microglial cells. J Biol Chem 276: 25946-25952.

Moller T, Hanisch UK, Ransom BR (2000) Thrombin-induced activation of cultured rodent microglia. J Neurochem 75: 1539-1547.

Moller T, Kann O, Prinz M, Kirchhoff F, Verkhratsky A, Kettenmann H (1997a) Endothelin-induced calcium signaling in cultured mouse microglial cells is mediated through ETB receptors. Neuroreport 8: 2127-2131.

Moller T, Nolte C, Burger R, Verkhratsky A, Kettenmann H (1997b) Mechanisms of C5a and C3a complement fragment-induced $[Ca2+]i$ signaling in mouse microglia. J Neurosci 17: 615-624.

Moorman SJ (1996) The inhibition of motility that results from contact between two oligodendrocytes in vitro can be blocked by pertussis toxin. Glia 16: 257-265.

Muller T, Moller T, Berger T, Schnitzer J, Kettenmann H (1992) Calcium entry through kainate receptors and resulting potassium-channel blockade in Bergmann glial cells. Science 256: 1563-1566.

Muller T, Moller T, Neuhaus J, Kettenmann H (1996) Electrical coupling among Bergmann glial cells and its modulation by glutamate receptor activation. Glia 17: 274-284.

Nett WJ, Oloff SH, McCarthy KD (2002) Hippocampal astrocytes in situ exhibit calcium oscillations that occur independent of neuronal activity. J Neurophysiol 87: 528-537.

Newman EA (2001) Propagation of intercellular calcium waves in retinal astrocytes and Muller cells. J Neurosci 21: 2215-2223.

Newman EA, Zahs KR (1997) Calcium waves in retinal glial cells. Science 275: 844-847.

Noda M, Nakanishi H, Nabekura J, Akaike N (2000) AMPA-kainate subtypes of glutamate receptor in rat cerebral microglia. J Neurosci 20: 251-258.

Nolte C, Moller T, Walter T, Kettenmann H (1996) Complement 5a controls motility of murine microglial cells in vitro via activation of an inhibitory G-protein and the rearrangement of the actin cytoskeleton. Neuroscience 73: 1091-1107.

Paemeleire K, Leybaert L (2000) ATP-dependent astrocyte-endothelial calcium signaling following mechanical damage to a single astrocyte in astrocyte-endothelial co-cultures. J Neurotrauma 17: 345-358.

Parpura V, Basarsky TA, Liu F, Jeftinija K, Jeftinija S, Haydon PG (1994) Glutamate-mediated astrocyte-neuron signaling. Nature 369:744-747.

Parri HR, Gould TM, Crunelli V (2001) Spontaneous astrocytic $Ca2+$ oscillations in situ drive NMDAR-mediated neuronal excitation. Nat Neurosci 4: 803-812.

Pasti L, Zonta M, Pozzan T, Vicini S, Carmignoto G (2001) Cytosolic calcium oscillations in astrocytes may regulate exocytotic release of glutamate. J Neurosci 21: 477-484.

Pende M, Holtzclaw LA, Curtis JL, Russell JT, Gallo V (1994) Glutamate regulates intracellular calcium and gene expression in oligodendrocyte progenitors through the activation of DL-alpha-amino-3-hydroxy-5-methyl-4-isoxazolepropionic acid receptors. Proc Natl Acad Sci U S A 91: 3215-3219.

Pizzo P, Burgo A, Pozzan T, Fasolato C (2001) Role of capacitative calcium entry on glutamate-induced calcium influx in type-I rat cortical astrocytes. J Neurochem 79: 98-109.

Rappert A, Biber K, Nolte C, Lipp M, Schubel A, Lu B, Gerard NP, Gerard C, Boddeke HW, Kettenmann H (2002) Secondary lymphoid tissue chemokine (CCL21) activates CXCR3 to trigger a Cl- current and chemotaxis in murine microglia. J Immunol 168: 3221-3226.

Rogers SW, Gregori NZ, Carlson N, Gahring LC, Noble M (2001) Neuronal nicotinic acetylcholine receptor expression by O2A/oligodendrocyte progenitor cells. Glia 33: 306-313.

Sanchez-Gomez MV, Matute C (1999) AMPA and kainate receptors each mediate excitotoxicity in oligodendroglial cultures. Neurobiol Dis 6: 475-485.

Sayah S, Jauneau AC, Patte C, Tonon MC, Vaudry H, Fontaine M (2003) Two different transduction pathways are activated by C3a and C5a anaphylatoxins on astrocytes. Brain Res Mol Brain Res 112: 53-60.

Scemes E, Suadicani SO, Spray DC (2000) Intercellular communication in spinal cord astrocytes: fine tuning between gap junctions and P2 nucleotide receptors in calcium wave propagation. J Neurosci 20: 1435-1445.

Schilling T, Repp H, Richter H, Koschinski A, Heinemann U, Dreyer F, Eder C (2002) Lysophospholipids induce membrane hyperpolarization in microglia by activation of IKCa1 Ca(2+)-dependent K(+) channels. Neuroscience 109: 827-835.

Schipke CG, Boucsein C, Ohlemeyer C, Kirchhoff F, Kettenmann H (2002) Astrocyte Ca2+ waves trigger responses in microglial cells in brain slices. FASEB J 16: 255-257.

Schipke CG, Ohlemeyer C, Matyash M, Nolte C, Kettenmann H, Kirchhoff F (2001) Astrocytes of the mouse neocortex express functional N-methyl-D- aspartate receptors. FASEB J 15: 1270-1272.

Shelton MK, McCarthy KD (2000) Hippocampal astrocytes exhibit Ca2+-elevating muscarinic cholinergic and histaminergic receptors in situ. J Neurochem 74: 555-563.

Simpson PB, Mehotra S, Lange GD, Russell JT (1997) High density distribution of endoplasmic reticulum proteins and mitochondria at specialized Ca2+ release sites in oligodendrocyte processes. J Biol Chem 272: 22654-22661.

Simpson PB, Russell JT (1996) Mitochondria support inositol 1,4,5-trisphosphate-mediated Ca2+ waves in cultured oligodendrocytes. J Biol Chem 271: 33493-33501.

Simpson PB, Russell JT (1997) Role of sarcoplasmic/endoplasmic-reticulum Ca2+-ATPases in mediating Ca2+ waves and local Ca2+-release microdomains in cultured glia. Biochem J 325 (Pt 1): 239-247.

Simpson PB, Russell JT (1998) Mitochondrial Ca2+ uptake and release influence metabotropic and ionotropic cytosolic Ca2+ responses in rat oligodendrocyte progenitors. J Physiol 508 (Pt 2): 413-426.

Steiner MR, Urso JR, Klein J, Steiner SM (2002) Multiple astrocyte responses to lysophosphatidic acids. Biochim Biophys Acta 1582: 154-160.

Stephens GJ, Marriott DR, Djamgoz MB, Wilkin GP (1993) Electrophysiological and biochemical evidence for bradykinin receptors on cultured rat cortical oligodendrocytes. Neurosci Lett 153: 223-226.

Stout CE, Costantin JL, Naus CC, Charles AC (2002) Intercellular calcium signaling in astrocytes via ATP release through connexin hemichannels. J Biol Chem 277: 10482-10488.

Suadicani SO, Pina-Benabou MH, Urban-Maldonado M, Spray DC, Scemes E (2003) Acute downregulation of Cx43 alters P2Y receptor expression levels in mouse spinal cord astrocytes. Glia 42: 160-171.

Tabuchi S, Kume K, Aihara M, Shimizu T (2000) Expression of lysophosphatidic acid receptor in rat astrocytes: mitogenic effect and expression of neurotrophic genes. Neurochem Res 25: 573-582.

Takeda M, Nelson DJ, Soliven B (1995) Calcium signaling in cultured rat oligodendrocytes. Glia 14: 225-236.

Toescu EC, Moller T, Kettenmann H, Verkhratsky A (1998) Long-term activation of capacitative Ca2+ entry in mouse microglial cells. Neuroscience 86: 925-935.

Toms NJ, Roberts PJ (1999) Group 1 mGlu receptors elevate [Ca2+]i in rat cultured cortical type 2 astrocytes: [Ca2+]i synergy with adenosine A1 receptors. Neuropharmacology 38: 1511-1517.

Tuschick S, Kirischuk S, Kirchhoff F, Liefeldt L, Paul M, Verkhratsky A, Kettenmann H (1997) Bergmann glial cells in situ express endothelinB receptors linked to cytoplasmic calcium signals. Cell Calcium 21: 409-419.

Venance L, Premont J, Glowinski J, Giaume C (1998) Gap junctional communication and pharmacological heterogeneity in astrocytes cultured from the rat striatum. J Physiol 510 (Pt 2): 429-440.

Verderio C, Bruzzone S, Zocchi E, Fedele E, Schenk U, De Flora A, Matteoli M (2001) Evidence of a role for cyclic ADP-ribose in calcium signaling and neurotransmitter release in cultured astrocytes. J Neurochem 78: 646-657.

Verderio C, Matteoli M (2001) Atp mediates calcium signaling between astrocytes and microglial cells: modulation by ifn-gamma. J Immunol 166: 6383-6391.

Verkhratsky AN, Trotter J, Kettenmann H (1990) Cultured glial precursor cells from mouse cortex express two types of calcium currents. Neurosci Lett 112: 194-198.

Walz W, Gimpl G, Ohlemeyer C, Kettenmann H (1994) Extracellular ATP-induced currents in astrocytes: involvement of a cation channel. J Neurosci Res 38: 12-18.

Walz W, Ilschner S, Ohlemeyer C, Banati R, Kettenmann H (1993) Extracellular ATP activates a cation conductance and a K+ conductance in cultured microglial cells from mouse brain. J Neurosci 13: 4403-4411.

Wang Z, Haydon PG, Yeung ES (2000) Direct observation of calcium-independent intercellular ATP signaling in astrocytes. Anal Chem 72: 2001-2007.

Whittemore ER, Korotzer AR, Etebari A, Cotman CW (1993) Carbachol increases intracellular free calcium in cultured rat microglia. Brain Res 59-64.

Wisden W, Seeburg PH (1993) Mammalian ionotropic glutamate receptors. Curr Opin Neurobiol 3: 291-298.

Ye ZC, Wyeth MS, Baltan-Tekkok S, Ransom BR (2003) Functional hemichannels in astrocytes: a novel mechanism of glutamate release. J Neurosci 23: 3588-3596.

Zhang L, McLarnon JG, Goghari V, Lee YB, Kim SU, Krieger C (1998) Cholinergic agonists increase intracellular Ca2+ in cultured human microglia. Neurosci Lett 255: 33-36.

Zonta M, Angulo MC, Gobbo S, Rosengarten B, Hossmann KA, Pozzan T, Carmignoto G (2003) Neuron-to-astrocyte signaling is central to the dynamic control of brain microcirculation. Nat Neurosci 6: 43-50.

12.5. Abbreviations

trans-ACPD	$(1S,3R)$-1-Aminocyclopentane-1,3-dicarboxylic acid
AMPA (R)	α-amino-3-hydroxy-5-methyl-4-isoxazole propionate (receptor)
BAPTA	1,2-*bis*-(o-minophenoxy)ethanie-N,N,N',N'-tetraacetic acid
C5a, C3a	Complement factor 5a, etc.
$[Ca^{2+}]_i$	Cytosolic free calcium concentration
CaSR	Calcium sensing receptor
CCL21	Chemokine CCL21
CCR	Chemokine receptor binding CC type chemokines
CNS	Central nervous system
CRAC	Calcium release activated channel
Cx	Connexins, various gap junction proteins
CXCR	Chemokine receptor binding CXC type chemokines
ET	Endothelin
GABA	γ-amino butyric acid
$GABA_ARs$	$GABA_A$ receptors
GluRs	Glutamate receptors
mGluRs	Metabotropic glutamate receptors
gp120	HIV envelop glycoprotein 120
IFN-γ	Interferon gamma

IL	Interleukin
InsP$_3$(R)	Inositol trisphosphate (receptor)
LPA	Lysophosphatidic acid
LPS	Lipopolysaccharide
MIP	Macrophage inflammatory protein
MRF	microglial response factor
NE	Norepinephrine
NMDA(R)	N-methyl-D-aspartate receptors
NO	Nitric oxide
PAR	Protease activated receptor
PTX	Pertussis toxin
TNFα	Tumor necrosis factor alpha
TTX	Tetrodotoxin

Chapter 13

Astrocyte gap junctions and glutamate-induced neurotoxicity

Christian Giaume*, William Même and Annette Koulakoff

INSERM U114, Collège de France, 11 Place Marcelin Berthelot 75005 Paris, France

*Corresponding author: christian.giaume@college-de-france.fr

Contents

13.1. Introduction

In brain, gap junctions are widely expressed in various cell types including neurons and glial cells. They are present between neurons at electrical synapses (Bennett, 1977) and provide the intercellular pathway for astrocytic networks (Giaume and McCarthy, 1996). We have recently reviewed the expression of gap junctions in the central nervous system and discussed their physiopathological relevance in several brain dysfunctions (Rouach et al., 2002b). In the present chapter, we focus on the expression and function of connexins (Cxs) in a major glial cell population, the astrocytes, that outnumber neurons and make up about 50% of human brain volume (Tower and Young, 1973). Data indicating that astrocytic connexins represent an identified target of neuroglial and glial-glial interactions and that changes in their properties and/or their pattern of expression may be relevant in physiopathological situations are described. With that objective, we concentrate on the role of glutamate, which plays a key role in neurotoxic processes, and as a working hypothesis we discuss the potential contribution of astrocyte gap junctional communication (GJC) in the homeostasis of this excitatory amino acid.

13.2. Connexins are the molecular constituents of intercellular channels at gap junctions

13.2.1. From connexins to gap junctions

In most tissues, intercellular channels localized at specialized membrane areas, termed gap junctions, provide the morphological basis for direct electrical and biochemical communication between adjacent cells, defining ionic and metabolic cell-to-cell coupling. A full gap junction channel spans two neighboring plasma membranes and is formed by the alignment of two hemi-channels, or connexons, that interact in the extracellular space and constitute a relatively large hydrated pore between the cytoplasm of coupled cells (Bennett et al., 1991; Bruzzone et al., 1996). Each connexon is a hexamer composed of subunit proteins, Cxs, which form a multigenic family whose members are defined and named according to their predicted molecular mass in kDa. Cxs are tetraspan membrane proteins with a topology characterized by cytoplasmic amino and carboxyl termini and a cytoplasmic loop intercalated between the second and third transmembrane domains. In addition, two extracellular loops allow the docking between facing Cxs borne by the adjacent membranes (Fig. 13.1A). So far, up to 20 Cxs have been identified in human or mouse based on genomic analysis, and orthologues are increasingly characterized in other vertebrates (Willecke et al., 2002). It has now been clearly demonstrated that most cells express multiple Cx isoforms, consequently a connexon can be built up by one or several Cxs forming homotypic or heterotypic connexons (Fig. 13.1B). In addition, an intercellular channel can assemble different types of connexons and contribute to the formation of either homotypic, heterotypic, or heteromeric channels (Fig. 13.1C).

13.2.2. Regulation of gap junction-mediated intercellular communication

As expected, the pattern of connexin expression in a specific cell type at a defined developmental stage results from regulation occurring at different levels (genomic, transcriptional, degradation and recycling). In addition, based on the charge and size selectivity defined by each Cx, the nature and the dynamics of the intercellular message exchanged between two cells through gap junction channels may vary. Indeed, it is expected that Cxs "speak a coded language" and have evolved diverse forms of intercellular communication among cells (Bruzzone and Giaume, 1999). First, channels composed of different Cxs are endowed with distinct biophysical and regulatory properties (Harris, 2001). Although Cxs do not form ion-selective channels in the classical sense, they exhibit a defined profile of selectivity for cations and anions (Veenstra, 2001). In addition, because gap junction channels are permeable to signaling molecules, channel selectivity may allow the discrimination and modulation of intercellular exchanges of second messengers and metabolites. Second, compatibility profiles have been established for number of Cxs (Bukauskas, 2001). They refer to the ability of Cxs to functionally interact with other members of the Cx family. Indeed, the relative homology in the primary sequences of extracellular loops has initially suggested that the formation of heterotypic channels would be favored. However, experimental data have shown that the establishment of functional gap junction channels depends on the ability of Cxs to discriminate between different partners. A consequence of this property is that the expression of different Cxs in a group of cells may provide a powerful means to determine cellular compartments in cellular groups of cells. Third, intercellular communication is also dictated by both covalent and non-covalent modifications of Cxs that affect the channel structure and gating properties. The combination of these three classes of channel properties (selectivity, compatibility, gating) demonstrates that the nature and the level of intercellular communication are highly dependent on the identity of the molecular constituents and give sense to the diversity of Cxs.

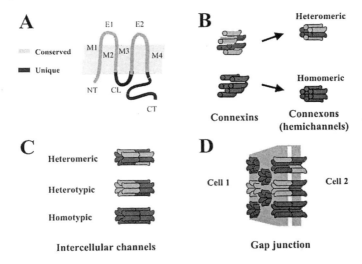

Figure 13.1. Connexins, connexons, intercellular channels and gap junctions. A. Membrane topology of a generic connexin (Cx) with four transmembrane domains (M1-M4), two extracellular loops (E1 and E2) and three cytoplasmic portions (amino terminal: NT; cytoplasmic loop, CL; carboxyl terminal, CT). B. Six Cxs oligomerize into connexons that can be either homomeric, if they contain one Cx type, or heteromeric, if multiple Cxs are assembled. C. Two connexons interact and align to form complete intercellular channels that can be heteromeric, heterotypic or homotypic. D. Cx channels cluster in specialized domains of the plasma membrane called gap junctions. Modified from (Bruzzone and Giaume, 1999).

13.2.3. Proteins associated with connexins

Cx channels have been considered for a long time as simple cell-to-cell channels with little interaction with other cellular constituents. Recently, the concept of a tight interaction of Cxs with protein scaffolding has emerged. Indeed, as other ionic channels or membrane receptors, Cx proteins interact with other cellular components and appear to be linked into a macromolecular domain, the Nexus complex (Spray et al., 1999; Duffy et al., 2002). Since the cytoplasmic amino terminal greatly varies between Cxs it is expected that Nexus components also vary. Among the different Cxs, the association of Cx43 with other proteins has been documented and a rather extended list of protein partners is available. For instance, zonula occludens-1, adherens junction associated protein β-catenin, tubulin and proto-ontogenic signaling protein Src have now been described to interact with Cx43 (Kanemitsu et al., 1997; Giepmans and Moolenaar, 1998; Toyofuku et al., 1998; Giepmans et al., 2001). Moreover, cholesterol-sphingolipid-rich micro domains working as membrane rafts involved in membrane trafficking and signal transduction have been reported to be associated with Cxs. Indeed, Cx43 co-localizes and interacts with calveolin-1, an integral raft protein (Schubert et al., 2002). Accordingly, structural and functional changes in gap junctions may depend on alteration in the affinities of protein-protein interactions involving Cx scaffolding partners. The cytoplasmic loop and carboxyl terminal domains confer most of the diversity among connexin subtypes. The occurrence of these variations that contain known signaling domains suggest that these two regions may be important in differential connexin function that could involve variation in protein-protein interactions (see Duffy et al., 2002).

13.2.4. Connexin hemichannels

Increasing evidence indicates that Cxs form not only full intercellular channels (Fig. 13.1D) but also functional hemichannels, or connexons, which can be open in defined conditions. Because connexons in non-junctional membranes were thought to share properties with those of intercellular channels it has been assumed that they were closed in normal conditions to prevent massive calcium influx or loss of cellular contents such as small metabolites. However, increasing evidence exists that several cell types exhibit opening of endogenous hemichannels induced by strong depolarization and/or bathing in low Ca^{2+} solutions (DeVries and Schwartz, 1992; O'Brien et al., 1998; Quist et al., 2000; Bruzzone et al., 2001; Romanello et al., 2001). Moreover, opening of hemichannels in response to metabolic inhibition was also described and was thought to contribute to cell death after ischemia in myocytes (Kondo et al., 2000) and astrocytes (Contreras et al., 2002). These observations indicate that the function of Cxs is not restricted to intercellular communication and that in particular conditions, e.g. pathological situations, they might be involved in cell permeation of low molecular weight signaling molecules.

13.3. Connexins and gap junction expression in glia

13.3.1. Distribution

The initial concept of a syncytial organization of glial cells proposed by Mugnaini was based on the observation at the ultrastructural level of numerous gap junctions linking astrocytes to astrocytes, as well as to oligodendrocytes and ependymal cells in white matter regions of the mammalian central nervous system (CNS) (Massa and Mugnaini, 1982; Mugnaini, 1986). This network of communicating cells has now been visualized in slices from different cerebral areas (hippocampus, striatum, cerebellum, cortex), after injection in a single astrocyte of low molecular weight tracer known to diffuse through gap junctions (Binmoller and Muller, 1992; Konietzko and Muller, 1994; Muller et al., 1996; D'Ambrosio et al., 1998). Ten to hundreds of dye-stained cells are thus revealed in a large area surrounding the injected cell; most of them (> 70%) are glial fibrillary acidic protein (GFAP)-positive astrocytes, as shown by immunocytochemical labeling. Indeed, the majority of astrocytic GJ is homologous, i.e. formed between contiguous astrocytes, and represent the structural basis of the organization of astrocytes in groups of cells able to cross-talk. Heterologous gap junctions between astrocytes and other cellular partners have also been described using several experimental approaches. Gap junctional coupling between astrocytes and oligodendrocytes is well documented and was observed in culture as well as *in vivo* (Zahs, 1998). Interestingly, the majority of GJ in oligodendrocytes are heterologous, with astrocyte as the second partner (Rash et al., 2001a). As these two cell types do not express the same repertoire of Cxs, GJ between astrocytes and oligodendrocytes are formed by hemi-channels containing different Cxs which may account for unidirectional intercellular coupling pathways (Robinson et al., 1993; Rash et al., 1997). The presence of GJ between astrocytes and neurons has also been reported in different situations. During development, there are several pieces of evidence indicating the presence of dye and/or electrical coupling between astrocytes and neurons in slices from cerebral tissue of young animals (P3 – P14) (Alvarez-Maubecin et al., 2000; Bittman et al., 2002) and between Purkinje cells and Bergmann glia in cerebellar slices from P14-P21 (Pakhotin and Verkhratsky, 2003). Such heterologous coupling was also shown in co-cultures of neurons and astrocytes raised from embryonic or newborn rat brain hemispheres (Froes et al., 1999) or human fetal hippocampus (Rozental et al., 2001b). In general, when an astrocyte was injected with Lucifer Yellow, dye transfer to neuron was frequently observed (in about 50% of cases), in addition to the extensive dye spreading to neighboring astrocytes. Dye loading of neurons led also to dye diffusion into astrocytes, although less frequently. However, in most cases, electrical coupling was found to be bidirectional. Interestingly, Froes et al. (1999) have observed that astrocyte-neuron coupling was transient and declined rapidly with neuronal maturation. Hence, this heterocellular coupling may be restricted to specific periods of development when direct exchanges of signaling molecules or metabolites might be important for neuronal maturation. The persistence of neuron-astrocyte coupling in the adult remains an open question although no evidence of gap junctions between these two cell types was found in an ultrastructural analysis using immunogold labeling on freeze-fracture replica (Rash et al., 2001b).

Gap junctions may also be formed between processes and lamellae of the same astrocyte, as shown at the ultrastructural level in the adult rat visual cortex (Rohlmann and Wolff, 1996). These reflexive gap junctions may represent up to a quarter of the gap junctions expressed by an astrocyte. Such reflexive gap junctions have also been described in astrocytes cultured at a low density so that most of them are "solitary" cells devoid of intercellular contacts (Wolff et al., 1998). It is noteworthy that they are found in close association with "mechanical" junctions connecting surface membranes and cytoskeletal elements. Although their function has not been unraveled, it has been hypothesized that they may contribute to the formation of microdomains which, may function independently of the soma. Such independent compartments may fulfill local, specific tasks in particular locations, e.g. in the astrocytic endfeet surrounding blood vessels where gap junctions are noticeably dense or in the processes enwrapping synapses (Giaume and McCarthy, 1996; Rohlmann and Wolff,1996).

Advances in the characterization of new members of the Cx family and availability of specific tools to identify them allowed investigation of the molecular composition of astrocytic gap junctions. As stated above, none of the Cxs are cell-specific, however, a given cell type expresses a set of specific Cxs. In the adult brain, astrocytic gap junctions are mainly composed of different combinations of Cx43, Cx30 and Cx26. All of them were unambiguously detected in adult rat brain and ultrastructurally identified as astrocytic gap junctions using immunogold labeling on freeze-fracture replica (Nagy and Rash, 2000). Their expression is differentially regulated during development and displays distinct regional distribution (reviewed in Nagy and Rash, 2000; Rouach et al., 2002b). Briefly, Cx43 appears early in the embryonic brain after neural tube closure and is detected in radial glial processes (Nadarajah et al., 1997). Its level increases during prenatal development, peaks at birth and the immunoreactive punctuate staining characteristic of the adult pattern is reached at different post-natal stages according to the functional maturation of the various brain areas, most often during the second postnatal week. The second major astrocytic Cx, Cx30, has a delayed onset of appearance: its mRNA becomes detectable in astrocytes during the second week of post-natal development in the rat (Dahl et al., 1996; Condorelli et al., 2002) while the protein expression was first detected at P16, reached a peak during the 4th PN week to remain at high levels during adulthood (Kunzelmann et al., 1999). In the adult, both Cx43 and Cx30 have a widespread distribution in grey matter astrocytes, with quantitative regional differences (Nagy et al., 1999). In contrast, white matter astrocytes do express Cx43 but lack Cx30. Finally, Cx26 is the least represented and appears restricted to subpopulations of astrocytes (Mercier and Hatton, 2001; Nagy et al., 2001). This pairing of identical or different Cxs in astrocytic GJ may confer their distinct coupling properties, thus allowing differential regulation of permeability in specific locations according to their Cx content.

13.3.2. Permeability properties

An important question concerning the role of gap junctions between astrocytes is the identification of the signals that are exchanged through this intercellular pathway. Since the permeability profile of Cx channels depends on their molecular constituents (Elfgang et al., 1995; Niessen et al., 2000), it is expected that the amount and the nature of ions or signaling molecules permeating astrocyte gap junctions are directly related to their identity. As described above, diversity of Cx expression in astrocytes suggests that intercellular exchanges are likely dependent on several types of gap junctional channels made by these Cxs. Although essential, up to now such a question was very difficult to address in situ due to technical limitations. However, the situation is much more favorable in vitro, since most gap junction channels in cultured astrocytes are made up of Cx43 as demonstrated by quantitative analysis showing that 95% of the electrical coupling is lacking in astrocytes of Cx43 knock-out mice (Scemes et al., 1998). Accordingly, cultured astrocytes have been used to determine which ions and signaling molecules can be exchanged between adjacent astrocytes through open Cx43 channels.

Although Cx43 channels are poorly selective for ions, double patch-clamp recordings have established that they favor the passage of cations versus anions (Beblo and Veenstra, 1997). Since astrocytes have been proposed to contribute to the ionic homeostasis of the extracellular medium the permeability of gap junctions have been proposed to contribute to this process in particular for K^+ (Ransom, 1995). Several studies have demonstrated that GJC are also involved in the intercellular homeostasis of Na^+ (Rose and Ransom, 1997) and Ca^{2+} (Venance et al., 1998). Besides ionic coupling, in these electrically inexcitable glial cells the role of gap junctions is likely to be even more critical in biochemical coupling. Indeed, there is now converging evidence indicating that intercellular exchange of signaling molecules occurs in cultured astrocytes and in glioma cell lines transfected with Cx43 (Table 13.1). From these works several potential implications of gap junctions in astrocytes functions can be proposed. First, the demonstration of the permeability of astrocytes gap junctions for inositol-1,4,5-trisphosphate (IP_3) (Leybaert and Sanderson, 2001) provides an argument in favor of their involvement in the propagation of intercellular calcium waves. Indeed, besides an extracellular component that is due to ATP release (Guthrie et al., 1999), an intercellular route through gap junction channels has been proposed to contribute to this calcium signaling process in which IP_3 plays a critical role (Venance et al., 1997; Hofer et al., 2002). Second, the permeability of astrocyte gap junctions to glucose and its metabolites, including lactate, indicates that this intercellular pathway may participate to metabolic trafficking between the source of energetic substrates and the main site of energy consumption, respectively, the blood circulation and neurons (Giaume et al., 1997). Third, transfection of C6 cells with Cx43 has allowed the demonstration that several nucleotides, in particular ATP and ADP, can be transferred through Cx43 channels (Goldberg et al., 1999; Goldberg et al., 2002). This observation indicates that junctional channels may contribute to the distribution of cellular metabolites and maintenance of the energy status over a glial cell population. Fourth, glutamate and glutamine were also shown to permeate Cx43 channels in astrocytes and in C6 cells (Tabernero et al., 1996; Goldberg et al., 1999; Goldberg et al., 2002). These observations are particularly relevant since after release from glutamatergic neurons, the neurotransmitter is rapidly inactivated by cellular uptake predominantly into astrocytes (Pellerin and Magistretti, 1994; Bergles and Jahr, 1998). Glutamate is then amidated to glutamine by the ATP-consuming reaction catalyzed by glutamine synthetase, an enzyme present in astrocytes but not in neurons. Glutamine is then released by astrocytes and taken up by neurons where its hydrolysis provides glutamate. Consequently, the regeneration of this neurotransmitter should not solely be considered as the result of the contribution of isolated and independent astrocytes but rather as groups of communicating astrocytes that can exchange glutamate and glutamine. As discussed below, permeability for this excitatory amino acid may play an important role in the interaction between astrocytes and neurons. Finally, gap junction channels in astrocytes were shown to propagate and amplify cell injury by allowing intercellular diffusion of death signals (Lin et al., 1998). Indeed, although overexpression of the human proto-oncogene bcl2 in C6 glioma cells increased their resistance to injury, the relative resistance of $bcl2^+$ cells to calcium overload, oxidative stress and metabolic inhibition was altered to that of more vulnerable cells, like $bcl2^-$ cells and astrocytes when they communicated via gap junctions. Through this pathway dying cells killed adjacent cells that would otherwise have escaped to injury. Although the nature of the death signals involved is not known, it has been proposed that such a process could account for the secondary propagation of brain injury, such as in cerebral ischemia (Lin et al., 1998).

Table 13.1. Permeability of gap junction channels to signaling molecules studied in astrocytes and C6 glioma cells transfected with Cx43

Cell models	Permeant molecules	Techniques	Block of gap junctional communication	References
Cultured cortical astrocytes	glucose glucose-6-phosphate lactate	SL/DT, radiolabeled compounds	octanol α−glycyrrhetinic acid arachidonic acid endothelin-1	Tabernero et al., 1996
Cultured cortical astrocytes	glutamate glutamine	SL/DT, radiolabeled compounds	octanol	Giaume et al., 1997
Cultured cortical astrocytes	inositol-trisphosphate	Calcium imaging	NT	Leybaert et al., 1998
C6 transfected with Cx43 Co-cultured with astrocytes	unidentified death signals	Cell viability (TUNEL) ATP cell content	Non transfected C6 cells	Lin et al., 1998
C6 transfected with Cx43	ADP, ATP glutathione glutamate	Capture of radiolabeled compounds	Non transfected C6 cells	Goldberg et al., 1999
C6 transfected with Cx43	ATP, ADP, AMP glutathione glutamate glucose	Layered culture system, radiolabeled compounds	Non transfected C6 cells	Goldberg et al., 2002

Abbreviations: SL\DT, scrape-loading/dye-transfer technique; TUNEL, Terminal deoxynucleotidyl transferase Uridine Nick End Labeling; NT, not tested; ADP, adenosine diphosphate; ATP, adenosine triphosphate; AMP adenosine monophosphate.

13.3.3. Modulation of gap junctional communication in astrocytes

GJC is controlled by external signals such as bioactive molecules released in normal as well as pathological situations. Indeed, this notion of a regulation of the amount and the extent of cell-to-cell communication supposes that the astrocytic network is not static, but rather dynamic. This demonstration was achieved by combining functional assays and immunodetection of astrocytic Cxs, mainly Cx43. Until now, most of the studies on the regulation of GJC have been conducted on primary cultures (for review see Rouach et al., 2002b). In the near future these findings should be tested in a more integrated situation since dye coupling between astrocytes studied from acute brain slices is reported to be extensive in several brain regions.

Like other classes of ionic membrane channels, gap junction channels are regulated on two temporal scales. One mechanism operates at the transcriptional level and represents a long-term regulation (hours and days) associated with changes in the number of junctional plaques and/or of channels per plaque. A second one, a short-term regulation (minutes) results from changes in the biophysical properties (opening-closing probabilities, duration of opening and unitary conductance) of channels already present at gap junctions. An exciting point is that Cx expression and GJC in astrocytes are targets for neurotransmitters, growth factors, peptides, cytokines and endogenous bioactive lipids indicating that astrocytic networks are subject to plasticity, controlled by products secreted by neurons as well as other brain cells types (astrocytes, microglia) and endothelial cells (for review see Rouach et al., 2002b). Besides the pharmacological demonstration of the regulation of GJC by exogenous application of different classes of compounds that act through the stimulation of membrane receptors and the activation of their associated signal transduction pathways, there are now several observations that point to more complex mechanisms. First, in human astrocytes pro-inflammatory treatment with IL-1β induces a reciprocal regulation of Cx43 and claudin-1, an integral membrane protein associated with the tight junction complex. The observation that gap and tight junctions proteins are inversely regulated indicates that claudin-1 may substitute for Cx43 at the scaffolding complex localized to astrocytes cell membranes in inflammatory situations (Duffy et al., 2000). Finally, treatments that are known to affect cytoskeletal elements such as aluminum, cytochalasin D or microinjection of anti-actin antibodies were reported to decrease Cx43 expression and GJC in cultured astrocytes (Theiss and Meller, 2002a, b; but see Cotrina et al., 1998a). Accordingly, the integrity of the cytoskeletal organization of intermediate filaments, GFAP and microfilaments (binding actin) seems to be fundamental for the translocation of Cxs from cytoplasmic compartments to cell membrane.

13.4. Characteristic of the glutamatergic system in astrocytes

Intracellular glutamate concentration ($[Glu]_i$) in astrocytes is estimated to be ~1 mM (Erecinska and Silver, 1990), a value that is somewhat lower than in neurons (10 mM) likely due to the activity of the glutamine synthetase. In contrast, the glutamate concentration in the extracellular space ($[Glu]_o$) is low and is maintained in the micromolar range (1-3 μM) in order to assure an efficient signal-to-noise ratio at glutamatergic synapses and to prevent excitotoxicity of neurons. This concentration gradient is maintained by uptake mechanisms of several subtypes of glutamate transporters expressed in both neurons and astrocytes. The latter have been shown to play a dominant role in the process of glutamate clearance in the vicinity of the synaptic cleft. Besides this buffering role, astrocytes also play a role in glutamate homeostasis by responding to the increase in Glu_o through the activation of membrane receptors, the generation and propagation of calcium waves that in turn can trigger glutamate release. The diagram in Figure 13.2 summarizes our knowledge of the glutamate system and takes into account the interaction between astrocytes and neurons.

13.4.1. Glutamate uptake

Under resting conditions, glutamate uptake in astrocytes is mainly mediated by Na^+-dependent systems since Na^+-independent uptake through chloride-dependent glutamate/cystine antiporters represents only a small proportion (<5%) of total glutamate uptake. So far, five distinct glutamate transporters have been cloned:

GLAST, GLT-1, EAAC1, EAAT4 and EAAT5. For all of them, the uptake of glutamate is coupled to a membrane transport system with one glutamate molecule co-transported with three Na^+ and one H^+ while one K^+ is counter-transported to the exterior (Barbour et al., 1988). These isoforms exhibit different patterns of expression depending on the cell type, the developmental stage and the brain region considered (Anderson and Swanson, 2000). For instance, EAAC1 is abundant in glutamatergic neurons in the striatum, cortex and hippocampus while the expression of EAAT5 seems to be restricted to photoreceptors and Müller cells. In contrast, GLAST and GLT-1 are considered to be more specific for astrocytes, GLT-1 being highly expressed in the hippocampus and the cerebral cortex, while GLAST is preferentially expressed in Bergmann glial cells from the molecular layer of the cerebellum. Finally, based on the use of transgenic animals lacking isoforms of the glutamate transporter family, it has been demonstrated that GLAST and GLT-1 are mainly responsible for extracellular glutamate clearance (Rothstein et al., 1996). Hence, astrocytic uptake is a major contributor to glutamate homeostasis.

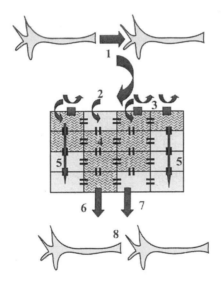

Figure 13.2. Astrocyte-neuron interactions and glutamate homeostasis (neurons are in yellow). The different numbered steps summarizing the contribution of astrocytes are listed in the following order. 1- release of glutamate at glutamate synapses, 2- activation of ionotropic and metabotropic receptors in astrocytes that triggers calcium waves in astrocytes, 3- glutamate uptake by astrocytic transporters, 4- propagation of intercellular calcium waves within a population of astrocytes; note that the propagation is not uniform, but follows preferential pathways excluding subpopulations of astrocytes, 5- permeability of astrocyte gap junctions to glutamate and glutamine that contributes to the equilibrium of $[Glu]_i$ despite a heterogeneous distribution of glutamate transporters, 6- calcium-dependent release of glutamate, 7- calcium-independent efflux of glutamate operating through the reversal of astrocytic glutamate receptors and/or through the activation of volume-sensitive organic osmolyte anion channels and/or through Cx43 hemichannels that could be open in define conditions, 8- activation of distal neurons by glutamate originating from astrocytes.

13.4.2. Glutamate receptors

Typically, glutamate receptors (GluRs) are divided in two main groups, referred as ionotropic and metabotropic receptors (mGluRs). The mGluRs are G-protein linked receptors that contain at least eight subtypes (mGluR1-8) grouped according to their sequence homology, pharmacological profile and signal-transduction mechanism. Group I mGluRs (mGluR1 and mGluR5) are coupled to the IP3-Ca^{2+} cascade as well as to various K^+ channels, whereas Group II (mGluR2 and mGluR3) and group III (mGluR4, 6, 7 and 8) are associated with ionic channels and negatively linked to adenylyl cyclase. Molecular and immunological studies have demonstrated the expression of mGluR2, mGluR3 and mGluR5 in astrocytes (Rothstein et al., 1996; Balazs et al., 1997; Schools and Kimelberg, 1999; Ulas et al., 2000). This finding is in agreement with functional assays demonstrating that in hippocampal astrocytes increase in intracellular calcium ion concentration ($[Ca^{2+}]_i$) occurs through the activation of Group I mGluRs (Shelton and McCarthy, 1999). Ionotropic GluRs are ligand-gated ion channels composed of N-methyl-D-aspartate (NMDA), α-amino-3-hydroxy-5-methyl-4-isoxazole propionate (AMPA) and kainate receptors. The assembly of four or five subunits that form homomeric or heteromeric complexes constitutes these receptors. The NMDA receptors are formed by subunits from the NR1 and NR2 type, while the assembly of GluR1-4 and GluR5-7 composes AMPA and kainate receptors, respectively. Functional AMPA/kainate receptors have been detected in several types of glial cells in culture as well as in acute brain slices, while the existence of functional NMDA receptors in astrocytes is still a matter of debate. In addition, a sub-population of astrocytes (Bergmann glial cells) expresses AMPA receptors that are not permeable to Ca^{2+} due to their low content of GluR2 (Muller et al., 1992), the subunit that confers Ca^{2+} permeability to AMPA receptors in neurons (Jonas et al., 1994). Altogether, these data demonstrate that astrocytes express a broad range of glutamate receptor types and that their activation generates complex changes in $[Ca^{2+}]_i$. Such changes in $[Ca^{2+}]_i$ have been shown to mediate the induction of immediate early genes (Condorelli et al., 1993) and to initiate long-range calcium signaling in astrocytes (Cornell-Bell et al., 1990) that could in turn affect neuronal signaling (Nedergaard, 1994; Parpura et al., 1994).

Recently, a segregated expression of glutamate receptors (AMPA) and glutamate transporters was reported for two distinct types of GFAP positive cells (Matthias et al., 2003). This work indicates that none of these cells coexpressed glutamate receptors and transporters revealing an astrocyte heterogeneity in regard to these two glutamate related processes.

13.4.3. Glutamate release

Although net glutamate influx occurs in astrocytes under normal conditions, glutamate release mechanisms have been identified in response to specific signaling pathways. This includes Ca^{2+}-dependent mechanisms induced by receptor-mediated rises in $[Ca^{2+}]_i$ in the presence of prostaglandin E2, ATP, bradykinin and glutamate itself (Parpura et al., 1994; Bezzi et al., 1998; Jeremic et al., 2001). Although the question of the vesicular nature of glutamate release is still a matter of debate, there is increasing evidence in favor of such hypothesis (Volterra and Bezzi, 2002). First, glutamate release operates in a graded manner at physiological $[Ca^{2+}]_i$ levels

(Parpura and Haydon, 2000) and its inhibition is achieved by buffering $[Ca^{2+}]_i$ with calcium chelators (Jeftinija et al., 1997). Second, patch-clamp recording of NMDA receptor-transfected cells used as "sensor" cells when co-cultured with astrocytes suggests that the release of glutamate occurs with quantal release events. This observation argues for a glutamate release by vesicular exocytosis (Pasti et al., 2001). Third, the main proteins involved in neuronal secretion, including synaptobrevin II, syntaxin and SNAP-25, have also been reported in astrocytes (Maienschein et al., 1999). Fourth, glutamate release is stimulated or blocked by compounds, including toxins, that interact with the exocytosis apparatus (Parpura et al., 1995; Bezzi et al., 1998; Araque et al., 2000). Alternatively, the millimolar concentration of glutamate present in the cytosol can represent a source for a non-vesicular process of glutamate release, which may involve two pathways. Glutamate release can result from a change in astrocytic volume regulation where the activation of volume-sensitive organic anion channels may allow the efflux of ions and amino acids including glutamate, following cell swelling (see Hansson et al, 2000). In addition, due to their electrogenic properties reversal of sodium-dependent glutamate transporters could also be responsible for glutamate release (Barbour et al., 1988). These two mechanisms of glutamate efflux involve distinct pathways since agonists that induce glutamate release do not cause swelling of astrocytes whereas, glutamate transport inhibitors do not suppress calcium-induced glutamate release (Bezzi et al., 1998). However, in order to result in a significant release of glutamate, that could affect neuronal properties, these two mechanisms require particular conditions of cell swelling or a level of membrane depolarization that are only reached in pathological situations.

13.4.4. Glutamate-induced intercellular calcium waves in astrocytes

The superfusion of a confluent astrocyte culture with glutamate was the first protocol used to observe the propagation of rises in $[Ca^{2+}]_i$ in a cell population (Cornell-Bell et al., 1990). Then, two pathways contributing to such long-range signaling process have been identified: one is mediated through gap junction channels (Finkbeiner, 1992; Venance et al., 1997) and the second is due to an extracellular component supported by ATP release (Hassinger et al., 1996; Guthrie et al., 1999). These two components can coexist and their balance may vary depending on the preparation, the brain region and the mode of stimulation used to trigger the induction of the waves (see Scemes, 2000; Charles and Giaume, 2002). In addition, glutamate was also shown to induce calcium waves either by direct focal application (Venance et al., 1997) or by electrical stimulation of neuronal glutamatergic afferents (Dani et al., 1992). Glutamate release from astrocytes was then visualized using an enzymatic assay demonstrating that this process occurs in a regenerative way as the consequence of the "passage" of a calcium wave (Innocenti et al., 2000). Finally, there is now growing evidence that increase in $[Ca^{2+}]_i$ in astrocytes generates neuronal calcium responses (Nedergaard, 1994; Parpura et al., 1994) and that a slow inward current is mediated in adjacent neurons both by NMDA and AMPA glutamate receptors (Araque et al., 1998). The latter observations performed in co-cultures have been corroborated by data obtained in acute hippocampal slices (Pasti et al., 1997; Parri et al., 2001).

13.5. Glutamate and gap junctions in astrocytes

13.5.1. Glutamate as a regulating factor of astrocyte gap junctions

Among number of neurotransmitters, glutamate has been shown to regulate the permeability of astrocytes gap junctions (Table 13.2) (see Rouach et al., 2002b). In cultures of cortical and striatal astrocytes, glutamate increases the level of GJC through a mechanism that involves the activation of AMPA/kainate receptors. Indeed, this effect is mimicked by kainate, AMPA and quisqualate while its is antagonized by 6-cyano-7-nitroquinoxaline-2-3-dione (CNQX) (Enkvist and McCarthy, 1994; Rouach et al., 2000). The facilitating effect of glutamate on GJC depends of the brain region from which the cells originate. It is observed in astrocytes cultured from the cortex and the hippocampus while it is not detected in those from the brain stem and the hypothalamus (Blomstrand et al., 1999a). This facilitation likely involves a short-term regulation of gap junction channels activity since the glutamate-induced increase in GJC is detected after treatment as short as 10 min, a time scale that is not compatible with an increased Cx43 expression. Long-term glutamate exposure cannot be examined since it is taken up by astrocytes and the inhibitor of glutamate uptake has a toxic effect when applied for 24 h. However, kainate exposure for 20 min and 24 h led to similar increase in GJC indicating that prolonged activation of AMPA/kainate receptors does not interfere with its initial effect on GJC (Rouach et al., 2000). In brain slices, the situation is somewhat different as shown by monitoring electrical coupling between two Bergmann glial cells in the cerebellum (Muller et al., 1996). In this preparation, kainate reduces by 30% the coupling response and this effect is not observed in the absence of external calcium, which is consistent with the absence of GluR2 subunit in Bergmann glial cells (Muller et al., 1992). Moreover, glutamate treatment of hippocampal slices for 1 h produces a dephosphorylation of Cx43, an epitope masking and gap junction internalization, as indicated by using several antibodies directed against different sequences of Cx43 (Nagy and Li, 2000). The effects of glutamate are prevented by 2-amino-5-phosphonovaleric acid, an antagonist of the NMDA receptor, suggesting that they are mediated through the activation of neuronal receptors.

There is another example of astrocyte GJC regulation by glutamatergic receptors that results from an indirect effect mediated through the activation of nearby neurons. Such mode of interaction was recently demonstrated in striatal co-cultures in which astrocytes do not respond to NMDA stimulation while neurons do. In this preparation, the co-stimulation of NMDA and muscarinic receptors expressed in neurons induces a 50% reduction of GJC in astrocytes (Rouach et al., 2002a). This inhibitory effect is mediated by the production of the transcellular messenger arachidonic acid by neurons and by its action on astrocyte gap junctions once metabolized through products of the cyclooxygenase pathway. In these co-cultures, the co-application of glutamate and the muscarinic agonist carbachol has no effect although a similar amount of arachidonic acid is produced by the neurons. This is likely due to the direct action of glutamate on astrocytes that *per se* results in an increase in GJC. Together, these results indicate that glutamate modulates astrocyte gap junctions by multiple mechanisms and that its action tightly depends on the expression of glutamate receptor subtypes and the targeted cellular type, astrocytes versus neurons.

Table 13.2. Regulatory effects of glutamate on astrocyte gap junctions

Preparations	Techniques	Treatments	Effect on astrocyte GJC	Pharmacology	References
Primary cultures astrocytes (rat cortex)	dye injections	glutamate (400 µM) kainate (400 µM) quisqualate (400 µM)	increase increase	block by CNQX (10 µM)	Enkvist and McCarthy, 1994
Bergmann glial cells in cerebellar slices (mouse P6 and P20)	double patch-clamp	kainate (1 mM)	inhibition	block by 0 external Ca^{2+}	Müller et al., 1996
Mixed astroglial-neuronal cultures (rat; hippocampus, cortex, brain stem, hypothalamus)	SL/DT	glutamate (100 µM)	Increase in cortical and hippocampal astrocytes No effect in brain stm and hypothalamus	NT	Blomstrand et al., 1999a
Mixed astroglial-neuronal cultures (rat hippocampus)	calcium imaging	glutamate (100 µM)	Increase in velocity and extent of intercellular calcium waves	NT	Blomstrand et al., 1999b
Hippocampal slices (adult rats)	immunocytochemistry	glutamate (1 mM)	Cx43 dephosphorylation epitope masking gap junctions internalization	NT	Nagy and Li, 2000
Co-culture of striatal astrocytes (mouse)	SL/DT	glutamate (400 µM) kainate (400 µM)	increase	Block by CNQX	Rouach et al., 2000
Co-culture of striatal astrocytes (mouse)	SL/DT dye injections	NMDA (100 µM) + Carbachol (1 mM)	decrease	Block by mepacrine, BSA, indomethacine Block by MK801, atropine	Rouach et al., 2002c

Abbreviations: CNQX, 6-cyano-7-nitroquinoxaline-2,3-dione disodium; SL/DT, scrape-loading/dye-transfer technique; NT, not tested; BSA, bovine serum albumin; NMDA, N-methyl-D-aspartate; MK801, (5R,10S) - (+) – 5 – methyl - 10,11 – dihydro - 5H-dibenzo[a,b] cyclohepten-5, 10-imine hydrogen maleate.

13.5.2. Glutamate permeability of connexin 43 channels

As indicated in Table 13.1, Cx43 channels have been shown to be permeable to glutamate and glutamine. This was demonstrated for astrocyte gap junctions, mainly composed of Cx43 channels and for the C6 glioma cell line transfected with Cx43 (Goldberg et al., 1999). These observations indicate that exchanges of this excitatory amino acid and its derivatives may occur between coupled astrocytes if sufficient concentration gradients are generated between connected cells, for instance as a consequence of local release or uptake of glutamate from individual astrocytes. Since the estimated $[Glu]_i$ is rather high (1-3 mM), such transmembrane trafficking has to be drastic and sustained in order to result in a significant difference in $[Glu]_i$ between adjacent astrocytes. However, until now, estimation of $[Glu]_i$ has been obtained from a whole populations of cells which likely have open gap junctions channels. These conditions suppose that glutamate and glutamine could be freely exchanged between cells, but it is expected that significant differences in $[Glu]_i$ could be observed in non-communicating astrocytes. Such cellular heterogeneity for a cytosolic factor, that can cross gap junctions, has already been demonstrated for Na^+ homeostasis (Rose and Ransom, 1997). Indeed, in coupled astrocytes $[Na^+]_i$ is high (10 mM) and is found to be similar in all confluent astrocytes. In contrast, when cells are uncoupled significant differences are measured in neighboring astrocytes indicating that they develop different levels of resting $[Na^+]_i$ when they are isolated from one another by uncoupling agents. It was thus concluded that in astrocytes, an apparent role for GJC is the intercellular exchange of Na^+ ions to equalize resting $[Na^+]_i$, in order to coordinate physiological responses that depend on the intracellular concentration of this ion (Rose and Ransom, 1997). Similarly, it can be postulated that [Glu]i homeostasis follows the same rule and that a consequence of the down-regulation of GJC is unmasking the functional heterogeneity of the glutamate system in astrocytes that could result from differences in uptake mechanism due to a heterogeneous expression of glutamate transporters (see Matthias et al., 2003) or in the molecular steps involved in the release process.

In addition, the participation of hemichannels in glutamate homeostasis should be kept in mind as a working hypothesis. Indeed, since an electrochemical gradient between the inside and the outside favors the outflow of glutamate, open Cx43 hemichannels could be involved in the release process of this amino acid. Recently, this hypothesis was confirmed since it was reported that functional hemichannels in astrocytes can provide a pathway for glutamate release (Ye et al., 2003). In addition, the existence of such pathway has already been shown for the release of ATP which participates to the propagation of intercellular calcium waves in astrocytes (Cotrina et al., 1998c; Stout et al., 2002). Due to the conditions that are required for the opening of Cx43 hemichannels in astrocytes (depolarization, low external calcium, metabolic inhibition) the role of such glutamate release is expected to be associated with pathological situations characterized by an increase in $[Glu]_e$ contributing to excitotoxicity.

In addition to glutamate (147 Da) other amino acids are potential candidates to be exchanged between coupled astrocytes since their molecular weights are small enough to pass through gap junction channels (<1.2 kDa). This was nicely demonstrated for glycine (75 Da) in bipolar cells of the retina indicating that the intercellular pathway provided by gap junction channels allows neurotransmitter coupling in the retina. Indeed, in cone-associated bipolar cells, the elevated glycine concentration does not result from high-affinity uptake or de novo synthesis but is obtained by neurotransmitter exchange through gap junctions with glycinergic amacrine cells (Vaney et al., 1998). According to this concept, the case of D-serine (105 Da) is particularly interesting because this amino acid is a well-known endogenous agonist of NMDA receptors and selectively binds to the glycine site (Schell et al., 1995), thus playing a role in glutamatergic transmission (Mothet et al., 2000). It is noteworthy that D-serine satisfies the major criteria for a glial-derived factor that can regulate NMDA receptors. Evidence includes i) the synthesis and storage of serine in astrocytes rather in neurons (Snyder and Ferris, 2000), ii) the selective localization of D-serine and its biosynthetic enzyme, serine racemase, in astrocytes and its release following glutamate activation, iii) the ability of D-serine to fully mimic the activity at the glycine site of NMDA receptors and the depression of NMDA transmission following selective degradation of D-serine (Baranano et al., 2001). Therefore, the permeability of gap junction channels in astrocytes could permit an even distribution of D-serine in a group of astrocytes that will compensate local changes in concentration due to its release or synthesis.

13.6. Role of astrocyte gap junctions in neuronal cell death

13.6.1. Neurodegenerative diseases and connexin expression in astrocytes

As recently reviewed, expression and function of astrocytic Cxs are associated with several brain dysfunction and pathologies such as epilepsy, ischemia and local inflammation [see (Rouach et al., 2002b)]. Moreover, this last decade, several attempts have been made to determine whether changes in gap junction properties in neurons, as well as in glial cells, are associated with at least two neurodegenerative diseases, Alzheimer's and Parkinson's diseases. Indeed, an elevation of Cx43 was described in human temporal cortex at sites of amyloid plaques in Alzheimer's disease. Cortical areas containing numerous amyloid plaques were found to exhibit increased immunostaining density for Cx43, with some plaques corresponding exactly to sites of intensified Cx43 immunoreactivity and Cx43 localized at ultrastructurally identified astrocytic gap junctions (Nagy et al., 1996). The immunoreactivity for Cx43 antibodies was changed in the caudate nucleus, but not in the globus pallidus. Indeed, in the caudate nucleus, Cx43 expression in astrocytes was increased in plaques and was associated with a large enhancement of GFAP staining. Moreover, analysis of Cx43 expression was carried out with a rat MPTP-model of Parkinson's disease (Rufer et al., 1996). In MPTP-treated animals, the level of Cx43 expression was transiently enhanced in the striatum in parallel with an increased number of GFAP positive cells. Unilateral administration of fibroblast growth factor-2, which has potent trophic effects on developing and impaired dopaminergic neurons in Parkinson's disease, resulted in a further increase in Cx43-positive puncta. However, similar information is lacking for the other main astrocytic Cx, i.e. Cx30, and for other Cxs that are expressed in lower amounts in astrocytes.

13.6.2. Positive and negative influences of astrocytic gap junctions on neuronal survival

In addition to the well-known role of astrocytes on neuronal survival (Mattson et al., 1997) there is recent experimental evidence arguing for a contribution of astrocytic GJC and Cxs expression to neuroprotection. Indeed, inhibitors of GJC in astrocytes, such as halothane and octanol, were shown to reduce the extent of brain injuries during ischemia and spreading depression (Rawanduzy et al., 1997; Saito et al., 1997). Moreover, immunohistological studies performed *in vivo* after kainic acid lesion indicate that massive neuronal loss, alone, or in conjunction with direct action of excitotoxins on astrocytes, resulted in an astrocytic reaction accompanied by a redistribution of Cx43 (Ochalski et al., 1995). Thus reorganization of GJC within the astrocytic networks may be neuroprotective by isolating the site of lesion from the healthy syncytium. The incidence of astrocytic GJC in neuroprotection has been directly investigated using co-culture systems and by comparing neuronal vulnerability to oxidative stress in the presence of communicating and non-communicating astrocytes (Blanc et al., 1998). In this study, the blockade of GJC in astrocytes following exposure to oxidative insults resulted in a markedly enhanced generation of intracellular peroxides and neuronal death. In addition, the peak elevation of neuronal Ca^{2+} induced by oxidative stress was larger following uncoupling treatment, suggesting that astrocytic GJC was also involved in Ca^{2+} homeostasis in neurons through a mechanism that remains to be elucidated. These observations suggest the existence of a link between astrocytic GJC and neuronal vulnerability induced by oxidative insults. Astroglial intercellular communication decreases neuronal vulnerability to injury by a mechanism involving stabilization of cellular Ca^{2+} homeostasis and dissipation of oxidative stress. Such contribution of astrocyte GJC to neuronal survival could be a more general property and be relevant in excitotoxicity. Indeed, co-cultures with non-communicating astrocytes have been recently shown to be less neuroprotective for glutamate-induced neurotoxicity (Naus et al., 2001). Blockade of astrocytes gap junctions with carbenoxolone in neuron-astrocyte co-cultures results in an increased number of dead neurons after treatment with glutamate (1 mM, 3 h) (Ozog et al., 2002). Complementing these observations, it has been recently shown that heterozygotic Cx43-null mice, deficient in astrocytic GJC (Naus et al., 1997), exhibited increased infarct volume 4 days after unilateral middle cerebral artery occlusion (Siushansian et al., 2001).

Conversely, GJC could also play an important role in the propagation of death signals in astrocytic networks, which secondarily may affect neuronal fate. Although GJC in astrocytes is significantly reduced during ischemic conditions, junctional channels were reported to remain open in dying astrocytes (Cotrina et al., 1998b), allowing free exchange of intracellular messengers between dying astrocytes. From this observation, it was proposed that astrocyte GJC may contribute to secondary expansion of ischemic lesions, which in turn could affect bystander neurons suggesting that GJC may connect ischemic astrocytes in an evolving infarct. Furthermore, in focal ischemia, analysis of Cx43 distribution has demonstrated changes in the location and phosphorylation status of this protein (Li et al., 1998), which suggests differential functional status of astrocytic gap junction channels at the ischemic center versus the periphery. Finally, GJC in astrocytes were shown to propagate and amplify cell injury by allowing intercellular diffusion of death signal (see above).

In conclusion, there are data in the literature that argue for a neuroprotective role of astrocytic GJC, but conversely there is evidence indicating that GJC could provide an intercellular mode for the extension of deleterious signals. In the case of a propagation of death signals, astrocyte viability should be primarily affected and this process will secondarily interfere with neuronal survival since a decrease in number of astrocytes reduces the efficiency of their neuroprotective role. Whether GJC in astrocytes has positive or negative consequences on neuronal survival in pathological situations remains a matter of debate. In numerous studies, the specificity of the tools used to suppress astrocytic GJC can be questioned and it cannot be excluded that gap junction uncouplers also inhibit GJC in neurons (see Rozental et al., 2001a). In addition, it is possible that the involvement of astrocyte GJC in neuronal survival likely depends on the model of neurotoxicity that is used and on the time at which neuronal death is investigated.

13.7. What is the role for astrocyte gap junctions in glutamate homeostasis and neuronal death?

Brain trauma or injury are known to be followed by a pathological increase in $[Glu]_o$ which originates from neurons, but also from astrocytes. Such enhanced concentration of excitatory amino acid plays a central role in mediating and expending neuronal degeneration. In neurons, extracellular glutamate activates an excitotoxic cascade due to uncontrolled activation of ionotropic and metabotropic glutamate receptors (Hansson et al., 2000). Although the complete sequence of molecular mechanisms leading to neuronal death is not fully understood, several events are known to be critical, in particular intracellular calcium overload. Indeed, increase in $[Glu]_o$ leads to a massive entry of calcium through glutamate receptors and voltage dependent calcium channels activated by sustained depolarization, together with calcium release from internal stores. This unusual increase in neuronal $[Ca^{2+}]_i$ results in uncontrolled activation of protein kinases, phospholipases, proteases and nitric oxide synthase (Hudspith, 1997) leading to subsequent proteolysis, lipid peroxidation and free radical formation that provoke the death of neurons. How do astrocytes actively participate in these processes and which of their properties play a key roles, are essential questions to answer in order to understand the weight of neuroglial interactions in neuronal death. For instance, it is noteworthy that neuronal vulnerability to glutamate is 100-fold greater in low-density rather than in rich astrocytes cultures (Rosenberg and Aizenman, 1989). The contribution of astrocytes to neuronal death is likely evolving with time, since after any type of brain injury, surviving astrocytes progressively acquire a new phenotype termed reactive astrocyte (Ridet et al., 1997). This is of particular interest since glutamate-induced neuronal death occurs in the acute phase of brain injury but also a large number of neurons suffer from a delayed death (Lynch and Dawson, 1994). This process is likely to be associated with both changes in the expression of numerous proteins and changes in astrocytic functions that may contribute to modification in neuroglial interactions. The situation of disruption of glutamate homeostasis that results from changes in the steps governing the glutamate system is summarized in Figure 13.3.

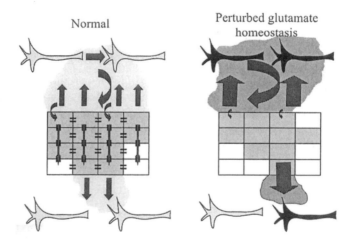

Figure 13.3. Summary diagrams comparing the various steps involved in glutamate homeostasis and neuroglial interaction in a normal versus a pathological situation. The sequences illustrated refer to those that have been detailed in Fig. 13.2. The size of the arrows indicates the changes in the contribution of the different steps and the red clouds illustrate the modification of glutamate concentration in the extracellular step. As mentioned in the text the propagation of intercellular waves is considered as maintained in pathological situation, this is in agreement with data indicating that the external pathway prevails when GJC is down-regulated. The arrows through gap junctions represent the intercellular permeability of gap junction channels to glutamate. In addition, glutamate could also occur through Cx43 open hemichannels and thus contribute to the increase in external concentration of this amino acid.

As a high level of GJC is a typical feature of astrocytes and several properties of Cx43 channels are directly linked to glutamate (permeability, regulation, neuroprotection), the understanding of their respective contribution to neuroglial interaction in normal and pathological situations is important and might help to open new perspectives and strategies in the attempt to prevent, or at least delay, neuronal death. Indeed, changes in astrocytic GJC could secondarily affect glutamate homeostasis and thereby have a rebound effect on neuronal survival. Accordingly, it is critical to define what are the existing links between gap junctions and astrocytic functions involved in the homeostasis of glutamate such as its uptake, intercellular trafficking, metabolism and release. Of course these links are likely to be indirect and they probably involve basic properties of astrocytes such as the regulation of $[Ca^{2+}]_i$, the release of metabolic intermediates (e.g., glutamine, lactate, alanine, etc.), or the scavenging of oxygen free radicals. In the future, the answer to these questions might be used as an alternative basis to develop new pharmacological strategies to exert neuroprotective treatment by targeting GJC and Cx expression in astrocytes, an alternative strategy that, up-to-now, has been poorly investigated.

Acknowledgements: The original work presented in this chapter was supported by a grant from the European Community N°QLK6-CT1999-02203.

13.8. References

Alvarez-Maubecin V, Garcia-Hernandez F, Williams JT, Van Bockstaele EJ (2000) Functional coupling between neurons and glia. J Neurosci 20:4091-4098.

Anderson CM, Swanson RA (2000) Astrocyte glutamate transport: review of properties, regulation, and physiological functions. Glia 32:1-14.

Araque A, Parpura V, Sanzgiri RP, Haydon PG (1998) Glutamate-dependent astrocyte modulation of synaptic transmission between cultured hippocampal neurons. Eur J Neurosci 10:2129-2142.

Araque A, Li N, Doyle RT, Haydon PG (2000) SNARE protein-dependent glutamate release from astrocytes. J Neurosci 20:666-673.

Balazs R, Miller S, Romano C, de Vries A, Chun Y, Cotman CW (1997) Metabotropic glutamate receptor mGluR5 in astrocytes: pharmacological properties and agonist regulation. J Neurochem 69:151-163.

Baranano DE, Ferris CD, Snyder SH (2001) Atypical neural messengers. Trends Neurosci 24:99-106.

Barbour B, Brew H, Attwell D (1988) Electrogenic glutamate uptake in glial cells is activated by intracellular potassium. Nature 335:433-435.

Beblo DA, Veenstra RD (1997) Monovalent cation permeation through the connexin40 gap junction channel. Cs, Rb, K, Na, Li, TEA, TMA, TBA, and effects of anions Br, Cl, F, acetate, aspartate, glutamate, and NO3. J Gen Physiol 109:509-522.

Bennett MV (1977) Electrical transmission: a functional analysis and comparison with chemical transmission. In: Cellular Biology of Neurons (Kandel E, ed), pp 357-416. Baltimore: Williams and Wilkins.

Bennett MV, Barrio LC, Bargiello TA, Spray DC, Hertzberg E, Saez JC (1991) Gap junctions: new tools, new answers, new questions. Neuron 6:305-320.

Bergles DE, Jahr CE (1998) Glial contribution to glutamate uptake at Schaffer collateral-commissural synapses in the hippocampus. J Neurosci 18:7709-7716.

Bezzi P, Carmignoto G, Pasti L, Vesce S, Rossi D, Rizzini BL, Pozzan T, Volterra A (1998) Prostaglandins stimulate calcium-dependent glutamate release in astrocytes. Nature 391:281-285.

Binmoller FJ, Muller CM (1992) Postnatal development of dye-coupling among astrocytes in rat visual cortex. Glia 6:127-137.

Bittman K, Becker DL, Cicirata F, Parnavelas JG (2002) Connexin expression in homotypic and heterotypic cell coupling in the developing cerebral cortex. J Comp Neurol 443:201-212.

Blanc EM, Bruce-Keller AJ, Mattson MP (1998) Astrocytic gap junctional communication decreases neuronal vulnerability to oxidative stress-induced disruption of Ca2+ homeostasis and cell death. J Neurochem 70:958-970.

Blomstrand F, Aberg ND, Eriksson PS, Hansson E, Ronnback L (1999a) Extent of intercellular calcium wave propagation is related to gap junction permeability and level of connexin-43 expression in astrocytes in primary cultures from four brain regions. Neuroscience. 92:255-265

Blomstrand F, Khatibi S, Muyderman H, Hansson E, Olsson T, Ronnback L (1999b) 5-Hydroxytryptamine and glutamate modulate velocity and extent of intercellular calcium signalling in hippocampal astroglial cells in primary cultures. Neuroscience 88:1241-1253.

Bruzzone R, Giaume C (1999) Connexins and information transfer through glia. Adv Exp Med Biol 468:321-337.

Bruzzone R, White TW, Paul DL (1996) Connections with connexins: the molecular basis of direct intercellular signaling. Eur J Biochem 238:1-27.

Bruzzone S, Guida L, Zocchi E, Franco L, De Flora A (2001) Connexin 43 hemi channels mediate Ca2+-regulated transmembrane NAD+ fluxes in intact cells. Faseb J 15:10-12.

Bukauskas FF (2001) Inducing de novo formation of gap junction channels. Methods Mol Biol 154:379-393.

Charles AC, Giaume, C. (2002) Intercellular calcium waves in astrocytes: underlying mechanisms and functional significance. In: The tripartite synapse: glia in synaptic transmission (Volterra A, Magistretti, P. and Haydon, P.G., ed), pp 110-126. Oxford: Oxford University Press.

Condorelli DF, Mudo G, Trovato-Salinaro A, Mirone MB, Amato G, Belluardo N (2002) Connexin-30 mRNA is up-regulated in astrocytes and expressed in apoptotic neuronal cells of rat brain following kainate-induced seizures. Mol Cell Neurosci 21:94-113.

Condorelli DF, Dell'Albani P, Amico C, Kaczmarek L, Nicoletti F, Lukasiuk K, Stella AM (1993) Induction of primary response genes by excitatory amino acid receptor agonists in primary astroglial cultures. J Neurochem 60:877-885.

Contreras JE, Sanchez HA, Eugenin EA, Speidel D, Theis M, Willecke K, Bukauskas FF, Bennett MV, Saez JC (2002) Metabolic inhibition induces opening of unapposed connexin 43 gap junction hemichannels and reduces gap junctional communication in cortical astrocytes in culture. Proc Natl Acad Sci U S A 99:495-500.

Cornell-Bell AH, Finkbeiner SM, Cooper MS, Smith SJ (1990) Glutamate induces calcium waves in cultured astrocytes: long-range glial signaling. Science 247:470-473.

Cotrina ML, Lin JH, Nedergaard M (1998a) Cytoskeletal assembly and ATP release regulate astrocytic calcium signaling. J Neurosci 18:8794-8804.

Cotrina ML, Kang J, Lin JH, Bueno E, Hansen TW, He L, Liu Y, Nedergaard M (1998b) Astrocytic gap junctions remain open during ischemic conditions. J Neurosci 18:2520-2537.

Cotrina ML, Lin JH, Alves-Rodrigues A, Liu S, Li J, Azmi-Ghadimi H, Kang J, Naus CC, Nedergaard M (1998c) Connexins regulate calcium signaling by controlling ATP release. Proc Natl Acad Sci U S A 95:15735-15740.

D'Ambrosio R, Wenzel J, Schwartzkroin PA, McKhann GM, 2nd, Janigro D (1998) Functional specialization and topographic segregation of hippocampal astrocytes. J Neurosci 18:4425-4438.

Dahl E, Manthey D, Chen Y, Schwarz HJ, Chang YS, Lalley PA, Nicholson BJ, Willecke K (1996) Molecular cloning and functional expression of mouse connexin-30,a gap junction gene highly expressed in adult brain and skin. J Biol Chem 271:17903-17910.

Dani JW, Chernjavsky A, Smith SJ (1992) Neuronal activity triggers calcium waves in hippocampal astrocyte networks. Neuron 8:429-440.

DeVries SH, Schwartz EA (1992) Hemi-gap-junction channels in solitary horizontal cells of the catfish retina. J Physiol 445:201-230.

Duffy HS, Delmar M, Spray DC (2002) Formation of the gap junction nexus: binding partners for connexins. J Physiol Paris 96:243-249.

Duffy HS, John GR, Lee SC, Brosnan CF, Spray DC (2000) Reciprocal regulation of the junctional proteins claudin-1 and connexin43 by interleukin-1beta in primary human fetal astrocytes. J Neurosci 20:RC114.

Elfgang C, Eckert R, Lichtenberg-Frate H, Butterweck A, Traub O, Klein RA, Hulser DF, Willecke K (1995) Specific permeability and selective formation of gap junction channels in connexin-transfected HeLa cells. J Cell Biol 129:805-817.

Enkvist MO, McCarthy KD (1994) Astroglial gap junction communication is increased by treatment with either glutamate or high K+ concentration. J Neurochem 62:489-495.

Erecinska M, Silver IA (1990) Metabolism and role of glutamate in mammalian brain. Prog Neurobiol 35:245-296.

Finkbeiner S (1992) Calcium waves in astrocytes-filling in the gaps. Neuron 8:1101-1108.

Froes MM, Correia AH, Garcia-Abreu J, Spray DC, Campos de Carvalho AC, Neto MV (1999) Gap-junctional coupling between neurons and astrocytes in primary central nervous system cultures. Proc Natl Acad Sci U S A 96:7541-7546.

Giaume C, McCarthy KD (1996) Control of gap-junctional communication in astrocytic networks. Trends Neurosci 19:319-325.

Giaume C, Tabernero A, Medina JM (1997) Metabolic trafficking through astrocytic gap junctions. Glia 21:114-123.

Giepmans BN, Moolenaar WH (1998) The gap junction protein connexin43 interacts with the second PDZ domain of the zona occludens-1 protein. Curr Biol 8:931-934.

Giepmans BN, Hengeveld T, Postma FR, Moolenaar WH (2001) Interaction of c-Src with gap junction protein connexin-43. Role in the regulation of cell-cell communication. J Biol Chem 276:8544-8549.

Goldberg GS, Lampe PD, Nicholson BJ (1999) Selective transfer of endogenous metabolites through gap junctions composed of different connexins. Nat Cell Biol 1:457-459.

Goldberg GS, Moreno AP, Lampe PD (2002) Gap junctions between cells expressing connexin 43 or 32 show inverse permselectivity to adenosine and ATP. J Biol Chem 277:36725-36730.

Guthrie PB, Knappenberger J, Segal M, Bennett MV, Charles AC, Kater SB (1999) ATP released from astrocytes mediates glial calcium waves. J Neurosci 19:520-528.

Hansson E, Muyderman H, Leonova J, Allansson L, Sinclair J, Blomstrand F, Thorlin T, Nilsson M, Ronnback L (2000) Astroglia and glutamate in physiology and pathology: aspects on glutamate transport, glutamate-induced cell swelling and gap-junction communication. Neurochem Int 37:317-329.

Harris AL (2001) Emerging issues of connexin channels: biophysics fills the gap. Q Rev Biophys 34:325-472.

Hassinger TD, Guthrie PB, Atkinson PB, Bennett MV, Kater SB (1996) An extracellular signaling component in propagation of astrocytic calcium waves. Proc Natl Acad Sci U S A 93:13268-13273.

Hofer T, Venance L, Giaume C (2002) Control and plasticity of intercellular calcium waves in astrocytes: a modeling approach. J Neurosci 22:4850-4859.

Hudspith MJ (1997) Glutamate: a role in normal brain function, anaesthesia, analgesia and CNS injury. Br J Anaesth 78:731-747.

Innocenti B, Parpura V, Haydon PG (2000) Imaging extracellular waves of glutamate during calcium signaling in cultured astrocytes. J Neurosci 20:1800-1808.

Jeftinija SD, Jeftinija KV, Stefanovic G (1997) Cultured astrocytes express proteins involved in vesicular glutamate release. Brain Res 750:41-47.

Jeremic A, Jeftinija K, Stevanovic J, Glavaski A, Jeftinija S (2001) ATP stimulates calcium-dependent glutamate release from cultured astrocytes. J Neurochem 77:664-675.

Jonas P, Racca C, Sakmann B, Seeburg PH, Monyer H (1994) Differences in Ca2+ permeability of AMPA-type glutamate receptor channels in neocortical neurons caused by differential GluR-B subunit expression. Neuron 12:1281-1289.

Kanemitsu MY, Loo LW, Simon S, Lau AF, Eckhart W (1997) Tyrosine phosphorylation of connexin 43 by v-Src is mediated by SH2 and SH3 domain interactions. J Biol Chem 272:22824-22831.

Kondo RP, Wang SY, John SA, Weiss JN, Goldhaber JI (2000) Metabolic inhibition activates a non-selective current through connexin hemichannels in isolated ventricular myocytes. J Mol Cell Cardiol 32:1859-1872.

Konietzko U, Muller CM (1994) Astrocytic dye coupling in rat hippocampus: topography, developmental onset, and modulation by protein kinase C. Hippocampus 4:297-306.

Kunzelmann P, Schroder W, Traub O, Steinhauser C, Dermietzel R, Willecke K (1999) Late onset and increasing expression of the gap junction protein connexin30 in adult murine brain and long-term cultured astrocytes. Glia 25:111-119.

Leybaert L, Sanderson MJ (2001) Intercellular calcium signaling and flash photolysis of caged compounds. A sensitive method to evaluate gap junctional coupling. Methods Mol Biol 154:407-430.

Li WE, Ochalski PA, Hertzberg EL, Nagy JI (1998) Immunorecognition, ultrastructure and phosphorylation status of astrocytic gap junctions and connexin43 in rat brain after cerebral focal ischaemia. Eur J Neurosci 10:2444-2463.

Lin JH, Weigel H, Cotrina ML, Liu S, Bueno E, Hansen AJ, Hansen TW, Goldman S, Nedergaard M (1998) Gap-junction-mediated propagation and amplification of cell injury. Nat Neurosci 1:494-500.

Lynch DR, Dawson TM (1994) Secondary mechanisms in neuronal trauma. Curr Opin Neurol 7:510-516.

Maienschein V, Marxen M, Volknandt W, Zimmermann H (1999) A plethora of presynaptic proteins associated with ATP-storing organelles in cultured astrocytes. Glia 26:233-244.

Massa PT, Mugnaini E (1982) Cell junctions and intramembrane particles of astrocytes and oligodendrocytes: a freeze-fracture study. Neuroscience 7:523-538.

Matthias K, Kirchhoff F, Seifert G, Huttmann K, Matyash M, Kettenmann H, Steinhauser C (2003) Segregated expression of AMPA-type glutamate receptors and glutamate transporters defines distinct astrocyte populations in the mouse hippocampus. J Neurosci 23:1750-1758.

Mattson MP, Barger SW, Furukawa K, Bruce AJ, Wyss-Coray T, Mark RJ, Mucke L (1997) Cellular signaling roles of TGF beta, TNF alpha and beta APP in brain injury responses and Alzheimer's disease. Brain Res Brain Res Rev 23:47-61.

Mercier F, Hatton GI (2001) Connexin 26 and basic fibroblast growth factor are expressed primarily in the subpial and subependymal layers in adult brain parenchyma: roles in stem cell proliferation and morphological plasticity? J Comp Neurol 431:88-104.

Mothet JP, Parent AT, Wolosker H, Brady RO, Jr., Linden DJ, Ferris CD, Rogawski MA, Snyder SH (2000) D-serine is an endogenous ligand for the glycine site of the N-methyl-D-aspartate receptor. Proc Natl Acad Sci U S A 97:4926-4931.

Mugnaini E (1986) Cell junctions of astrocytes, ependymal and related cells in the mammal central nervous system, with emphasis on the hypothesis of a generalized syncytium of supporting cells. In: Astrocytes (A FSaV, ed), pp 329-371. New York: Academic Press.

Muller T, Moller T, Neuhaus J, Kettenmann H (1996) Electrical coupling among Bergmann glial cells and its modulation by glutamate receptor activation. Glia 17:274-284.

Muller T, Moller T, Berger T, Schnitzer J, Kettenmann H (1992) Calcium entry through kainate receptors and resulting potassium-channel blockade in Bergmann glial cells. Science 256:1563-1566.

Nadarajah B, Jones AM, Evans WH, Parnavelas JG (1997) Differential expression of connexins during neocortical development and neuronal circuit formation. J Neurosci 17:3096-3111.

Nagy JI, Li WE (2000) A brain slice model for in vitro analyses of astrocytic gap junction and connexin43 regulation: actions of ischemia, glutamate and elevated potassium. Eur J Neurosci 12:4567-4572.

Nagy JI, Rash JE (2000) Connexins and gap junctions of astrocytes and oligodendrocytes in the CNS. Brain Res Brain Res Rev 32:29-44.

Nagy JI, Li W, Hertzberg EL, Marotta CA (1996) Elevated connexin43 immunoreactivity at sites of amyloid plaques in Alzheimer's disease. Brain Res 717:173-178.

Nagy JI, Patel D, Ochalski PA, Stelmack GL (1999) Connexin30 in rodent, cat and human brain: selective expression in gray matter astrocytes, co-localization with connexin43 at gap junctions and late developmental appearance. Neuroscience 88:447-468.

Nagy JI, Li X, Rempel J, Stelmack G, Patel D, Staines WA, Yasumura T, Rash JE (2001) Connexin26 in adult rodent central nervous system: demonstration at astrocytic gap junctions and colocalization with connexin30 and connexin43. J Comp Neurol 441:302-323.

Naus CC, Ozog MA, Bechberger JF, Nakase T (2001) A neuroprotective role for gap junctions. Cell Commun Adhes 8:325-328.

Naus CC, Bechberger JF, Zhang Y, Venance L, Yamasaki H, Juneja SC, Kidder GM, Giaume C (1997) Altered gap junctional communication, intercellular signaling, and growth in cultured astrocytes deficient in connexin43. J Neurosci Res 49:528-540.

Nedergaard M (1994) Direct signaling from astrocytes to neurons in cultures of mammalian brain cells. Science 263:1768-1771.

Niessen H, Harz H, Bedner P, Kramer K, Willecke K (2000) Selective permeability of different connexin channels to the second messenger inositol 1,4,5-trisphosphate. J Cell Sci 113 (Pt 8):1365-1372.

O'Brien J, Bruzzone R, White TW, Al-Ubaidi MR, Ripps H (1998) Cloning and expression of two related connexins from the perch retina define a distinct subgroup of the connexin family. J Neurosci 18:7625-7637.

Ochalski PA, Sawchuk MA, Hertzberg EL, Nagy JI (1995) Astrocytic gap junction removal, connexin43 redistribution, and epitope masking at excitatory amino acid lesion sites in rat brain. Glia 14:279-294.

Ozog MA, Siushansian R, Naus CC (2002) Blocked gap junctional coupling increases glutamate-induced neurotoxicity in neuron-astrocyte co-cultures. J Neuropathol Exp Neurol 61:132-141.

Parpura V, Haydon PG (2000) Physiological astrocytic calcium levels stimulate glutamate release to modulate adjacent neurons. Proc Natl Acad Sci U S A 97:8629-8634.

Parpura V, Fang Y, Basarsky T, Jahn R, Haydon PG (1995) Expression of synaptobrevin II, cellubrevin and syntaxin but not SNAP-25 in cultured astrocytes. FEBS Lett 377:489-492.

Parpura V, Basarsky TA, Liu F, Jeftinija K, Jeftinija S, Haydon PG (1994) Glutamate-mediated astrocyte-neuron signalling. Nature 369:744-747.

Parri HR, Gould TM, Crunelli V (2001) Spontaneous astrocytic Ca2+ oscillations in situ drive NMDAR-mediated neuronal excitation. Nat Neurosci 4:803-812.

Pasti L, Volterra A, Pozzan T, Carmignoto G (1997) Intracellular calcium oscillations in astrocytes: a highly plastic, bidirectional form of communication between neurons and astrocytes in situ. J Neurosci 17:7817-7830.

Pasti L, Zonta M, Pozzan T, Vicini S, Carmignoto G (2001) Cytosolic calcium oscillations in astrocytes may regulate exocytotic release of glutamate. J Neurosci 21:477-484.

Pakhotin P, Verkhratsky A (2003) Electrical synapses between Bergmann glia cells and Purkinje neurones in rat cerebellar slices. J Physiol:O44.

Pellerin L, Magistretti PJ (1994) Glutamate uptake into astrocytes stimulates aerobic glycolysis: a mechanism coupling neuronal activity to glucose utilization. Proc Natl Acad Sci U S A 91:10625-10629.

Ransom BR (1995) Gap junctions. In: Neuroglia (Kettenmann HaR, B.R., ed), pp 299-318. Oxford: Oxford University Press.

Quist AP, Rhee SK, Lin H, Lal R (2000) Physiological role of gap-junctional hemichannels. Extracellular calcium-dependent isosmotic volume regulation. J Cell Biol 148:1063-1074.

Rash JE, Yasumura T, Dudek FE, Nagy JI (2001a) Cell-specific expression of connexins and evidence of restricted gap junctional coupling between glial cells and between neurons. J Neurosci 21:1983-2000.

Rash JE, Duffy HS, Dudek FE, Bilhartz BL, Whalen LR, Yasumura T (1997) Grid-mapped freeze-fracture analysis of gap junctions in gray and white matter of adult rat central nervous system, with evidence for a "panglial syncytium" that is not coupled to neurons. J Comp Neurol 388:265-292.

Rash JE, Yasumura T, Davidson KG, Furman CS, Dudek FE, Nagy JI (2001b) Identification of cells expressing Cx43, Cx30, Cx26, Cx32 and Cx36 in gap junctions of rat brain and spinal cord. Cell Commun Adhes 8:315-320.

Rawanduzy A, Hansen A, Hansen TW, Nedergaard M (1997) Effective reduction of infarct volume by gap junction blockade in a rodent model of stroke. J Neurosurg 87:916-920.

Ridet JL, Malhotra SK, Privat A, Gage FH (1997) Reactive astrocytes: cellular and molecular cues to biological function. Trends Neurosci 20:570-577.

Robinson SR, Hampson EC, Munro MN, Vaney DI (1993) Unidirectional coupling of gap junctions between neuroglia. Science 262:1072-1074.

Rohlmann A, Wolff JR (1996) Subcellular topography and plasticity of gap junction distribution. In: Gap Junctions in the Nervous System (R. SDCaD, ed), pp 175-192. Austin: R.G. Landes Company.

Romanello M, Pani B, Bicego M, D'Andrea P (2001) Mechanically induced ATP release from human osteoblastic cells. Biochem Biophys Res Commun 289:1275-1281.

Rose CR, Ransom BR (1997) Gap junctions equalize intracellular Na+ concentration in astrocytes. Glia 20:299-307.

Rosenberg PA, Aizenman E (1989) Hundred-fold increase in neuronal vulnerability to glutamate toxicity in astrocyte-poor cultures of rat cerebral cortex. Neurosci Lett 103:162-168.

Rothstein JD, Dykes-Hoberg M, Pardo CA, Bristol LA, Jin L, Kuncl RW, Kanai Y, Hediger MA, Wang Y, Schielke JP, Welty DF (1996) Knockout of glutamate transporters reveals a major role for astroglial transport in excitotoxicity and clearance of glutamate. Neuron 16:675-686.

Rouach N, Glowinski J, Giaume C (2000) Activity-dependent neuronal control of gap-junctional communication in astrocytes. J Cell Biol 149:1513-1526.

Rouach N, Tence M, Glowinski J, Giaume C (2002a) Costimulation of N-methyl-D-aspartate and muscarinic neuronal receptors modulates gap junctional communication in striatal astrocytes. Proc Natl Acad Sci U S A 99:1023-1028.

Rouach N, Avignone E, Meme W, Koulakoff A, Venance L, Blomstrand F, Giaume C (2002b) Gap junctions and connexin expression in the normal and pathological central nervous system. Biol Cell 94:457-475.

Rozental R, Srinivas M, Spray DC (2001a) How to close a gap junction channel. Efficacies and potencies of uncoupling agents. Methods Mol Biol 154:447-476.

Rozental R, Andrade-Rozental AF, Zheng X, Urban M, Spray DC, Chiu FC (2001b) Gap junction-mediated bidirectional signaling between human fetal hippocampal neurons and astrocytes. Dev Neurosci 23:420-431.

Rufer M, Wirth SB, Hofer A, Dermietzel R, Pastor A, Kettenmann H, Unsicker K (1996) Regulation of connexin-43, GFAP, and FGF-2 is not accompanied by changes in astroglial coupling in MPTP-lesioned, FGF-2-treated parkinsonian mice. J Neurosci Res 46:606-617.

Saito R, Graf R, Hubel K, Fujita T, Rosner G, Heiss WD (1997) Reduction of infarct volume by halothane: effect on cerebral blood flow or perifocal spreading depression-like depolarizations. J Cereb Blood Flow Metab 17:857-864.

Scemes E (2000) Components of astrocytic intercellular calcium signaling. Mol Neurobiol 22:167-179.

Scemes E, Dermietzel R, Spray DC (1998) Calcium waves between astrocytes from Cx43 knockout mice. Glia 24:65-73.

Schell MJ, Molliver ME, Snyder SH (1995) D-serine, an endogenous synaptic modulator: localization to astrocytes and glutamate-stimulated release. Proc Natl Acad Sci U S A 92:3948-3952.

Schools GP, Kimelberg HK (1999) mGluR3 and mGluR5 are the predominant metabotropic glutamate receptor mRNAs expressed in hippocampal astrocytes acutely isolated from young rats. J Neurosci Res 58:533-543.

Schubert AL, Schubert W, Spray DC, Lisanti MP (2002) Connexin family members target to lipid raft domains and interact with caveolin-1. Biochemistry 41:5754-5764.

Shelton MK, McCarthy KD (1999) Mature hippocampal astrocytes exhibit functional metabotropic and ionotropic glutamate receptors in situ. Glia 26:1-11.

Siushansian R, Bechberger JF, Cechetto DF, Hachinski VC, Naus CC (2001) Connexin43 null mutation increases infarct size after stroke. J Comp Neurol 440:387-394.

Snyder SH, Ferris CD (2000) Novel neurotransmitters and their neuropsychiatric relevance. Am J Psychiatry 157:1738-1751.

Spray DC, Duffy HS, Scemes E (1999) Gap junctions in glia. Types, roles, and plasticity. Adv Exp Med Biol 468:339-359.

Stout CE, Costantin JL, Naus CC, Charles AC (2002) Intercellular calcium signaling in astrocytes via ATP release through connexin hemichannels. J Biol Chem 277:10482-10488.

Tabernero A, Giaume C, Medina JM (1996) Endothelin-1 regulates glucose utilization in cultured astrocytes by controlling intercellular communication through gap junctions. Glia 16:187-195.

Theiss C, Meller K (2002a) Microinjected anti-actin antibodies decrease gap junctional intercellular commmunication in cultured astrocytes. Exp Cell Res 281:197-204.

Theiss C, Meller K (2002b) Aluminum impairs gap junctional intercellular communication between astroglial cells in vitro. Cell Tissue Res 310:143-154.

Tower DB, Young OM (1973) The activities of butyrylcholinesterase and carbonic anhydrase, the rate of anaerobic glycolysis, and the question of a constant density of glial cells in cerebral cortices of various mammalian species from mouse to whale. J Neurochem 20:269-278.

Toyofuku T, Yabuki M, Otsu K, Kuzuya T, Hori M, Tada M (1998) Direct association of the gap junction protein connexin-43 with ZO-1 in cardiac myocytes. J Biol Chem 273:12725-12731.

Ulas J, Satou T, Ivins KJ, Kesslak JP, Cotman CW, Balazs R (2000) Expression of metabotropic glutamate receptor 5 is increased in astrocytes after kainate-induced epileptic seizures. Glia 30:352-361.

Vaney DI, Nelson JC, Pow DV (1998) Neurotransmitter coupling through gap junctions in the retina. J Neurosci 18:10594-10602.

Veenstra RD (2001) Determining ionic permeabilities of gap junction channels. Methods Mol Biol 154:293-311.

Venance L, Stella N, Glowinski J, Giaume C (1997) Mechanism involved in initiation and propagation of receptor-induced intercellular calcium signaling in cultured rat astrocytes. J Neurosci 17:1981-1992.

Venance L, Premont J, Glowinski J, Giaume C (1998) Gap junctional communication and pharmacological heterogeneity in astrocytes cultured from the rat striatum. J Physiol (Lond) 510:429-440.

Volterra A, Bezzi P (2002) Release of transmitters from glial cells. In: The tripartite synapse: glial in synaptic transmission (Volterra A, Magistretti, P. and Haydon, P.G., ed), pp 164-182. OXford: Oxford University Press.

Willecke K, Eiberger J, Degen J, Eckardt D, Romualdi A, Guldenagel M, Deutsch U, Sohl G (2002) Structural and functional diversity of connexin genes in the mouse and human genome. Biol Chem 383:725-737.

Wolff JR, Stuke K, Missler M, Tytko H, Schwarz P, Rohlmann A, Chao TI (1998) Autocellular coupling by gap junctions in cultured astrocytes: a new view on cellular autoregulation during process formation. Glia 24:121-140.

Ye ZC, Wyeth MS, Baltan-Tekkok S, Ransom BR (2003) Functional hemichannels in astrocytes: a novel mechanism of glutamate release. J Neurosci. 239:3588-3596.

Zahs KR (1998) Heterotypic coupling between glial cells of the mammalian central nervous system. Glia 24:85-96.

13.9. Abbreviations

AMPA	α-amino-3-hydroxy-5-methyl-4-isoxazole propionate
CNQX	6-cyano-7-nitroquinoxaline-2-3-dione
CNS	Central nervous system
Cxs	Connexins
EAAC1	Glutamate transporters
EAAT4	Glutamate transporters
EAAT5	Glutamate transporters
GFAP	Glial fibrillary acidic protein
GJC	Gap junctional communication
GLAST	Glutamate transporters
GLT-1	Glutamate transporters
GluRs	Glutamate receptors
$[Glu]_i$	Intracellular glutamate concentration
$[Glu]_o$	Extracellular glutamate concentration
IP_3	Inositol-1,4,5-trisphosphate
mGluRs	Metabotropic receptors
NMDA	N-methyl-D-aspartate
$[X^{\pm}]_i$	Intracellular concentration of ion X
$[X^{\pm}]_o$	Extracellular concentration of ion X

Chapter 14

Mechanism and significance of astrocytic Ca^{2+} signaling

Gregory Arcuino, Marisa Cotrina and Maiken Nedergaard*

Center for Aging and Developmental Biology, University of Rochester School of Medicine
Rochester, NY 14642, USA

Corresponding author: nedergaard@urmc.rochester.edu

Contents

---

14. 1. Introduction

Astrocytes are remarkably multifunctional cells. One of their main tasks is to rapidly scavenge transmitters released during synaptic activity. Astrocytes also express neurotransmitter receptors and respond to neuronal activity by increases in intracellular Ca^{2+} concentrations ($[Ca^{2+}_i]$). In turn, stimulated astrocytes release glutamate, which by both pre- and post- synaptic mechanisms modulates synaptic strength. The ability of astrocytes to sense neuronal activity and respond by increases in $[Ca^{2+}_i]$, has been a topic of intense research for the last few years. Here we review the mechanisms of astrocytic Ca^{2+} signaling.

Astrocytes are electrically non-excitable cells, which communicate by transient increases in $[Ca^{2+}_i]$, that is largely based on the low resting level of $[Ca^{2+}_i]$, 50-250 nM, combined with the ability to rapidly mobilize intracellular Ca^{2+} stores resulting in increments in $[Ca^{2+}_i]$ in the μM range (Fatatis and Russell, 1992; Duffy and MacVicar, 1994; Peuchen et al., 1996). Ca^{2+} signaling is common to many cell types and denotes a high degree of conservancy among electrically non-excitable cell types. Several of the mechanisms discussed here with regard to astrocytic Ca^{2+} signaling may therefore be general to cell types outside the central nervous system (CNS).

14.1.1. Ca^{2+} permeable membrane channels

The influx of Ca^{2+} from extracellular space can be accomplished by voltage-gated and ligand-gated Ca^{2+} channels that are well founded components in neuronal membrane. Though there is some evidence that voltage-gated Ca^{2+} channels do exist in cultured astrocytes (MacVicar, 1984) and during pathological conditions (Fern, 1998; Westenbroek et al., 1998), it is controversial whether they are expressed in acute slices (Carmignoto et al., 1998). Astrocytes in culture and in situ express alpha-amino-3-hydroxy-5-methyl-4-isoxazole-4-propionic acid (AMPA), ionotropic glutamate receptor (GluR) subunits 1-4 (Fan et al., 1999; Shelton and McCarthy, 1999), though culture conditions can influence receptor expression (Janssens and Lesage, 2001). In culture AMPA receptor channels are demonstrated to possess a 6-cyano-7-nitroquinoxaline-2,3-dione (CNQX)- and cyclothiazide-sensitive Ca^{2+} current when activated (Fan et al., 1999), indicating low GluR2 subunit expression. However, in situ though astrocytic AMPA receptor expression can be demonstrated, functional Ca^{2+} permeability is lacking probably due to GluR2 subunit expression. In the cerebellum this is not the case with Bergmann glial cells where AMPA receptors clearly respond with currents to synaptic glutamate release (Iino et al., 2001). Metabotropic glutamate receptors (mGluR) that are linked to inositol-1,4,5-trisphosphate (IP_3) sensitive intracellular Ca^{2+} stores appear to represent the primary mechanism of astrocytic Ca^{2+} mobilization. Histological expression of ionotropic nucleotide receptors of the relatively recently described purinergic P2X class of ATP receptors has been reported for astrocytes in situ (Franke et al., 2001). Electrophysiology of astrocytes in cultures reveals that adenosine 5'-triphosphate (ATP) and P2X agonists induce activation of a non-selective cation channel that permits the influx of Na^+, K^+, and Ca^{2+}, and possible efflux of glutamate (Walz et al., 1994). However, it still remains to be established whether astrocytes in intact brain express $P2X_7$ receptors.

14.1.2. Intracellular Ca^{2+} stores

The primary mechanism for Ca^{2+} mobilization in astrocytes is through intracellular stores, with the glial endoplasmic reticulum (ER) as the primary Ca^{2+} storage organelle (Peuchen et al., 1996). Ca^{2+} release from these internal stores is regulated by receptor channels of which IP_3 (IP_3 R) and ryanodine (RyR) types have been most extensively studied. Both channel types are primarily activated by Ca^{2+} itself in addition to the receptor ligand (Berridge et al., 2000). The astrocyte ER can have a complex patterning of compartments with segregated, regulated stores linked to either IP_3Rs or RyRs (Golovina and Blaustein, 1997). Receptor-mediated Ca^{2+} signaling relative to these ryanodine-sensitive stores has not been well characterized. Recent studies demonstrate that a modulator of RyR's, cyclic ADP-ribose, can influence astrocytic Ca^{2+} signaling and down stream effectors (Verderio et al., 2001; Matyash et al., 2002). The Ca^{2+} signaling cascade involving phosphoinositide hydrolysis by G-protein activated phospholipase C (PLC) is the most widely studied, and since astrocytes express metabotropic receptors for major brain transmitters like glutamate and ATP that are coupled to this cascade (Venance et al., 1997), it is most likely the major mechanism for receptor mediated Ca^{2+} mobilization in astrocytes.

14.2. Astrocytic Ca²⁺ signaling

Generally, dynamic spatial and temporal Ca^{2+} signaling patterns in cells are shaped by a combination of factors (Berridge et al., 2000): i) amplification of the initial intracellular Ca^{2+} concentration increase, ii) spatial buffering of the Ca^{2+}, and iii) extrusion of the Ca^{2+} to regain "baseline" $[Ca^{2+}]_i$. These factors most likely contribute to two distinct types of Ca^{2+} signaling modalities that astrocytes display: $[Ca^{2+}]_i$ oscillations and propagating intercellular $[Ca^{2+}]_i$ waves (Wang et al., 1997). $[Ca^{2+}]_i$ oscillations are repetitive monophasic increases in cytosolic Ca^{2+} limited to a single cell. These oscillations can be evoked by exposure to several different transmitters, including glutamate and ATP. $[Ca^{2+}]_i$ oscillations can also be triggered by removal of extracellular Ca^{2+}, or by exposure of cultured astrocytes to hypo-osmotic solutions (Zanotti and Charles, 1997; Darby et al., 2003) . An extensive literature has documented that $[Ca^{2+}]_i$ oscillations involve activation of phospholipase A (PLA), IP_3 production, and release of intracellular stores, rather than influx of Ca^{2+} through membrane channels in astrocytes (Verkhratsky et al., 1998).

What are the implications of astrocytic Ca^{2+} oscillations? Since astrocytic Ca^{2+} increases can trigger glutamate signaling in adjacent neurons (Araque et al., 1998), an appealing hypothesis is that a repetitive pattern of Ca^{2+} increases contributes to transient episodes of glutamate release. Astrocytic glutamate release may, by activation of presynaptic mGluR, inhibit neuronal glutamate release and thereby function as a negative feedback mechanism, which dampens local excitation. Astrocytic Ca^{2+} oscillations may also participate in activity-dependent increases in cerebral blood flow by release of a diffusible agent, possibly prostaglandins (Zonta et al., 2003), supporting again the idea of astrocytic Ca^{2+} oscillations as a major mechanism to control the release of neuromodulatory transmitters.

But astrocytes not only produce Ca^{2+} oscillations in response to neuronal activity. Two studies have uncovered spontaneous Ca^{2+} oscillations in thalamic (Parri and Crunelli, 2001) and hippocampal (Nett et al., 2002) astrocytes in situ. These reports proposed that astrocytes can display intrinsic activity, e.g. Ca^{2+} oscillations that cannot be blocked by a combination of several different receptor antagonists, including inhibitors of glutamate and purinergic receptors(Nett et al., 2002). The challenge now is to decipher the functional significance of these spontaneous, neuron-independent astrocytic activities.

An important aspect of frequency-coded information is the requirement for specific cellular "decoders" that are capable of translating the Ca^{2+} information into a cellular response. The two most studied Ca^{2+}-sensitive proteins that are involved in decoding Ca^{2+} signals are camodulin kinase and protein kinase C (PKC) although only the latter has been evaluated in astrocytes. Thus, it seems that glutamate-induced astrocytic Ca^{2+} oscillations depend on the periodic translocation and activation of PKC which, in turn, responds to the oscillating diacylglycerol and Ca^{2+} concentrations (Codazzi et al., 2001).

While the role of astrocytic Ca^{2+} oscillations is still poorly understood, Ca^{2+} oscillations in early developing neurons have been associated with neuronal differentiation (Gu and Spitzer, 1995) , axonal growth (Gomez and Spitzer, 1999), and establishment of neuronal networks (Yuste et al., 1992).

14.2.1. Propagating Ca^{2+} waves

The second type of astrocytic Ca^{2+} signaling is propagating Ca^{2+} waves. Cornell-Bell and co-workers were the first to describe that astrocytes in culture generated propagating Ca^{2+} waves when exposed to glutamate (Cornell-Bell et al., 1990). The discovery that astrocytes possess a mechanism for long-distance communication had profound impact on the field and further questioned the traditional view that astrocytes are passive support cells. Later, studies showed that astrocytic Ca^{2+} waves evoked increases in neuronal cytosolic Ca^{2+}, suggesting that astrocytes may participate directly in neurotransmission(Nedergaard, 1994; Parpura et al., 1994). It was subsequently confirmed that astrocytic Ca^{2+} signaling modulates the strength of synaptic transmission; stimulation of astrocytes led to a decrease in synaptic failure rate between pairs of synaptically-coupled interneurons and CA1 pyramidal cells in acute slice preparation (Kang et al., 1998). Astrocytic Ca^{2+} waves modulate the firing frequency of both ganglion cells in dissected eyecup retinas (Newman and Zahs, 1998) and in hippocampal cultures (Araque et al., 1998). Similarly, Schwann cells regulate neuromuscular transmission in pathway that requires intracellular Ca^{2+} signaling (Robitaille, 1998). Together these observations identified a new signaling loop between neurons and astrocytes; astrocytes can modulate the Ca^{2+} level, and thereby the firing pattern, of neurons in their surroundings. In turn, neurons can trigger astrocytic Ca^{2+} signaling by releasing glutamate (Dani et al., 1992; Giaume and Venance, 1998)

14.2.2. Mechanism of astrocytic Ca^{2+} waves

The advent of Ca^{2+} sensing dyes opened the field of brain signaling to the exciting prospect that astrocytes in addition to neurons may play a role in brain signaling. Research into astrocytic Ca^{2+} signaling has been intensively cultivated over the past decade and a half. Ca^{2+} waves in cultured astrocytes can be stimulated by focal electrical stimulation, mechanical stimulation, decreased extracellular Ca^{2+} levels, or by local application of transmitters, glutamate or ATP (Cornell-Bell et al., 1990; Dani et al., 1992; Nedergaard, 1994; Zanotti and Charles, 1997; Arcuino et al., 2002). High levels of neuronal activity in organotypic slices have also induced astrocyte Ca^{2+} waves (Dani et al., 1992). Our current understanding of the mechanism driving the propagation of astrocytic Ca^{2+} waves is mainly a result of observations gathered from experiments using mechanical or focal electrical stimulation in astrocyte cultures. Of course, the mechanistic models ascribed to Ca^{2+} wave propagation have undergone some changes, and they continue to evolve. Though models may have conflicting aspects there are standard observations that hold fast. Generally, Ca^{2+} waves propagate with a velocity of around 20 μm/s and expand over a maximum radius ranging from around 300 to 400 μm (Tashiro et al., 2002), which includes between 30 and 60 astrocytes per wave (Cornell-Bell et al., 1990). Also, Ca^{2+} waves require activation of phospholipase C (PLC), with subsequent events leading to IP$_3$ production and release of Ca^{2+} from IP$_3$ sensitive internal stores (Boitano et al., 1992; Sheppard et al., 1997; Venance et al., 1997).

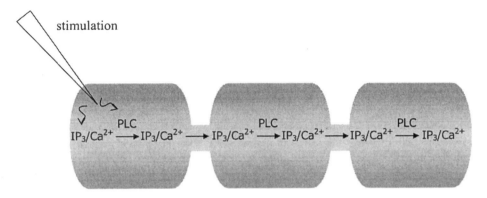

stimulation

Figure 14.1. Gap junction conducted regenerative Ca^{2+} wave propagation model. Ca^{2+} wave propagation is mediated by increased IP_3/Ca^{2+} in the stimulated cell, followed by gap junction conducted diffusion of IP_3/Ca^{2+} into neighboring cells and regenerative mobilization of IP_3/Ca^{2+} in these cells. PLC, phospholipase C.

14.2.3. Gap junction mediated, regenerative Ca^{2+} waves

Initially, it was proposed that propagation of Ca^{2+} waves was conducted through the diffusion of IP_3 and/or Ca^{2+} through gap junctions (Sanderson et al., 1990) (Fig. 14.1) Diffusion of IP_3 alone may release Ca^{2+} from IP_3 sensitive stores, or Ca^{2+} diffusion can initiate Ca^{2+}- induced Ca^{2+} release. Whether both act together or alone, in the end PLC activation is required for propagation to continue. All together these processes expand from cell to cell in a regenerative manner. The supportive crux for this model depended on the inability of a connexin (Cx)-deficient glioma cell line, C6, to propagate Ca^{2+} waves. Following transfection of the gap junction subunit Cx43, the C6 cells gained the ability to propagate Ca^{2+} waves greater than 200 μm in diameter (Zanotti and Charles, 1997). Subsequent studies confirmed these results by demonstrating that exogenous expression of another connexin subtype, Cx32, in C6 glioma or HeLa cells significantly potentiated the diameter of Ca^{2+} wave propagation (Cotrina et al., 1998; Paemeleire et al., 2000; Fry et al., 2001).

14.2.4. ATP mediated regenerative Ca^{2+} waves

Whether gap junctions were even involved in Ca^{2+} wave propagation was first presented by a study demonstrating that physically isolated astrocytes can still engage in Ca^{2+} waves, suggesting that an extracellular element mediated Ca^{2+} signaling (Hassinger et al., 1996). Using pharmacologic approaches, several labs demonstrated that ATP was the diffusible messenger, the extracellular element (Cotrina et al., 1998; Cotrina et al., 2000; Fam et al., 2000; Wang et al., 2000) (Fig. 14.2). Similar studies also demonstrated that ATP mediates Ca^{2+} waves in other systems like epithelium (Hansen et al., 1993; Homolya et al., 2000), liver (Patel et al., 1999), heart (Kaneko et al., 2000), and osteoblasts (Jorgensen et al., 1997; Romanello et al., 2001). Though there are reported differences in culture or in situ, astrocytes express $P2Y_1$, $P2Y_2$, $P2Y_4$ and P2X receptors (John et al., 1999; Moran-Jimenez and Matute, 2000; Franke et al., 2001; Zhu and Kimelberg, 2001) and it is therefore likely that multiple purinergic receptor subtypes are involved in Ca^{2+} wave propagation in astrocytes. So the current revised model for Ca^{2+} wave propagation is that the extracellular element ATP is produced in a regenerative manner that depends on increases in cytosolic Ca^{2+} (Guthrie et al., 1999). Nevertheless, the model did not explain why the waves had a maximal radius of a few hundred micrometers. A truly regenerative wave would only stop short of the edge of the culture.

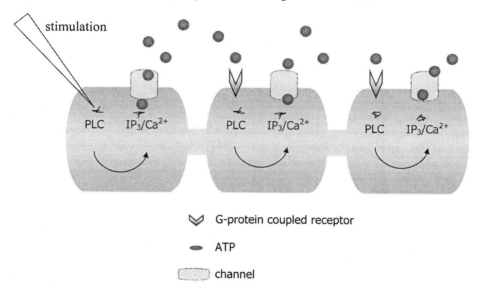

Figure 14.2. Regenerative ATP release model of Ca^{2+} wave propagation. Ca^{2+} wave propagation is mediated by ATP release in the stimulated cell, followed by P2Y receptor mediated increases in cytosolic Ca^{2+} in neighboring cells, which then trigger additional ATP release in these cells. PLC, phospholipase C

14.2.5. Non-regenerative Ca^{2+} waves mediated by point source ATP release

The previous models of Ca^{2+} wave propagation, whether solely mediated by IP_3 and or Ca^{2+} diffusion through gap junctions or by a combination of this and activation of purinergic receptors resulting from extracellular ATP release, are both regenerative in nature. The observation that has been most counter-intuitive to these regenerative models is the limited propagation of the Ca^{2+} wave. If Ca^{2+} wave propagation were truly regenerative then the wave would only be bounded by the absence of cells. Yet, in cultures of astrocytes, Ca^{2+} wave propagation does not spread throughout the entire culture. Based upon this observation, we hypothesized that ATP is released by a single cell only and that "Ca^{2+} wave propagation" reflects simple diffusion of ATP from a point source only. To test this hypothesis, we utilized the observation that lowering extracellular Ca^{2+} concentration elicits spontaneous Ca^{2+} waves in cultured astrocytes. We loaded the cultures with the Ca^{2+} indicator fluo-3 and added propidium iodide to the extracellular solution in high concentrations (1-2 mM). Our rationale was that cells that allow efflux of ATP would also allow influx of a large cation, propidium (MW=562). Using confocal microscopy, we monitored the generation of spontaneous Ca^{2+} waves and simultaneous uptake of propidium. We observed that only the cell in the epicenter of the wave took up propidium, whereas surrounding cells increased cytosolic Ca^{2+} concentration, but excluded propidium (Fig. 14.3)(Arcuino et al., 2002). These observations suggest that only the cells that initiated the wave released ATP, whereas surrounding cells did not release additional ATP. To further test the idea that ATP is released from a single cell only, we next analyzed the distance by which waves travel across a cell-free lane. We observed that a Ca^{2+} wave initiated on one side propagates just as far across the cell free lane as the side that is not separated (Fig. 14.4). Thus, ATP released from cells that secondarily engaged in Ca^{2+} waves do not contribute to wave expansion. Together, this set of observations indicates that ATP is released from only a single cell (Fig. 14.5).

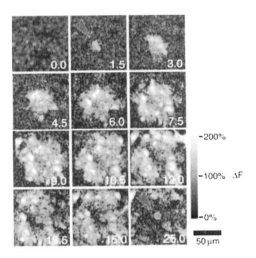

Figure 14.3. Astrocytic Ca^{2+} signaling is associated with a transient increase in membrane permeability and uptake of propidium in a single cell. Sequence of images (in seconds) demonstrating the time course of propidium uptake in the cell that triggers a Ca^{2+} wave. Propidium uptake is superimposed upon a time series of confocal images displaying relative increases in fluo-3 emission (ΔF). A single cell located in the epicenter of the Ca^{2+} wave displays uptake of propidium (red arrowhead). Scale bar is 50 μm.

14.2.6. Do gap junction "hemichannels" mediate ATP release?

The concentration of cytosolic ATP in astrocytes is around 2-4 mM (Berridge et al., 2000)). Several lines of work have over the past few years provided evidence for channel-mediated release of ATP and it has been suggested that gap junction, Cx, hemichannels mediate the release. An important argument for the involvement of Cxs in ATP release is the observation that over expression of eitherCx43, Cx32, or Cx26 is associated with a 3- to 10-fold increase in receptor stimulated ATP release (Cotrina et al., 1998). The Cx-mediated potentiation of ATP release has been observed in several cell lines, including HeLa, C6 and N2A cells. Other lines of evidence have suggested that anion channel blockers decrease ATP release, but most importantly, removal to extracellular Ca^{2+} potentiates ATP release. Lowering of extracellular ATP is known to be associated with opening of Cx hemichannels detected by dye indicator uptake. Interestingly, we found that ATP release was a linear function of the number of cells with propidium uptake. Combined, these observations suggest that Cx hemichannels mediate ATP release. However, it is in this regard important to note that over expression of Cx's are associated with a marked alteration in gene expression. The possibility exists, that transfection with cDNA for Cx proteins induce the expression of another channel with a pore diameter large enough to allow passage of ATP. In that case, Cxs potentiate ATP release, but do not directly mediate the efflux (Cotrina et al., 2000). Combining single channel recordings with bioluminescence imaging of ATP release is expected to provide the final proof (or disprove), that Cx hemichannels allow efflux of cytosolic ATP.

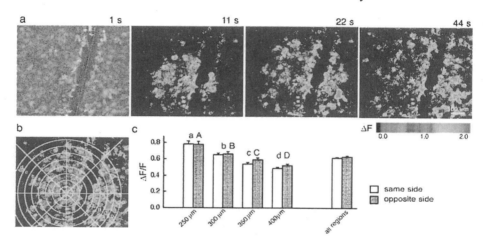

Figure 14.4. The effect of a cell free lane on mechanically induced astrocytic Ca^{2+} signaling. (a) Sequential expansion of Ca^{2+} wave (1-44 seconds). The Ca^{2+} wave was evoked on the left side of the cell free lane (yellow asterisk). Relative increases in intracellular Ca^{2+} (ΔF) were superimposed upon a fluo-3 image collected before stimulation. (b) Grid used for quantification of ΔF. The grid was positioned with its center on top of the stimulation site and consisted of concentric rings each increasing their radii by 50 μm. ΔF was calculated in these radially defined sections (a,b,c,d) and compared with matching regions on the opposite side of the cell free lane (A,B,C,D). (c) Histogram comparing ΔF in matched sections at increasing distance from the point of stimulation (n = 44-67). "All regions" indicates ΔF (mean ± SEM) in a total of 242 matched regions analyzed. No difference between regions on either side of the cell free lane was evident.

Another line of work have suggested that ATP release is mediated by exocytosis of ATP containing vesicles. The major evidence for exocytosis of ATP is that co-localization of ATP with proteins involved in vesicular release (Verkhratsky et al., 1998). The co-existence of both channel and vesicular release is possible, because the two pathways are not mutually exclusive.

Based on these observations in culture we propose a new model of astrocytic Ca^{2+} wave propagation: Astrocytic Ca^{2+} waves are a manifestation of ATP diffusion from a point source release site subsequently activating purinergic receptors on neighboring cells, and is spatially restricted because ATP release is from a central single cell and is non-regenerative in neighboring cell (Fig. 14.5).

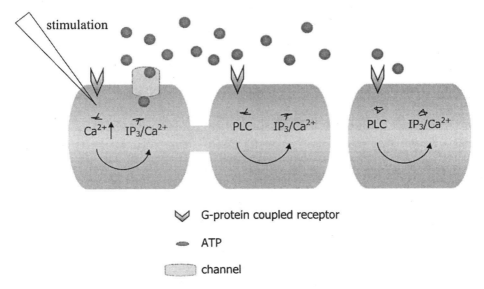

$\vee$ G-protein coupled receptor

$-$ ATP

$\boxed{}$ channel

Figure 14.5. Point source ATP release model of Ca^{2+} wave propagation. Ca^{2+} wave propagation is mediated by ATP release in the stimulated cell, followed by P2Y receptor mediated increases in cytosolic Ca^{2+} in neighboring cells. PLC, phospholipase C.

14.2.7. Astrocytes in intact tissue support propagation of Ca^{2+} waves

The studies discussed so far on Ca^{2+} wave propagation were based on observation in cultured astrocytes or organotypic slices. Ca^{2+} waves have also been observed in the retina following mechanical stimulation (Newman, 2001) and a recent report documented that intact brain tissue supported the propagation of Ca^{2+} waves (Schipke et al., 2002). Electrical field stimulation (4 s at 10 Hz) triggered Ca^{2+} waves, which migrated with a velocity of 14 μm/s and expanded more than 500 μm in coronal slices from 5- to 8-day-old mice. The characteristics of these Ca^{2+} waves in brain slices were strikingly similar to astrocytic Ca^{2+} waves in vitro. For example, depletion of internal Ca^{2+} stores with thapsigargin attenuated the waves, while removal of extracellular Ca^{2+} potentiated wave propagation. Most importantly, purinergic receptor blockers strongly inhibited the expansion of long-distance Ca^{2+} wave in the slice preparation (Schipke et al., 2002).

So, astrocytes in brain slices support the idea that Ca^{2+} wave propagation depends on purinergic receptors. However, it remains an open question whether Ca^{2+} waves are initiated by physiological stimuli in brain slices. In fact, several lines of evidence may point to the opposite conclusion because intense neuronal or local application of neurotransmitters trigger astrocytic Ca^{2+} oscillations, but not propagating Ca^{2+} waves (Porter and McCarthy, 1996; Pasti et al., 1997; Kang et al., 1998). Because induction of astrocytic Ca^{2+} waves requires powerful stimulation, this type of signaling might relate to pathophysiological events, rather than normal brain physiology.

14.3. Trophic effects of purinergic signaling

Morphogenic effects of extracellular purines on both astrocytes and neurons have been described (Neary et al., 1996; Rathbone et al., 1998). Similarly, a direct trophic effect of purines on human neuroblastoma cells (Wang et al., 1990), PC12 cells(Soltoff et al., 1998) and myenteric neuronal cells (Schafer et al., 1995), has been demonstrated. Nucleotides can act synergistically with polypeptides, like basic fibroblast growth factor (Abbracchio et al., 1995). We recently asked whether ATP released from glia enhanced neuronal maturation. We used C6 cell culture with and without expression of Cxs as a tool to manipulate the extracellular levels of purines. The steady-state extracellular concentration of ATP in C6 cells expressing either Cx43 or Cx32 is approximately 20-100-fold higher than in cultures of Cx-deficient C6 clones (Cotrina et al., 2000). We found that neurons in co-culture with Cx-expressing C6 cells had significantly longer neurites than when co-cultured with Cx-deficient C6-mock cells. The purinergic receptor blockers, reactive blue and suramin, abolished the trophic effects of surrounding glia, indicating that the increased levels of extracellular ATP promoted neuronal maturation (Cotrina et al., 2000). The trophic effects of purines may in part, explain why developing neurons in culture form inefficient synapses that require glial signals to become functional (Pfrieger and Barres, 1997; Pfrieger, 2003). Others have reported that exposure of cultured astrocytes to non-degradable ATP analogs resulted in stellation of glial fibrillary acidic protein (GFAP)-positive cells in a concentration-dependent manner and a suramin-sensitive increase in the mean length of GFAP-positive processes (Neary et al., 1994). Intriguingly, activation of purinergic receptors in several systems is associated with increases of cyclic adenosine monophosphate (cAMP) (Insel et al., 1996; Klinker et al., 1996; Merten et al., 1998). Elevation of cAMP itself is sufficient to promote survival of spinal motor neurons and several lines of evidence suggest that cAMP enhances trophic responsiveness (Hanson et al., 1998). Indeed, cAMP elevation enhances brain-derived neurotrophic factor responsiveness of ganglion cells by recruiting trkB to the plasma membrane (Meyer-Franke et al., 1998).

Together, these studies suggest that astrocytic release of ATP, in addition to its role in rapid signaling events, also may have long-term effects upon intact maturation and integrity of astrocyte-neuronal networks.

14.4. Perspectives

The concept that glia, not only neurons, are active participants in brain signaling has emerged in the past decade and has been fueled by work from laboratories demonstrating glial-neuronal interactions. Glutamatergic and purinergic receptor-mediated Ca^{2+} signaling between interacting glia and neurons has been observed in cell co-cultures, organotypic brain slices, in situ peripheral nerve preps, and acute brain slices. Several lines of work demonstrate receptor mediated Ca^{2+} increases traveling as a Ca^{2+} wave amongst astrocytes and support the notion that glia cells are active participants in the processing and coordination of brain signals. These Ca^{2+} waves are mediated by ATP efflux as demonstrations in astrocytic cultures reveal an extracellular, non-gap junction mediated, component of Ca^{2+} wave propagation, where Ca^{2+} waves can engage cells that are physically isolated from the centrally stimulated cell and where these Ca^{2+} waves are attenuated by the presence of purinergic receptor antagonists. Much has been gleaned from culture work. Beyond this frontier lay exciting and obvious questions: How is astrocytic Ca^{2+} signaling manifest in vivo? Are there astrocytic Ca^{2+} oscillations and waves that are a part of physiological events in the brain of a whole animal? We can begin to answer these questions with the advent of relatively new imaging technologies such as multi-photon laser scanning microscopy. This imaging technology coupled with new Ca^{2+} sensitive green fluorescent protein variants, the chameleons, is expected to provide a window into astrocytic Ca^{2+} signaling in live, intact animals.

14.5. References

Abbracchio MP, Ceruti S, Langfelder R, Cattabeni F, Saffrey MJ, Burnstock G (1995) Effects of ATP analogues and basic fibroblast growth factor on astroglial cell differentiation in primary cultures of rat striatum. Int J Dev Neurosci 13:685-693.

Araque A, Parpura V, Sanzgiri RP, Haydon PG (1998) Glutamate-dependent astrocyte modulation of synaptic transmission between cultured hippocampal neurons. Eur J Neurosci 10:2129-2142.

Arcuino G, Lin JH, Takano T, Liu C, Jiang L, Gao Q, Kang J, Nedergaard M (2002) Intercellular calcium signaling mediated by point-source burst release of ATP. Proc Natl Acad Sci U S A 99:9840-9845.

Berridge MJ, Lipp P, Bootman MD (2000) The versatility and universality of calcium signalling. Nat Rev Mol Cell Biol 1:11-21.

Boitano S, Dirksen ER, Sanderson MJ (1992) Intercellular propagation of calcium waves mediated by inositol trisphosphate. Science 258:292-295.

Carmignoto G, Pasti L, Pozzan T (1998) On the role of voltage-dependent calcium channels in calcium signaling of astrocytes in situ. J Neurosci 18:4637-4645.

Codazzi F, Teruel MN, Meyer T (2001) Control of astrocyte Ca(2+) oscillations and waves by oscillating translocation and activation of protein kinase C. Curr Biol 11:1089-1097.

Cornell-Bell AH, Finkbeiner SM, Cooper MS, Smith SJ (1990) Glutamate induces calcium waves in cultured astrocytes: long-range glial signaling. Science 247:470-473.

Cotrina ML, Lin JH, Lopez-Garcia JC, Naus CC, Nedergaard M (2000) ATP-mediated glia signaling. J Neurosci 20:2835-2844.

Cotrina ML, Lin JH, Alves-Rodrigues A, Liu S, Li J, Azmi-Ghadimi H, Kang J, Naus CC, Nedergaard M (1998) Connexins regulate calcium signaling by controlling ATP release. Proc Natl Acad Sci U S A 95:15735-15740.

Dani JW, Chernjavsky A, Smith SJ (1992) Neuronal activity triggers calcium waves in hippocampal astrocyte networks. Neuron 8:429-440.

Darby M, Kuzmiski JB, Panenka W, Feighan D, MacVicar BA (2003) ATP released from astrocytes during swelling activates chloride channels. J Neurophysiol 89:1870-1877.

Duffy S, MacVicar BA (1994) Potassium-dependent calcium influx in acutely isolated hippocampal astrocytes. Neuroscience 61:51-61.

Fam SR, Gallagher CJ, Salter MW (2000) P2Y(1) purinoceptor-mediated Ca(2+) signaling and Ca(2+) wave propagation in dorsal spinal cord astrocytes. J Neurosci 20:2800-2808.

Fan D, Grooms SY, Araneda RC, Johnson AB, Dobrenis K, Kessler JA, Zukin RS (1999) AMPA receptor protein expression and function in astrocytes cultured from hippocampus. J Neurosci Res 57:557-571.

Fatatis A, Russell JT (1992) Spontaneous changes in intracellular calcium concentration in type I astrocytes from rat cerebral cortex in primary culture. Glia 5:95-104.

Fern R (1998) Intracellular calcium and cell death during ischemia in neonatal rat white matter astrocytes in situ. J Neurosci 18:7232-7243.

Franke H, Grosche J, Schadlich H, Krugel U, Allgaier C, Illes P (2001) P2X receptor expression on astrocytes in the nucleus accumbens of rats. Neuroscience 108:421-429.

Fry T, Evans JH, Sanderson MJ (2001) Propagation of intercellular calcium waves in C6 glioma cells transfected with connexins 43 or 32. Microsc Res Tech 52:289-300.

Giaume C, Venance L (1998) Intercellular calcium signaling and gap junctional communication in astrocytes. Glia 24:50-64.

Golovina VA, Blaustein MP (1997) Spatially and functionally distinct Ca2+ stores in sarcoplasmic and endoplasmic reticulum. Science 275:1643-1648.

Gomez TM, Spitzer NC (1999) In vivo regulation of axon extension and pathfinding by growth-cone calcium transients. Nature 397:350-355.

Gu X, Spitzer NC (1995) Distinct aspects of neuronal differentiation encoded by frequency of spontaneous Ca2+ transients. Nature 375:784-787.

Guthrie PB, Knappenberger J, Segal M, Bennett MV, Charles AC, Kater SB (1999) ATP released from astrocytes mediates glial calcium waves. J Neurosci 19:520-528.

Hansen M, Boitano S, Dirksen ER, Sanderson MJ (1993) Intercellular calcium signaling induced by extracellular adenosine 5'-triphosphate and mechanical stimulation in airway epithelial cells. J Cell Sci 106 (Pt 4):995-1004.

Hanson MG, Jr., Shen S, Wiemelt AP, McMorris FA, Barres BA (1998) Cyclic AMP elevation is sufficient to promote the survival of spinal motor neurons in vitro. J Neurosci 18:7361-7371.

Hassinger TD, Guthrie PB, Atkinson PB, Bennett MV, Kater SB (1996) An extracellular signaling component in propagation of astrocytic calcium waves. Proc Natl Acad Sci U S A 93:13268-13273.

Homolya L, Steinberg TH, Boucher RC (2000) Cell to cell communication in response to mechanical stress via bilateral release of ATP and UTP in polarized epithelia. J Cell Biol 150:1349-1360.

Iino M, Goto K, Kakegawa W, Okado H, Sudo M, Ishiuchi S, Miwa A, Takayasu Y, Saito I, Tsuzuki K, Ozawa S (2001) Glia-synapse interaction through Ca2+-permeable AMPA receptors in Bergmann glia. Science 292:926-929.

Insel PA, Firestein BL, Xing M, Post SR, Jacobson JP, Balboa MA, Hughes RJ (1996) P2-purinoceptors utilize multiple signalling pathways in MDCK-D1 cells. J Auton Pharmacol 16:311-313.

Janssens N, Lesage AS (2001) Glutamate receptor subunit expression in primary neuronal and secondary glial cultures. J Neurochem 77:1457-1474.

John GR, Scemes E, Suadicani SO, Liu JS, Charles PC, Lee SC, Spray DC, Brosnan CF (1999) IL-1beta differentially regulates calcium wave propagation between primary human fetal astrocytes via pathways involving P2 receptors and gap junction channels. Proc Natl Acad Sci U S A 96:11613-11618.

Jorgensen NR, Geist ST, Civitelli R, Steinberg TH (1997) ATP- and gap junction-dependent intercellular calcium signaling in osteoblastic cells. J Cell Biol 139:497-506.

Kaneko T, Tanaka H, Oyamada M, Kawata S, Takamatsu T (2000) Three distinct types of Ca(2+) waves in Langendorff-perfused rat heart revealed by real-time confocal microscopy. Circ Res 86:1093-1099.

Kang J, Jiang L, Goldman SA, Nedergaard M (1998) Astrocyte-mediated potentiation of inhibitory synaptic transmission. Nat Neurosci 1:683-692.

Klinker JF, Wenzel-Seifert K, Seifert R (1996) G-protein-coupled receptors in HL-60 human leukemia cells. Gen Pharmacol 27:33-54.

MacVicar BA (1984) Voltage-dependent calcium channels in glial cells. Science 226:1345-1347.

Matyash M, Matyash V, Nolte C, Sorrentino V, Kettenmann H (2002) Requirement of functional ryanodine receptor type 3 for astrocyte migration. Faseb J 16:84-86.

Merten MD, Saleh A, Kammouni W, Marchand S, Figarella C (1998) Characterization of two distinct P2Y receptors in human tracheal gland cells. Eur J Biochem 251:19-24.

Meyer-Franke A, Wilkinson GA, Kruttgen A, Hu M, Munro E, Hanson MG, Jr., Reichardt LF, Barres BA (1998) Depolarization and cAMP elevation rapidly recruit TrkB to the plasma membrane of CNS neurons. Neuron 21:681-693.

Moran-Jimenez MJ, Matute C (2000) Immunohistochemical localization of the P2Y(1) purinergic receptor in neurons and glial cells of the central nervous system. Brain Res Mol Brain Res 78:50-58.

Neary JT, Baker L, Jorgensen SL, Norenberg MD (1994) Extracellular ATP induces stellation and increases glial fibrillary acidic protein content and DNA synthesis in primary astrocyte cultures. Acta Neuropathol (Berl) 87:8-13.

Neary JT, Rathbone MP, Cattabeni F, Abbracchio MP, Burnstock G (1996) Trophic actions of extracellular nucleotides and nucleosides on glial and neuronal cells. Trends Neurosci 19:13-18.

Nedergaard M (1994) Direct signaling from astrocytes to neurons in cultures of mammalian brain cells. Science 263:1768-1771.

Nett WJ, Oloff SH, McCarthy KD (2002) Hippocampal astrocytes in situ exhibit calcium oscillations that occur independent of neuronal activity. J Neurophysiol 87:528-537.

Newman EA (2001) Propagation of intercellular calcium waves in retinal astrocytes and Muller cells. J Neurosci 21:2215-2223.

Newman EA, Zahs KR (1998) Modulation of neuronal activity by glial cells in the retina. J Neurosci 18:4022-4028.

Paemeleire K, Martin PE, Coleman SL, Fogarty KE, Carrington WA, Leybaert L, Tuft RA, Evans WH, Sanderson MJ (2000) Intercellular calcium waves in HeLa cells expressing GFP-labeled connexin 43, 32, or 26. Mol Biol Cell 11:1815-1827.

Parpura V, Basarsky TA, Liu F, Jeftinija K, Jeftinija S, Haydon PG (1994) Glutamate-mediated astrocyte-neuron signalling. Nature 369:744-747.

Parri HR, Crunelli V (2001) Pacemaker calcium oscillations in thalamic astrocytes in situ. Neuroreport 12:3897-3900.

Pasti L, Volterra A, Pozzan T, Carmignoto G (1997) Intracellular calcium oscillations in astrocytes: a highly plastic, bidirectional form of communication between neurons and astrocytes in situ. J Neurosci 17:7817-7830.

Patel S, Robb-Gaspers LD, Stellato KA, Shon M, Thomas AP (1999) Coordination of calcium signalling by endothelial-derived nitric oxide in the intact liver. Nat Cell Biol 1:467-471.

Peuchen S, Clark JB, Duchen MR (1996) Mechanisms of intracellular calcium regulation in adult astrocytes. Neuroscience 71:871-883.

Pfrieger FW (2003) Outsourcing in the brain: do neurons depend on cholesterol delivery by astrocytes? Bioessays 25:72-78.

Pfrieger FW, Barres BA (1997) Synaptic efficacy enhanced by glial cells in vitro. Science 277:1684-1687.

Porter JT, McCarthy KD (1996) Hippocampal astrocytes in situ respond to glutamate released from synaptic terminals. J Neurosci 16:5073-5081.

Rathbone MP, Middlemiss P, Andrew C, Caciagli F, Ciccarelli R, Di Iorio P, Huang R (1998) The trophic effects of purines and purinergic signaling in pathologic reactions of astrocytes. Alzheimer Dis Assoc Disord 12 Suppl 2:S36-45.

Robitaille R (1998) Modulation of synaptic efficacy and synaptic depression by glial cells at the frog neuromuscular junction. Neuron 21:847-855.

Romanello M, Pani B, Bicego M, D'Andrea P (2001) Mechanically induced ATP release from human osteoblastic cells. Biochem Biophys Res Commun 289:1275-1281.

Sanderson MJ, Charles AC, Dirksen ER (1990) Mechanical stimulation and intercellular communication increases intracellular Ca2+ in epithelial cells. Cell Regul 1:585-596.

Schafer KH, Saffrey MJ, Burnstock G (1995) Trophic actions of 2-chloroadenosine and bFGF on cultured myenteric neurones. Neuroreport 6:937-941.

362 Glial ⟺ Neuronal Signaling

Schipke CG, Boucsein C, Ohlemeyer C, Kirchhoff F, Kettenmann H (2002) Astrocyte Ca2+ waves trigger responses in microglial cells in brain slices. Faseb J 16:255-257.
Shelton MK, McCarthy KD (1999) Mature hippocampal astrocytes exhibit functional metabotropic and ionotropic glutamate receptors in situ. Glia 26:1-11.
Sheppard CA, Simpson PB, Sharp AH, Nucifora FC, Ross CA, Lange GD, Russell JT (1997) Comparison of type 2 inositol 1,4,5-trisphosphate receptor distribution and subcellular Ca2+ release sites that support Ca2+ waves in cultured astrocytes. J Neurochem 68:2317-2327.
Soltoff SP, Avraham H, Avraham S, Cantley LC (1998) Activation of P2Y2 receptors by UTP and ATP stimulates mitogen-activated kinase activity through a pathway that involves related adhesion focal tyrosine kinase and protein kinase C. J Biol Chem 273:2653-2660.
Tashiro A, Goldberg J, Yuste R (2002) Calcium oscillations in neocortical astrocytes under epileptiform conditions. J Neurobiol 50:45-55.
Venance L, Stella N, Glowinski J, Giaume C (1997) Mechanism involved in initiation and propagation of receptor-induced intercellular calcium signaling in cultured rat astrocytes. J Neurosci 17:1981-1992.
Verderio C, Bruzzone S, Zocchi E, Fedele E, Schenk U, De Flora A, Matteoli M (2001) Evidence of a role for cyclic ADP-ribose in calcium signalling and neurotransmitter release in cultured astrocytes. J Neurochem 78:646-657.
Verkhratsky A, Orkand RK, Kettenmann H (1998) Glial calcium: homeostasis and signaling function. Physiol Rev 78:99-141.
Walz W, Gimpl G, Ohlemeyer C, Kettenmann H (1994) Extracellular ATP-induced currents in astrocytes: involvement of a cation channel. J Neurosci Res 38:12-18.
Wang DJ, Huang NN, Heppel LA (1990) Extracellular ATP shows synergistic enhancement of DNA synthesis when combined with agents that are active in wound healing or as neurotransmitters. Biochem Biophys Res Commun 166:251-258.
Wang Z, Haydon PG, Yeung ES (2000) Direct observation of calcium-independent intercellular ATP signaling in astrocytes. Anal Chem 72:2001-2007.
Wang Z, Tymianski M, Jones OT, Nedergaard M (1997) Impact of cytoplasmic calcium buffering on the spatial and temporal characteristics of intercellular calcium signals in astrocytes. J Neurosci 17:7359-7371.
Westenbroek RE, Bausch SB, Lin RC, Franck JE, Noebels JL, Catterall WA (1998) Upregulation of L-type Ca2+ channels in reactive astrocytes after brain injury, hypomyelination, and ischemia. J Neurosci 18:2321-2334.
Yuste R, Peinado A, Katz LC (1992) Neuronal domains in developing neocortex. Science 257:665-669.
Zanotti S, Charles A (1997) Extracellular calcium sensing by glial cells: low extracellular calcium induces intracellular calcium release and intercellular signaling. J Neurochem 69:594-602.
Zhu Y, Kimelberg HK (2001) Developmental expression of metabotropic P2Y(1) and P2Y(2) receptors in freshly isolated astrocytes from rat hippocampus. J Neurochem 77:530-541.
Zonta M, Sebelin A, Gobbo S, Fellin T, Pozzan T, Carmignoto G (2003) Glutamate-mediated cytosolic calcium oscillations regulate a pulsatile prostaglandin release from cultured rat astrocytes. J Physiol 553:407-414.

14.6. Abbreviations

AMPA	Alpha-amino-3-hydroxy-5-methyl-4-isoxazole-4-propionic acid
ATP	Adenosine 5'-triphosphate
$[Ca^{2+}]_i$	Intracellular Ca^{2+} concentrations
cAMP	Cyclic adenosine monophosphate
CNQX	6-cyano-7-nitroquinoxaline-2,3-dione
CNS	Central nervous system

Cx	Connexin
ER	Endoplasmic reticulum
GFAP	Glial fibrillary acidic protein
GluR	Glutamate receptors
IP_3	Inositol-1,4,5-trisphosphate
IP_3R	IP_3 receptors
mGluR	Metabotropic GluR
PKC	Protein kinase C
PLA	Phospholipase A
PLC	Phospholipase C
RyR	Ryanodine receptor

Chapter 15

Glutamate-mediated bi-directional signaling between neurons and astrocytes

Vladimir Parpura

Department of Cell Biology and Neuroscience, and
Center for Nanoscale Science and Engineering
University of California Riverside, CA 92521 USA

Corresponding author: vlad@citrus.ucr.edu

Contents

15.1. Introduction

Functional plasticity is an important property of the central nervous system (CNS). A major site for this plasticity is at the chemical synapse. Here, neurons and astrocytes intermingle forming a morphologically intimate relationship (Chapters 3 and 4) where astrocytes are favorably positioned to exchange signals with neurons (Figure 15.1). Ca^{2+} entry though voltage-gated channels into the presynaptic terminal signals to the secretory machinery, which allows the release of neurotransmitter stored in synaptic vesicles into the synaptic cleft. Released neurotransmitter then signals to the postsynaptic neuron by activating its receptors (Figure 15.1, arrow 1). Under certain circumstances, neurotransmitter can 'spillover' from the synaptic cleft and reach neurotransmitter receptors in adjacent astrocytes (Figure 15.1, arrow 2), eliciting astrocytic increases in intracellular Ca^{2+} ion concentration $[Ca^{2+}]_i$. These evoked and/or spontaneous elevations of $[Ca^{2+}]_i$ in astrocytes can cause the release of a neurotransmitter, e.g., glutamate, from astrocytes, which signals to the presynaptic nerve terminal to modulate synaptic neurotransmission and/or released glutamate can affect postsynaptic cells (Figure 15.1, arrows 3 and 4). Additional signaling can occur between astrocytes in the form of intercellular Ca^{2+} waves (Figure 15.1, arrows 5; Chapters 12-14). In this chapter the focus is on glutamate-mediated bi-directional signaling between neurons and astrocytes.

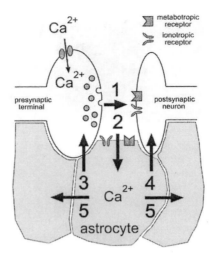

Figure 15.1. Diagram of glutamate-mediated bi-directional astrocyte-neuron signaling. After arrival of action potentials at a presynaptic terminal and opening of voltage gated Ca^{2+} channels, glutamate stored in synaptic vesicles (filled circles) is released into the synaptic cleft and in turn signals to postsynaptic neuron by acting on ionotropic/metabotropic receptors (1). A portion of the released glutamate can reach astrocytes surrounding the synapse, that can stimulate their receptors (2) leading to increase in astrocytic intracellular Ca^{2+} levels. Additionally, glutamate can be taken-up by astrocytes via plasma membrane glutamate transporters. The increase of $[Ca^{2+}]_i$ in a single astrocyte can spread to adjacent astrocytes in the form of a wave of elevated $[Ca^{2+}]_i$, a phenomenon predominately mediated by ATP (5). Through Ca^{2+} - dependent glutamate release, astrocytes can signal to neuronal pre- (3) and post- synaptic (4) sites.

15.2. Neuron-astrocyte signaling

The pioneering work of Orkand et al. (1966) has shown the existence of neuron-glia signaling. Using the mud puppy optic nerve as a model, they showed that electrical impulses delivered to nerve fibers caused depolarization of surrounding glia. The membrane potential changes recorded in glia were interpreted as being physiological since the authors obtained similar results in anesthetized mud puppies. Glial depolarization during neuronal activity has also been detected in the leech CNS (Baylor and Nicholls, 1969) and in mammals (Ransom and Goldring, 1973). The mechanism underlying this type of signaling is an accumulation of K^+ in the extracellular space as a result of neuronal activity. Since astrocytes are electrically coupled to one another (Chapter 13), the conduction properties of such coupled cells can be much the same as they would be if the cells were a syncytium. If several astrocytes are depolarized by an increased extracellular K^+ ($[K^+]_o$), they draw a charge from neighboring cells creating a current flow.

The pre-requisite for the existence of receptor-mediated neuron-astrocyte signaling is that astrocytes express receptors for neuroligands. Indeed, astrocytes express many ion channels (Chapters 6-8) and receptors for neuroligands (Chapter 12), such as serotonin, acetylcholine (ACh), bradykinin, glutamate and norepinephrine (Hosli et al., 1982; Hosli et al., 1988; Stephens et al., 1993;

Steinhäuser et al., 1994; Jalonen et al., 1997; Sharma and Vijayaraghavan, 2001). Activation of these neuroligand receptors can result in mobilization of Ca^{2+} from internal stores (Cornell-Bell et al., 1990; Jensen and Chiu, 1990; Charles et al., 1991; Finkbeiner, 1992). Cornell-Bell et al. (1990) made a seminal observation that extracellular glutamate can elicit increases in $[Ca^{2+}]_i$ of cultured hippocampal astrocytes. These increases of $[Ca^{2+}]_i$ had distinct patterns (Figure 15.2), either sustained oscillators with constant or decreasing frequencies, or damped-oscillators and step responders. Besides oscillatory $[Ca^{2+}]_i$ changes (Movie 15.1; see legend, end of text), in some cases, they observed the spread of increased $[Ca^{2+}]_i$ within single excited astrocytes, and also between adjacent cells in the form of waves (Movie 15.2; see legend, end of text), whose radii were glutamate concentration-dependent. At low concentrations of glutamate (< 1 μM) intracellular waves were recorded, while at higher concentrations (1-10 μM) these intracellular waves started to propagate to the surrounding cells. At even higher concentrations (10-100 μM) intercellular waves propagated over long distances (several hundred μm). However, at 1 mM of glutamate the cellular responses were step-like increases in $[Ca^{2+}]_i$, and there were no waves. This study opened a possibility that astrocytes could receive signals from neurons mediated by glutamate and that information from neurons could be graded by the amount of released glutamate from neurons and encoded by astrocytes through the pattern and the frequency of their $[Ca^{2+}]_i$ changes. Indeed, the use of $[Ca^{2+}]_i$ changes for encoding information transfer by astrocytes is still speculative and remains to be experimentally addressed. Nonetheless, glutamate-mediated neuron-astrocyte signaling has been experimentally tested as described below. An additional outcome of the Cornel-Bell at al. study was to present the possibility of long-range signaling between astrocytes based on Ca^{2+} waves, discussed elsewhere in this volume (Chapters 12-14).

Given that astrocytes depolarize in conditions of high neuronal activity and express receptors for neuroligands, the activation of which can lead to $[Ca^{2+}]_i$ increases, astrocytes should be able to "sense" synaptic transmission. Dani et al. (Dani et al., 1992) have demonstrated that neuronal activity can trigger $[Ca^{2+}]_i$ increases and intercellular waves in an astrocytic network mediated by glutamate released from synaptic terminals. In this work the authors used organotypic slice cultures of rat hippocampus. These slices readily load with cell permeable form of Ca^{2+} indicator, fluo-3, the fluorescence of which was observed with a confocal microscope equipped with time-lapse video recording. They used an extracellular pipette to electrically stimulate mossy fibers originating in dentate gyrus of hippocampus (Figure 15.3). These fibers project onto CA3 pyramidal neurons that are organized in palisades and surrounded by astrocytes. Using low frequency stimulation (8 Hz) of mossy fibers, the authors observed $[Ca^{2+}]_i$ increases in both neurons and astrocytes within the CA3 area. Whilst neuronal $[Ca^{2+}]_i$ reached steady state levels within several seconds, the astrocytic population, located in stratum radiatum, lucidum and oriens, and also intermingled among pyramidal cell somata, started to show substantial increases in $[Ca^{2+}]_i$ after several seconds of mossy fiber stimulation. When high frequency (50 Hz) mossy fiber stimulation was used, the astrocytic response could be observed within a 2 second minimal latency of the stimulus onset (Figure 15.3 and Movie 15.3). Additionally, sustained neuronal stimulation at low frequency (8 Hz) induced $[Ca^{2+}]_i$ oscillation in astrocytic somata and processes. These oscillations exhibited periodicity/frequency similar to those seen in cultured astrocytes (Table 15.1), although they were less regular. The identity of astrocytes in slices was defined by post-recording immunocytochemisty using glial fibrillary acidic proteins (GFAP) as an astrocytic marker. Since all astrocytic $[Ca^{2+}]_i$ responses to neuronal stimulation could be blocked by kynurenic acid, a glutamate receptor (GluR) antagonist, the straight forward explanation of this study is that the astrocytes in hippocampal organotypic slice cultures respond to the glutamate released from neurons, thus demonstrating glutamate-mediated neuron-astrocyte signaling.

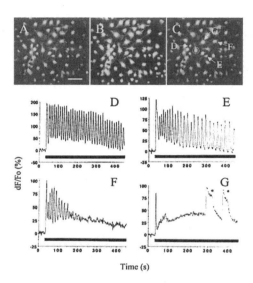

Figure 15.2. Extracellular glutamate induces $[Ca^{2+}]_i$ variations in cultured hippocampal astrocytes. Fluorescent intensity of astrocytes loaded with Ca^{2+} indicator fluo-3 at rest (A) increased after addition of extracellular glutamate (B), indicating the increase in $[Ca^{2+}]_i$. C) is the same image as in A), but with added arrows and letters marking the astrocytes for which traces are shown in D-G). Astrocytes showed different patterns of $[Ca^{2+}]_i$ increases due to glutamate application (100 μM, solid bar just above abscissae): sustained oscillations with constant frequency (D) and with decreasing frequency (E), damped-oscillations (F), and the step-like increases in $[Ca^{2+}]_i$ (G). The cell in (G) participated in two intercellular $[Ca^{2+}]_i$ waves, appearing in its trace as two peaks (asterisks), initiated in the cell shown by a dotted circle in (C). The time-lapse sequence of this experiment is shown in Movie 15.2 (see legend, end of text). Fluo-3 fluorescence is expressed as dF/Fo (%), where Fo represents a baseline fluorescence, and dF represents a change from the baseline. Scale bar, 200 μm. Modified from Cornell-Bell et al., 1990. Data courtesy of Dr. Stephen J. Smith, Stanford University.

The long-standing question of whether astrocytes can respond to neuronal transmitter release in acute slices was addressed by Porter and McCarthy (1996). Using acutely isolated hippocampal slices they observed that electrical stimulation of Schaffer collaterals (2 s, 50 Hz) caused increases in $[Ca^{2+}]_i$ in astrocytes located in the stratum radiatum of the CA1 region. This effect was mediated by metabotropic GluR (mGluRs). Additional experiments suggested that at higher levels of neuronal activity both metabotropic and ionotropic GluRs (iGluRs) on astrocytes were involved in neuron-astrocyte signaling.

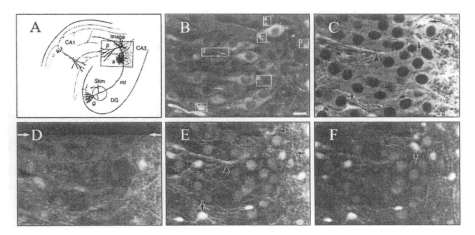

Figure 15.3. High frequency (50 Hz) electrical stimulation of mossy fibers evokes $[Ca^{2+}]_i$ responses in CA3 region astrocytes. A) Drawing shows positioning of stimulating electrode (Stim) and imaged area (rectangular area) shown in B-F with respect to microanatomy of transverse hippocampal slice. Stimulating electrode is placed in dentate gyrus (DG) to depolarize axons of granule cells (g), which synapse onto pyramidal neurons (p) in CA3 region. Cell bodies of pyramidal neurons form palisades (dotted outlines) and are surrounded by astrocytes (a). B) Resting fluorescence observed within CA3 region after loading slices with Ca^{2+} indicator fluo-3 (32 frame average). Note the stratum pyramidale (palisades) formed by neuronal somata (left 2/3 of the image), while stratum lucidum lies to the far right. The squares numbered 1-5 indicate astrocytes, while 6 indicates a neuron. C) GFAP immunofluorescent reactivity of the field shown in B) acquired after the Ca^{2+}imaging sequence shown in D-F (single frames). Arrows and arrowhead indicate astrocytic somata and processes, respectively. D) The earliest response in CA3 region following electrical stimulation of dentate gyrus. The arrows indicate the active horizontal scan line at the time of stimulus onset (t = 0 s). Thus, the portion of the image above the line represents fluorescence before stimulation, while the portion of the image below the line reports on fluorescence intensities after electrical stimulation, showing $[Ca^{2+}]_i$ increases in pyramidal cell bodies and fine neuronal processes. E) After an additional 2 s of stimulation (t = 4 s), the pyramidal cell bodies exhibited large $[Ca^{2+}]_i$ increases, but also many GFAP-positive cell bodies and processes showed $[Ca^{2+}]_i$ increases. Arrows and arrowhead in (E) and (F) correspond to those in (C). F) After 4 s of stimulation (t = 6 s) almost all astrocytes within the imaging area responded with $[Ca^{2+}]_i$ increases. Scale bar, 20 μm. The time-lapse sequence of this experiment is provided in Movie 15.3 (see legend, end of text). Modified from Dani et al., 1992. Data courtesy of Dr. Stephen J. Smith, Stanford University.

The responsiveness of astrocytes to synaptically released glutamate is not restricted to hippocampal astrocytes. Pasti et al. (1997) using acute slices from both visual cortex and hippocampus, have demonstrated that astrocytes can respond to neuronal activity by $[Ca^{2+}]_i$ oscillations mediated through mGluRs (Table 15.1). The frequency of these astrocytic $[Ca^{2+}]_i$ oscillations was correlated to the level of synaptic activity, since the increased frequency or intensity of stimuli applied to presynaptic afferents caused an increase in the frequency of astrocytic $[Ca^{2+}]_i$ oscillations. Additionally, astrocytes *in situ* exhibited changes in $[Ca^{2+}]_i$ oscillations. Namely, in their preceding work in culture, Pasti et al (1995) observed a long-lasting increase in the frequency of $[Ca^{2+}]_i$ oscillations when astrocytes were challenged by multiple applications of a mGluR agonist (1S, 3R)-1-aminocyclopentane-1, 3-dicarboxlylic acid (t-ACPD). Similarly, astrocytes *in situ* adjacent to repeatedly stimulated neurons exhibited increases in $[Ca^{2+}]_i$ oscillation frequency. This increase in the frequency of $[Ca^{2+}]_i$ oscillations was postulated to represent a form of cellular learning in astrocytes. The functional consequences of this type of cellular learning, however, still need experimental testing. Since increases in their $[Ca^{2+}]_i$ stimulates glutamate release from astrocytes (Parpura et al., 1994; Hassinger et al., 1995; Jeftinija et al., 1996; Pasti et al., 1997; Bezzi et al., 1998) (see section 15.3), it is tempting to speculate that increased frequency of $[Ca^{2+}]_i$ oscillations could lead to increased glutamate release from astrocytes.

Zonta et al. (2003b) showed that astrocytes play a role in coupling neuronal activity to vascular tone in cerebral cortex. Using acute slices they demonstrated that astrocytic mGluRs serve as sensors of neuronal activity. The activation of these receptors led to $[Ca^{2+}]_i$ elevations in astrocytes and consequent vasodilatation, a process in which a cyclooxygenase product was involved. Perhaps, the release of prostaglandin E_2 (PGE$_2$) from astrocytes, regulated by their glutamate-induced $[Ca^{2+}]_i$ oscillations, could be the underlying mechanism for this phenomenon (Zonta et al., 2003a). Thus, glutamate-mediated neuron-astrocyte signaling participates in the control of brain microcirculation.

Glutamate is not the only mediator of neuron-astrocyte signaling. Because astrocytes respond to many neurotransmitters with $[Ca^{2+}]_i$ mobilization, this raises the possibility of widespread neuron-astrocytes signaling in the CNS. Recent results indicate, for example, that synaptically released ACh evokes $[Ca^{2+}]_i$ elevations in astrocytes in hippocampal slices through the activation of astrocytic metabotropic ACh receptors (Araque et al., 2002).

Besides neuron-astrocyte signaling mediated via spillover of synaptically released neurotransmitters, this signaling could occur through direct synapse-like, or even classical synaptic connections. There are direct inputs from neurons through synapse-like, synaptoid contacts (see Chapter 4, Figure 4.12), where axonal projections end on pituicytes, stellate astrocyte-like glia (Wittkowski and Brinkmann, 1974; van Leeuwen et al., 1983; Buijs et al., 1987). Stimulation of pituitary stalk led to depolarization of pituicytes *in situ*, an effect mediated by γ-aminobutyric acid (GABA) and dopamine receptors on this glial cell type (Mudrick-Donnon et al., 1993). Similar contacts exist on septohippocampal astrocytes that receive inputs from norepinephrine terminals (Milner et al., 1995). This possibility of neuron-astrocyte signaling via synaptoid contacts is exciting since it would warrant sensitivity of astrocytic responses to the neuronal activity at the level of neurotransmitter release due to a single action potential, as opposed to the repetitive stimulation necessary for spillover to occur. Finally, direct glutamatergic and GABAergic synapses on oligodendrocyte precursor cells were observed in the hippocampus (Bergles et al., 2000; Lin and Bergles, 2004). Although similar synaptic connections onto astrocytes have not been reported so far, the existence of multiple transmitters mediating transfer of information from neuron to astrocytes using different routes, spillover and synaptoid, suggests high level of complexity and specificity in neuron-astrocyte communication. For example, it is feasible that the spillover of glutamate from synapses conveys entirely different information than the spillover of synaptically released ACh, or perhaps directly released norepinephrine through a synaptoid contact.

Table 15.1. Astrocytic [Ca^{2+}]$_i$ oscillations

Preparation	Animal	Brain region	periodicity (s)	peaks/min	frequency (Hz)	Stimulus	Reference
dissociated cell culture	rat * (Sprague-Dawley)	hippocampus	9 to 23		0.043-0.111	glutamate (100 µM)	(Cornell-Bell et al., 1990) text, p 247
dissociated cell culture	rat (Wistar)	visual cortex		4.8	0.08	glutamate (20 µM)	(Pasti et al., 1995) Table I
				4.1	0.068	t-ACPD (10 µM)	
dissociated cell culture	rat (Wistar)	cortex	~84 to 132		0.008-0.012	L-quisqualate (3 µM)	(Pasti et al., 2001) Figure 1
				~2.12	0.035	t-ACPD (20 µM)+ AMPA (2 µM)	Figure 2
dissociated cell culture	rat (Wistar)	cortex		~1.6-2.17	0.027-0.036	L-quisqualate (10 µM)	(Zonta et al., 2003a) Figures 1 and 2
organotypic slice culture	rat (Sprague-Dawley)	hippocampus, CA3	16 to 30		0.033-0.063	**Mf (8Hz)	(Dani et al., 1992) text, p 432
acute slice	rat (Wistar)	hippocampus, CA1		0.66 to 1.55	0.011-0.026	t-ACPD (2-10 µM)	(Pasti et al., 1997) Table 1
				1.41 to 2.58	0.023-0.043	**Sc (0.1-1 Hz)	text, p 7823 and Figure 6
		visual cortex		1.05	0.0175	t-ACPD (2-10 µM)	Table 1
acute slice	rat	ventrobasal thalamus	99 to 333		0.003 - 0.01	spontaneous	(Parri et al., 2001) text, p 803
acute slice	rat	ventrobasal thalamus	10 to 300		0.003 - 0.1	spontaneous***	(Parri and Crunelli, 2001) text, p 3898
acute slice	rat	ventrobasal thalamus	~70		0.014	spontaneous	(Parri and Crunelli, 2003) text, p 981
acute slice	mouse (C57/BL6)	hippocampus, CA1		0.44 to 1.56	0.007 - 0.026	spontaneous	(Nett et al., 2002) Figure 1

t-ACPD, (1S, 3R)-1-aminocyclopentane-1, 3-dicarboxlyic acid; AMPA, α-amino-3-hydroxy-5-methyl-isoxazole propionate; Mf, Mossy fibers; Sc, Schaffer collateral. * Dr. Stephen J. Smith, personal communication; ** Mf and Sc are glutamatergic neurotransmission; *** a subset of these astrocytes exhibit rhythmic, i.e. pacemaker, oscillations with the average frequency of 0.019 Hz (10-90% range, 0.012-0.02Hz)

15.3. Ca²⁺- dependent release of glutamate from astrocytes

So far, we have seen that astrocytes can respond to neuronal stimuli by changing their Ca^{2+} homeostasis, e.g., neurotransmitters caused $[Ca^{2+}]_i$ elevations in astrocytes. One emerging consequence of these $[Ca^{2+}]_i$ elevations is that astrocytes can release glutamate. There are several mechanisms that had been implicated in the release of glutamate from astrocytes, as discussed in Chapters 13 and 16. Here, I focus on Ca^{2+}- dependent release of glutamate from astrocytes, which is an integral part of bi-directional communications between neurons and astrocytes.

The first evidence for Ca^{2+}-dependent glutamate release from astrocytes originated from purified cortical astrocytic culture (Parpura et al., 1994). There, bradykinin caused $[Ca^{2+}]_i$ elevations and consequent glutamate release from astrocytes (Figure 15. 4). This novel release pathway is not a peculiarity of the cell culture system, since its existence has been confirmed in acute hippocampal slices as well (Bezzi et al., 1998). Ca^{2+}- dependent glutamate release from astrocytes exhibits characteristics similar to those of exocytotic process at presynaptic terminals; it shows Ca^{2+} dependency, and astrocytes express proteins involved in exocytosis and in mediating glutamate accumulation by acidic/vesicular intracellular compartments.

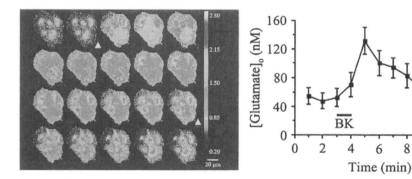

Figure 15.4. Bradykinin causes $[Ca^{2+}]_i$ elevations in cultured astrocytes originating from visual cortex (Left), and also stimulates glutamate release from these cells (Right). Left panel: Ca^{2+} levels in astrocytes were monitored using a Ca^{2+} indicator fura-2. Images were acquired 5 seconds apart, with sequence staring from top left corner and ending at the bottom right corner. Bradykinin was added to astrocytes (top arrowhead) and washed away after 65 seconds (bottom arrowhead), causing a transient $[Ca^{2+}]_i$ elevations in these cells. Color scale is a pseudocolor representation shown in the form of the ratio of fura-2 emission at 510 nm due to sequential excitation at 350 and 380 nm. Astrocytic resting $[Ca^{2+}]_i$ was ~ 100 nM, while the peak response was up to ~ 1 μM. Bradykinin (BK) causes release of glutamate from astrocytes (right; modified from Parpura et al., 1994). The superfusate from astrocytes was collected at 1-minute intervals and levels of extracellular glutamate were measured using high-performance liquid chromatography. Points and bars indicate means ± s.e.m.

15.3.1. Ca $^{2+}$ dependency

[Ca^{2+}]$_i$ elevations in astrocytes were sufficient and necessary to cause glutamate release (Parpura et al., 1994), because the addition of Ca^{2+} ionophore ionomycin to astrocytes in the presence of external calcium ions, but not in their absence, caused glutamate release from these cells. Subsequently, other stimuli that directly increased astrocytic [Ca^{2+}]$_i$, such as mechanical stimulation (Parpura et al., 1994; Araque et al., 1998a; Araque et al., 1998b), photostimulation (Parpura et al., 1994) and photolysis of Ca^{2+} cages (Araque et al., 1998b; Parpura and Haydon, 2000), all caused glutamate release as well. Additionally, the manipulations of [Ca^{2+}]$_i$ in astrocytes using the calcium chelator, BAPTA (Araque et al., 1998a; Bezzi et al., 1998), or pre-incubation of cells with thapsigargin, an inhibitor of Ca^{2+}-ATPase specific for internal stores (Araque et al., 1998a), led to reduction of evoked glutamate release from astrocytes. Thus, unlike in neurons, it seems that the internal stores represent a predominant source of Ca^{2+} necessary for glutamate release from astrocytes. This is consistent with their reported absence or inactivity of voltage-gated calcium channels (Carmignoto et al., 1998). However, since astrocytes express various voltage-gated calcium channels (MacVicar, 1984; Latour et al., 2003) and transient receptor potential genes (Pizzo et al., 2001), the source of calcium ions in this release will have to be studied in detail. Indeed, recent work suggests a dual source for Ca^{2+}, both the release of calcium ions from internal stores and their entry from extracellular space, in exocytotic glutamate release from astrocytes (Hua et al., 2002; 2004).

The amount of Ca^{2+} in synaptic terminals is critical for shaping synaptic transmission due to Ca^{2+} regulation of neurotransmitter release at the terminal. Seminal work by Dodge and Rahamimoff (1967) had established the quantitative relationship between the neuronal calcium levels and the neurotransmitter release by determining the slope of this relationship on a logarithm-logarithm plot, commonly referred as the Hill coefficient. This coefficient indicates the cooperativity of calcium ions in the release of neurotransmitter at synaptic terminals, and since then have been reported to be between 2 and 4 (Augustine and Eckert, 1984; Smith et al., 1985; Stanley, 1986; Zhong and Wu, 1991; Trudeau et al., 1998). Such basic quantitative assessment of the secretory apparatus in astrocytes has been recently initiated (Parpura and Haydon, 2000), showing that: (i) the threshold level of [Ca^{2+}]$_i$ necessary to stimulate glutamate release from astrocytes is much lower than that in neurons ([Ca^{2+}]$_i$ elevations from resting ~ 80 nM to only 140 nM caused glutamate release), and that (ii) the Hill coefficient for glutamate release is 2.1-2.7, suggesting multiple Ca^{2+} binding sites in glutamate release from astrocytes.

15.3.2. Exocytotic secretory machinery

Glutamate release from astrocytes is stimulated by α-latrotoxin, a component of black widow spider venom (Parpura et al., 1995b). Because α-latrotoxin also induces vesicular fusion and neuronal transmitter release (Ushkaryov et al., 1992; Petrenko, 1993), these data suggest that astrocytes may release transmitters using a mechanism similar to the neuronal secretory process. Indeed, astrocytes express the protein components of the soluble N-ethyl maleimide-sensitive fusion protein attachment protein receptors (SNARE) known to mediate exocytosis at presynaptic terminals: synaptobrevin 2 and its non-neuronal homologue cellubrevin, syntaxin 1 and SNAP-23, a non-neuronal homologue of SNAP-25 (Parpura et al., 1995a; Jeftinija et al., 1997; Hepp et al., 1999; Maienschein et al., 1999; Araque et al., 2000; Pasti et al., 2001) (Figure 15.5). *Clostridial* toxins can specifically cleave some of these proteins in astrocytes (Parpura et al., 1995a; Jeftinija et al., 1997), for example, tetanus toxin cleaves synaptobrevin 2. These toxins also inhibit Ca^{2+}-dependent release of glutamate from these cells (Jeftinija et al., 1997; Bezzi et al., 1998; Araque et al., 2000; Pasti et al., 2001) (also see Figure 15.5 A-B). A Ca^{2+} sensor for glutamate release in astrocytes is most likely synaptotagmin, consistent with the presence of neurexins, as indicated by the action of α-latrotoxin, and with the Hill coefficient for glutamate release reported above. Some additional proteins of neuronal secretory machinery, such as synapsin I and rab3a were also found in astrocytes (Maienschein et al., 1999). Rab 3a displays a partial co-localization with glutamate puncta as revealed by indirect immunocytochemisty (Anlauf and Derouiche, 2002). An immnoelectron microscopic study demonstrated that these exocytotic proteins can be associated with electron lucent or dense-core vesicular structures, although their diameters were less uniform than those reported in neurons (Maienschein et al., 1999) (also see Figure 15.5 G). Consistent with the possibility that astrocytes can exhibit release via dense-core vesicles, a Ca^{2+}-dependent release of secretogranin II, a marker for dense-core vesicles, has been demonstrated (Calegari et al., 1999). Additionally, exocytotic release of atrial natriuretic peptide with concomitant uptake of the membrane recycling dye FM 4-64 has been recently reported, confirming the presence of exocytosis though dense-core vesicles in cultured astrocytes (Krzan et al., 2003) (also see Figure 15.5 F).

The storage of glutamate in synaptic vesicles requires the presence of V-type H^+-ATPase (V-ATPase) and vesicular glutamate transporters (VGLUTs). Astrocytic Ca^{2+}-dependent glutamate release can be blocked with bafilomycin A_1 (Araque et al., 2000; Bezzi et al., 2001; Pasti et al., 2001) that specifically interferes with V-ATPase leading to alkalinization of the vesicular lumen, and collapse of the proton gradient necessary for VGLUTs to transport glutamate into vesicles (Figure 15.5 A and B). Recently, there has been a report indicating the presence of a VGLUT 3 isoform in subpopulations of inhibitory neurons, cholinergic and monoaminergic neurons and some glia (Fremeau et al., 2002)(also see Figure 15.5 E). Additionally, the expression of VGLUTs 1, 2 and 3 in cultured and freshly- isolated astrocytes from rat visual cortices, exhibits a punctate subcellular localization pattern consistent with their vesicular association. Since pharmacological inhibition of VGLUTs via allosteric modulation using Rose Bengal (Figure 15.5 A and B) greatly reduces Ca^{2+}-dependent exocytotic release of glutamate from astrocytes, these proteins can play a functional role in astrocytic glutamate release in the CNS (Ni et al., 2003; Montana et al., 2004).

The process of exocytosis relies on an increase of $[Ca^{2+}]_i$ that, through actions on a fusion complex, causes quantal release of neurotransmitter due to vesicular fusion. Indeed, quantal-like events were recorded from astrocytes using biosensor cells expressing functional N-methyl D-Aspartate receptors (NMDARs) as a detection system, consistent with vesicular exocytosis (Pasti et al., 2001).

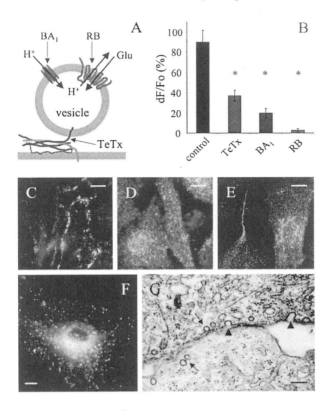

Figure 15.5. Exocytosis underlies Ca^{2+}-dependent glutamate release from cultured astrocytes. A) A drawing of exocytotic process in astrocytes. Astrocytes express SNARE proteins synaptobrevin 2 (red), syntaxin (green) and SNAP-23 (blue). They also express the vacuolar type H^+-ATPase (V-ATPase, brown) and vesicular glutamate transporters (VGLUTs, pink), that are necessary for acidification of vesicles and filling them with glutamate, respectively. B) Pre-treatment of astrocytes with Tetanus toxin (TeTx), pre-incubation with Bafilomycin A_1 (BA_1), or application of Rose Bengal (RB), reduced mechanically-induced Ca^{2+}-dependent glutamate release from astrocytes (Montana et al., 2004). Levels of extracellular glutamate were fluorescently monitored using an L-glutamate dehydrogenase (GDH)-linked assay (Innocenti et al., 2000) and represented as dF/Fo. Bars represent means ± s.e.m Asterisks indicate significant changes of measurements as compared with the control group (* $p<0.01$). Subcellular localization of synaptobrevin 2 (C), β-subunit of V-ATPase (D), and VGLUT 3 (E) in astrocytes. Synaptobrevin 2 was primarily located at the leading edge of the cells, although there were some puncta present throughout the entire cell body. Staining with anti-V-ATPase or anti-VGLUT 3 showed a punctate pattern of immunoreactivity that was present throughout the entire cell body and processes. E) Astrocytes exposed to the co-application of a recycling dye RH-414 (40 μM) and bradykinin, known to cause Ca^{2+}- dependent glutamate release (see Figure 15.4), followed by a wash, accumulated RH-414, exhibiting a punctate pattern of its fluorescence throughout entire cell body. F) An electron micrograph showing the contact between two astrocytes. There are several clear vesicles (arrows) close to the plasma membrane, which exhibits some omega shapes consistent with vesicles fusing with or pinching off the plasma membrane (arrowheads). Scale bars in C-F, 10 μm, and 200 nm in G. Micrograph courtesy of Dr. Srdija Jeftinija, Iowa State University.

Exocytotic cues I discussed above support the existence of vesicular exocytosis in astrocytes. A conclusive demonstration, however, will require the direct observation of vesicular fusions to the plasma membrane, and visualization of spatio-temporal characteristics of exocytosis in astrocytes including the location and morphological correlates of the release sites *in situ*.

Of importance for our further discussion regarding bi-directional signaling, however, is the fate of glutamate released from astrocytes, i.e., its actions on adjacent cells, particularly neurons, and the existence of glutamate-mediated astrocyte-neuron signaling, described below.

15.4. Glutamate-mediated astrocyte-neuron signaling

Intracellular Ca^{2+} elevations in astrocytes can lead to subsequent intracellular Ca^{2+} elevations in adjacent neurons (Charles, 1994; Nedergaard, 1994; Parpura et al., 1994; Hassinger et al., 1995; Jeftinija et al., 1996; Pasti et al., 1997; Bezzi et al., 1998; Parri et al., 2001). There are two mechanisms implicated in this astrocyte-neuron signaling, heterocellular gap junctions (Nedergaard, 1994) and the release of glutamate from astrocytes (Parpura et al., 1994; Hassinger et al., 1995; Jeftinija et al., 1996; Pasti et al., 1997; Araque et al., 1998a; Araque et al., 1998b; Bezzi et al., 1998; Sanzgiri et al., 1999; Araque et al., 2000; Parri et al., 2001).

Astrocyte-neuron signaling remained speculative until Nedergard (Nedergaard, 1994) demonstrated this phenomenon in hippocampal culture. She stimulated astrocytes using micropipettes to increase $[Ca^{2+}]_i$ in a single astrocyte that then spread to adjacent astrocytes in the form of Ca^{2+} wave. When the leading edge of a Ca^{2+} wave reached a co-cultured neuron, the neuron exhibited an increase in $[Ca^{2+}]_i$. This intercellular signaling was blocked in the presence of octanol and heptanol, lending support for possible gap junctional involvement in this process. Indeed, the existence of gap junctions between neurons and glia has been demonstrated by Peracchia (1981) in crayfish. Also, direct heterocellular coupling of neurons and glia of mammalian origin, have been demonstrated in co-cultured cells from cerebral hemispheres (Froes et al., 1999), and in acute slices from locus coeruleus (Alvarez-Maubecin et al., 2000).

Parpura et al. (1994) used three different means to stimulate cultured astrocytes from visual cortex, neuroligand bradykinin, mechanical and photostimulation. Each of these stimuli raised $[Ca^{2+}]_i$ in astrocytes and caused glutamate-dependent elevation of neuronal $[Ca^{2+}]_i$. Since similar results were obtained for all three stimuli, discussion here focuses on experiments using bradykinin. This neuroligand caused increase of $[Ca^{2+}]_i$ in astrocytes (Figure 15.4), but not in neurons alone. However, when neurons were co-cultured with astrocytes, application of bradykinin caused increase in astrocytic and neuronal $[Ca^{2+}]_i$ (Figure 15.6). This astrocyte-neuron signaling could be prevented by GluR antagonists. Broad spectrum antagonist, D-glutamylglycine (DGG) prevented bradykinin-induced Ca^{2+} accumulations in neurons, without altering astrocytic Ca^{2+} responses to bradykinin (Figure 15.6 A-E). These data suggested that bradykinin elevates neuronal Ca^{2+} via glutamate released from astrocytes in response to bradykinin. To study the pharmacology of receptors, further confocal microscopy was employed (Figure 15.6 F). Bradykinin reliably caused accumulation of Ca^{2+} in neurons, that was prevented by NMDAR antagonist D-2-amino-phosphonopentanoic acid (D-AP5), but not by an α-amino-3-hydroxy-5-

methyl-isoxazole propionate (AMPA) receptor antagonist 6-cyano-7-nitroquinoxaline-2,3-dione (CNQX), or an mGluR antagonist 2-amino-3-phosphonopropionic acid (L-AP3). Consistent with the role of NMDARs in mediating this effect, removal of extracellular Mg^{2+} and addition of glycine augmented the bradykinin-induced neuronal Ca^{2+} elevations, and this augmented response was also sensitive to D-AP5. These results showed that $[Ca^{2+}]_i$ increases in astrocytes lead to glutamate release that in turn signals to adjacent neurons. The existence of this pathway was confirmed by others in hippocampal astrocyte-neuron co-cultures (Hassinger et al., 1995; Araque et al., 1998a; Araque et al., 1998b), and in acute hippocampal (Pasti et al., 1997; Bezzi et al., 1998) and ventrobasal thalamic slices (Parri et al., 2001).

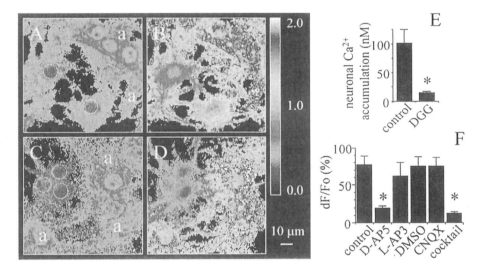

Figure 15.6. Bradykinin causes a glutamate-mediated accumulation of internal Ca^{2+} in neurons co-cultured with astrocytes. The $[Ca^{2+}]_i$ in neocortical neurons (dotted circles in A and C) and astrocytes (a in A and C) was monitored using fura-2. A) Mixed culture at rest. B) Application of bradykinin caused an elevation in $[Ca^{2+}]_i$ in astrocytes and neurons. However, when co-cultures were bathed in DGG (C), application of bradykinin did not significantly alter neuronal $[Ca^{2+}]_i$ calcium levels, even though bradykinin elevated the astrocytic $[Ca^{2+}]_i$ (D). Color scale indicates pseudocolor representation of $[Ca^{2+}]_i$, by fura-2 emission ratio ranging from 0 to 2.0. In E) the mean bradykinin-evoked internal Ca^{2+} accumulations (peak value subtracted from resting) in neurons are shown (in control and when pre-incubated with DGG). Bradykinin elevated neuronal $[Ca^{2+}]_i$ when neurons were co-cultured with astrocytes, and DGG blocked this response. F) GluR pharmacology was studied using confocal microscopy and the Ca^{2+} indicator fluo-3. Bradykinin-induced elevations of internal Ca^{2+} in neurons were reduced by D-AP5, but not by CNQX or L-AP3. Cocktail contained all three GluR inhibitors. DMSO is a carrier for CNQX. *Significant at $p < 0.01$. Bars: means ± s.e.m. Modified from Parpura et al., 1994.

Hassinger et al. (1995) used mechanical stimulation of astrocytes to increase $[Ca^{2+}]_i$ in single astrocytes. Similar to Nedergaard's experimental observations, as a Ca^{2+} wave approached a neuron, there was an increase of neuronal $[Ca^{2+}]_i$. However, this effect was mediated through ionotropic non-NMDA and NMDA GluRs, further implicating glutamate-mediated astrocyte-neuron signaling. Additionally, using simultaneous measurements of $[Ca^{2+}]_i$ changes in astrocytes and neurons, and electrical activity in neurons, when the authors recorded neuronal $[Ca^{2+}]_i$ increases due to astrocytic stimulation, they also recorded increased neuronal electrical excitability, e.g., depolarization of neuronal resting membrane potential that led to firing action potentials. Similar increases in electrical excitability of neurons leading to initiation of action potentials were observed by Araque et al. (1999). These authors employed voltage-clamp recordings to assess electrical responses in neurons due to increase in astrocytic $[Ca^{2+}]_i$, and revealed that the neuronal depolarization caused by glutamate released from astrocytes is carried out by a slow-inward current mediated by the activation of ionotropic non-NMDA and NMDA GluRs (Araque et al., 1998a).

Thus, astrocytes can receive neuronal signals that can stimulate astrocytic receptors to cause an increase in $[Ca^{2+}]_i$. In turn, Ca^{2+}-dependent astrocytic glutamate release can serve to signal adjacent neurons. This implies that astrocytes could be integral elements in the computational power of the CNS. To have a full partnership in this possible bi-directional communication between neurons and astrocytes, astrocytes should be able to initiate astrocyte-neuron signaling based on their intrinsic activity. Additionally, glutamate-mediated astrocyte-neuron signaling should be governed by physiological levels of $[Ca^{2+}]_i$ in astrocytes.

Using freshly prepared slices from ventrobasal thalamus and Ca^{2+} imaging, Parri et al. (2001) showed that astrocytes *in situ* display intrinsic $[Ca^{2+}]_i$ oscillations. Spontaneous astrocytic $[Ca^{2+}]_i$ oscillations were not driven by neuronal activity since they could not be blocked by tetrodotoxin. Astrocytes *in situ* displaying spontaneous $[Ca^{2+}]_i$ oscillations could initiate Ca^{2+} waves in adjacent astrocytes, and also cause NMDAR-mediated neuronal excitability, electrophysiologically recorded as inward currents in thalamocortical neurons. Even though they observed that this spontaneous activity decreased significantly within two weeks postnatally, it is possible that some of these oscillations and consequent astrocyte-neuron signaling would persist in adult animals. Although astrocytes mainly showed oscillations of irregular amplitudes and frequencies, a subset of spontaneously active astrocytes exhibited rhythmic, i.e., pacemaker $[Ca^{2+}]_i$ oscillations (Parri and Crunelli, 2001). Nett et al. (2002) also recorded spontaneous $[Ca^{2+}]_i$ oscillations in a large subpopulation (~65%) of astrocytes in acute hippocampal slices. The frequency of spontaneous $[Ca^{2+}]_i$ oscillations recorded in these three studies were in good agreement with frequencies of pharmacologically- or synaptically- evoked oscillations recorded in cultured astrocytes and astrocytes in organotypic slice cultures and acute slices (Table 15.1).

Whether the release of glutamate from astrocytes and the consequent signaling to neurons is used as a physiological signaling pathway or recruited only under pathophysiological conditions was addressed by Parpura and Haydon (2000). In order to study the relationship between $[Ca^{2+}]_i$ levels in astrocytes and consequent Ca^{2+}-dependent glutamate release from astrocytes, there are two critical experimental conditions that must be met: (i) it is essential that the experimental stimulus selectively increases $[Ca^{2+}]_i$ in astrocytes, and (ii) the assay system must selectively detect released glutamate. It has been shown that mechanical (Charles et al., 1991), electrical (Innocenti et al., 2000) or photostimulation (Parpura et al., 1994) of a single astrocyte evokes an elevation of $[Ca^{2+}]_i$ within stimulated and surrounding astrocytes. Although all three forms of stimulation have been shown to cause the release of glutamate from astrocytes (Parpura et al., 1994; Araque et al., 1998a; Araque et al., 1998b; Innocenti et al., 2000), they do not allow quantitative control of the $[Ca^{2+}]_i$. To overcome this problem, we have worked with a method in which we used UV photolysis to release Ca^{2+} from a UV-sensitive cage (Araque et al., 1998b; Parpura and Haydon, 1999a, b, 2000). To measure glutamate release from astrocytes, we monitored glutamate-mediated responses in reporter cells, single neurons, using whole-cell voltage-clamp.

We used hippocampal neurons grown in microisland cultures (Figures 15.7) (Furshpan et al., 1986; Bekkers and Stevens, 1991; Parpura and Haydon, 2000). In this method, a single neuron is cultured on top of an island of astrocytes. A single neuron can form a synapse with itself (autapse). In this configuration the same neuron that is electrically stimulated to evoke transmitter release shows synaptic currents. In our cultures, we detected functional autapses in 62% of neurons. The majority of autaptically connected cells exhibited an inhibitory (77%), while a minority (23%) showed excitatory transmission. We have never found a neuron that made both inhibitory (GABAergic) and excitatory (glutamatergic) connections. Therefore, this type of culture enhanced the resolution of our experiments because we could record from inhibitory neurons and study glutamate-mediated astrocyte-neuron signaling without glutamate contamination from neurotransmission.

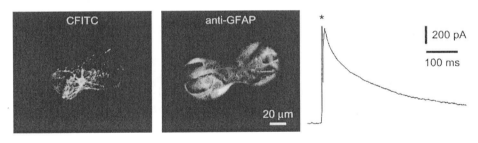

Figure 15.7. Microisland in cell culture. Left panel shows a single hippocampal neuron labeled with fluorescein-conjugated C fragment of tetanus toxin (CFITC), while central panel shows the associated island of hippocampal astrocytes labeled with anti-GFAP (rhodamine-conjugated secondary antibody). Right panel shows an inhibitory autaptic current (asterisk indicates artifact due to application of a depolarizing step in the neuron). Left and central panels are modified from Parpura and Haydon, 2000.

The experimental paradigm is presented in Figure 15.8. Astrocytes and neurons were co-loaded with cell permeant forms of Ca^{2+} indicator fluo-3 and Ca^{2+} cage o-nitrophenyl (NP)-EGTA, and visually located using wide field epi-fluorescence microscopy. One concern with the co-loading approach is that both astrocytes and neurons were loaded, which could obscure any attempt to study glutamate-mediated responses in the neurons, because of possible direct effects of UV flashes on neurons. However, because we recorded from neurons in the whole-cell configuration mode we overcame this problem by dialysis of NP-EGTA/fluo-3 out of neuron prior to delivery of UV flashes. Following the loading procedure, implementation of a simple 10-minute dialysis protocol insured the absence of NP-EGTA/fluo-3 in the neuron. Since astrocytes underneath the dialyzed neuron still contained NP-EGTA, photolysis led to selective stimulation of astrocytes that increased their $[Ca^{2+}]_i$, and caused the neuronal SIC (Figure 15.8 D). In agreement with previous studies in mass culture (Araque et al., 1998a), photolytically induced SIC amplitudes were greatly reduced when the microisland cultures were treated with the combination of the NMDAR antagonist D-AP5, and ionotropic non-NMDA GluR antagonist, CNQX (Figure 15.8E). Therefore, the photolysis-induced neuronal SIC is a result of Ca^{2+}-dependent release of glutamate from astrocytes.

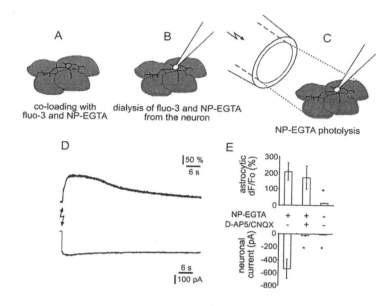

Figure 15.8. Photolytic elevation of astrocytic $[Ca^{2+}]_i$ causes NMDA and AMPA receptor-dependent neuronal slow-inward currents (SIC). A) Cells in mixed hippocampal culture were co-loaded with the cell permeant forms of Ca^{2+} indicator fluo-3 and the Ca^{2+} cage NP-EGTA. B) Both fluo-3 and NP-EGTA were dialyzed out from single neurons on top of astrocytic islands using a pipette in a whole-cell patch clamp configuration as indicated by a loss of fluo-3 fluorescence. Astrocytes remained loaded with NP-EGTA and fluo-3. Their resting $[Ca^{2+}]_i$ (A and B; in blue) was elevated (C; in red) when NP-EGTA was photolysed using UV pulses delivered through a UV transmitting optical fiber (C, D; lightning bolt) to cause an increase in astrocytic $[Ca^{2+}]_i$ (C, D). D) Simultaneous recordings of astrocytic $[Ca^{2+}]_i$ (top trace) and neuronal currents (bottom trace) indicate that the increase in astrocytic $[Ca^{2+}]_i$ is sufficient to cause glutamate-mediated SIC in neurons. In contrast, UV stimulation of unloaded astrocytes, neither elevated astrocytic $[Ca^{2+}]_i$ nor caused a neuronal SIC (E). D-AP5/CNQX significantly attenuated the ability of photolytic Ca^{2+} elevations in astrocytes to cause neuronal SICs (E). Changes in astrocytic $[Ca^{2+}]_i$ are represented as dF/Fo (%). *Significant at p<0.05. D) is modified from Parpura and Haydon, 2000.

Simultaneous recording of $[Ca^{2+}]_i$ in astrocytes and consequent glutamate-mediated neuronal currents allowed us to determine whether Ca^{2+}-dependent glutamate release operates within the physiological $[Ca^{2+}]_i$ levels seen in astrocytes. One such experiment where two UV flashes were provided to the sample is shown in

Figure 15.9. The initial flash elevated astrocytic $[Ca^{2+}]_i$ from about 100 to 200 nM and caused a SIC. A second UV flash, which caused a further increase in $[Ca^{2+}]_i$, led to an augmentation of the SIC recorded in the neuron. On average, the first UV flash elevated the astrocytic $[Ca^{2+}]_i$ from a resting level of about 84 nM to 140 nM, and induced effects on neurons resulting in sizable SIC amplitudes (-391 ± 139 pA). These modest changes of astrocytic $[Ca^{2+}]_i$, which caused glutamate release sufficient to stimulate adjacent neurons, were within range of $[Ca^{2+}]_i$ normally seen in astrocytes when they are stimulated by endogenous agonists norepinephrine, glutamate or dopamine (all at 50 μM). This suggests that Ca^{2+}- dependent glutamate release from astrocytes constitutes physiologically relevant signaling that can be used in the CNS for information transfer and neuronal modulation.

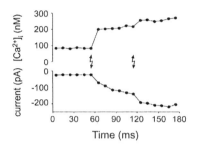

Figure 15.9. Simultaneous recordings of astrocytic $[Ca^{2+}]_i$ and neuronal currents can be used to reveal the relationship between astrocytic $[Ca^{2+}]_i$ and consequent glutamate release. UV pulses (lighting bolts) caused a step-like increase in astrocytic $[Ca^{2+}]_i$ (top trace) and an increase in the amplitude of the inward current recorded from the adjacent neuron (bottom trace). Modified from Parpura and Haydon, 2000.

15.4.1. Modulation of synaptic transmission by astrocytes

The ultrastructure of the CNS suggests that astrocytes might regulate synaptic neurotransmission. Astrocytes enwrap nerve terminals (Peters et al., 1991; Grosche et al., 1999; Ventura and Harris, 1999), which makes them perfectly positioned to exchange information with synapses. As discussed above, it has been demonstrated that astrocytes can respond to glutamatergic synaptic activation (Dani et al., 1992; Porter and McCarthy, 1996). Additionally, astrocytes can modulate synaptic neurotransmission by releasing glutamate (Araque et al., 1998a; Araque et al., 1998b; Kang et al., 1998; Newman and Zahs, 1998; Fiacco and McCarthy, 2004). There are two particularly illustrative studies in which astrocytes were shown to act on synapses and modulate spontaneous (Araque et al., 1998b) and action-potential evoked synaptic transmission (Araque et al., 1998a). Araque et al (1998b) used UV photolysis of a Ca^{2+} cage to raise the $[Ca^{2+}]_i$ in astrocytes while monitoring miniature excitatory and inhibitory postsynaptic currents (mEPSCs and mIPSCs) in adjacent neurons (Figure 15.10). Single astrocytes were microinjected with NP-EGTA together with the fluorescent dye fluoro-ruby to identify the injected cell. Following the recovery of cells after injection, fluoro-ruby- and NP-EGTA- containing astrocytes were localized based on their fluoro-ruby florescence. Once an astrocyte of interest was located, an optical fiber was brought into the field of view and used to deliver UV light. Photolysis of NP-EGTA that reliably increased intracellular $[Ca^{2+}]_i$ caused an increase in the frequency of mEPSCs and mIPSC. This increase in frequency was transient, lasted for about 1-2 minutes and was not accompanied by significant changes in the mPSC amplitudes, suggesting involvement of a presynaptic mechanism underlying this effect. D-AP5 blocked the ability of photolytically-induced Ca^{2+} elevations in astrocytes to raise mPSC frequency, indicating that the astrocytic modulatory effect on frequency of mPSCs is caused by glutamate released from astrocytes that selectively activates NMDARs located at presynaptic sites.

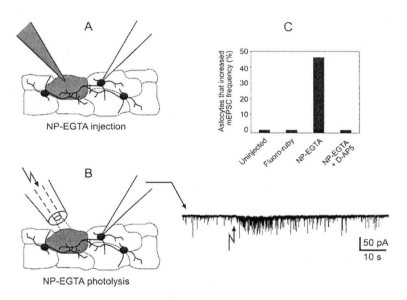

Figure 15.10. Intracellular Ca^{2+} elevations in astrocytes are sufficient to increase the frequency of mEPSCs. A) Single astrocytes were microinjected with the Ca^{2+} cage NP-EGTA (together with the fluorescent dye fluoro-ruby to identify the injected cell) that was photolysed using UV pulses (B, lighting bolts) delivered through a UV transmitting optical fiber. Following recovery after injection, the astrocyte at rest (A, blue), was stimulated by photolysis, which reliably increased intracellular Ca^{2+} (B, red) as monitored using fluo-3. In parallel experiments analyzing the effects on neuronal currents, photolysis reliably evoked an increase in the frequency of mEPSCs (B, trace; C). In contrast, UV stimulation of either uninjected astrocytes or fluoro-ruby injected astrocytes, did not change the mEPSC frequency. D-AP5 blocked the ability of photolytic astrocytic $[Ca^{2+}]_i$ elevations to raise mEPSC frequency. Trace in (B) and graph (C) are modified from Araque et al., 1998b.

To assess the role of astrocytes in evoked synaptic transmission, Araque et al. (1998a) recorded in the whole-cell patch-clamp configuration from one neuron while electrically stimulating another with an extracellular patch pipette (Figure 15.11). After obtaining the basal measurement of synaptic transmission, single astrocytes were mechanically stimulated to cause an increase in their $[Ca^{2+}]_i$ that spread to adjacent astrocytes in a form of Ca^{2+} wave. This stimulus, which induces a wave of elevated $[Ca^{2+}]_i$ among astrocytes, produced a corresponding spread of extracellular glutamate (Innocenti et al., 2000) (also see Movies 15.4 and 15.5; see legends, end of text), and reduced the amplitude of action potential-evoked PSCs. The transient decrease in evoked synaptic transmission lasted tens of seconds and was recorded both in excitatory and inhibitory transmissions, mediated through presynaptic mGluRs. Modulation of inhibitory synaptic transmission was mediated by (S)-α-methyl-4-carboxyphenylglycine (MCPG)-sensitive mGluRs, while excitatory synaptic transmission depression was due to the activation of (S)-2-amino-2-methyl-4-phosphonobutanoic acid (MAP-4)-sensitive group of mGluRs.

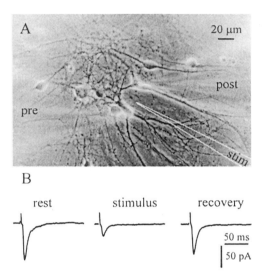

Figure 15.11. Astrocytes modulate evoked synaptic transmission. A) Micrograph of cultured hippocampal cells and an experimental arrangement. While the currents of the postsynaptic neuron (post) evoked by extracellular presynaptic stimulation (pre) were recorded, an adjacent astrocyte was mechanically stimulated (stim) to evoke a Ca^{2+} wave propagating between neighboring astrocytes (see Movie 15.4; see legend, end of text) and a consequent extracellular glutamate wave (see Movie 15.5) B) Following astrocytic stimulation, the amplitudes of excitatory postsynaptic currents were transiently decreased for about 1 min. B) is modified from Araque et al., 1998a. Micrograph courtesy of Dr. Louis-Eric Trudeau, University of Montreal.

Besides the ability of astrocytes to modulate synaptic transmission via releasing glutamate, another well documented role of astrocytes related to glutamate signaling is that of re-uptake of glutamate via plasma membrane glutamate transporters (Chapter 9). Current evidence suggests that astrocytes express vast numbers of transporters that are quite efficient in eliminating extracellular glutamate. This can in effect shape excitatory neurotransmission in cultured hippocampal cells (Mennerick and Zorumski, 1994; Tong and Jahr, 1994) as well as *in situ* at auditory nerve calyceal somatic synapses in the nucleus magnocellularis (Otis et al., 1996) and Schaffer collateral - commissural synapses of hippocampus (Bergles and Jahr, 1998).

Taken together these studies indicate the potential for astrocytes in the control of synaptic neurotransmission. Therefore, there is a possibility that astrocyte-neuron signaling may play a role in synaptic plasticity, especially in long-term potentiation (LTP) and long-term depression (LTD). Astrocytes, in their capacity to release glutamate and modulate synaptic transmission, could represent a site for the regulation of these modes of synaptic plasticity, although this hypothetical scenario remains to be established. However, electrophysiological studies using acute hippocampal (Sastry et al., 1988; Janigro et al., 1997; Ma and Zhao, 2002; Yang et al., 2003) or spinal cord (Ma and Zhao, 2002) slices have suggested involvement of glial cells in long-term plasticity. Furthermore, using molecular genetics approaches, in mice devoid of GFAP, it was found that cerebellar LTD was impaired, while regular excitatory transmission was unaltered (Shibuki et al., 1996). These data support the notion that astrocytic intermediate filament protein GFAP is required for the induction and maintenance of LTD. In a different study (McCall et al., 1996), GFAP-null mice displayed an enhancement of LTP in the CA1 region of hippocampus. Similarly, deletion of the astrocytic Ca^{2+}- binding protein S100B in mice resulted in enhancement of LTP in the hippocampal CA1 region (Yang et al., 2003), while over expression of this protein altered synaptic plasticity and impaired spatial learning (Gerlai et al., 1995). These studies represent a direct demonstration that a primary defect in astrocytic proteins affects neuronal physiology.

15.5. Glutamate is not the only mediator of bi-directional signaling

Glutamate is just one of many mediators of bi-directional signaling between neurons and astrocytes. For example, β-adrenergic stimulation of cultured astrocytes can lead to release of homocysteic acid (Do et al., 1997), an endogenous NMDAR agonist. This opens an intriguing possibility that putative noradrenergic terminals making synaptoid contacts could stimulate astrocytes to release homocysteic acid, which can in turn act on adjacent neurons through activation of their NMDAR. In addition to β-adrenergic stimulation, astrocytes in hippocampal slices can respond to norepinephrine with an increase in $[Ca^{2+}]_i$ mediated through α1-receptors (Duffy and MacVicar, 1995), further supporting a role for norepinephrine in neuron-astrocyte communication in CNS.

Besides homocysteic acid, another example of a gliotransmitter that acts on NMDARs as an endogenous ligand is D-serine (Schell et al., 1995). Astrocytes express serine racemase, an enzyme synthesizing D-serine (Wolosker et al., 1999), which can in turn be released (Mothet et al., 2000) and contributes to the physiological activation of NMDARs of retinal ganglion cells (Stevens et al., 2003), as well as to the hippocampal LTP (Yang et al., 2003) through its actions on the glycine site of neuronal NMDARs.

ATP can be released from astrocytes and plays roles in astrocyte-astrocyte signaling, being a prime molecule to support intercellular Ca^{2+} waves (Guthrie et al., 1991; Cotrina et al., 2000; Arcuino et al., 2002; Stout et al., 2002; also see Chapter 14), in astrocyte-microglia (Verderio and Matteoli, 2001) and astrocyte-endothelial cell signaling (Braet et al., 2001; also see Chapter 12, section 12.1.11). Additionally, ATP plays a role in astrocyte-neuron signaling in whole mount retina (Newman, 2003). There, stimulated astrocytes release ATP into extracellular space, where it was converted by ectoenzymes to adenosine. Subsequent activation of adenosine receptors located on retinal ganglion cells led to hyperpolarization of these cells and reduction in spontaneous firing rate of those neurons exhibiting spontaneous spike activity. Similarly, ATP released from astrocytes can cause tonic and activity-dependent suppression of excitatory synaptic transmission in hippocampal cultures (Koizumi et al., 2003) and acute slices (Zhang et al., 2003). ATP can be co-released with other neurotransmitters at nerve terminals (Redman and Silinsky, 1994; von Kugelgen et al., 1994; Sperlagh et al., 1998; Poelchen et al., 2001), and it mediates neuron-astrocyte signaling in cell cultures of cerebral cortices (Jeremic et al., 2001). Additionally, ATP can stimulate Ca^{2+}-dependent glutamate release from astrocytes (Jeremic et al., 2001), and, likewise, glutamate can stimulate ATP release (Queiroz et al., 1997), findings that support another possible heterocellular cross-talk pathway.

ACh spillover from synaptic transmission can lead to $[Ca^{2+}]_i$ increases in astrocytes in hippocampal slices, and this ACh-mediated neuron-astrocyte signaling is mediated by astrocytic muscarinic receptors (Araque et al., 2002). Recent findings indict that astrocytes also express nicotinic ACh receptors (nAChRs), particularly those with $\alpha 7$ subunits (Sharma and Vijayaraghavan, 2001). Since activation of both types of AChRs on astrocytes can lead to $[Ca^{2+}]_i$ increases, it is tempting to speculate that this would lead to Ca^{2+}-dependent release of glutamate and signaling back to neurons. Additional complexity in ACh-mediated heterocellular signaling arises from the finding that glial cells of the mollusk *Lymnea stagnalis* express an nAChR-like protein, ACh binding protein (AChBP) (Smit et al., 2001). Presynaptic release of ACh induces secretion of AChBP through glial secretory pathway. Since AChBP is lacking nAChR domains to form a transmembrane ion channel, its release caused the suppression of cholinergic transmission. Whether a similar system for the cessation of cholinergic synaptic transmission exists in the mammalian CNS in not known. If so, it would be interesting to know how AChBP-like molecules would complement or compete with the fast actions of ACh-esterase in the clearance of ACh from synaptic clefts.

Stimulation of GABAergic interneurons in hippocampal slices can cause $[Ca^{2+}]_i$ elevations in adjacent astrocytes mediated though $GABA_BR$ activation (Kang et al., 1998). Modulation of neuronal activity by glia cells in retina also involves GABAergic transmission (Newman and Zahs, 1998). Namely, stimulation of intercellular astrocytic Ca^{2+} waves in retina leads to changes in light-evoked spike activity in retinal ganglion cells. This modulatory effect is mediated by glutamatergic, GABAergic and glycinergic transmission.

Taurine can be released from cultured cell line astrocytes by β-adrenergic stimulation and this release is independent of changes in $[Ca^{2+}]_i$ (Shain et al., 1989). Additionally, swelling of primary astrocytes cultured from cerebral cortices caused release of glutamate, aspartate and taurine (Kimelberg et al., 1990). However, the best available example of the regulation of neuronal activity mediated by taurine is in the hypothalamo-neurohypophysial system (also see Chapter 4). There osmotic regulation of activity in supraoptic nucleus neurons, whose axons terminate in the posterior pituitary, depends in part on activation of neuronal glycine receptors (GlyR) by taurine released from adjacent astrocytes (Hussy et al., 1997; Deleuze et al., 1998). Indeed, taurine immunoreactivity has been shown in the supraoptic nucleus (Decavel and Hatton, 1995) and posterior pituitary (Pow, 1993; Miyata et al., 1997), where taurine is prominently located in astrocytes and astrocyte-like pituicytes, respectively. Upon exposure to hypoosmotic media, pituicytes released taurine (Miyata et al., 1997), which can activate GlyR located at adjacent nerve terminals of vasopressin releasing magnocellular neurons (Hussy et al., 2001). Taurine-induced activation of GlyRs leads to reduction of firing in supraoptic neurons and reduction in the release of vasopressin near fenestrated capillaries, resulting in reduction of its anti-diuretic actions.

Activation of astrocytic CXC chemokine receptor 4 (CXCR4) caused release of tumor necrosis factor α (TNFα) that can then stimulate glutamate release from astrocytes which subsequently acts on neuronal NMDARs (Bezzi et al., 2001). This pathway can be amplified by surrounding activated microglia cells and lead to neurotoxicity. Thus, this signaling may have importance for HIV infections. In the CNS, only microglia are productively infected by HIV-1. Activated microglia can release HIV-1 coat protein gp120 (that can activate CXCR4) and lead to apoptotic neuronal death (Kaul et al., 2001). Thus, the outlined signaling pathway may provide fertile ground for therapeutic intervention in the prevention of dementia that can develop in HIV infected individuals as a result of neuronal loss. Additionally, TNFα when released from astrocytes can cause an increase in the surface expression of neuronal AMPARs, and, thus, this factor plays a role in controlling synaptic strength (Beattie et al., 2002).

Hypothalamic astrocytes regulate luteinizing hormone-releasing hormone (LHRH), a neuropeptide important in the control of sexual development, from LHRH neurons. This astrocytic regulation is seen at the level of plastic rearrangements in the median eminence, and also in activating astrocyte-astrocyte and astrocyte-neuron signaling (Ojeda et al., 2000). Two peptides, transforming growth factor α and the neuroregulins are produced and released by hypothalamic astrocytes to stimulate autocrine/paracrine activation of erbB receptor complexes on astrocytes. This receptor activation leads to production of PGE_2, which then binds to receptors on LHRH neurons causing release of LHRH. Furthermore, the co-activation of astrocytic AMPARs and mGluRs enhances astrocytic capability to utilize erbB pathway (Dziedzic et al., 2003). This presents the intriguing possibility that this neuroendocrine system may utilize glutamatergic neuron-astrocyte signaling as a regulatory mechanism to coordinate astroglial input to LHRH neurons during sexual development.

15.6. Concluding remarks

The intent of this chapter was to put forward the findings supporting the existence of bi-directional, primarily glutamate-mediated, astrocyte-neuron signaling. A brief summary follows. After the arrival of the action potential to the presynaptic terminal, the neurotransmitter, e.g., glutamate is released. A portion of the glutamate is taken up by surrounding astrocytes and released upon physiological increases in astrocytic $[Ca^{2+}]_i$. The released glutamate from astrocytes can then act on adjacent neurons, experimentally recorded as (i) an increase of neuronal $[Ca^{2+}]_i$, (ii) SIC, (iii) an increase in the frequency of mPSCs and (iv) a reduction in evoked synaptic transmission. What is going on here? This looks much like an "eclectic collection", where the release of glutamate from astrocytes can cause almost anything that an experimentalist would test. However, this might be explainable if the localization of glutamate release sites on astrocytes in respect to synaptic sites could dictate the nature of astrocytic effects on neurons. Therefore, it would be advantageous in future work to address the location of the release sites on astrocytes. Here, the resolution available in cell culture systems seems like an ideal starting point, but the potential findings will have to be validated in the brain tissue, acute slices and *in vivo*.

Are astrocytes out of the neuronal shadow? Initially termed "star cells" due to their morphological appearance, astrocytes are no longer dismissed as just a neuronal metabolic support. Although their astrocytic nurturing activities are very important for brain functions (Chapter 11), this is no longer the sole reason for researchers' excitement about astrocytes. Another area of interest is the recognition that astrocytes may have communication skills that can complement those of neurons. Experimental evidence supports a lively chat between neurons and astrocytes. Indeed, the astrocytes posses the necessary equipment for such communication. They have listening devices, i.e. receptors for different neurotransmitters (Chapters 6 and 7), and can also talk back to neurons, by releasing different neuroligands. They can even initiate conversation through spontaneous intracellular Ca^{2+} oscillations and subsequent transmittance of information to neurons. It appears that this astrocyte-neuron relationship is now more like a partnership established to achieve brain functions. One intriguing question to be addressed in the near future is how this intercellular communication and cross-talk between not only astrocytes and neurons, but also other glial cells, vasculature and immune cells to name a few, are orchestrated in the service of efficient brain operation. Perhaps one way is to start explaining the role of these heterocellular communications in behavioral outputs. An attempt in this direction has already been made (Laming et al., 1998). It will be necessary to take experiments out of Petri dishes and rigorously test hypotheses on freely-moving animals and humans. Of course, as a pre-requisite to testing hypotheses, or making educated guesses, we will first have to collect and catalogue information regarding the involvement of heterocellular signaling in brain (patho) physiology. It should then become possible to intervene in brain operations by specifically targeting brain areas and intercellular communication channels in health and disease. However, this might be wishful thinking and far-reaching at the present time. Thus, it does not hurt to remind ourselves of a proverb: *Festina lente.*

Acknowledgements. The author's research is supported by a grant from DOD/DARPA/DMEA under Award No. DMEA90-02-2-0216 and the Whitehall Foundation (award 2000-05-17). Thanks are due to the laboratory members Vedrana Montana and Dr. Steven E. Rosenwald for providing some of their unpublished data. I thank Dr. Sarjeet S. Gill, University of California Riverside for kindly providing the antibody against β-subunit of V-ATPase. I am grateful to Dr. Stephen J. Smith, Stanford University, for providing materials for some figures and movies, and Dr. Srdija Jeftinja, Iowa State University, and Dr. Louis-Eric Trudeau, University of Montreal, for providing their micrographs. I also thank Dr. Glenn I. Hatton, Dr. Srdija Jeftinija and Todd A. Ponzio for their comments on earlier versions of this manuscript, and for engaging discussions related to this chapter. The author is an Institute for Complex Adaptive Matter Senior Fellow.

Movie legends

Movie 15.1. Glutamate-induced $[Ca^{2+}]_i$ oscillations in cultured hippocampal astrocytes. Astrocytes were loaded with Ca^{2+} indicator fluo-3 and visualized using wide-filed fluorescence microscopy. Application of glutamate (at time 0; 100 μM) to the cells at rest caused oscillations in their $[Ca^{2+}]_i$, seen as the transient changes in the intensity of fluo-3 emission. The digital clock indicates time in seconds. Movie provided by the courtesy of Dr. Stephen J. Smith, Stanford University.

Movie 15.2. Waves of $[Ca^{2+}]_i$ elevations propagating between glutamate-stimulated astrocytes. This movie represents a time-lapse recording of the data presented in Figure 15.2. Extracellular addition of glutamate (100 µM) to the astrocytes at rest initiates $[Ca^{2+}]_i$ oscillations in cultured hippocampal astrocytes. At ~248 seconds after the application of glutamate began, there were two consecutive intercellular $[Ca^{2+}]_i$ waves. These waves appeared to be initiated in the cell located in the center of the filed (Figure 15.2 C, dotted circle) and then propagated towards the upper right quadrant of the imaging filed. The speed of these waves is about 19 µm/s. The digital clock indicates time in seconds. Movie provided by the courtesy of Dr. Stephen J. Smith, Stanford University.

Movie 15.3. Neuron-astrocyte signaling. This movie is a video frame rate time-lapse imaging of the experiment outlined in the Figure 15.3. At the onset of imaging, when cells are at their resting $[Ca^{2+}]_i$, one can observe neuronal bodies forming palisades (stratum pyramidale). The onset of the electrical stimulation (50 Hz, 6 seconds), that appears like a flash of increased fluorescence intensity, caused quick neuronal responses, followed briefly after with responses of many astrocytic processes and bodies. Please consult Figure 15.3 C for the location of GFAP immunopositive astrocytes in this video clip. Movie courtesy of Dr. Stephen J. Smith, Stanford University.

Movie 15.4. Mechanical stimulation of a single astrocyte elicits a propagating intercellular wave of elevated $[Ca^{2+}]_i$ in cultured astrocytes. Astrocytes were loaded with a Ca^{2+} indicator fluo-3. To evoke radially propagating waves of elevated $[Ca^{2+}]_i$ in astrocytes, we used a patch pipette to establish a mechanical contact, monitored as an increase in pipette resistance. Image size, 211 x 167 µm. Speed of wave propagation, ~ 15 µm/s.

Movie 15.5. Ca^{2+}- dependent glutamate release from cultured astrocytes. Mechanical stimulation of a single astrocyte elicits a propagating wave of elevated extracellular glutamate from astrocytes in culture. We fluorescently monitored glutamate using NADH generated from glutamate through a GDH-linked assay. Image size, 211 x 167 µm. Speed of wave propagation, ~ 15 µm/s.

15.7. References

Alvarez-Maubecin V, Garcia-Hernandez F, Williams JT, Van Bockstaele EJ (2000) Functional coupling between neurons and glia. J Neurosci 20:4091-4098.
Anlauf E, Derouiche A (2002) Exocytosis markers label glutamate-containing vesicles in cultured astrocytes. Glia Suppl 1:33.
Araque A, Parpura V, Sanzgiri RP, Haydon PG (1998a) Glutamate-dependent astrocyte modulation of synaptic transmission between cultured hippocampal neurons. Eur J Neurosci 10:2129-2142.
Araque A, Sanzgiri RP, Parpura V, Haydon PG (1998b) Calcium elevation in astrocytes causes an NMDA receptor-dependent increase in the frequency of miniature synaptic currents in cultured hippocampal neurons. J Neurosci 18:6822-6829.
Araque A, Sanzgiri RP, Parpura V, Haydon PG (1999) Astrocyte-induced modulation of synaptic transmission. Can J Physiol Pharmacol 77:699-706.
Araque A, Li N, Doyle RT, Haydon PG (2000) SNARE protein-dependent glutamate release from astrocytes. J Neurosci 20:666-673.
Araque A, Martin ED, Perea G, Arellano JI, Buno W (2002) Synaptically released acetylcholine evokes Ca2+ elevations in astrocytes in hippocampal slices. J Neurosci 22:2443-2450.

Arcuino G, Lin JH, Takano T, Liu C, Jiang L, Gao Q, Kang J, Nedergaard M (2002) Intercellular calcium signaling mediated by point-source burst release of ATP. Proc Natl Acad Sci U S A 99:9840-9845.

Augustine GJ, Eckert R (1984) Divalent cations differentially support transmitter release at the squid giant synapse. J Physiol 346:257-271.

Baylor DA, Nicholls JG (1969) Changes in extracellular potassium concentration produced by neuronal activity in the central nervous system of the leech. J Physiol 203:555-569.

Beattie EC, Stellwagen D, Morishita W, Bresnahan JC, Ha BK, Von Zastrow M, Beattie MS, Malenka RC (2002) Control of synaptic strength by glial TNFalpha. Science 295:2282-2285.

Bekkers JM, Stevens CF (1991) Excitatory and inhibitory autaptic currents in isolated hippocampal neurons maintained in cell culture. Proc Natl Acad Sci U S A 88:7834-7838.

Bergles DE, Jahr CE (1998) Glial contribution to glutamate uptake at Schaffer collateral-commissural synapses in the hippocampus. J Neurosci 18:7709-7716.

Bergles DE, Roberts JD, Somogyi P, Jahr CE (2000) Glutamatergic synapses on oligodendrocyte precursor cells in the hippocampus. Nature 405:187-191.

Bezzi P, Carmignoto G, Pasti L, Vesce S, Rossi D, Rizzini BL, Pozzan T, Volterra A (1998) Prostaglandins stimulate calcium-dependent glutamate release in astrocytes. Nature 391:281-285.

Bezzi P, Domercq M, Brambilla L, Galli R, Schols D, De Clercq E, Vescovi A, Bagetta G, Kollias G, Meldolesi J, Volterra A (2001) CXCR4-activated astrocyte glutamate release via TNFalpha: amplification by microglia triggers neurotoxicity. Nat Neurosci 4:702-710.

Braet K, Paemeleire K, D'Herde K, Sanderson MJ, Leybaert L (2001) Astrocyte-endothelial cell calcium signals conveyed by two signalling pathways. Eur J Neurosci 13:79-91.

Buijs RM, van Vulpen EH, Geffard M (1987) Ultrastructural localization of GABA in the supraoptic nucleus and neural lobe. Neuroscience 20:347-355.

Calegari F, Coco S, Taverna E, Bassetti M, Verderio C, Corradi N, Matteoli M, Rosa P (1999) A regulated secretory pathway in cultured hippocampal astrocytes. J Biol Chem 274:22539-22547.

Carmignoto G, Pasti L, Pozzan T (1998) On the role of voltage-dependent calcium channels in calcium signaling of astrocytes in situ. J Neurosci 18:4637-4645.

Charles AC (1994) Glia-neuron intercellular calcium signaling. Dev Neurosci 16:196-206.

Charles AC, Merrill JE, Dirksen ER, Sanderson MJ (1991) Intercellular signaling in glial cells: calcium waves and oscillations in response to mechanical stimulation and glutamate. Neuron 6:983-992.

Cornell-Bell AH, Finkbeiner SM, Cooper MS, Smith SJ (1990) Glutamate induces calcium waves in cultured astrocytes: long-range glial signaling. Science 247:470-473.

Cotrina ML, Lin JH, Lopez-Garcia JC, Naus CC, Nedergaard M (2000) ATP-mediated glia signaling. J Neurosci 20:2835-2844.

Dani JW, Chernjavsky A, Smith SJ (1992) Neuronal activity triggers calcium waves in hippocampal astrocyte networks. Neuron 8:429-440.

Decavel C, Hatton GI (1995) Taurine immunoreactivity in the rat supraoptic nucleus: prominent localization in glial cells. J Comp Neurol 354:13-26.

Deleuze C, Duvoid A, Hussy N (1998) Properties and glial origin of osmotic-dependent release of taurine from the rat supraoptic nucleus. J Physiol 507 (Pt 2):463-471.

Do KQ, Benz B, Sorg O, Pellerin L, Magistretti PJ (1997) beta-Adrenergic stimulation promotes homocysteic acid release from astrocyte cultures: evidence for a role of astrocytes in the modulation of synaptic transmission. J Neurochem 68:2386-2394.

Dodge FA, Jr., Rahamimoff R (1967) Co-operative action a calcium ions in transmitter release at the neuromuscular junction. J Physiol 193:419-432.

Duffy S, MacVicar BA (1995) Adrenergic calcium signaling in astrocyte networks within the hippocampal slice. J Neurosci 15:5535-5550.

Dziedzic B, Prevot V, Lomniczi A, Jung H, Cornea A, Ojeda SR (2003) Neuron-to-glia signaling mediated by excitatory amino acid receptors regulates ErbB receptor function in astroglial cells of the neuroendocrine brain. J Neurosci 23:915-926.

Fiacco TA, McCarthy KD (2004) Intracellular astrocyte calcium waves in situ increase the frequency of spontaneous AMPA receptor currents in CA1 pyramidal neurons. J Neurosci 24:722-732.

Finkbeiner S (1992) Calcium waves in astrocytes-filling in the gaps. Neuron 8:1101-1108.

Fremeau RT, Jr., Burman J, Qureshi T, Tran CH, Proctor J, Johnson J, Zhang H, Sulzer D, Copenhagen DR, Storm-Mathisen J, Reimer RJ, Chaudhry FA, Edwards RH (2002) The identification of vesicular glutamate transporter 3 suggests novel modes of signaling by glutamate. Proc Natl Acad Sci U S A 99:14488-14493.

Froes MM, Correia AH, Garcia-Abreu J, Spray DC, Campos de Carvalho AC, Neto MV (1999) Gap-junctional coupling between neurons and astrocytes in primary central nervous system cultures. Proc Natl Acad Sci U S A 96:7541-7546.

Furshpan EJ, Landis SC, Matsumoto SG, Potter DD (1986) Synaptic functions in rat sympathetic neurons in microcultures. I. Secretion of norepinephrine and acetylcholine. J Neurosci 6:1061-1079.

Gerlai R, Wojtowicz JM, Marks A, Roder J (1995) Overexpression of a calcium-binding protein, S100 beta, in astrocytes alters synaptic plasticity and impairs spatial learning in transgenic mice. Learn Mem 2:26-39.

Grosche J, Matyash V, Moller T, Verkhratsky A, Reichenbach A, Kettenmann H (1999) Microdomains for neuron-glia interaction: parallel fiber signaling to Bergmann glial cells. Nat Neurosci 2:139-143.

Guthrie PB, Segal M, Kater SB (1991) Independent regulation of calcium revealed by imaging dendritic spines. Nature 354:76-80.

Hassinger TD, Atkinson PB, Strecker GJ, Whalen LR, Dudek FE, Kossel AH, Kater SB (1995) Evidence for glutamate-mediated activation of hippocampal neurons by glial calcium waves. J Neurobiol 28:159-170.

Hepp R, Perraut M, Chasserot-Golaz S, Galli T, Aunis D, Langley K, Grant NJ (1999) Cultured glial cells express the SNAP-25 analogue SNAP-23. Glia 27:181-187.

Hosli L, Hosli E, Zehntner C, Lehmann R, Lutz TW (1982) Evidence for the existence of alpha- and beta-adrenoceptors on cultured glial cells--an electrophysiological study. Neuroscience 7:2867-2872.

Hosli L, Hosli E, Della Briotta G, Quadri L, Heuss L (1988) Action of acetylcholine, muscarine, nicotine and antagonists on the membrane potential of astrocytes in cultured rat brainstem and spinal cord. Neurosci Lett 92:165-170.

Hua X, Rosenwald SR, Parpura V (2002) Calcium-dependent glutamate release involves two classes of endoplasmic reticulum (ER) Ca^{2+} stores in astrocytes. Soc Neurosci Abst, 527.3.

Hua X, Malarkey EB, Sunjara V, Rosenwald SR, Li W-h, Parpura V (2004) Ca^{2+}- dependent glutamate release involves two classes of endoplasmic reticulum Ca^{2+} stores in astrocytes. J Neurosci Res In Press.

Hussy N, Deleuze C, Pantaloni A, Desarmenien MG, Moos F (1997) Agonist action of taurine on glycine receptors in rat supraoptic magnocellular neurones: possible role in osmoregulation. J Physiol 502 (Pt 3):609-621.

Hussy N, Bres V, Rochette M, Duvoid A, Alonso G, Dayanithi G, Moos FC (2001) Osmoregulation of vasopressin secretion via activation of neurohypophysial nerve terminals glycine receptors by glial taurine. J Neurosci 21:7110-7116.

Innocenti B, Parpura V, Haydon PG (2000) Imaging extracellular waves of glutamate during calcium signaling in cultured astrocytes. J Neurosci 20:1800-1808.

Jalonen TO, Margraf RR, Wielt DB, Charniga CJ, Linne ML, Kimelberg HK (1997) Serotonin induces inward potassium and calcium currents in rat cortical astrocytes. Brain Res 758:69-82.

Janigro D, Gasparini S, D'Ambrosio R, McKhann G, 2nd, DiFrancesco D (1997) Reduction of K+ uptake in glia prevents long-term depression maintenance and causes epileptiform activity. J Neurosci 17:2813-2824.

Jeftinija SD, Jeftinija KV, Stefanovic G (1997) Cultured astrocytes express proteins involved in vesicular glutamate release. Brain Res 750:41-47.

Jeftinija SD, Jeftinija KV, Stefanovic G, Liu F (1996) Neuroligand-evoked calcium-dependent release of excitatory amino acids from cultured astrocytes. J Neurochem 66:676-684.

Jensen AM, Chiu SY (1990) Fluorescence measurement of changes in intracellular calcium induced by excitatory amino acids in cultured cortical astrocytes. J Neurosci 10:1165-1175.

Jeremic A, Jeftinija K, Stevanovic J, Glavaski A, Jeftinija S (2001) ATP stimulates calcium-dependent glutamate release from cultured astrocytes. J Neurochem 77:664-675.

Kang J, Jiang L, Goldman SA, Nedergaard M (1998) Astrocyte-mediated potentiation of inhibitory synaptic transmission. Nat Neurosci 1:683-692.

Kaul M, Garden GA, Lipton SA (2001) Pathways to neuronal injury and apoptosis in HIV-associated dementia. Nature 410:988-994.

Kimelberg HK, Goderie SK, Higman S, Pang S, Waniewski RA (1990) Swelling-induced release of glutamate, aspartate, and taurine from astrocyte cultures. J Neurosci 10:1583-1591.

Koizumi S, Fujishita K, Tsuda M, Shigemoto-Mogami Y, Inoue K (2003) Dynamic inhibition of excitatory synaptic transmission by astrocyte-derived ATP in hippocampal cultures. Proc Natl Acad Sci U S A 100:11023-11028.

Krzan M, Stenovec M, Kreft M, Pangrsic T, Grilc S, Haydon PG, Zorec R (2003) Calcium-dependent exocytosis of atrial natriuretic peptide from astrocytes. J Neurosci 23:1580-1583.

Laming PR, Sykova E, Reichenbach A, Hatton GI, Bauer H (Eds.) Glial cells and their role in behaviour. Cambridge University Press, Cambridge, U.K. 1998

Latour I, Hamid J, Beedle AM, Zamponi GW, Macvicar BA (2003) Expression of voltage-gated Ca2+ channel subtypes in cultured astrocytes. Glia 41:347-353.

Lin SC, Bergles DE (2004) Synaptic signaling between GABAergic interneurons and oligodendrocyte precursor cells in the hippocampus. Nat Neurosci 7:24-32.

Ma JY, Zhao ZQ (2002) The involvement of glia in long-term plasticity in the spinal dorsal horn of the rat. Neuroreport 13:1781-1784.

MacVicar BA (1984) Voltage-dependent calcium channels in glial cells. Science 226:1345-1347.

Maienschein V, Marxen M, Volknandt W, Zimmermann H (1999) A plethora of presynaptic proteins associated with ATP-storing organelles in cultured astrocytes. Glia 26:233-244.

McCall MA, Gregg RG, Behringer RR, Brenner M, Delaney CL, Galbreath EJ, Zhang CL, Pearce RA, Chiu SY, Messing A (1996) Targeted deletion in astrocyte intermediate filament (Gfap) alters neuronal physiology. Proc Natl Acad Sci U S A 93:6361-6366.

Mennerick S, Zorumski CF (1994) Glial contributions to excitatory neurotransmission in cultured hippocampal cells. Nature 368:59-62.

Milner TA, Kurucz OS, Veznedaroglu E, Pierce JP (1995) Septohippocampal neurons in the rat septal complex have substantial glial coverage and receive direct contacts from noradrenaline terminals. Brain Res 670:121-136.

Miyata S, Matsushima O, Hatton GI (1997) Taurine in rat posterior pituitary: localization in astrocytes and selective release by hypoosmotic stimulation. J Comp Neurol 381:513-523.

Montana V, Ni Y, Sunjara V, Hua X, Parpura V (2004) Vesicular glutamate transporter-dependent glutamate release from astrocytes. J Neurosci In Press.

Mothet JP, Parent AT, Wolosker H, Brady RO, Jr., Linden DJ, Ferris CD, Rogawski MA, Snyder SH (2000) D-serine is an endogenous ligand for the glycine site of the N-methyl-D-aspartate receptor. Proc Natl Acad Sci U S A 97:4926-4931.

Mudrick-Donnon LA, Williams PJ, Pittman QJ, MacVicar BA (1993) Postsynaptic potentials mediated by GABA and dopamine evoked in stellate glial cells of the pituitary pars intermedia. J Neurosci 13:4660-4668.

Nedergaard M (1994) Direct signaling from astrocytes to neurons in cultures of mammalian brain cells. Science 263:1768-1771.

Nett WJ, Oloff SH, McCarthy KD (2002) Hippocampal astrocytes in situ exhibit calcium oscillations that occur independent of neuronal activity. J Neurophysiol 87:528-537.

Newman EA (2003) Glial cell inhibition of neurons by release of ATP. J Neurosci 23:1659-1666.

Newman EA, Zahs KR (1998) Modulation of neuronal activity by glial cells in the retina. J Neurosci 18:4022-4028.

Ni Y, Sunjara V, Parpura V (2003) Expression of vesicular glutamate transporters in cultured astrocytes. FASEB J 17:A457 Part 451 Suppl.

Ojeda SR, Ma YJ, Lee BJ, Prevot V (2000) Glia-to-neuron signaling and the neuroendocrine control of female puberty. Recent Prog Horm Res 55:197-223; discussion 223-194.

Orkand RK, Nicholls JG, Kuffler SW (1966) Effect of nerve impulses on the membrane potential of glial cells in the central nervous system of amphibia. J Neurophysiol 29:788-806.

Otis TS, Wu YC, Trussell LO (1996) Delayed clearance of transmitter and the role of glutamate transporters at synapses with multiple release sites. J Neurosci 16:1634-1644.

Parpura V, Haydon PG (1999a) "Uncaging" using optical fibers to deliver UV light directly to the sample. Croat Med J 40:340-345.

Parpura V, Haydon PG (1999b) UV photolysis using a micromanipulated optical fiber to deliver UV energy directly to the sample. J Neurosci Methods 87:25-34.

Parpura V, Haydon PG (2000) Physiological astrocytic calcium levels stimulate glutamate release to modulate adjacent neurons. Proc Natl Acad Sci U S A 97:8629-8634.

Parpura V, Fang Y, Basarsky T, Jahn R, Haydon PG (1995a) Expression of synaptobrevin II, cellubrevin and syntaxin but not SNAP-25 in cultured astrocytes. FEBS Lett 377:489-492.

Parpura V, Basarsky TA, Liu F, Jeftinija K, Jeftinija S, Haydon PG (1994) Glutamate-mediated astrocyte-neuron signalling. Nature 369:744-747.

Parpura V, Liu F, Brethorst S, Jeftinija K, Jeftinija S, Haydon PG (1995b) Alpha-latrotoxin stimulates glutamate release from cortical astrocytes in cell culture. FEBS Lett 360:266-270.

Parri HR, Crunelli V (2001) Pacemaker calcium oscillations in thalamic astrocytes in situ. Neuroreport 12:3897-3900.

Parri HR, Crunelli V (2003) The role of Ca^{2+} in the generation of spontaneous astrocytic Ca^{2+} oscillations. Neuroscience 120:979-992.

Parri HR, Gould TM, Crunelli V (2001) Spontaneous astrocytic Ca^{2+} oscillations in situ drive NMDAR-mediated neuronal excitation. Nat Neurosci 4:803-812.

Pasti L, Pozzan T, Carmignoto G (1995) Long-lasting changes of calcium oscillations in astrocytes. A new form of glutamate-mediated plasticity. J Biol Chem 270:15203-15210.

Pasti L, Volterra A, Pozzan T, Carmignoto G (1997) Intracellular calcium oscillations in astrocytes: a highly plastic, bidirectional form of communication between neurons and astrocytes in situ. J Neurosci 17:7817-7830.

Pasti L, Zonta M, Pozzan T, Vicini S, Carmignoto G (2001) Cytosolic calcium oscillations in astrocytes may regulate exocytotic release of glutamate. J Neurosci 21:477-484.

Peracchia C (1981) Direct communication between axons and sheath glial cells in crayfish. Nature 290:597-598.

Peters A, Palay SL, Webster Hd (1991) The fine structure of the nervous system, 3rd Edition. New York-Oxford: Oxford University Press.

Petrenko AG (1993) alpha-Latrotoxin receptor. Implications in nerve terminal function. FEBS Lett 325:81-85.

Pizzo P, Burgo A, Pozzan T, Fasolato C (2001) Role of capacitative calcium entry on glutamate-induced calcium influx in type-I rat cortical astrocytes. J Neurochem 79:98-109.

Poelchen W, Sieler D, Wirkner K, Illes P (2001) Co-transmitter function of ATP in central catecholaminergic neurons of the rat. Neuroscience 102:593-602.

Porter JT, McCarthy KD (1996) Hippocampal astrocytes in situ respond to glutamate released from synaptic terminals. J Neurosci 16:5073-5081.

Pow DV (1993) Immunocytochemistry of amino-acids in the rodent pituitary using extremely specific, very high titre antisera. J Neuroendocrinol 5:349-356.

Queiroz G, Gebicke-Haerter PJ, Schobert A, Starke K, von Kugelgen I (1997) Release of ATP from cultured rat astrocytes elicited by glutamate receptor activation. Neuroscience 78:1203-1208.

Ransom BR, Goldring S (1973) Slow depolarization in cells presumed to be glia in cerebral cortex of cat. J Neurophysiol 36:869-878.

Redman RS, Silinsky EM (1994) ATP released together with acetylcholine as the mediator of neuromuscular depression at frog motor nerve endings. J Physiol 477 (Pt 1):117-127.

Sanzgiri RP, Araque A, Haydon PG (1999) Prostaglandin E(2) stimulates glutamate receptor-dependent astrocyte neuromodulation in cultured hippocampal cells. J Neurobiol 41:221-229.

Sastry BR, Goh JW, May PB, Chirwa SS (1988) The involvement of nonspiking cells in long-term potentiation of synaptic transmission in the hippocampus. Can J Physiol Pharmacol 66:841-844.

Schell MJ, Molliver ME, Snyder SH (1995) D-serine, an endogenous synaptic modulator: localization to astrocytes and glutamate-stimulated release. Proc Natl Acad Sci U S A 92:3948-3952.

Shain W, Connor JA, Madelian V, Martin DL (1989) Spontaneous and beta-adrenergic receptor-mediated taurine release from astroglial cells are independent of manipulations of intracellular calcium. J Neurosci 9:2306-2312.

Sharma G, Vijayaraghavan S (2001) Nicotinic cholinergic signaling in hippocampal astrocytes involves calcium-induced calcium release from intracellular stores. Proc Natl Acad Sci U S A 98:4148-4153.

Shibuki K, Gomi H, Chen L, Bao S, Kim JJ, Wakatsuki H, Fujisaki T, Fujimoto K, Katoh A, Ikeda T, Chen C, Thompson RF, Itohara S (1996) Deficient cerebellar long-term depression, impaired eyeblink conditioning, and normal motor coordination in GFAP mutant mice. Neuron 16:587-599.

Smit AB, Syed NI, Schaap D, van Minnen J, Klumperman J, Kits KS, Lodder H, van der Schors RC, van Elk R, Sorgedrager B, Brejc K, Sixma TK, Geraerts WP (2001) A glia-derived acetylcholine-binding protein that modulates synaptic transmission. Nature 411:261-268.

Smith SJ, Augustine GJ, Charlton MP (1985) Transmission at voltage-clamped giant synapse of the squid: evidence for cooperativity of presynaptic calcium action. Proc Natl Acad Sci U S A 82:622-625.

Sperlagh B, Sershen H, Lajtha A, Vizi ES (1998) Co-release of endogenous ATP and [3H]noradrenaline from rat hypothalamic slices: origin and modulation by alpha2-adrenoceptors. Neuroscience 82:511-520.

Stanley EF (1986) Decline in calcium cooperativity as the basis of facilitation at the squid giant synapse. J Neurosci 6:782-789.

Steinhäuser C, Jabs R, Kettenmann H (1994) Properties of GABA and glutamate responses in identified glial cells of the mouse hippocampal slice. Hippocampus 4:19-35.

Stephens GJ, Marriott DR, Djamgoz MB, Wilkin GP (1993) Electrophysiological and biochemical evidence for bradykinin receptors on cultured rat cortical oligodendrocytes. Neurosci Lett 153:223-226.

Stevens ER, Esguerra M, Kim PM, Newman EA, Snyder SH, Zahs KR, Miller RF (2003) D-serine and serine racemase are present in the vertebrate retina and contribute to the physiological activation of NMDA receptors. Proc Natl Acad Sci U S A 100:6789-6794.

Stout CE, Costantin JL, Naus CC, Charles AC (2002) Intercellular calcium signaling in astrocytes via ATP release through connexin hemichannels. J Biol Chem 277:10482-10488.

Tong G, Jahr CE (1994) Block of glutamate transporters potentiates postsynaptic excitation. Neuron 13:1195-1203.

Trudeau LE, Fang Y, Haydon PG (1998) Modulation of an early step in the secretory machinery in hippocampal nerve terminals. Proc Natl Acad Sci U S A 95:7163-7168.

Ushkaryov YA, Petrenko AG, Geppert M, Sudhof TC (1992) Neurexins: synaptic cell surface proteins related to the alpha-latrotoxin receptor and laminin. Science 257:50-56.

van Leeuwen FW, Pool CW, Sluiter AA (1983) Enkephalin immunoreactivity in synaptoid elements on glial cells in the rat neural lobe. Neuroscience 8:229-241.

Ventura R, Harris KM (1999) Three-dimensional relationships between hippocampal synapses and astrocytes. J Neurosci 19:6897-6906.

Verderio C, Matteoli M (2001) ATP mediates calcium signaling between astrocytes and microglial cells: modulation by IFN-gamma. J Immunol 166:6383-6391.

von Kugelgen I, Allgaier C, Schobert A, Starke K (1994) Co-release of noradrenaline and ATP from cultured sympathetic neurons. Neuroscience 61:199-202.

Wittkowski W, Brinkmann H (1974) Changes of extent of neuro-vascular contacts and number of neuro-glial synaptoid contacts in the pituitary posterior lobe of dehydrated rats. Anat Embryol (Berl) 146:157-165.

Wolosker H, Sheth KN, Takahashi M, Mothet JP, Brady RO, Jr., Ferris CD, Snyder SH (1999) Purification of serine racemase: biosynthesis of the neuromodulator D-serine. Proc Natl Acad Sci U S A 96:721-725.

Yang Y, Ge W, Chen Y, Zhang Z, Shen W, Wu C, Poo M, Duan S (2003) Contribution of astrocytes to hippocampal long-term potentiation through release of D-serine. Proc Natl Acad Sci U S A 100:15194-15199.

Zhang JM, Wang HK, Ye CQ, Ge W, Chen Y, Jiang ZL, Wu CP, Poo MM, Duan S (2003) ATP released by astrocytes mediates glutamatergic activity-dependent heterosynaptic suppression. Neuron 40:971-982.

Zhong Y, Wu CF (1991) Altered synaptic plasticity in Drosophila memory mutants with a defective cyclic AMP cascade. Science 251:198-201.

Zonta M, Sebelin A, Gobbo S, Fellin T, Pozzan T, Carmignoto G (2003a) Glutamate-mediated cytosolic calcium oscillations regulate a pulsatile prostaglandin release from cultured rat astrocytes. J Physiol 553:407-414.

Zonta M, Angulo MC, Gobbo S, Rosengarten B, Hossmann KA, Pozzan T, Carmignoto G (2003b) Neuron-to-astrocyte signaling is central to the dynamic control of brain microcirculation. Nat Neurosci 6:43-50.

15.8. Abbreviations

ACh	Acetylcholine
AChBP	ACh binding protein
AMPA	α-amino-3-hydroxy-5-methyl-isoxazole propionate
ATP	Adenosine 5'-triphosphate
BAPTA	1,2-bis(2-aminophenoxy)ethane-N,N,N',N'-tetraacetic acid
CNQX	6-cyano-7-nitroquinoxaline-2,3-dione
CNS	Central nervous system
CXCR4	CXC Chemokine receptor 4
D-AP5	D-2-amino-phosphonopentanoic acid
DGG	D-glutamylglycine
DMSO	Dimethyl sulfoxide
EGTA	Ethylene glycol-bis(2-aminoethyl)-N,N, N',N'-tetraacetic acid
GABA	γ-aminobutyric acid
GDH	L-glutamate dehydrogenase
GFAP	Glial fibrillary acidic protein
GluR	Glutamate receptor
GlyR	Glycine receptor
HIV-1	Human immunodeficiency virus 1
iGluR	Ionotropic glutamate receptor
L-AP3	2-amino-3-phosphonopropionic acid
LHRH	Luteinizing hormone-releasing hormone
LTD	Long-term depression
LTP	Long-term potentiation
MAP-4	(S)-2-amino-2-methyl-4-phosphonobutanoic acid
MCPG	(S)-α-methyl-4-carboxyphenylglycine
mEPSC	Miniature excitatory postsynaptic currents
mGluR	Metabotropic glutamate receptor
mIPSC	Miniature inhibitory postsynaptic currents
mPSC	Miniature postsynaptic currents
nAChR	Nicotinic acetylcholine receptors
NAD^+	β-nicotinamide adenine dinucleotide
NMDAR	N-methyl D-aspartate receptors
NP-EGTA	o-nitrophenyl-EGTA
PGE_2	Prostaglandin E_2
SIC	Slow inward current
SNAP-23/25	Synaptosome-associated protein of 23 or 25 kDa
SNARE	Soluble N-ethyl maleimide-sensitive fusion protein attachment protein receptor
t-ACPD	(1S, 3R)-1-aminocyclopentane-1, 3-dicarboxlylic acid
TNFα	Tumor Necrosis Factor α
UV	Ultraviolet
V-ATPase	Vacuolar-type H^+-ATPase
VGLUT	Vesicular glutamate transporter
$[X]_i$	Intracellular concentration of ion/molecule X
$[X]_o$	Extracellular concentration of ion/molecule X

Chapter 16

The regulated release of transmitters from astrocytes

Daniel S. Evanko, Jai-Yoon Sul, Qi Zhang and Philip G. Haydon*

Department of Neuroscience, University of Pennsylvania School of Medicine
Philadelphia, PA 19104 USA

Corresponding author: pghaydon@mail.med.upenn.edu

Contents

16.1. Introduction

Research over the past decade has given us novel insights into the diverse roles played by astrocytes in the functioning of numerous processes within the central nervous system (CNS) that have been the focus of several recent reviews (Anderson and Swanson, 2000; Carmignoto, 2000; Hussy et al., 2000; Araque et al., 2001; Haydon, 2001; Mazzanti et al., 2001; Cotrina and Nedergaard, 2002; Chen and Swanson, 2003). This review focuses on recent observations concerning the mechanisms of release of chemical transmitters from astrocytes. Two observations in 1994 led to a significant breakthrough in our thinking about astrocyte function (Nedergaard, 1994; Parpura et al., 1994). These studies showed that calcium elevations in astrocytes could lead to delayed neuronal calcium elevations. However, the mechanisms believed to underlie astrocyte-to-neuron signaling were quite distinct. While Nedergaard concluded that gap junctions mediate astrocyte-to-neuron signaling, Parpura et al. found evidence to support the notion that glutamate released from the astrocyte leads to an N-methyl-D-Aspartate receptor (NMDAR)-dependent elevation of neuronal calcium. Although additional support for the role of gap junctions has come from studies in the locus coeruleus (Alvarez-Maubecin et al., 2000), there is greater evidence to support the concept that it is the extracellular release of chemical transmitters from astrocytes that mediates astrocyte-to-neuron signaling.

Neuronal signaling via release of chemical transmitters is one of the foundations of CNS function. Astrocytes play a critical role in clearing neurotransmitters from the vicinity of neurons during neuron-to-neuron signaling through the use of transporters specific to different neurotransmitters (Anderson and Swanson, 2000). These transporters make use of voltage potential and ion gradients across the astrocyte cell membrane to move glutamate, aspartate, taurine, GABA and glycine up large chemical gradients. For instance, the extracellular concentration of L-glutamate is estimated to vary from 0.6 µM to 10 µM, while its concentration in glial cells is 0.1-5 mM (Attwell et al., 1993). This results in concentration gradients ranging from 10- to 10,000-fold. This can provide a large potential driving force for release of these neurotransmitters if the permeability of the plasma membrane to these substances is increased.

One condition during which permeability is known to increase is ischemia. Release of excitatory amino acids (EAAs) during ischemia is one of the primary causes of post-ischemic neuronal cell death. Although EAAs are also released from presynaptic nerve terminals, the amount of the EAA, glutamate, released from astrocytes exposed to hypoxic conditions is greater than that released from neurons (Ogata et al., 1992). Understanding the mechanisms of EAA release from astrocytes during this pathological condition could aid significantly in reducing brain damage following trauma to the brain. The two primary means proposed for release of EAAs and other transmitters from astrocytes during ischemia are cell swelling-induced opening of anion channels and transporter reversal (Phillis and O'Regan, 2003).

In addition to using the prominent chemical gradient to drive the release of neurotransmitters, there is increasing evidence that astrocytes use a Ca^{2+}-dependent vesicular release mechanism triggered by increases in intracellular calcium. This mechanism is much like that used by neurons to release neurotransmitters at synapses. Unlike transporter reversal or anion channel-mediated release of substances down a concentration gradient, this mode of release utilizes active transport of neurotransmitters into vesicles. These vesicles store the neurotransmitters until the appropriate stimulus triggers fusion with the plasma membrane and release of the vesicular contents into the extracellular space. This process lends itself well to activation and modulation by specific extracellular stimuli that increase intracellular calcium within the astrocyte via receptor activation of calcium mobilization. This concept of bidirectional signaling between neurons and astrocytes via common messaging molecules is supported by the observation that astrocytes and neurons respond to many of the same neurotransmitters (Porter and McCarthy, 1997). Although astrocytes may possess neurotransmitter receptors due to their need to adjust their metabolic and support functions to the type and level of neuronal activity in their vicinity, this receptor expression could also suggest a more active role for astrocytes in neuronal signaling.

The ability of glia to release numerous neuroactive compounds following non-pathological external stimuli has been recognized for some time (Martin, 1992). Although astrocytes can release neurotransmitters via many mechanisms it is not yet clear which mechanisms are utilized in specific situations or the functional significance of these release pathways. Here we focus on the release of chemical transmitters from astrocytes and, in particular, on the release of glutamate. Table 16.1 summarizes a sequence of reports that have documented that astrocytes do indeed release chemical transmitters. It is clear from this table that a diversity of transmitters is released and that it is likely that many mechanisms serve to release these transmitters. A breakthrough in elucidating the purpose of astrocyte neurotransmitter release came when Parpura et al. showed that one of these transmitters, glutamate, could modulate signaling in neurons following its release from neighboring astrocytes (Parpura et al., 1994). The role of astrocytes in modulating signaling by neurons has since been demonstrated repeatedly

(Nedergaard, 1994; Parpura et al., 1994; Rigo et al., 1994; Pasti et al., 1997; Araque et al., 1998; Kang et al., 1998; Araque et al., 1999; Duffy and MacVicar, 1999; Sanzgiri et al., 1999; Parpura and Haydon, 2000; Parri et al., 2001; Pasti et al., 2001; Araque et al., 2002; Mazzanti and Haydon, 2003). Glutamate is now recognized as a signal used by astrocytes to alter signaling between neurons. It is likely that other neurotransmitters released from astrocytes also affect neuronal signaling. Understanding these release pathways will be necessary for understanding the role of astrocytes in information processing in the CNS.

16.2. Astrocyte plasma membrane transporters

Significant amounts of various neurotransmitters are released by presynaptic terminals during neuronal activity. Uptake of these transmitters from the synaptic cleft is essential for termination of synaptic transmission; furthermore, if these transmitters are not removed they will accumulate and could cause EAA-induced excitotoxicity to neurons and/or diffuse over great distances where they could induce unwanted synaptic modulation. Na^+-dependent transporters located in the astrocytic plasma membrane remove transmitters from the extracellular milieu adjacent to the astrocytic cell membrane, thus leading to a rapid clearing from the synaptic cleft. These transporters are dependent on the membrane potential and the ionic transmembrane gradient created by a Na^+/K^+ ATPase. Astrocytes possess transporters for glutamate/aspartate, glycine, taurine and, in some situations, GABA (Gadea and Lopez-Colome, 2001a, b, c). Little is known about the taurine transporter in general, or the glycine transporter in regards to transmitter release, while the GABA transporter is rare in glia. Thus, our discussion is limited to the glutamate transporters prevalent in glia.

The glial L-glutamate transporter (GLT-1), or excitatory amino acid transporter 2 (EAAT2), and L-glutamate/L-aspartate transporter (GLAST-1), or excitatory amino acid transporter 1 (EAAT1), transporter proteins are found exclusively in glial cells. EAAT2 is restricted to astrocytes throughout the central nervous system while the highest concentrations of EAAT1 are found in Bergmann glia of the cerebellum (Gadea and Lopez-Colome, 2001c). The subcellular localization of the glutamate transporters both supports the vital role of these transporters in clearing transmitter from areas of synaptic transmission and demonstrates how release from astrocytes through the transporters would result in potent synaptic stimulation. For example, EAAT1 and EAAT2 are preferentially located in astrocytic membranes facing synapses, axons and spines rather than those facing capillaries, pia or stem dendrites (Chaudhry et al., 1995). Of the other excitatory amino acid transporters, EAAT3 and EAAT4 have only been found in neurons, where expression appears to be largely restricted to the cell body and dendrites, while EAAT5 is found only in the retina (Seal and Amara, 1999; Gadea and Lopez-Colome, 2001c).

Understanding the physiology and role of astrocytes in neuronal signaling via release of neurotransmitters requires an understanding of the uptake pathway and the constraints it places on astrocyte function. Uptake of glutamate is coupled to the inward transport of 2 or 3 Na^+ and one H^+, in conjunction with the outward movement of one K^+ (Zerangue and Kavanaugh, 1996). L-glutamate or L-aspartate transport is accompanied by an inward Cl⁻ flux, which is responsible for 95% of the current elicited by EAAT4 but which is only a small component of the current elicited by EAAT1 and EAAT2 (Seal and Amara, 1999). The function of this current, and more particularly the small Cl⁻ current associated with transporters present in glia, is unknown. The importance of these transmitter uptake pathways to synaptic function most certainly imposes constraints on the physiology of the astrocyte. Because the glutamate transporters are electrogenic, uptake of transmitter would be significantly impaired if the membrane potential of the astrocyte departed from a large negative potential. Thus it is not surprising that the astrocytic membrane potential is relatively stable at about -80 mV and that these non-neuronal cells do not generate action potentials.

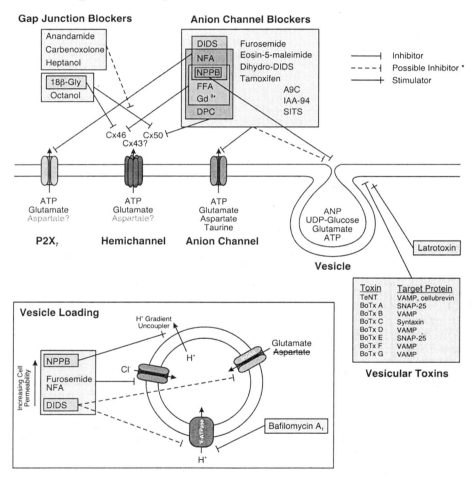

Potentcies

P2X, - NFA ≥ NPPB > DIDS >> DPC,Tamoxifen

Cx46 - NPPB ≥ 18β-Gly, FFA, Gd ³⁺ (Ineffective - Octanol, NFA, DPC, Furosemide, DIDS, SITS, Tamoxifen, A9C, IAA-94)

Cx50 - NFA, NPPB, DPC, FFA, 18β-Gly ≥ Octanol ≥ Gd ³⁺ (Ineffective - Furosemide, DIDS, SITS, Tamoxifen, A9C, IAA-9)

Figure 16.1. Pathways of neurotransmitter release in astrocytes and reagents used to identify them. Schematic representation of the four potential physiological pathways of neurotransmitter release from astrocytes. Many of the common reagents used to determine the identity of a release pathway are shown. The arrow type represents whether a compound is an inhibitor, possible inhibitor, stimulator or if no hard evidence is available. Since the potencies of some gap junction blockers for specific hemichannels have not been determined they are shown as possible inhibitors. Ability of compounds to inhibit vesicle loading is dependent upon cell permeability. The estimated relative permeabilities of several compounds demonstrated to inhibit vesicles are shown based on an examination of their structures. Potencies of some compounds on $P2X_7$, Cx46 and Cx50 are also presented. See text for descriptions and references. (* Nearly all anion channel inhibitors have the potential to inhibit vesicle transport by blocking the vesicular chloride channel. However, only membrane permeable inhibitors will be able to reach the vesicular channels. All gap junction blockers are possible hemichannel blockers but they display a pronounced dependency on connexin subtype which has not been tested for most compounds.)

Table 16.1. List of reports showing the release of transmitters from astrocytes

Reference	Glut	Asp	Taurine	ATP	ANP	UDP-Glucose	Proposed Mechanism
(Kimelberg et al., 1990)	X	X	X				Anion Channel
(Jackson and Strange, 1993)			X				Anion Channel
(Parpura et al., 1994)	X						Ca^{2+} Dependent
(Longuemare and Swanson, 1995)		X					Transporter Rev
(Parpura et al., 1995b)	X						Vesicular
(Jeftinija et al., 1996)	X	X					Vesicular
(Jeftinija et al., 1997)	X						Vesicular
(Queiroz et al., 1997)				X			Non-Vesicular
(Bezzi et al., 1998)	X						Ca^{2+} Dependent
(Cotrina et al., 1998)				X			Hemichannels
(Deleuze et al., 1998)			X				Anion Channel
(Rutledge et al., 1998)		X					Anion Channel
(Basarsky et al., 1999)	X						Anion Channel
(Harden and Lazarowski, 1999)				X			
(Maienschein et al., 1999)				X			Vesicular
(Queiroz et al., 1999)				X			Non-Vesicular
(Araque et al., 2000)	X						Vesicular
(Parpura and Haydon, 2000)	X						Ca^{2+} Dependent
(Bres et al., 2000)			X				Anion Channel
(Innocenti et al., 2000)	X						Vesicular
(Wang et al., 2000)				X			Ca^{2+} Independent
(Jeremic et al., 2001)	X	X					Ca^{2+} Dependent
(Pasti et al., 2001)	X						Vesicular
(Bal-Price et al., 2002)	X			X			Vesicular
(Mongin and Kimelberg, 2002)		X		X			Anion Channel
(Stout et al., 2002)				X			Hemichannels
(Darby et al., 2003)				X			Transporter
(Duan et al., 2003)	X	X					$P2X_7$
(Krzan et al., 2003)					X		Vesicular
(Lazarowski et al., 2003)				X		X	Vesicular
(Ye et al., 2003)	X						Hemichannels

One of the only situations in which the membrane potential does not remain stable is during ischemia when astrocytes undergo membrane depolarization, increased intracellular Na^+ and extracellular K^+ as well as decreased intracellular ATP. It was suggested that this could lead to reversal of the plasma membrane transporters and efflux of glutamate and other transmitters. This proved to be true; blocking glycolytic and oxidative metabolism in primary astrocyte cultures led to energy failure and the production of a net efflux of exogenously pre-loaded D-aspartate (Longuemare and Swanson, 1995). This efflux could be blocked by preloading the cells with competitive inhibitors of Na^+-dependent uptake, demonstrating that release was indeed via Na^+-dependent transporters. When reversal occurs, the transporters release neurotransmitters in a process that does not require Ca^{2+} or ATP. Because inward glutamate transport is coupled to outward K^+ movement it could be predicted that an elevated extracellular K^+ concentration would reduce part of the force driving uptake and lead to a net efflux of glutamate. To determine whether it would be possible to get net glutamate release with extracellular K^+ levels that are attainable *in vivo*, astrocyte cultures were exposed to $[K^+]_o$ from 4 to 80 mM and examined for net glutamate and aspartate release. However, no such release was observed (Longuemare and Swanson, 1997). It was determined that intact astrocytes compensate for the increased $[K^+]_o$ with compensatory reductions in $[Na^+]_i$ (Longuemare et al., 1999). Thus, astrocytes appear to actively shield themselves from changes in the extracellular ionic environment that could result in transport reversal. Although reverse transport is unlikely to operate under physiological conditions, under pathological conditions transporters operating in reverse likely release significant quantities of glutamate and contribute to excitotoxicity (Rossi et al., 2000).

In addition to uptake pathways that are capable of reversal and consequent transmitter release, astrocytes also possess intrinsic neurotransmitter release pathways. Four pathways for neurotransmitter release have received significant attention: (1) anion transporters; (2) hemi-channels; (3) P_2X receptors, and (4) Ca^{2+}-dependent exocytosis. Each of these mechanisms is discussed below.

16.3. Anion channel-mediated release

Release of neurotransmitters from astrocytes was first noted following exposure to hypotonic media to induce cell swelling. These conditions simulate those of ischemia and resulted in cell swelling and release of glutamate, aspartate and taurine from astrocytes in culture (Kimelberg et al., 1990). This release was almost completely blocked by several anion transport inhibitors, some lipoxygenase blockers and certain polyunsaturated fatty acids. Furthermore, whole-cell patch clamp measurements demonstrated that swelling rapidly increased the outwardly-rectified Cl⁻ conductance approximately 100-fold (Kimelberg et al., 1990). The relative permeability of taurine to Cl⁻ was determined to be 0.2, indicating that negatively charged amino acids could make up a significant fraction of released anions (Jackson and Strange, 1993). Though these results demonstrate that EAAs are released from astrocytes via cell swelling-induced anion transport, it is not clear that this mechanism can operate under physiological conditions. Volume-dependent aspartate release appears to require large changes in cell volume that are unlikely to occur in astrocytes under normal conditions (Rutledge and Kimelberg, 1996). The question has been raised as to whether this pathway would ever be gated under physiological conditions since large changes in osmolarity are normally used to trigger release in experimental studies. However, a recent study has shown that ATP released during cell swelling can collaborate with a hypo-osmotic change to amplify the release of aspartate and potentially that of ATP (Mongin and Kimelberg, 2002). In experiments with moderately and substantially swollen astrocytes (5% and 35% reduction in medium osmolarity, respectively) ATP was found to greatly potentiate aspartate release. Thus, even changes in osmolarity as low as 14 mosM can, in the presence of 10 μM ATP, lead to significant EAA release.

Changes in light transmittance can be used as an indirect indication of cell volume changes. This technique was used to examine the cellular swelling associated with spreading depression (SD), a wave of neuronal and glial depolarization and swelling. Incubation of hippocampal or neocortical brain slices in Ca^{2+}-free solution failed to stop SD even though it did abolish Ca^{2+} wave propagation (Basarsky et al., 1998). A subsequent study demonstrated that preincubation of the slice with 100 μM of the Cl^- channel inhibitor 5-nitro-2-(3-phenyl-propylamino)benzoic acid (NPPB) could slow recovery to initial light transmittance levels after the peak of the SD waveform. Recovery at 30 sec post peak was reduced from 47% to 2% of complete recovery, indicating a role for the channels in regulating cell volume decrease following SD-induced swelling in Ca^{2+}-free solution (Basarsky et al., 1999). Furthermore, although removal of Ca^{2+} resulted in a 5-fold reduction in the onset slope of SD, as measured by the change in intrinsic optical signals, preincubation of the slice with 100 μM of the Cl^- channel inhibitor NPPB resulted in a further 60% reduction in the slope of SD. To determine if glutamate release was influenced by NPPB, glutamate released into the superfusate was measured after SD onset. Glutamate release underwent a 10-fold decrease upon incubation in Ca^{2+}-free solution. However, preincubation with NPPB resulted in a further 60% decrease in glutamate release without affecting release of GABA, indicating that the 60% decrease by NPPB was likely through its action on astrocytes and not on neurons. These results were interpreted as demonstrative of a large neuronal vesicular release component in SD that was blocked by removal of Ca^{2+}, while cellular swelling seemed to contribute a small glutamate release component that was required for propagation. It is unclear what portion of the vesicular release component was from astrocytes and what was from neurons. However, since glial cells account for half of cell volume in the brain it is likely that a significant portion of the cellular swelling observed during SD is due to astrocytes. If NPPB were acting solely on plasma membrane Cl^- flux then glutamate release triggered by cellular swelling of astrocytes appears to be a significant component of SD.

Unlike the well-known neurotransmitter glutamate, the amino acid taurine is a major osmolyte used by cells to regulate cell volume during changes in extracellular osmolarity. However, it also possesses agonist properties on glycine and GABA receptors of neurons in the paraventricular and supraoptic nuclei that regulate whole-body fluid balance by releasing the neurohormones vasopressin and oxytocin into the blood (Hussy et al., 1997). Glial cells near these neurons possess high concentrations of taurine, the release of which can be triggered by hypo-osmotic medium. Although osmotic reductions of more than 15% resulted in only a transient release of taurine, which was probably due to regulatory volume decrease, smaller changes in extracellular osmolarity resulted in sustained release of taurine (Deleuze et al., 1998). Release was not dependent on extracellular Ca^{2+} or Na^+ and could be blocked by the anion channel blockers, 4,4'-diisothiocyanato-stilbene-2,2'-disulfonate (DIDS) and diphenylamin-2-carboxylate (DPC), indicating that release was probably through anion channels. Further characterization of the pharmacology of the hypothetical anion channel involved in the release of taurine indicated that it did not conform to typical anion channels and was completely insensitive to the broadly inhibitory compound tamoxifen (Bres et al., 2000). These studies demonstrate that physiological changes in extracellular osmolarity can induce release of taurine from astrocytes. The exact mechanism of this taurine release is still unclear but appears to be an as-yet uncharacterized anion channel.

Hypo-osmotic saline has been proven to induce the release of EAAs from astrocytes. However, experiments that rely largely on the use of anion transport inhibitors are extremely difficult to interpret due to uncertainties about the non-specific effects of these compounds (Figure 16.1). Loading of neurotransmitters into synaptic vesicles requires transmitter-specific transporters that make use of a proton gradient across the vesicle membrane. This proton gradient is driven by ATP-dependent proton pumps known as V-ATPases (Nelson et al., 2000). The proton gradient across the vesicle membrane requires anions to be transported into the vesicles to prevent the formation of an insurmountable electrical gradient that would prevent the transport of further protons or positively charged neurotransmitters (Pothos et al., 2002). Vesicles possess chloride channels that transport Cl⁻ into the vesicles to alleviate the charge imbalance (Maycox et al., 1990). Vesicular chloride channels are sensitive to some of the same anion transport inhibitors that are used to block plasma membrane ion transport. This has been demonstrated by soaking intact muscles in hypertonic solution containing 30 μM of the anion transport inhibitor NPPB. This was able to block the vesicular chloride channel, resulting in inhibition of ACh uptake into synaptic vesicles (Van der Kloot, 2003). Hartinger and Jahn (1993) used another anion channel blocker, DIDS, to examine the role of Cl⁻ in glutamate loading of purified vesicles. This group proposed that the inhibitor exerted its effect by binding to a Cl⁻ binding site on the glutamate transporter itself, resulting in the inhibition of vesicle loading. Other anion channel blockers, such as eosin-5-maleimide, furosemide, niflumic acid (NFA) and dihydro-DIDS, were also found to be inhibitory but less so than DIDS. DIDS has also been shown to inhibit the ATPase proton pump in vesicles, though with a lower potency, while NPPB uncouples the H^+ gradient across a membrane (Xie et al., 1983; Lukacs et al., 1991; Hartinger and Jahn, 1993). However, short incubation periods in whole cell studies may not be problematic for some inhibitors such as DIDS that are largely membrane-impermeant (Passow, 1986). NPPB, unlike DIDS, is membrane permeable. It is thought to exert its uncoupling effect via a dissociable proton and a strong electron withdrawing moiety coupled to a large hydrophobic group that provides solubility in the membrane bilayer and has been shown to uncouple mitochondria in intact cells (Lukacs et al., 1991). A recent study demonstrated that the stimulation-evoked increase in vesicle size in chromaffin cells was inhibited by NPPB as well as the vacuolar-type H^+-ATPase inhibitor bafilomycin A_1, confirming the action of this anion channel blocker on vesicular trafficking (Pothos et al., 2002).

Further complicating use of these anion channels blockers in the study of neurotransmitter release is the recent finding that many are also very efficient blockers of hemichannels, which is another possible neurotransmitter release mechanism (Eskandari et al., 2002). Gd^{3+}, NPPB, flufenamic acid (FFA), niflumic acid (NFA) and DPC were found to be potent inhibitors of connexin50 (Cx50) hemichannels while anthracene-9-carboxylate (A9C), furosemide, R(+)-[(6,7-dichloro-2-cyclopentyl-2,3-dihydro-2-methyl-1-oxo-1H-inden-5-yl)-oxy]acetic acid (IAA-94), DIDS, 4-acetamido-4'-isothiocyanato-stilbene-2,2'-disulfonate (SITS) and tamoxifen were not. Cx46 hemichannels showed similar sensitivities with the exception of NFA and DPC, which were ineffective. An earlier study demonstrated that Cx38 hemichannels could also be blocked by FFA and NFA (Zhang et al., 1998). The various sensitivities of individual Cxs to each anion channel blocker further complicate their use unless the identity of each channel subtype in a cell is known. However, astrocytes seem to express primarily Cx43 (also, see Chapter 13). The specificities of the channel blockers for these hemichannel connexins have yet to be determined (Dermietzel et al., 1991; Giaume et al., 1991). Such cross-reactivities of the anion channel blockers could cause concern in studies that utilize anion channel blockers to demonstrate that neurotransmitter is released through plasma membrane anion channels.

In an attempt to distinguish between an anion transporter-mediated release pathway and vesicle-mediated release, cultured astrocytes were treated with the clostridial toxin, tetanus toxin, which can cleave the SNARE protein synaptobrevin II (Mongin and Kimelberg, 2002). Tetanus toxin was shown to have no effect on the release of aspartate in response to hypo-osmotic challenge. However, it should be noted that tetanus toxin requires binding to neuron specific receptors for efficient internalization that do not appear to be present on astrocytes, making it difficult to interpret these studies (Araque et al., 1998; Herreros et al., 2000). However, there are distinct properties of this release pathway which suggest that it is distinct from the exocytotic pathway of EAA release. One method that can be used to distinguish non-vesicular from vesicular release of glutamate is to utilize the fact that uptake into synaptic vesicles is specific for L-glutamate as opposed to L-aspartate or D-glutamate (Naito and Ueda, 1985; Bellocchio et al., 2000) while release from anion channels or transporter reversal relies on the concentration gradient of glutamate or aspartate to drive release. Thus, even though reagent specificity makes it difficult to determine which particular mechanism mediates the hypo-osmolarity-induced release of EAAs from astrocytes, the observed aspartate release during hypo-osmotic conditions strongly suggests a mechanism distinct from exocytosis. Moreover, elevations of astrocytic calcium are necessary and sufficient for the release of glutamate, but do not appear to be necessary for the release of aspartate (Mongin and Kimelberg, 2002). It is likely that the release of EAAs evoked by hypo-osmotic saline is through a mechanism distinct from vesicle-mediated exocytosis. Thus, EAAs can be released by an exocytosis-independent pathway in response to hypo-osmotic saline.

16.4. Hemichannel-mediated release

Gap junctions in astrocytes are thought to link individual cells into a functional syncytium capable of concerted action (Chapters 14). These gap junctions are composed of connexons or hemichannels in the membranes of two adjacent cells that dock together to form a pore between the cell interiors. Each hemichannel is an oligomer of six protein subunits termed connexins. The most prevalent connexin in astrocytes is Cx43. In recent years it has been appreciated that hemichannels not incorporated into gap junctions are able to mediate the flux of molecules between the intracellular cytosol and the extracellular space (Evans and Martin, 2002). Antibodies targeted to the extracellular loops of Cx43 have been shown to inhibit dye uptake in Ca^{2+}-deficient medium. This demonstrates that low $[Ca^{2+}]_o$ can function by opening membrane hemichannels (Hofer and Dermietzel, 1998). Interestingly, dye uptake varied in a clonal fashion as spatially segregated groups of cells were highly labeled while other groups showed no dye uptake. This indicates that specific groups of astrocytes can be much more sensitive to low $[Ca^{2+}]_o$ than other astrocytes. At first glance it would seem unlikely that a channel with a pore diameter as large as about 2 nm and that is able to permit passage molecules up to about 1 kDa would mediate the regulated release of transmitters from astrocytes (Lal and Lin, 2001). However, there is compelling evidence to support this concept. Studies of ATP release from glial cells showed that the expression of Cx43 in gap junction-deficient glioma cell lines, which express low levels of connexins, leads to an augmentation of P2Y receptor-evoked ATP release (Cotrina et al., 1998). Release was facilitated by removal of Cl⁻ or Ca^{2+} from the bath medium and was blocked by Cl⁻ channel inhibitors. Although this study demonstrated that artificially expressing connexins in astrocytes can mediate ATP release it suggested little about whether this release mechanism also occurs *in vivo*. Two subsequent studies demonstrated that connexins can mediate the release of ATP and/or glutamate from astrocytes via natively-expressed connexins. Stout et al., using whole-cell patch clamp methods, demonstrated low $[Ca^{2+}]_o$ stimulated currents characteristic of connexin hemichannels in *Xenopus* oocytes (Stout et al., 2002). Low $[Ca^{2+}]_o$ or induction of an intracellular Ca^{2+} wave facilitated the reversible uptake of the dye, Lucifer yellow. The ability of astrocytes to release hemichannel-permeant and -impermeant dyes matched observations on known hemichannels and release also demonstrated the expected pharmacological profile of hemichannels. The same results were observed in regards to release of ATP. Release was not blocked by the anion channel blocker DIDS. As mentioned earlier, DIDS, unlike several other anion channel blockers, does not block connexin hemichannels composed of Cx46 or Cx50. However, DIDS has not been tested with Cx43, the connexin which forms the hemichannels used in this study.

Ye et al. proposed that hemichannels can also mediate the release of glutamate from astrocytes, albeit under conditions of lowered external calcium (Ye et al., 2003). Hippocampal astrocytes in nominal divalent cation-free solution exhibited significant release of glutamate and aspartate that could be blocked by multivalent cations and gap junction blockers. 10 to 40% of maximal glutamate release could be triggered by $[Ca^{2+}]_o$ in the range of 500 to 100 µM. The results paralleled those obtained by examining Lucifer yellow uptake in astrocytes. Controls indicated that release was not mediated by transporter reversal, anion channels, P2X₇ purinergic receptor pores or intracellular Ca^{2+} mobilization. The release of aspartate as well as glutamate and the extensive controls used in this study provide highly convincing evidence that glutamate can be released through hemichannels in astrocytes. The major question at this point is whether or not the low $[Ca^{2+}]_o$ conditions used in these studies occur *in vivo* and, if so, whether they account for a physiologically significant fraction of ATP or glutamate release. There are a few studies that indicate that hemichannels may be able to open under physiological conditions. Application of hemichannel blockers to the retina hyperpolarized Cx26-containing horizontal cells, thus leading to modulation of cone cells (Kamermans et al., 2001). A second study demonstrated that cells expressing Cx43 could undergo a significant and reversible increase in cell volume after a reduction in $[Ca^{2+}]_o$ from 1.8 to 1.6 mM and this increase could be blocked by gap junction blockers (Quist et al., 2000). These studies lend increased support for the notion that hemichannel-mediated release of neurotransmitters is physiologically significant.

When trying to interpret the data from these studies within a physiological context, three significant concerns arise. First, the manipulation of Cx43 expression changes the expression of thousands of other genes (Spray, 2003). Thus, although the expression of Cx43 can augment the release of transmitter, it is not clear whether this is a direct effect of Cx43 expression or is an action mediated by the one or more of the thousands of other genes that are up- or down-regulated. Recent studies that do not rely on changing connexin expression obviate this problem. Second, the specificity of the pharmacological agents used to block hemichannels is a known concern. It may be possible to address this concern through the use of a dominant-negative Cx43- Enhanced Green Fluorescent Protein (EGFP) that has been shown to inhibit synchronization of calcium transients through gap junctions in cardiomyocytes (Oyamada et al., 2002). Finally, there is serious concern about the gating mechanism of the hemichannel. Some studies of the release of transmitter required nominally divalent cation free saline, which raises the question as to whether this release pathway could be used in a physiological setting. However, recent studies have shown that synaptic activity can deplete the extracellular space of Ca^{2+}. The Ca^{2+} flux through synaptically-activated NMDA receptors leads to depletion of extracellular Ca^{2+} sufficient to reduce the subsequent amount of transmitter released at the same synapse (Rusakov and Fine, 2003). Could the activity of neuronal calcium-permeant channels deplete the external calcium level sufficiently to induce gating of astrocytic hemichannels? To summarize, mounting evidence supports the notion that hemichannels are capable of releasing transmitters from astrocytes. However, significant attention needs to be focused on the conditions that would permit hemi-channel gating so that it is possible to determine whether this pathway can be gated under physiological conditions.

16.5. P2X₇ receptor-mediated release

The most recently discovered mechanism of neurotransmitter release by astrocytes utilizes a unique form of ATP receptor known as the $P2X_7$ or P2Z receptor. $P2X_7$ receptors exist as large homomeric complexes that can function as ATP-gated channels with an amplified response in low divalent cation solution (North and Surprenant, 2000). The channels formed appear to vary in a cell-type dependent manner from large channels permeable to molecules up to 900 Da in size to small channels that can provide ion selectivity. These receptors have been localized to a number of CNS-specific cell types including astrocytes (Kukley et al., 2001). In the first study to demonstrate a $P2X_7$-based channel activity, astrocytes in primary culture were shown to express $P2X_7$ receptors that mediated an ATP-induced inward current, as assessed by patch clamp (Duan et al., 2003). This current was inhibited by the P2X receptor antagonist pyridoxal phosphate-6-azophenyl-2'-4'-disulfonic acid (PPADS) as well as the anion channel blocker DIDS. 3'-O-(4-benzoyl)benzoyl ATP (BzATP), a potent activator of $P2X_7$ receptors, was able to induce a small astrocyte uptake of Lucifer yellow in standard medium but a large increase in uptake with incubation in Ca^{2+}/Mg^{2+}-free medium. Efflux of glutamate and aspartate could be induced by application of ATP. There was significant efflux with 1 mM ATP in standard medium or 10 mM ATP in Ca^{2+}/Mg^{2+}-free medium. Because release was amplified by removal of Ca^{2+} from the medium it is unlikely to be mediated by Ca^{2+}-dependent vesicular release. This was further supported by preincubating the cells with the calcium chelator BAPTA-AM which usually completely blocks Ca^{2+}-dependent vesicle mediated release.

This novel means of transmitter release is yet one more pathway that must be explored in any new studies of astrocytic release mechanisms. Since P2X$_7$ receptor-based channels are inhibited by many of the same anion channel blockers that are used to determine anion channel-mediated release it is possible that transmitter release heretofore believed to be mediated by anion channels is in fact mediated by P2X$_7$ receptors. However, in future studies it will be a simple matter to test for the existence of a P2X$_7$ pathway with specific activators and inhibitors of P2X$_7$.

16.6. Vesicle-mediated exocytotic release

All eukaryotic cells utilize secretory vesicles to transport new membrane and proteins to the plasma membrane during a process known as constitutive exocytosis. Most cell types also possess a second pathway of regulated exocytosis in which secretory vesicles fuse with the plasma membrane in response to a stimulus, usually an increase in intracellular calcium. The most extensively studied form of regulated exocytosis is the release of neurotransmitters from presynaptic nerve terminals via synaptic vesicles. In addition to secretory vesicles, many non-neuronal cells also contain small vesicles that have been designated synaptic-like microvesicles (SLMVs) (Burgoyne and Morgan, 2003). All of these pathways utilize much of the same core machinery to control vesicle docking and fusion. This machinery includes the three SNARE proteins syntaxin, SNAP-25 (or SNAP-23) and synaptobrevin/VAMP (Burgoyne and Morgan, 2003). Not only do all cells contain the machinery for exocytosis but non-neuronal cells have also been shown to utilize this pathway in the release of neurotransmitters. Ahnert-Hilger demonstrated that SLMVs in pancreatic β-cells release the neurotransmitter GABA which may function to regulate surrounding cells (Ahnert-Hilger et al., 1996). Since exocytosis is an ubiquitous pathway for release of extracellular substances it is probable that this pathway is utilized by astrocytes to release neurotransmitters that modulate neuronal activity.

Although all of the mechanisms of neurotransmitter release considered thus far either require or are enhanced by a fall in extracellular osmolarity or $[Ca^{2+}]_e$, this is not the case for the vesicle-mediated release of neurotransmitters. The first evidence that vesicles can mediate the release of neurotransmitters from astrocytes came from the finding that bradykinin induced elevations in intracellular calcium could stimulate the release of glutamate. This glutamate release subsequently caused an NMDA-mediated increase in neuronal calcium (Parpura et al., 1994). Examination of the mechanism of bradykinin-induced EAA release from astrocytes showed that glutamate transporter inhibitors failed to block EAA release while α-latrotoxin, a compound that stimulates exocytosis in neurons, increased the amount of glutamate release (Parpura et al., 1995b; Jeftinija et al., 1996). Further support for a vesicular mode of glutamate release came from the use of clostridial toxins that specifically block vesicle release by cleaving proteins required for vesicle docking with the plasma membrane. Pretreatment of astrocytes with botulinum toxins A or B, toxins that specifically block exocytosis in neurons by cleavage of SNAP-25 or synaptobrevin/VAMP respectively, decreased the bradykinin-induced and baseline release of glutamate (Jeftinija et al., 1997). In addition to bradykinin, PGE$_2$ was found to stimulate the calcium-dependent release of glutamate from astrocytes in culture and in acute brain slices (Bezzi et al., 1998). Release was inhibited by the anion channel blocker furosemide, which has not been demonstrated to block hemichannels, as well as the blocker of neuronal exocytotic release, tetanus neurotoxin (TeNT).

If release of glutamate is being specifically blocked by clostridial toxins then astrocytes should express the synaptic proteins that are the substrates of these toxins. In fact, astrocytes in culture express a large complement of synaptic proteins including synaptobrevin II, synaptotagmin I, synaptophysin, rab3a, synapsin I, SNAP-23, SNAP-25, syntaxin I and cellubrevin (Parpura et al., 1995a; Jeftinija et al., 1997; Maienschein et al., 1999). Synaptic protein expression was highest within the first few days after plating and generally declined with time in culture, suggesting that long-term culture of astrocytes may result in the loss of vesicle-mediated release of transmitters that exists *in vivo* (Maienschein et al., 1999). Recent results from our laboratory demonstrate the presence of numerous synaptic proteins in freshly-isolated astrocytes as determined by RT-PCR and immunocytochemistry, further supporting their existence within astrocytes *in vivo*. Additionally this study has demonstrated the presence of a vesicular glutamate transporter within astrocytic processes adjacent to synapses in adult hippocampal synapses (Zhang et al., Submitted).

A question raised by the observation of synaptobrevin II/VAMP2 in astrocytes is why TeNT, which acts through cleavage of this synaptic protein, takes so much longer to exert its effect on neurotransmitter release from astrocytes than from neurons (Schiavo et al., 1992). For example, Bezzi et al. found that inhibition by TeNT (2 µg/ml) took 8 hrs for detection and reached 70% inhibition only after 20 hrs of exposure, while TeNT blocks synaptic release of neurotransmitters from neurons in a matter of minutes (Bezzi et al., 1998). Also curious is the observed selective labeling of neurons, but not astrocytes, by a FITC-labeled C-terminal fragment of tetanus toxin (Araque et al., 1998). These results may be explained by the discovery that efficient internalization of TeNT requires binding of the C-terminal half of TeNT to a neural-specific receptor on the plasma membrane followed by internalization via synaptic vesicle endocytosis (Matteoli et al., 1996; Herreros et al., 2000). Bypassing the problem of efficient neurotoxin uptake in astrocytes by direct injection of botulinum neurotoxin B (BoNT/B), a toxin that specifically blocks exocytosis in neurons by cleavage of synaptobrevin, can quickly reduce synaptobrevin immunofluorescence and block glutamate release while leaving calcium responses unaffected (Araque et al., 2000). The same study also demonstrated that the vacuolar-type H^+-ATPase inhibitor bafilomycin A_1 can reduce the Ca^{2+}-dependent release of glutamate from astrocytes. Although there is substantial evidence demonstrating that TeNT is not efficiently internalized into astrocytes, it appears that BoNT can be actively internalized into astrocytes (Verderio et al., 1999). Treatment of astrocyte cultures with BoNT/F for 2 hours resulted in 20-70% cleavage of cellubrevin 19 hours later.

Actual visualization of calcium-mediated release of glutamate from astrocytes showed that an intercellular Ca^{2+} wave traveling at 10-30 µm/sec induced a wave of regenerative glutamate release that propagated at the same speed (Innocenti et al., 2000). The glutamate wave was unaffected by inhibitors of glutamate transport or replacement of extracellular sodium with lithium (Innocenti et al., 2000). Further evidence of the fast kinetics of Ca^{2+}-dependent glutamate release from astrocytes was provided by the use of HEK 293 cells expressing the NMDA receptor as glutamate sensors when plated over astrocytes (Pasti et al., 2001). $[Ca^{2+}]_i$ oscillations in astrocytes triggered synchronous oscillations in sensor cells via NMDAR activation which were inhibited by TeNT or bafilomycin without affecting the astrocytic $[Ca^{2+}]_i$ oscillations. There is little question that astrocytes are able to release glutamate in response to external stimuli that raise intracellular calcium. Since glutamate can be released via this pathway, other neurotransmitters could also be released.

Glutamate is not the only neurotransmitter found to be released from astrocytes via Ca^{2+}-dependent exocytosis. Though technically a neuropeptide rather than a neurotransmitter, atrial natriuretic peptide (ANP), has been identified in neurons and astrocytes in the CNS. Myocardial cells are known to release ANP by exocytosis of clathrin-coated vesicles (Klein et al., 1993). To examine the mechanism of release in astrocytes pro-ANP was fused with a fluorescent protein and visualized during an increase in $[Ca^{2+}]_i$ (Krzan et al., 2003). Recycling dye FM 4-64 was also used to monitor incorporation of new vesicle membrane into the plasma membrane. The labeled ANP produced fluorescent puncta in the cells. The number of puncta decreased when $[Ca^{2+}]_i$ was increased, while the fluorescence attributable to FM 4-64 increased, suggesting that ANP is released via Ca^{2+}-dependent exocytosis. UDP-glucose, a potential new extracellular signaling molecule in astrocytes and other cells that activates the $P2Y_{14}$ receptor was found to be released along with ATP (Lazarowski et al., 2003). It is hypothesized that release of ATP and UDP-glucose is mediated by the pathway of constitutive exocytosis via secretory granules that deliver glycoproteins to the plasma membrane and which can be activated by mechanical stimulation via a change of extracellular media.

Nitric oxide was found to induce a rapid release of ATP and glutamate from cultured astrocytes that was inhibited by intracellular calcium chelators and long-term incubation with botulinum toxin C but was unaffected by glutamate transport inhibitors (Bal-Price et al., 2002). ATP has been found in secretory granules within astrocytes where its accumulation was blocked by bafilomycin A_1 (Coco et al., 2003). It appears that vesicular release of ATP may be via a pathway distinct from that of glutamate release. Although TeNT almost completely blocked glutamate release it only partially inhibited ATP release. Ca^{2+}-stimulated release of glutamate was much higher than that of ATP (Coco et al., 2003). Despite the small effect of TeNT on ATP release the substrates of the clostridial toxins have been found in association with ATP-storing organelles (Maienschein et al., 1999)

Although there is a great deal of evidence to support Ca^{2+}-dependent vesicular release of glutamate from astrocytes it is highly probable that other pathways also come into play. For example, treatment of organotypic hippocampal slices with an inhibitor of glutamate uptake led to a rapid increase in extracellular glutamate (Jabaudon et al., 1999). The increase was Ca^{2+}-independent, could not be blocked by clostridial toxins and appeared to originate from glia. However, the overwhelming evidence for a vesicular release pathway for glutamate and increasing evidence for the release of other substances indicates that this is a significant mode of release from astrocytes. More significant in terms of astrocyte modulation of neuronal function is the ability of vesicular release of transmitters to be easily modulated by intracellular calcium signaling. This lends itself very well to cross-talk between neurons and astrocytes and may form a basis for new levels of control of neuronal signaling.

16.7. Future perspectives

Clearly there is a plethora of mechanisms that mediate the regulated release of neurotransmitters from astrocytes in the CNS. Release can be triggered by extracellular stimuli ranging from receptor-mediated agonists, to changes in osmolarity, to the extracellular levels of specific ions. However, questions remain. Which of these stimuli occur during normal physiological operation of the brain and which are relevant only during pathological conditions such as ischemia? Is it also possible that processes that are dominant during trauma also operate at a reduced level in a physiological setting and contribute to the mechanisms that are the primary mediators of glial modulation of neurons via the regulated release of neurotransmitters?

One of the biggest obstacles to addressing these questions is the availability of specific reagents. As can be seen in Figure 16.1 there is a great deal of cross-reactivity in the chemical inhibitors currently being used to try and discriminate between the different release pathways. Some of the available compounds may be suitable for use once they have been adequately characterized but unfortunately very few studies have been done to determine their specificities. This is very much the case with over half of the anion channel inhibitors and all of the gap junction inhibitors. Although the clostridial toxins have been well characterized and are very specific to vesicular release they can be difficult to use, particularly in experiments in tissue. Until the reagents that exist are well characterized as to their specificities or new highly specific compounds or methods are developed it will remain extremely difficult to determine exactly what pathways are being used by astrocytes to release neurotransmitters *in vivo*.

Acknowledgments.   Supported by grants from the NINDS, R37NS37585 and R01NS43142

16.8. References

Ahnert-Hilger G, Stadtbaumer A, Strubing C, Scherubl H, Schultz G, Riecken EO, Wiedenmann B (1996) gamma-Aminobutyric acid secretion from pancreatic neuroendocrine cells. Gastroenterology 110:1595-1604.

Alvarez-Maubecin V, Garcia-Hernandez F, Williams JT, Van Bockstaele EJ (2000) Functional coupling between neurons and glia. J Neurosci 20:4091-4098.

Anderson CM, Swanson RA (2000) Astrocyte glutamate transport: review of properties, regulation, and physiological functions. Glia 32:1-14.

Araque A, Carmignoto G, Haydon PG (2001) Dynamic signaling between astrocytes and neurons. Annu Rev Physiol 63:795-813.

Araque A, Parpura V, Sanzgiri RP, Haydon PG (1998) Glutamate-dependent astrocyte modulation of synaptic transmission between cultured hippocampal neurons. Eur J Neurosci 10:2129-2142.

Araque A, Sanzgiri RP, Parpura V, Haydon PG (1999) Astrocyte-induced modulation of synaptic transmission. Can J Physiol Pharmacol 77:699-706.

Araque A, Li N, Doyle RT, Haydon PG (2000) SNARE protein-dependent glutamate release from astrocytes. J Neurosci 20:666-673.

Araque A, Martin ED, Perea G, Arellano JI, Buno W (2002) Synaptically released acetylcholine evokes Ca2+ elevations in astrocytes in hippocampal slices. J Neurosci 22:2443-2450.

Attwell D, Barbour B, Szatkowski M (1993) Nonvesicular release of neurotransmitter. Neuron 11:401-407.

Bal-Price A, Moneer Z, Brown GC (2002) Nitric oxide induces rapid, calcium-dependent release of vesicular glutamate and ATP from cultured rat astrocytes. Glia 40:312-323.

Basarsky TA, Feighan D, MacVicar BA (1999) Glutamate release through volume-activated channels during spreading depression. J Neurosci 19:6439-6445.

Basarsky TA, Duffy SN, Andrew RD, MacVicar BA (1998) Imaging spreading depression and associated intracellular calcium waves in brain slices. J Neurosci 18:7189-7199.

Bellocchio EE, Reimer RJ, Fremeau RT, Jr., Edwards RH (2000) Uptake of glutamate into synaptic vesicles by an inorganic phosphate transporter. Science 289:957-960.

Bezzi P, Carmignoto G, Pasti L, Vesce S, Rossi D, Rizzini BL, Pozzan T, Volterra A (1998) Prostaglandins stimulate calcium-dependent glutamate release in astrocytes. Nature 391:281-285.

Bres V, Hurbin A, Duvoid A, Orcel H, Moos FC, Rabie A, Hussy N (2000) Pharmacological characterization of volume-sensitive, taurine permeable anion channels in rat supraoptic glial cells. Br J Pharmacol 130:1976-1982.

Burgoyne RD, Morgan A (2003) Secretory granule exocytosis. Physiol Rev 83:581-632.

Carmignoto G (2000) Reciprocal communication systems between astrocytes and neurones. Prog Neurobiol 62:561-581.

Chaudhry FA, Lehre KP, van Lookeren Campagne M, Ottersen OP, Danbolt NC, Storm-Mathisen J (1995) Glutamate transporters in glial plasma membranes: highly differentiated localizations revealed by quantitative ultrastructural immunocytochemistry. Neuron 15:711-720.

Chen Y, Swanson RA (2003) Astrocytes and brain injury. J Cereb Blood Flow Metab 23:137-149.

Coco S, Calegari F, Pravettoni E, Pozzi D, Taverna E, Rosa P, Matteoli M, Verderio C (2003) Storage and release of ATP from astrocytes in culture. J Biol Chem 278:1354-1362.

Cotrina ML, Nedergaard M (2002) Astrocytes in the aging brain. J Neurosci Res 67:1-10.

Cotrina ML, Lin JH, Alves-Rodrigues A, Liu S, Li J, Azmi-Ghadimi H, Kang J, Naus CC, Nedergaard M (1998) Connexins regulate calcium signaling by controlling ATP release. Proc Natl Acad Sci U S A 95:15735-15740.

Darby M, Kuzmiski JB, Panenka W, Feighan D, MacVicar BA (2003) ATP released from astrocytes during swelling activates chloride channels. J Neurophysiol 89:1870-1877.

Deleuze C, Duvoid A, Hussy N (1998) Properties and glial origin of osmotic-dependent release of taurine from the rat supraoptic nucleus. J Physiol 507 (Pt 2):463-471.

Dermietzel R, Hertberg EL, Kessler JA, Spray DC (1991) Gap junctions between cultured astrocytes: immunocytochemical, molecular, and electrophysiological analysis. J Neurosci 11:1421-1432.

Duan S, Anderson CM, Keung EC, Chen Y, Swanson RA (2003) P2X7 receptor-mediated release of excitatory amino acids from astrocytes. J Neurosci 23:1320-1328.

Duffy S, MacVicar BA (1999) Modulation of neuronal excitability by astrocytes. Adv Neurol 79:573-581.

Eskandari S, Zampighi GA, Leung DW, Wright EM, Loo DD (2002) Inhibition of gap junction hemichannels by chloride channel blockers. J Membr Biol 185:93-102.

Evans WH, Martin PE (2002) Gap junctions: structure and function (Review). Mol Membr Biol 19:121-136.

Gadea A, Lopez-Colome AM (2001a) Glial transporters for glutamate, glycine, and GABA III. Glycine transporters. J Neurosci Res 64:218-222.

Gadea A, Lopez-Colome AM (2001b) Glial transporters for glutamate, glycine, and GABA: II. GABA transporters. J Neurosci Res 63:461-468.

Gadea A, Lopez-Colome AM (2001c) Glial transporters for glutamate, glycine and GABA I. Glutamate transporters. J Neurosci Res 63:453-460.

Giaume C, Fromaget C, el Aoumari A, Cordier J, Glowinski J, Gros D (1991) Gap junctions in cultured astrocytes: single-channel currents and characterization of channel-forming protein. Neuron 6:133-143.

Harden TK, Lazarowski ER (1999) Release of ATP and UTP from astrocytoma cells. Prog Brain Res 120:135-143.

Hartinger J, Jahn R (1993) An anion binding site that regulates the glutamate transporter of synaptic vesicles. J Biol Chem 268:23122-23127.

Haydon PG (2001) GLIA: listening and talking to the synapse. Nat Rev Neurosci 2:185-193.

Herreros J, Lalli G, Schiavo G (2000) C-terminal half of tetanus toxin fragment C is sufficient for neuronal binding and interaction with a putative protein receptor. Biochem J 347 Pt 1:199-204.

Hofer A, Dermietzel R (1998) Visualization and functional blocking of gap junction hemichannels (connexons) with antibodies against external loop domains in astrocytes. Glia 24:141-154.

Hussy N, Deleuze C, Desarmenien MG, Moos FC (2000) Osmotic regulation of neuronal activity: a new role for taurine and glial cells in a hypothalamic neuroendocrine structure. Prog Neurobiol 62:113-134.

Hussy N, Deleuze C, Pantaloni A, Desarmenien MG, Moos F (1997) Agonist action of taurine on glycine receptors in rat supraoptic magnocellular neurones: possible role in osmoregulation. J Physiol 502 (Pt 3):609-621.

Innocenti B, Parpura V, Haydon PG (2000) Imaging extracellular waves of glutamate during calcium signaling in cultured astrocytes. J Neurosci 20:1800-1808.

Jabaudon D, Shimamoto K, Yasuda-Kamatani Y, Scanziani M, Gahwiler BH, Gerber U (1999) Inhibition of uptake unmasks rapid extracellular turnover of glutamate of nonvesicular origin. Proc Natl Acad Sci U S A 96:8733-8738.

Jackson PS, Strange K (1993) Volume-sensitive anion channels mediate swelling-activated inositol and taurine efflux. Am J Physiol 265:C1489-1500.

Jeftinija SD, Jeftinija KV, Stefanovic G (1997) Cultured astrocytes express proteins involved in vesicular glutamate release. Brain Res 750:41-47.

Jeftinija SD, Jeftinija KV, Stefanovic G, Liu F (1996) Neuroligand-evoked calcium-dependent release of excitatory amino acids from cultured astrocytes. J Neurochem 66:676-684.

Jeremic A, Jeftinija K, Stevanovic J, Glavaski A, Jeftinija S (2001) ATP stimulates calcium-dependent glutamate release from cultured astrocytes. J Neurochem 77:664-675.

Kamermans M, Fahrenfort I, Schultz K, Janssen-Bienhold U, Sjoerdsma T, Weiler R (2001) Hemichannel-mediated inhibition in the outer retina. Science 292:1178-1180.

Kang J, Jiang L, Goldman SA, Nedergaard M (1998) Astrocyte-mediated potentiation of inhibitory synaptic transmission. Nat Neurosci 1:683-692.

Kimelberg HK, Goderie SK, Higman S, Pang S, Waniewski RA (1990) Swelling-induced release of glutamate, aspartate, and taurine from astrocyte cultures. J Neurosci 10:1583-1591.

Klein RM, Kelley KB, Merisko-Liversidge EM (1993) A clathrin-coated vesicle-mediated pathway in atrial natriuretic peptide (ANP) secretion. J Mol Cell Cardiol 25:437-452.

Krzan M, Stenovec M, Kreft M, Pangrsic T, Grilc S, Haydon PG, Zorec R (2003) Calcium-dependent exocytosis of atrial natriuretic peptide from astrocytes. J Neurosci 23:1580-1583.

Kukley M, Barden JA, Steinhauser C, Jabs R (2001) Distribution of P2X receptors on astrocytes in juvenile rat hippocampus. Glia 36:11-21.

Lal R, Lin H (2001) Imaging molecular structure and physiological function of gap junctions and hemijunctions by multimodal atomic force microscopy. Microsc Res Tech 52:273-288.

Lazarowski ER, Shea DA, Boucher RC, Harden TK (2003) Release of cellular UDP-glucose as a potential extracellular signaling molecule. Mol Pharmacol 63:1190-1197.

Longuemare MC, Swanson RA (1995) Excitatory amino acid release from astrocytes during energy failure by reversal of sodium-dependent uptake. J Neurosci Res 40:379-386.

Longuemare MC, Swanson RA (1997) Net glutamate release from astrocytes is not induced by extracellular potassium concentrations attainable in brain. J Neurochem 69:879-882.

Longuemare MC, Rose CR, Farrell K, Ransom BR, Waxman SG, Swanson RA (1999) K(+)-induced reversal of astrocyte glutamate uptake is limited by compensatory changes in intracellular Na+. Neuroscience 93:285-292.

Lukacs GL, Nanda A, Rotstein OD, Grinstein S (1991) The chloride channel blocker 5-nitro-2-(3-phenylpropyl-amino) benzoic acid (NPPB) uncouples mitochondria and increases the proton permeability of the plasma membrane in phagocytic cells. FEBS Lett 288:17-20.

Maienschein V, Marxen M, Volknandt W, Zimmermann H (1999) A plethora of presynaptic proteins associated with ATP-storing organelles in cultured astrocytes. Glia 26:233-244.

Martin DL (1992) Synthesis and release of neuroactive substances by glial cells. Glia 5:81-94.

Matteoli M, Verderio C, Rossetto O, Iezzi N, Coco S, Schiavo G, Montecucco C (1996) Synaptic vesicle endocytosis mediates the entry of tetanus neurotoxin into hippocampal neurons. Proc Natl Acad Sci U S A 93:13310-13315.

Maycox PR, Hell JW, Jahn R (1990) Amino acid neurotransmission: spotlight on synaptic vesicles. Trends Neurosci 13:83-87.

Mazzanti M, Haydon PG (2003) Astrocytes selectively enhance N-type calcium current in hippocampal neurons. Glia 41:128-136.

Mazzanti M, Sul JY, Haydon PG (2001) Glutamate on demand: astrocytes as a ready source. Neuroscientist 7:396-405.

Mongin AA, Kimelberg HK (2002) ATP potently modulates anion channel-mediated excitatory amino acid release from cultured astrocytes. Am J Physiol Cell Physiol 283:C569-578.

Naito S, Ueda T (1985) Characterization of glutamate uptake into synaptic vesicles. J Neurochem 44:99-109.

Nedergaard M (1994) Direct signaling from astrocytes to neurons in cultures of mammalian brain cells. Science 263:1768-1771.

Nelson N, Perzov N, Cohen A, Hagai K, Padler V, Nelson H (2000) The cellular biology of proton-motive force generation by V-ATPases. J Exp Biol 203 Pt 1:89-95.

North RA, Surprenant A (2000) Pharmacology of cloned P2X receptors. Annu Rev Pharmacol Toxicol 40:563-580.

Ogata T, Nakamura Y, Shibata T, Kataoka K (1992) Release of excitatory amino acids from cultured hippocampal astrocytes induced by a hypoxic-hypoglycemic stimulation. J Neurochem 58:1957-1959.

Oyamada Y, Zhou W, Oyamada H, Takamatsu T, Oyamada M (2002) Dominant-negative connexin43-EGFP inhibits calcium-transient synchronization of primary neonatal rat cardiomyocytes. Exp Cell Res 273:85-94.

Parpura V, Haydon PG (2000) Physiological astrocytic calcium levels stimulate glutamate release to modulate adjacent neurons. Proc Natl Acad Sci U S A 97:8629-8634.

Parpura V, Fang Y, Basarsky T, Jahn R, Haydon PG (1995a) Expression of synaptobrevin II, cellubrevin and syntaxin but not SNAP-25 in cultured astrocytes. FEBS Lett 377:489-492.

Parpura V, Basarsky TA, Liu F, Jeftinija K, Jeftinija S, Haydon PG (1994) Glutamate-mediated astrocyte-neuron signalling. Nature 369:744-747.

Parpura V, Liu F, Brethorst S, Jeftinija K, Jeftinija S, Haydon PG (1995b) Alpha-latrotoxin stimulates glutamate release from cortical astrocytes in cell culture. FEBS Lett 360:266-270.

Parri HR, Gould TM, Crunelli V (2001) Spontaneous astrocytic Ca2+ oscillations in situ drive NMDAR-mediated neuronal excitation. Nat Neurosci 4:803-812.

Passow H (1986) Molecular aspects of band 3 protein-mediated anion transport across the red blood cell membrane. Rev Physiol Biochem Pharmacol 103:61-203.

Pasti L, Volterra A, Pozzan T, Carmignoto G (1997) Intracellular calcium oscillations in astrocytes: a highly plastic, bidirectional form of communication between neurons and astrocytes in situ. J Neurosci 17:7817-7830.

Pasti L, Zonta M, Pozzan T, Vicini S, Carmignoto G (2001) Cytosolic calcium oscillations in astrocytes may regulate exocytotic release of glutamate. J Neurosci 21:477-484.

Phillis JW, O'Regan MH (2003) Characterization of modes of release of amino acids in the ischemic/reperfused rat cerebral cortex. Neurochem Int 43:461-467.

Porter JT, McCarthy KD (1997) Astrocytic neurotransmitter receptors in situ and in vivo. Prog Neurobiol 51:439-455.

Pothos EN, Mosharov E, Liu KP, Setlik W, Haburcak M, Baldini G, Gershon MD, Tamir H, Sulzer D (2002) Stimulation-dependent regulation of the pH, volume and quantal size of bovine and rodent secretory vesicles. J Physiol 542:453-476.

Queiroz G, Gebicke-Haerter PJ, Schobert A, Starke K, von Kugelgen I (1997) Release of ATP from cultured rat astrocytes elicited by glutamate receptor activation. Neuroscience 78:1203-1208.

Queiroz G, Meyer DK, Meyer A, Starke K, von Kugelgen I (1999) A study of the mechanism of the release of ATP from rat cortical astroglial cells evoked by activation of glutamate receptors. Neuroscience 91:1171-1181.

Quist AP, Rhee SK, Lin H, Lal R (2000) Physiological role of gap-junctional hemichannels. Extracellular calcium-dependent isosmotic volume regulation. J Cell Biol 148:1063-1074.

Rigo JM, Belachew S, Lefebvre PP, Leprince P, Malgrange B, Rogister B, Kettenmann H, Moonen G (1994) Astroglia-released factor shows similar effects as benzodiazepine inverse agonists. J Neurosci Res 39:364-376.

Rossi DJ, Oshima T, Attwell D (2000) Glutamate release in severe brain ischaemia is mainly by reversed uptake. Nature 403:316-321.

Rusakov DA, Fine A (2003) Extracellular Ca2+ depletion contributes to fast activity-dependent modulation of synaptic transmission in the brain. Neuron 37:287-297.

Rutledge EM, Kimelberg HK (1996) Release of [3H]-D-aspartate from primary astrocyte cultures in response to raised external potassium. J Neurosci 16:7803-7811.

Rutledge EM, Aschner M, Kimelberg HK (1998) Pharmacological characterization of swelling-induced D-[3H]aspartate release from primary astrocyte cultures. Am J Physiol 274:C1511-1520.

Sanzgiri RP, Araque A, Haydon PG (1999) Prostaglandin E(2) stimulates glutamate receptor-dependent astrocyte neuromodulation in cultured hippocampal cells. J Neurobiol 41:221-229.

Schiavo G, Benfenati F, Poulain B, Rossetto O, Polverino de Laureto P, DasGupta BR, Montecucco C (1992) Tetanus and botulinum-B neurotoxins block neurotransmitter release by proteolytic cleavage of synaptobrevin. Nature 359:832-835.

Seal RP, Amara SG (1999) Excitatory amino acid transporters: a family in flux. Annu Rev Pharmacol Toxicol 39:431-456.

Spray DC (2003) Neural gene alterations in mice lacking Cx43, the major astrocytic gap junction protein. J Neurochem 85:S27.

Stout CE, Costantin JL, Naus CC, Charles AC (2002) Intercellular calcium signaling in astrocytes via ATP release through connexin hemichannels. J Biol Chem 277:10482-10488.

Van der Kloot W (2003) A chloride channel blocker reduces acetylcholine uptake into synaptic vesicles at the frog neuromuscular junction. Brain Res 961:287-289.

Verderio C, Coco S, Rossetto O, Montecucco C, Matteoli M (1999) Internalization and proteolytic action of botulinum toxins in CNS neurons and astrocytes. J Neurochem 73:372-379.

Wang Z, Haydon PG, Yeung ES (2000) Direct observation of calcium-independent intercellular ATP signaling in astrocytes. Anal Chem 72:2001-2007.

Xie XS, Stone DK, Racker E (1983) Determinants of clathrin-coated vesicle acidification. J Biol Chem 258:14834-14838.

Ye ZC, Wyeth MS, Baltan-Tekkok S, Ransom BR (2003) Functional hemichannels in astrocytes: a novel mechanism of glutamate release. J Neurosci 23:3588-3596.

Zerangue N, Kavanaugh MP (1996) Flux coupling in a neuronal glutamate transporter. Nature 383:634-637.

Zhang Y, McBride DW, Jr., Hamill OP (1998) The ion selectivity of a membrane conductance inactivated by extracellular calcium in Xenopus oocytes. J Physiol 508 (Pt 3):763-776.

16.9. Abbreviations

A9C	Anthracene-9-carboxylate
ANP	Atrial natriuretic peptide
BoNT	Botulinum neurotoxin
BzATP	3'-O-(4-benzoyl)benzoyl ATP
CNS	Central nervous system
Cx	Connexin
DIDS	4,4'-diisothiocyanato-stilbene-2,2'-disulfonate
DPC	Diphenylamin-2-carboxylate
EAA	Excitatory amino acid
FFA	Flufenamic acid
GABA	γ-aminobutyric acid
IAA-94	R(+)-[(6,7-dichloro-2-cyclopentyl-2,3-dihydro-2-methyl-1-oxo-1H-inden-5-yl)-oxy]acetic acid
NFA	Niflumic acid
NMDA	N-methyl-D-aspartate
NPPB	5-nitro-2-(3-phenyl-propylamino)benzoic acid
PPADS	Pyridoxal phosphate-6-azophenyl-2'-4'-disulfonic acid
SD	Spreading depression
SITS	4-acetamido-4'-isothiocyanato-stilbene-2,2'-disulfonate
SLMVs	Synaptic-like microvesicles
TeNT	Tetanus neurotoxin
$[X^{\pm}]_i$	Intracellular concentration of ion X
$[X^{\pm}]_o$	Extracellular concentration of ion X

Chapter 17

Role of astrocytes in the formation, maturation and maintenance of synapses

Michal Slezak and Frank W. Pfrieger*

Max-Planck/CNRS Group, UPR 2356, Centre de Neurochimie 5
rue Blaise Pascal, F-67084 Strasbourg, France

Corresponding author: fw-pfrieger@gmx.de

Contents

17.1. Introduction
17.2. Synaptic birth control by astrocytes
17.3. Astrocytes help synapses mature
17.4. Glia let synapses live or die
17.5. Conclusion and further directions
17.6. References
17.7. Abbreviations

17. 1. Introduction

Views on the functions of astrocytes have changed within the last few years and mainstream neuroscientists have begun to acknowledge that these cells, once considered as mere filling mass, have a profound influence on neurons (for reviews see Laming et al., 2000; Araque et al., 2001; Bezzi and Volterra, 2001; Castonguay et al., 2001; Haydon, 2001; Volterra et al., 2002). A look at recent reviews on synaptogenesis (Lee and Sheng, 2000; Zhang and Benson, 2000; Dresbach et al., 2001; Featherstone and Broadie, 2000; Sanes and Lichtman, 2001; Garner et al., 2002; Ahmari and Smith, 2002; Cohen-Cory, 2002; Jin, 2002; Okabe, 2002; Zito and Svoboda, 2002; Scheiffele, 2003) reveals, however, that this fundamental process is still considered to be merely a play between two neuronal partners. Here, we summarize evidence suggesting that this may not hold true, and that there is a third actor on stage - the astrocyte. As with other types of liaisons, the life of a synapse can be divided into three sequential phases: 1) the establishment of a physical contact, 2) a maturation process, which endows the synapse with its characteristic properties and 3) a stabilization or elimination phase, where only selected connections are maintained. Here, we discuss the contribution of astrocytes to each phase (Fig. 17.1). Their roles in other aspects of neuronal development have been summarized elsewhere (Peles and Salzer, 2000; Wang and Barres, 2000; Gomes et al., 2001; Klambt et al., 2001; Lemke, 2001; Campbell and Götz, 2002; Du and Dreyfus, 2002; Mirsky et al., 2002; Nadarajah and Parnavelas, 2002; Oland and Tolbert, 2003).

17.2. Synaptic birth control by astrocytes

The idea that glial cells, namely astrocytes, play a role in the formation of synaptic contacts stems from a conspicuous temporal correlation between synaptogenesis and the differentiation of glial cells (Pfrieger and Barres, 1996). In rodents, for example, astrocytes are generated between the last embryonic and first postnatal week, whereas massive synaptogenesis starts in the second postnatal week and continues for two to three weeks (Vaughn, 1989; Jacobson, 1991; Pfrieger and Barres, 1996; Sauvageot and Stiles, 2002). The prolonged time course of synaptogenesis contrasts with the notion that synaptic contacts are formed within an hour or so (Friedman et al., 2000; Gomperts et al., 2000). Why then, does the synapse number increase so slowly *in vivo*? This could either be due to gradual stabilization of rapidly forming synapses or the existence of factors that limit the extent of synaptogenesis. Rakic and colleagues have postulated such a (humoral) factor based on their finding that synaptogenesis starts synchronously in different areas of the monkey brain (Rakic et al., 1986).

Do glial cells, in particular astrocytes, provide such factors? Studies on the neuromuscular junction (NMJ) have shown that processes of Schwann cells (SCs) guide the growth of nerve fibers *in vivo* (Son and Thompson, 1995a; Son and Thompson, 1995b; O'Malley et al., 1999; Herrera et al., 2000; Macleod et al., 2001; Love et al., 2003, for review see Son et al., 1996), but it is not clear whether they are necessary for NMJ formation. Similarly, the role of astrocytes in synaptogenesis *in vivo* is still unclear. Controlled ablation of astrocytes (Messing, 1998; Sofroniew et al., 1999; Cui et al., 2001) in living animals causes neurodegeneration, thus precluding an analysis of their role in synapse development.

An alternative approach to address this topic is offered by culture preparations, where synaptogenesis can be monitored in the presence or absence of glia. In co-cultures of neurons and muscle cells from frogs, ultrastructurally defined NMJs with no contact to SCs have been found (Weldon and Cohen, 1979; Nakajima et al., 1987). On the other hand, there is evidence that SCs secrete so far unidentified factor(s) that enable NMJ formation in cultured human muscle cells (Guettier-Sigrist et al., 2000).

The formation of synaptic contacts between central nervous system (CNS) neurons has been studied in several culture preparations. Neuronal cell lines represent a convenient approach, since they are glia-free by definition. Hartley and colleagues monitored synaptogenesis in NT2N cells, a neuron-like cell line, by electron microscopy, electrophysiological recordings and immunocytochemical staining (Hartley et al., 1999). These cells formed few and immature glutamatergic synapses when cultured without glia in serum-containing medium, whereas in the presence of astrocytes, synapse formation was enhanced. However, astrocytes also influenced neuronal outgrowth leaving the specificity of the synaptogenic effect unclear. The role of astrocytes in synapse formation has also been studied in neurons derived from stem cells of adult rat hippocampus (Toda et al., 2000; Song et al., 2002). Electrophysiological recordings showed that culturing these cells in the presence of soluble factors from glial cells strongly enhance the number of cells that showed synaptic activity. However, again this effect may have been due to stronger neuronal survival or neurite outgrowth. Finally, several groups observed effects of astrocytes on synapse formation or function in primary cultures of neurons from different areas of the rat brain including spinal cord (Li et al., 1999), striatum (Rouget et al., 1993), cortex (Nakanishi et al., 1994; van den Pol and Spencer, 2000), hippocampus (Verderio et al., 1999; van den Pol and Spencer, 2000) and hypothalamus (van den Pol and Spencer, 2000). These authors cultured neurons from embryonic or newborn tissue, where the number of astrocytes is still low. Again, however, the results do not establish a glial effect on synaptogenesis, since these culture preparations do not allow separation of direct effects on synapse formation from changes in neurite outgrowth, neuronal differentiation or survival.

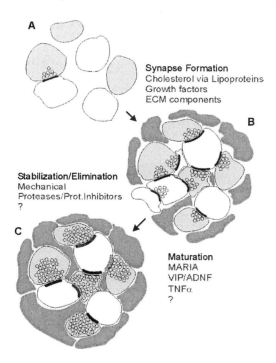

Figure 17.1. Diagram illustrating the different stages of synapse development and the possible role of astrocytes (in green) in rodents. **A**. In the embryonic stage, before astrocytes are generated, neuronal processes (presynaptic elements in yellow; postsynaptic elements in white) form few and immature synapses. **B**. The massive increase in number of synapses during the first postnatal weeks may be enabled by astrocyte-derived components, such as ECM components, growth factors and cholesterol contained in lipoproteins. Maturation process is mediated by factors, such as MARIA, VIP/ADNF, TNFα, but there are more likely additional, yet unknown factors (?) involved in this process. **C**. Excess synapses may be eliminated by astrocytic processes invading the synaptic cleft or by release of proteases that digest synapse-stabilizing components. On the other hand, astrocyte-derived signals may help to stabilize surviving synapses and to induce their functional maturation. Also, there might be other undetermined factors (?) that can assist in either elimination or stabilization process. Different colors of lines graphically representing synapses in C indicate different composition of postsynaptic receptor complex (variety of different receptors and density proteins) in different synapses. Note the increase of synaptic vesicles (circles within presynaptic terminals) in maturation and stabilization processes (compare A-C).

A series of recent studies provided direct evidence that astrocytes strongly enhance synapse formation. This has been made possible by the establishment of a method to highly (>99.5%) purify a specific type of CNS neuron, the retinal ganglion cell (RGC), from postnatal rats (Barres et al., 1988). Purified RGCs can be cultured for several weeks in a defined medium that supports survival and growth under glia-free conditions (Meyer-Franke et al., 1995). This culture model made it possible to assess rigorously the glial influence on synapse formation. In a first study, Pfrieger and Barres (1997) showed by electron microscopy that cultured RGCs form ultrastructurally defined synapses in the complete absence of glia or their natural partners from the superior colliculus. This shows that synapse formation per se is an intrinsic property of these neurons and does not require external signals. However, addition of glial cells strongly enhanced the level of synaptic activity (Pfrieger and Barres, 1997). Two subsequent studies on single RGCs growing in microcultures (Fig. 17.2) showed in parallel that a factor released by astrocytes enhances the number of synapses by sevenfold (Nägler et al., 2001; Ullian et al., 2001) (17.3). This effect was not due to changes in neurite outgrowth and, since it was observed in individual neurons, it was independent of changes in neuron density. Finally in 2001, our group identified the major synaptogenic factor contained in glia-conditioned medium (GCM): quite surprisingly, it turned out to be cholesterol (Mauch et al., 2001) (Fig. 17.4). So far, it is not clear, how cholesterol induced these effects. It may act as a synaptogenic signal, for example after conversion to a steroid, serve as building material for synaptic components, or allow for the formation of microdomains (rafts) and thus enhance cellular processes that are essential for synaptogenesis (Pfrieger, 2003b). Our observation that cholesterol enhances synapse development also raises the question of why neurons should depend on glia-derived cholesterol rather than produce it by themselves (Pfrieger, 2003a). A possible explanation is that cholesterol synthesis is energetically expensive. The synthesis of one cholesterol molecule requires 18 acetyl-CoA, 18 ATP and 29 NADPH molecules. Neurons may not be able to afford this costly pathway, since they need to spend their energy sources on their chief function: the generation of electrical signals. It has been shown that the mature cortex devotes about 85% of the glucose-derived energy to glutamatergic synaptic transmission (Sibson et al., 1998; for reviews see Attwell and Laughlin, 2001; Bonvento et al., 2002). Finally, the need for external cholesterol supply may be limited to axonal and dendritic compartments that are distal from the soma.

Do other astrocyte-derived molecules promote synaptogenesis? It is well known that astrocytes synthesize components of the extracellular matrix (ECM) (Fitch and Silver, 1997; Dow and Wang, 1998; Garwood et al., 2001) and growth factors including glial cell line-derived neurotrophic factor, cilliary neurotrophic factor and neurotrophins (Rudge et al., 1992; Friedman et al., 1998; Dougherty et al., 2000; Ivanova and Beyer, 2001; Oku et al., 2002; for reviews see Gomes et al., 2001; Du and Dreyfus, 2002). These factors influence the growth and arborization of neurites and enhance the formation of synapses (Martinez et al., 1998; Vicario-Abejon et al., 1998; Siegel et al., 2000; Alsina et al., 2001, for reviews see Snider and Lichtman, 1996; Poo, 2001; Vicario-Abejon et al., 2002).

The studies summarized above suggest a role of glia in synaptogenesis (Fig. 17.1). It appears that neurons can form synapses without the help of glia. However, the massive synaptogenesis during postnatal weeks may be limited by the availability of cholesterol, which must be provided by astrocytes. Other glial factors may enhance synapse formation as well. Their identification relies on cultures of isolated neurons, where effects on survival, growth and synapse formation can be strictly separated. Finally, it remains to be tested which glia-derived factors contribute to synaptogenesis in vivo.

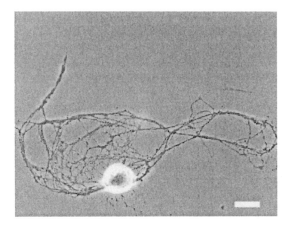

Figure 17.2. Phase-contrast micrograph of a rat retinal ganglion cell growing for a week under serum- and glia-free conditions on a small microisland of poly-D-lysine. Scale bar, 20μm.

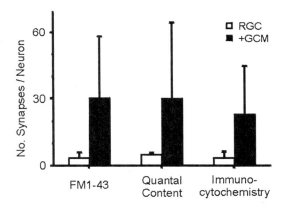

Figure 17.3. Bar graph summarizing evidence by three different experimental approaches that factors released by glial cells enhance the number of synapses formed by single RGCs in microculture (for details see Nägler et al., 2001). Bars indicate data from retinal ganglion cells tested in absence (open bars, RGC) or presence (filled bars, +GCM) of glia-conditioned medium. Error bars indicate standard deviations.

17.3. Astrocytes help synapses mature

Synapse maturation denotes a process, during which newly formed connections acquire their characteristic transmission properties, like fast postsynaptic currents or strong facilitation during stimulation. This involves changes in the number of vesicles in the presynaptic terminal, in the composition of the exocytosis machinery and in the density of postsynaptic receptors (for reviews see Cohen-Cory, 2002; Atwood and Karunanithi, 2002). Why should astrocytes control synapse maturation? The increasing evidence that astrocytes play an active role in synaptic transmission (see Araque et al., 2001; Bezzi and Volterra, 2001; Haydon, 2001) suggests that the development of synapses and the astrocytic processes that surround them must be coordinated by reciprocal signals. Recent studies indicate that astrocytes indeed promote postsynaptic maturation.

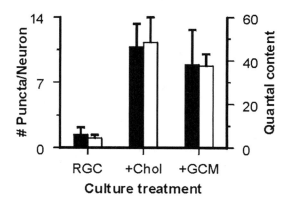

Figure 17.4. Cholesterol- and GCM-induced increases in the number of synapses in single RGCs. Number of synapsin- and glutamate receptor interacting protein-positive puncta per neuron (filled bars, left axis) and quantal content of evoked excitatory postsynaptic currents (open bars, right axis) in glia-free microcultures (n for RGC filled/open bars = 10/4) and in the presence of cholesterol (10 μg/ml, +Chol, n = 25/16) or of GCM (+GCM, n = 12/36). Error bars indicate SEM. For details see Mauch et al. (2001)

Mars and colleagues studied the differentiation of NMJs in spinal cord-muscle co-cultures and found that their development runs in parallel with SC differentiation (Mars et al., 2001). Electrophysiological recordings from purified RGCs in culture showed that glial cells enhance the size of miniature postsynaptic currents (Pfrieger and Barres, 1997; Nägler et al., 2001; Ullian et al., 2001). These events were independent of action potential-evoked transmission and due to release of individual quanta (or vesicles). In principle, the observed increase could be due to a higher intravesicular transmitter concentration or an enhanced postsynaptic receptor clustering. Ullian et al. (2001) showed that the presence of glial cells enhances the size of whole-cell currents that are evoked by application of glutamate by threefold. This observation points to a postsynaptic effect. Importantly, Nägler et al. (2001) observed a delay of at least 24 hours between addition of glia and the increase in the size of miniature synaptic currents. This clearly indicates a maturation effect rather than mere modulation of transmission, which may involve a decrease in receptor desensitization due to glial uptake of transmitter (Oliet, 2002) or an increase in vesicular transmitter content due to supply of transmitter precursor glutamine (Hertz et al., 2000; Broer and Brookes, 2001).

What glia-derived signals promote postsynaptic differentiation? Several candidates have appeared on the scene recently. Tumor necrosis factor α (TNFα), one of the best studied cytokines in the brain (Wang and Shuaib, 2002), is released by glial cells, but also by neurons (Allan and Rothwell, 2000). Beattie et al. (2001) showed that glia-derived TNFα causes an increase in the density of α-amino-3-hydroxy-5-methyl-4-isoxazole propionate (AMPA)-type glutamate receptors of hippocampal neurons *in vitro* and in acute slices. In many synapses, AMPA receptors are inserted after N-methyl-D-aspartate (NMDA) receptors and this represents a crucial step during their functional maturation (Liao et al., 1995; Durand et al., 1996; for reviews see Atwood and Wojtowicz, 1999; Malinow and Malenka, 2002). Application and removal of TNFα induced a rapid increase (within minutes) and decline (within hours) of the glutamate receptor density at synapses, suggesting that its continued presence is necessary to maintain functional transmission. We should mention that TNFα is probably not involved in the GCM-induced increase in the size of miniature postsynaptic currents in RGC cultures, since this effect developed with a much slower time course (Nägler et al., 2001). In any case, the finding of Beattie and colleagues reminds us to take cytokines into account when considering glia-derived signals that influence synapse development. Their pleiotropic action via a broad spectrum of intercellular pathways would allow for elaborate effects on synapses.

Another puzzling pathway by which glia may influence postsynaptic receptor clustering has been proposed by Blondel et al. (2000). They showed that vasoactive intestinal polypeptide (VIP) is necessary for the development of synapses in cultures of hippocampal neurons from embryonic rats. An antibody against activity-dependent neurotrophic factor (ADNF), which is released from astrocytes upon treatment with VIP (Gozes and Brenneman, 2000), completely blocked the action of VIP suggesting that VIP acts on synapses via astrocyte-derived ADNF. This factor strengthened glutamatergic synaptic transmission by increasing the density of NR2A and NR2B subunits of postsynaptic NMDA receptors without changing their mRNA expression. Changes in the receptor subunit composition of postsynaptic transmitter receptors modify the transmission properties of synapses (Hestrin, 1992) and are part of the maturation process (Tovar and Westbrook, 1999). Finally, Blondel et al. (2000) showed that ADNF stimulates the release of neurotrophin-3 (NT-3), which by itself can induce presynaptic differentiation (Collin et al., 2001). Taken together, the results suggest that VIP, released by neurons in an activity-dependent manner, induces release of ADNF from astrocytes, which in turn acts back on neurons and enhances postsynaptic receptor density directly or by stimulating release and autocrine actions of NT-3. Clearly, more studies are required to determine the relevance of such a complex neuron-glia interplay *in vivo*.

A glia-derived signal that controls the expression of specific transmitter receptors has been detected in the chick retina (Belmonte et al., 2000). Cultured Müller glia secrete a protein that raises the expression of the M2 subtype of muscarinic acetylcholine receptors (AChRs) in cultured retinal neurons by seven-fold within 24 hours. Interestingly, injection of a partially purified preparation of the factor, termed muscarinic acetylcholine receptor-inducing activity (MARIA), in eggs induced premature expression of M2 with a normal cellular distribution pattern. Moreover, MARIA acted selectively on M2, but not on other AChR subunits. The effects of MARIA, whose identity is unknown, may help to explain why during retinal development the M2 receptor appears after differentiation of Müller glia.

Finally, recent studies suggest a link between glial cells and the most prominent synaptogenic factor, agrin, a motoneuron-derived signal that is essential for the formation of NMJs (Sanes and Lichtman, 1999) and that may play a role in synaptogenesis in the CNS (Böse et al., 2000). SCs appear to produce and secrete agrin isoforms with receptor-clustering activity during development and after nerve injury (Yang et al., 2001) suggesting that these glial cells may influence the maintenance of NMJs and their reestablishment after injury. Notably, there is evidence that a SC-derived molecule promotes NMJ maturation, but its identity has remained unknown (Koenig et al., 1998). Lesuisse et al. (2000) observed that growing rat hippocampal neurons in contact with mouse glia reduce mRNA encoding for agrin, while soluble factors from mouse glia halve the expression of a specific isoform, but leave the total level of agrin unaffected. This suggests that contact and soluble factors from glia differentially affect agrin expression in hippocampal neurons.

Cholesterol, which enhances the formation of synapses, does not fully mimic the GCM-induced increase in the size of miniature postsynaptic currents (Mauch et al., 2001), suggesting that other factors play a role. Experiments on microcultures showed that the size of autaptic currents, which are functionally equivalent to miniature postsynaptic currents, is much larger in co-cultures with direct neuron-glia contact than in cultures treated with soluble factors (Nägler et al., 2001). This suggests that contact with astrocytes influences postsynaptic maturation.

Do astrocytes enhance presynaptic maturation? Nägler et al. (2001) observed that soluble glial factors enhance the efficacy of transmitter release. Those experiments with FM1-43, a styryl dye that has been used extensively to monitor transmitter release (Cochilla et al., 1999; Cousin and Robinson, 1999; Ryan, 2001), showed that treatment of RGC microcultures with GCM accelerates stimulation-induced destaining of FM1-43 labeled puncta (Fig. 17.5). Assuming that these puncta represent functional presynaptic release sites this result provides clear evidence that glial signals enhance release efficacy. Further evidence for such an effect comes from electrophysiological recordings. GCM treatment enhanced the frequency of spontaneously and asynchronously occurring synaptic events by 10- and 200-fold respectively (Fig. 17.6). The disproportionately large increase in asynchronous release indicates that glia also enhance release efficacy from individual terminals. If GCM increased only the number of synapses without affecting their efficacy, then both parameters should have grown by the same factor. The enhancement in asynchronous release was fully mimicked by cholesterol (Mauch et al., 2001) suggesting that this component raises not only the number of synapses, but also their release capacity, possibly by promoting the formation of vesicles or by enhancing the functionality of the release apparatus (Mitter et al., 2003; for review see Pfrieger, 2003b).

Synapse maturation involves changes in the composition of voltage-activated calcium channels in presynaptic terminals. These channels are located close to the sites of exocytosis and induce the fast and local rise in calcium concentration that triggers transmitter release. There are different classes of voltage-gated calcium channels with distinct biophysical properties and many studies have shown that terminals of different synapses are endowed with characteristic sets of calcium channels (Pfrieger et al., 1992; for review see Meir et al., 1999). Do astrocytes influence the establishment of these calcium channel patterns? In principle, this appears possible, since glial cells also guide channel clustering at nodes of Ranvier (for reviews see Martini, 2001; Pedraza et al., 2001; Rasband and Trimmer, 2001; Girault and Peles, 2002). Mazzanti and Haydon (2003) showed recently that contact with astrocytes strongly enhances N-type calcium currents in immature hippocampal neurons *in vitro*, but it is not clear, whether this also affected the presynaptic pool of channels. Barker and colleagues (Li et al., 1999) observed in cultured hippocampal neurons that contact with astrocytes accelerated the developmental increase in N-type calcium currents and induced a persistent increase in P/Q type currents. Ullian et al. (2001) reported a glia-induced increase in the density of whole-cell voltage-activated calcium currents of cultured RGCs, whereas Nägler et al. (2001) did not observe such a change. In any case, bypass of presynaptic calcium channels by application of a calcium ionophore still revealed a large glia-induced increase in transmitter release (Ullian et al., 2001). This indicates that GCM enhanced the capacity of terminals for transmitter release independently of calcium influx.

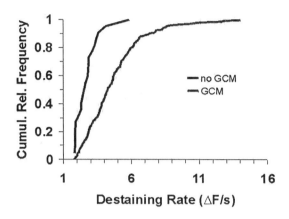

Figure 17.5. Effects of glial factors on transmitter release. Cumulative relative frequency plot of rates at which individual FM1-43 labeled release sites loose fluorescence upon extracellular electrical stimulation. Note that GCM-treatment strongly enhances the rates (ΔF/s represents change in fluorescence per second) indicating a direct effect of glial factors on release efficacy (for details see Nägler et al., 2001).

The reports summarized above suggest that signals from astrocytes regulate specific aspects of pre- and postsynaptic maturation, including the receptor density and subunit composition as well as the efficacy of transmitter release (Fig. 17.1). Interestingly, information on the reverse effect, namely that the acquisition of specific properties at synapses regulates the differentiation of surrounding astrocytic processes (Yamada et al., 2000) is still scarce.

17.4. Glia let synapses live or die

After synapses are formed, only some of them are strengthened and maintained, whereas the others are eliminated (Fig. 17.1). This process occurs during development, as well as in the adult nervous system during remodeling of neuronal circuits (Trachtenberg et al., 2002; Grutzendler et al., 2002; Walsh and Lichtman, 2003). Classic examples of synapse elimination have been described in the peripheral nervous system (PNS), where peripheral targets, including muscle cells, are initially innervated by multiple fibers. Subsequently, all fibers but one are eliminated (Purves and Lichtman, 1980; Sanes and Lichtman, 1999). Similarly, synapses between CNS neurons are produced in excess and subsequently eliminated. A prominent case is the Purkinje cell, which initially receives multiple climbing fibers inputs, but ends up with a single fiber input. Bulk elimination of synapses occurs also in those areas of the visual system, where specific columns or layers receive inputs from only one eye or respond to only specific visual cues. There is good evidence that electrical activity is a decisive factor in the selection process, but the molecular mechanisms of maintenance and elimination are still not well understood (for reviews see Sanes and Lichtman, 1999; Lichtman and Colman, 2000; Personius and Balice-Gordon, 2000; Cohen-Cory, 2002).

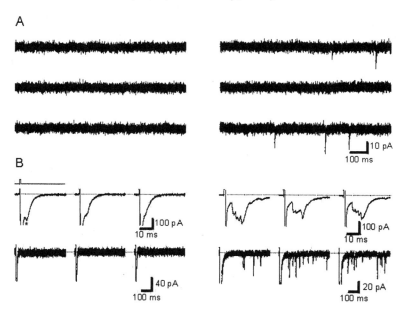

Figure 17.6. Effects of glial factors on synaptic activity in RGC microcultures. Current traces of spontaneous (A) and evoked (B) excitatory postsynaptic currents in RGCs cultured under glia-free condition (left panels) and in the presence of GCM (right panels). Note that GCM enhances asynchronous release (B) to a stronger degree than the spontaneous release (A). This provides further evidence that GCM enhances release efficacy from individual terminals (for details see Nägler et al., 2001).

In the following paragraphs, we summarize experimental evidence that astrocytes help to maintain synapses and that they actively participate in their elimination. A first hint came from long-term *in vivo* observations in parasympathetic ganglia that changes in glial cells accompany changes in the structural arrangement of synaptic connections (Pomeroy and Purves, 1988). Evidence that glia may be necessary to maintain connections has been provided by Trachtenberg and Thompson (1997). They showed *in vivo* that injection of neuregulin in neonatal rats, which induces SC proliferation and growth by activation of ErbB receptors (Adlkofer and Lai, 2000), causes retraction of SCs from NMJs, weakening of synaptic efficacy, withdrawal of nerve fibers and dispersal of acetylcholine receptor clusters within days. These effects were reversible and did not occur in adult muscles, probably due to loss of neuregulin sensitivity in SCs (Trachtenberg and Thompson, 1997). The preserving effect of SCs is further confirmed by observations in transgenic animals that lack SCs due to a defect in neuregulin signaling. ErbB2-knockout mice establish NMJs, albeit with morphologic defects, but fail to maintain them later on (Lin et al., 2000; for review see Garratt et al., 2000). Lack of NMJs causes immediate death after birth due to respiratory failure. A similar phenotype occurs in mice lacking agrin (Gautam et al., 1996; DeChiara et al., 1996).

The role of astrocytes in the maintenance of CNS synapses is less clear. Ablation of astrocytes *in vivo* causes loss of connections, but this may be the consequence rather than the cause of massive neurodegeneration (Cui et al., 2001). A hint that soluble glial signals may be necessary for synapses maintenance comes from Barres and colleagues (Ullian et al., 2001), who addressed the question in cultures of purified RGCs. They observed that removal of astrocytic feeding layers from RGCs causes a decrease in quantal content of evoked synaptic responses and in the number of synapses detected by double-staining with pre- and postsynaptic markers. However, it is not clear whether these effects were caused by a selective loss of synapses or indirectly, for example by degeneration of axons and dendrites. Removal of GCM from RGCs in microcultures did not cause a decrease in synaptic activity (K. Nägler, F.W. Pfrieger, unpublished observation). Together, there is convincing evidence that SCs are necessary to maintain NMJs, but there is much less information on whether astrocytes play a similar role at CNS synapses.

Do glia exert the opposite effect and actively eliminate synapses? Despite the fact that elimination of NMJs is well studied, the role of SCs in this process is not clear. Culican et al. (1998) observed in living mice that during elimination of supernumerary NMJs, terminal SCs retract, together with nerve endings, after the disassembly of postsynaptic receptor clusters, indicating that they are present when elimination is induced. On the other hand, Hirata et al. (1997) observed changes in the ratio of axons to terminal SCs at rat NMJs during postnatal development. They concluded that SCs are not involved in synapse elimination. Still, there is evidence that Schwann cells invade the synaptic cleft and remove terminals (see below).

Another classic example of synapse elimination can be found in the cerebellum, where the number of climbing fiber inputs to Purkinje cells is reduced to one during development. Earlier studies showed that transplantation of mature astrocytes to cerebellar explant cultures, where the number of astrocytes and granule cells has been reduced pharmacologically, decreases the number of somatic synapses (Meshul and Seil, 1988). Indirect evidence that climbing fiber innervation of Purkinje cells is regulated by Bergmann glia comes from a recent study (Iino et al., 2001). These authors created transgenic animals in which the calcium permeability of AMPARs in Bergmann glia could be manipulated in a temporally controlled manner. Elimination of calcium conductance in Bergmann glia of postnatal animals caused a retraction of glial processes from Purkinje cells and left 25% of the neurons innervated by multiple climbing fibers (Iino et al., 2001). Notably, Purkinje cells had already attained monosynaptic innervation, before glial retraction was induced, suggesting that removal of the glial sheath allowed for reinnervation. A crucial, but unanswered question is, whether removal of glial processes at an earlier stage would prevent the elimination of climbing fiber inputs.

Sims and Gilmore (2000) showed that irradiation of spinal cord in newborn rats induced invasion of SCs and loss of synapses in spinal cord gray matter suggesting that SCs eliminate synapses. However, it is not clear whether synapses were eliminated by invading synapses or by the expulsion of astrocytes. Finally, hormone-

or activity-dependent synapse elimination occurs in different brain areas in the adult stage. That these changes are accompanied by extension and retraction of astrocytic processes and that astrocytes are possibly main targets of hormones (Jordan, 1999) provokes the hypothesis that astrocytes play an active role in synapse elimination (for reviews see Hatton, 1997; Garcia-Segura et al., 1999; Mong and McCarthy, 1999; Laming et al., 2000; Theodosis and Poulain, 2001; Jones and Greenough, 2002).

How could astrocytes eliminate synapses? They could simply remove them mechanically (Fig. 17.1). Early electron microscopic studies on NMJs revealed that during reorganization, glial processes enter the synaptic cleft and phagocytose presynaptic terminals (Korneliussen and Jansen, 1976; Rosenthal and Taraskevich, 1977; Ronnevi, 1978). Similarly, Tweedle and Hatton observed that formation and elimination of synapses in the rat supraoptic nucleus in response to different degrees of hydration are accompanied by retraction and extension of glial processes (Tweedle and Hatton, 1984).

The invasion of glial cells into the cleft may be controlled by components of the ECM. It has been shown that a specific form of laminin, called s-laminin or laminin 11 (Patton, 2000), prevents the entry of Schwann cell processes into the cleft of NMJs (Patton et al., 1998). Thus, it appears that synapses destined for elimination loose components that guarantee their stability. This may be brought about by the release of proteolytic enzymes from astrocytes. A recent study showed that matrix metalloproteinase-3 (MMP-3) can remove agrin from the basal lamina of NMJs (VanSaun and Werle, 2000). The fact that MMP-3 can be produced by glia and that its release is regulated by electrical activity suggests that before entering synapses, glial cells secrete proteases, which eliminate synapse-stabilizing proteins in the ECM.

Another mechanism by which glial cells may induce synapse elimination was proposed by Nelson et al. (1995). They hypothesized that Hebbian plasticity of synaptic connections is due to elimination of non-stimulated synapses. They assumed that stimulation of postsynaptic neurons leads to release of proteases from this neuron and that on the other hand, signals accompanying neurotransmitter release stimulate astrocytes to secrete protease inhibitors. This would protect electrically active synapses and lead to the elimination of non-protected ones (Nelson et al., 1995). So far, this hypothesis awaits further testing. In any case, however, the balance of proteases and protease inhibitors released by glia (Lafon-Cazal et al., 2003) and neurons is likely to play a major role in synapse stabilization and elimination (Festoff et al., 2001).

17.5. Conclusion and further directions

Here, we have summarized evidence for a role of astrocytes in synapse formation, maintenance and elimination. We should note that the present hypotheses rely mainly on studies on culture preparations and that the molecular mechanisms of these interactions are still largely unknown. Progress in this area depends on two issues. First, we need to identify the astrocyte-derived signals that control synapse development. This may require new culture preparations that allow one to assess synaptogenesis in neurons in the presence or absence of glial cells. Second, we need to develop new animal models that allow for genetic manipulation of astrocytes in a temporally controlled manner in vivo. We should add that the large diversity of synapses suggests that not all synapses are created equal. Thus, some synapses may require glial signals for their development, whereas others may not. Along these lines, we need to know more about the functional specialization of astrocytic processes that surround different synapses. In any case, the idea that synaptogenesis is a purely neuronal affair appears outdated and needs to be replaced by a more integrative approach that encompasses glial cells in this fundamental process.

Acknowledgements. Research in our laboratory is supported by the Centre Nationale de la Recherche Scientifique, the Max-Planck-Gesellschaft, the Fondation Pour La Recherche Medicale, the Fondation Electricité de France, the Ara Parseghian Medical Research Foundation, the Region Alsace and the Deutsche Forschungsgemeinschaft.

17.6. References

Adlkofer K, Lai C (2000) Role of neuregulins in glial cell development. GLIA 29: 104-111.

Ahmari SE, Smith SJ (2002) Knowing a nascent synapse when you see it. Neuron 34: 333-336.

Allan SM, Rothwell NJ (2000) Cortical death caused by striatal administration of AMPA and interleukin-1 is mediated by activation of cortical NMDA receptors. J Cereb Blood Flow Metab 20: 1409-1413.

Alsina B, Vu T, Cohen-Cory S (2001) Visualizing synapse formation in arborizing optic axons *in vivo*: dynamics and modulation by BDNF. Nat Neurosci 4: 1093-1101.

Araque A, Carmignoto G, Haydon PG (2001) Dynamic signaling between astrocytes and neurons. Annu Rev Physiol 63: 795-813.

Attwell D, Laughlin SB (2001) An energy budget for signaling in the grey matter of the brain. J Cereb Blood Flow Metab 21: 1133-1145.

Atwood HL, Karunanithi S (2002) Diversification of synaptic strength: presynaptic elements. Nat Rev Neurosci 3: 497-516.

Atwood HL, Wojtowicz JM (1999) Silent synapses in neural plasticity: current evidence. Learn Mem 6: 542-571.

Barres BA, Silverstein BE, Corey DP, Chun LLY (1988) Immunological, morphological, and electrophysiological variation among retinal ganglion cells purified by panning. Neuron 1: 791-803.

Beattie EC, Stellwagen D, Morishita W, Bresnahan JC, Ha BK, Von Zastrow M, Beattie MS, Malenka RC (2002) Control of synaptic strength by glial TNFalpha. Science 295: 2282-2285.

Belmonte KE, McKinnon LA, Nathanson NM (2000) Developmental expression of muscarinic acetylcholine receptors in chick retina: selective induction of M2 muscarinic receptor expression in ovo by a factor secreted by muller glial cells. J Neurosci 20: 8417-8425.

Bezzi P, Volterra A (2001) A neuron-glia signalling network in the active brain. Curr Opin Neurobiol 11: 387-394.

Blondel O, Collin C, McCarran WJ, Zhu S, Zamostiano R, Gozes I, Brenneman DE, McKay RD (2000) A glia-derived signal regulating neuronal differentiation. J Neurosci 20: 8012-8020.

Bonvento G, Sibson N, Pellerin L (2002) Does glutamate image your thoughts? Trends Neurosci 25: 359-364.

Böse CM, Qiu D, Bergamaschi A, Gravante B, Bossi M, Villa A, Rupp F, Malgaroli A (2000) Agrin controls synaptic differentiation in hippocampal neurons. J Neurosci 20: 9086-9095.

Broer S, Brookes N (2001) Transfer of glutamine between astrocytes and neurons. J Neurochem 77: 705-719.

Campbell K, Götz M (2002) Radial glia: multi-purpose cells for vertebrate brain development. Trends Neurosci 25: 235-238.

Castonguay A, Levesque S, Robitaille R (2001) Glial cells as active partners in synaptic functions. Prog Brain Res 132: 227-240.

Cochilla AJ, Angleson JK, Betz WJ (1999) Monitoring secretory membrane with FM1-43 fluorescence. Annu Rev Neurosci 22: 1-10.

Cohen-Cory S (2002) The developing synapse: construction and modulation of synaptic structures and circuits. Science 298: 770-776.

Collin C, Vicario-Abejon C, Rubio ME, Wenthold RJ, McKay RD, Segal M (2001) Neurotrophins act at presynaptic terminals to activate synapses among cultured hippocampal neurons. Eur J Neurosci 13: 1273-1282.

Cousin MA, Robinson PJ (1999) Mechanisms of synaptic vesicle recycling illuminated by fluorescent dyes. J Neurochem 73: 2227-2239.

Cui W, Allen ND, Skynner M, Gusterson B, Clark AJ (2001) Inducible ablation of astrocytes shows that these cells are required for neuronal survival in the adult brain. GLIA 34: 272-282.

Culican SM, Nelson CC, Lichtman JW (1998) Axon withdrawal during synapse elimination at the neuromuscular junction is accompanied by disassembly of the postsynaptic specialization and withdrawal of Schwann cell processes. J Neurosci 18: 4953-4965.

DeChiara TM, Bowen DC, Valenzuela DM, Simmons MV, Poueymirou WT, Thomas S, Kinetz E, Compton DL, Rojas E, Park JS, Smith C, DiStefano PS, Glass DJ, Burden SJ, Yancopoulos GD (1996) The receptor tyrosine kinase MuSK is required for neuromuscular junction formation in vivo. Cell 85: 501-512.

Dougherty KD, Dreyfus CF, Black IB (2000) Brain-derived neurotrophic factor in astrocytes, oligodendrocytes, and microglia/macrophages after spinal cord injury. Neurobiol Dis 7: 574-585.

Dow KE, Wang W (1998) Cell biology of astrocyte proteoglycans. Cell Mol Life Sci 54: 567-581.

Dresbach T, Qualmann B, Kessels MM, Garner CC, Gundelfinger ED (2001) The presynaptic cytomatrix of brain synapses. Cell Mol Life Sci 58: 94-116.

Du YZ, Dreyfus CF (2002) Oligodendrocytes as providers of growth factors. J Neurosci Res 68: 647-654.

Durand GM, Kovalchuk Y, Konnerth A (1996) Long-term potentiation and functional synapse induction in developing hippocampus. Nature 381: 71-75.

Featherstone DE, Broadie K (2000) Surprises from Drosophila: genetic mechanisms of synaptic development and plasticity. Brain Res Bull 53: 501-511.

Festoff BW, Suo Z, Citron BA (2001) Plasticity and stabilization of neuromuscular and CNS synapses: interactions between thrombin protease signaling pathways and tissue transglutaminase. Int Rev Cytol 211: 153-177.

Fitch MT, Silver J (1997) Glial cell extracellular matrix: boundaries for axon growth in development and regeneration. Cell Tissue Res 290: 379-384.

Friedman HV, Bresler T, Garner CC, Ziv NE (2000) Assembly of new individual excitatory synapses: time course and temporal order of synaptic molecule recruitment. Neuron 27: 57-69.

Friedman WJ, Black IB, Kaplan DR (1998) Distribution of the neurotrophins brain-derived neurotrophic factor, neurotrophin-3, and neurotrophin-4/5 in the postnatal rat brain: an immunocytochemical study. Neuroscience 84: 101-114.

Garcia-Segura LM, Naftolin F, Hutchison JB, Azcoitia I, Chowen JA (1999) Role of astroglia in estrogen regulation of synaptic plasticity and brain repair. J Neurobiol 40: 574-584.

Garner CC, Zhai RG, Gundelfinger ED, Ziv NE (2002) Molecular mechanisms of CNS synaptogenesis. Trends Neurosci 25: 243-251.

Garratt AN, Britsch S, Birchmeier C (2000) Neuregulin, a factor with many functions in the life of a schwann cell. Bioessays 22: 987-996.

Garwood J, Rigato F, Heck N, Faissner A (2001) Tenascin glycoproteins and the complementary ligand DSD-1-PG/ phosphacan--structuring the neural extracellular matrix during development and repair. Restor Neurol Neurosci 19: 51-64.

Gautam M, Noakes PG, Moscoso L, Rupp F, Scheller RH, Merlie JP, Sanes JR (1996) Defective neuromuscular synaptogenesis in agrin-deficient mutant mice. Cell 85: 525-535.

Girault JA, Peles E (2002) Development of nodes of Ranvier. Curr Opin Neurobiol 12: 476-485.

Glowa JR, Panlilio LV, Brenneman DE, Gozes I, Fridkin M, Hill JM (1992) Learning impairment following intracerebral administration of the HIV envelope protein gp120 or a VIP antagonist. Brain Res 570: 49-53.

Gomes FC, Spohr TC, Martinez R, Moura N, V (2001) Cross-talk between neurons and glia: highlights on soluble factors. Braz J Med Biol Res 34: 611-620.

Gomperts SN, Carroll R, Malenka RC, Nicoll RA (2000) Distinct roles for ionotropic and metabotropic glutamate receptors in the maturation of excitatory synapses. J Neurosci 20: 2229-2237.

Gozes I, Brenneman DE (2000) A new concept in the pharmacology of neuroprotection. J Mol Neurosci 14: 61-68.

Gozes I, Glowa J, Brenneman DE, McCune SK, Lee E, Westphal H (1993) Learning and sexual deficiencies in transgenic mice carrying a chimeric vasoactive intestinal peptide gene. J Mol Neurosci 4: 185-193.

Grutzendler J, Kasthuri N, Gan WB (2002) Long-term dendritic spine stability in the adult cortex. Nature 420: 812-816.

Guettier-Sigrist S, Coupin G, Warter JM, Poindron P (2000) Cell types required to efficiently innervate human muscle cells *in vitro*. Exp Cell Res 259: 204-212.

Hartley RS, Margulis M, Fishman PS, Lee VM, Tang CM (1999) Functional synapses are formed between human NTera2 (NT2N, hNT) neurons grown on astrocytes. J Comp Neurol 407: 1-10.

Hatton GI (1997) Function-related plasticity in hypothalamus. Annu Rev Neurosci 20: 375-397.

Haydon PG (2001) GLIA: listening and talking to the synapse. Nat Rev Neurosci 2: 185-193.

Herrera AA, Qiang H, Ko CP (2000) The role of perisynaptic Schwann cells in development of neuromuscular junctions in the frog (Xenopus laevis). J Neurobiol 45: 237-254.

Hertz L, Yu AC, Kala G, Schousboe A (2000) Neuronal-astrocytic and cytosolic-mitochondrial metabolite trafficking during brain activation, hyperammonemia and energy deprivation. Neurochem Int 37: 83-102.

Hestrin S (1992) Developmental regulation of nmda receptor-mediated synaptic currents at a central synapse. Nature 357: 686-689.

Hirata K, Zhou C, Nakamura K, Kawabuchi M (1997) Postnatal development of Schwann cells at neuromuscular junctions, with special reference to synapse elimination. J Neurocytol 26: 799-809.

Iino M, Goto K, Kakegawa W, Okado H, Sudo M, Ishiuchi S, Miwa A, Takayasu Y, Saito I, Tsuzuki K, Ozawa S (2001) Glia-synapse interaction through Ca2+-permeable AMPA receptors in Bergmann glia. Science 292: 926-929.

Ivanova T, Beyer C (2001) Pre- and postnatal expression of brain-derived neurotrophic factor mRNA/protein and tyrosine protein kinase receptor B mRNA in the mouse hippocampus. Neurosci Lett 307: 21-24.

Jacobson M (1991) Developmental Neurobiology. New York: Plenum Press.

Jin Y (2002) Synaptogenesis: insights from worm and fly. Curr Opin Neurobiol 12: 71-79.

Jones TA, Greenough WT (2002) Behavioural experience-dependent plasticity of glial-neuronal interactions. In: The Tripartite Synapse: Glia in Synaptic Transmission (Volterra A, Magistretti PJ, Haydon PG, eds), pp 248-265. Oxford: Oxford University Press.

Jordan CL (1999) Glia as mediators of steroid hormone action on the nervous system: An overview. J Neurobiol 40: 434-445.

Klambt C, Hummel T, Granderath S, Schimmelpfeng K (2001) Glial cell development in Drosophila. Int J Dev Neurosci 19: 373-378.

Koenig J, de La PS, Chapron J (1998) The Schwann cell at the neuromuscular junction. J Physiol Paris 92: 153-155.

Korneliussen H, Jansen JK (1976) Morphological aspects of the elimination of polyneuronal innervation of skeletal muscle fibres in newborn rats. J Neurocytol 5: 591-604.

Lafon-Cazal M, Adjali O, Galeotti N, Poncet J, Jouin P, Homburger V, Bockaert J, Marin P (2003) Proteomic analysis of astrocytic secretion in the mouse. Comparison with the cerebrospinal fluid proteome. J Biol Chem., in press.

Laming PR, Kimelberg H, Robinson S, Salm A, Hawrylak N, Muller C, Roots B, Ng K (2000) Neuronal-glial interactions and behaviour. Neurosci Biobehav Rev 24: 295-340.

Lee SH, Sheng M (2000) Development of neuron-neuron synapses. Curr Opin Neurobiol 10: 125-131.

Lemke G (2001) Glial control of neuronal development. Annu Rev Neurosci 24: 87-105.

Lesuisse C, Qiu D, Bose CM, Nakaso K, Rupp F (2000) Regulation of agrin expression in hippocampal neurons by cell contact and electrical activity. Brain Res Mol Brain Res 81: 92-100.

Li YX, Schaffner AE, Barker JL (1999) Astrocytes regulate the developmental appearance of GABAergic and glutamatergic postsynaptic currents in cultured embryonic rat spinal neurons. Eur J Neurosci 11: 2537-2551.

Liao D, Hessler NA, Malinow R (1995) Activation of postsynaptically silent synapses during pairing- induced LTP in CA1 region of hippocampal slice. Nature 375: 400-404.

Lichtman JW, Colman H (2000) Synapse elimination and indelible memory. Neuron 25: 269-278.

Lin W, Sanchez HB, Deerinck T, Morris JK, Ellisman M, Lee KF (2000) Aberrant development of motor axons and neuromuscular synapses in erbB2-deficient mice. Proc Natl Acad Sci U S A 97: 1299-1304.

Love FM, Son YJ, Thompson WJ (2003) Activity alters muscle reinnervation and terminal sprouting by reducing the number of schwann cell pathways that grow to link synaptic sites. J Neurobiol 54: 566-576.

Macleod GT, Dickens PA, Bennett MR (2001) Formation and function of synapses with respect to Schwann cells at the end of motor nerve terminal branches on mature amphibian (Bufo marinus) muscle. J Neurosci 21: 2380-2392.

Malinow R, Malenka RC (2002) AMPA receptor trafficking and synaptic plasticity. Annu Rev Neurosci 25: 103-126.

Mars T, Yu KJ, Tang XM, Miranda AF, Grubic Z, Cambi F, King MP (2001) Differentiation of glial cells and motor neurons during the formation of neuromuscular junctions in cocultures of rat spinal cord explant and human muscle. J Comp Neurol 438: 239-251.

Martinez A, Alcantara S, Borrell V, Del Rio JA, Blasi J, Otal R, Campos N, Boronat A, Barbacid M, Silos-Santiago I, Soriano E (1998) TrkB and TrkC signaling are required for maturation and synaptogenesis of hippocampal connections. J Neurosci 18: 7336-7350.

Martini R (2001) The effect of myelinating Schwann cells on axons. Muscle Nerve 24: 456-466.

Mauch DH, Nägler K, Schumacher S, Göritz C, Müller EC, Otto A, Pfrieger FW (2001) CNS synaptogenesis promoted by glia-derived cholesterol. Science 294: 1354-1357.

Mazzanti M, Haydon PG (2003) Astrocytes selectively enhance N-type calcium current in hippocampal neurons. GLIA 41: 128-136.

Meir A, Ginsburg S, Butkevich A, Kachalsky SG, Kaiserman I, Ahdut R, Demirgoren S, Rahamimoff R (1999) Ion channels in presynaptic nerve terminals and control of transmitter release. Physiol Rev 79: 1019-1088.

Meshul CK, Seil FJ (1988) Transplanted astrocytes reduce synaptic density in the neuropil of cerebellar cultures. Brain Res 441: 23-32.

Messing A (1998) Transgenic studies of peripheral and central glia. Int J Dev Biol 42: 1019-1024.

Meyer-Franke A, Kaplan MR, Pfrieger FW, Barres BA (1995) Characterization of the signaling interactions that promote the survival and growth of developing retinal ganglion cells in culture. Neuron 15: 805-819.

Mirsky R, Jessen KR, Brennan A, Parkinson D, Dong Z, Meier C, Parmantier E, Lawson D (2002) Schwann cells as regulators of nerve development. J Physiol Paris 96: 17-24.

Mitter D, Reisinger C, Hinz B, Hollmann S, Yelamanchili SV, Treiber-Held S, Ohm TG, Herrmann A, Ahnert-Hilger G (2003) The synaptophysin/synaptobrevin interaction critically depends on the cholesterol content. J Neurochem 84: 35-42.

Mong JA, McCarthy MM (1999) Steroid-induced developmental plasticity in hypothalamic astrocytes: implications for synaptic patterning. J Neurobiol 40: 602-619.

Nadarajah B, Parnavelas JG (2002) Modes of neuronal migration in the developing cerebral cortex. Nat Rev Neurosci 3: 423-432.

Nakajima Y, Glavinovic MI, Miledi R (1987) *In vitro* formation of neuromuscular junctions between adult Rana muscle fibres and embryonic Xenopus neurons. Proc R Soc Lond B Biol Sci 230: 425-441.

Nakanishi K, Okouchi Y, Ueki T, Asai K, Isobe I, Eksioglu YZ, Kato T, Hasegawa Y, Kuroda Y (1994) Astrocytic contribution to functioning synapse formation estimated by spontaneous neuronal intracellular Ca^{2+} oscillations. Brain Research 659: 169-178.

Nägler K, Mauch DH, Pfrieger FW (2001) Glia-derived signals induce synapse formation in neurones of the rat central nervous system. J Physiol 533: 665-679.

Nelson PG, Fields RD, Liu Y (1995) Neural activity, neuron-glia relationships, and synapse development. Perspect Dev Neurobiol 2: 399-407.

O'Malley JP, Waran MT, Balice-Gordon RJ (1999) *In vivo* observations of terminal Schwann cells at normal, denervated, and reinnervated mouse neuromuscular junctions. J Neurobiol 38: 270-286.

Okabe S (2002) Birth, growth and elimination of a single synapse. Anat Sci Int 77: 203-210.

Oku H, Ikeda T, Honma Y, Sotozono C, Nishida K, Nakamura Y, Kida T, Kinoshita S (2002) Gene expression of neurotrophins and their high-affinity Trk receptors in cultured human Muller cells. Ophthalmic Res 34: 38-42.

Oland LA, Tolbert LP (2003) Key interactions between neurons and glial cells during neural development in insects. Annu Rev Entomol 48: 89-110.

Oliet SH (2002) Functional consequences of morphological neuroglial changes in the magnocellular nuclei of the hypothalamus. J Neuroendocrinol 14: 241-246.

Patton BL (2000) Laminins of the neuromuscular system. Microsc Res Tech 51: 247-261.

Patton BL, Chiu AY, Sanes JR (1998) Synaptic laminin prevents glial entry into the synaptic cleft. Nature 393: 698-701.

Pedraza L, Huang JK, Colman DR (2001) Organizing principles of the axoglial apparatus. Neuron 30: 335-344.

Peles E, Salzer JL (2000) Molecular domains of myelinated axons. Curr Opin Neurobiol 10: 558-565.

Personius KE, Balice-Gordon RJ (2000) Activity-dependent editing of neuromuscular synaptic connections. Brain Res Bull 53: 513-522.

Pfrieger FW (2003a) Outsourcing in the brain: do neurons depend on cholesterol delivery by astrocytes? Bioessays 25: 72-78.

Pfrieger FW (2003b) Role of cholesterol in synapse formation and function. Biochim Biophys Acta 1610: 271-280.

Pfrieger FW, Barres BA (1996) New views on synapse-glia interactions. Curr Opin Neurobiol 6: 615-621.

Pfrieger FW, Barres BA (1997) Synaptic efficacy enhanced by glial cells. Science 277: 1684-1687.

Pfrieger FW, Veselovsky NS, Gottmann K, Lux HD (1992) Pharmacological characterization of calcium currents and synaptic transmission between thalamic neurons *in vitro*. J Neurosci 12: 4347-4357.

Pomeroy SL, Purves D (1988) Neuron/glia relationships observed over intervals of several months in living mice. J Cell Biol 107: 1167-1175.

Poo MM (2001) Neurotrophins as synaptic modulators. Nat Rev Neurosci 2: 24-32.

Purves D, Lichtman JW (1980) Elimination of synapses in the developing nervous system. Science 210: 153-157.

Rakic P, Bourgeois JP, Eckenhoff MF, Zecevic N, Goldman-Rakic PS (1986) Concurrent overproduction of synapses in diverse regions of the primate cerebral cortex. Science 232: 232-235.

Rasband MN, Trimmer JS (2001) Developmental clustering of ion channels at and near the node of Ranvier. Dev Biol 236: 5-16.

Ronnevi LO (1978) Origin of the glial processes responsible for the spontaneous postnatal phagocytosis of boutons on cat spinal motoneurons. Cell Tissue Res 189: 203-217.

Rosenthal JL, Taraskevich PS (1977) Reduction of multiaxonal innervation at the neuromuscular junction of the rat during development. J Physiol 270: 299-310.

Rouget M, Araud D, Seite R, Prochiantz A, Autillo Touati A (1993) Astrocyte-regulated synaptogenesis: an *in vitro* ultrastructural study. Neurosci Lett 150: 85-88.

Rudge JS, Alderson RF, Pasnikowski E, Mcclain J, Ip NY, Lindsay RM (1992) Expression of ciliary neurotrophic factor and the neurotrophins - nerve growth-factor, brain-derived neurotrophic factor and neurotrophin-3 in cultured rat hippocampal astrocytes. Eur J Neurosci 4: 459-471.

Ryan TA (2001) Presynaptic imaging techniques. Curr Opin Neurobiol 11: 544-549.

Sanes JR, Lichtman JW (1999) Development of the vertebrate neuromuscular junction. Annu Rev Neurosci 22: 389-442.

Sanes JR, Lichtman JW (2001) Induction, assembly, maturation and maintenance of a postsynaptic apparatus. Nat Rev Neurosci 2: 791-805.

Sauvageot CM, Stiles CD (2002) Molecular mechanisms controlling cortical gliogenesis. Curr Opin Neurobiol 12: 244-249.

Scheiffele P (2003) Cell-Cell Signaling During Synapse Formation in the CNS. Annu Rev Neurosci 26: 485-508.

Sibson NR, Dhankhar A, Mason GF, Rothman DL, Behar KL, Shulman RG (1998) Stoichiometric coupling of brain glucose metabolism and glutamatergic neuronal activity. Proc Natl Acad Sci U S A 95: 316-321.

Siegel SG, Patton B, English AW (2000) Ciliary neurotrophic factor is required for motoneuron sprouting. Exp Neurol 166: 205-212.

Sims TJ, Gilmore SA (2000) Schwann cell-induced loss of synapses in the central nervous system. Brain Res 882: 221-225.

Snider WD, Lichtman JW (1996) Are neurotrophins synaptotrophins? Mol Cell Neurosci 7: 433-442.

Sofroniew MV, Bush TG, Blumauer N, Lawrence K, Mucke L, Johnson MH (1999) Genetically-targeted and conditionally-regulated ablation of astroglial cells in the central, enteric and peripheral nervous systems in adult transgenic mice. Brain Res 835: 91-95.

Son YJ, Thompson WJ (1995a) Nerve sprouting in muscle is induced and guided by processes extended by Schwann cells. Neuron 14: 133-141.

Son YJ, Thompson WJ (1995b) Schwann cell processes guide regeneration of peripheral axons. Neuron 14: 125-132.

Son YJ, Trachtenberg JT, Thompson WJ (1996) Schwann cells induce and guide sprouting and reinnervation of neuromuscular junctions. Trends Neurosci 19: 280-285.

Song H, Stevens CF, Gage FH (2002) Astroglia induce neurogenesis from adult neural stem cells. Nature 417: 39-44.

Theodosis DT, Poulain DA (2001) Maternity leads to morphological synaptic plasticity in the oxytocin system. Prog Brain Res 133: 49-58.

Toda H, Takahashi J, Mizoguchi A, Koyano K, Hashimoto N (2000) Neurons generated from adult rat hippocampal stem cells form functional glutamatergic and GABAergic synapses *in vitro*. Exp Neurol 165: 66-76.

Tovar KR, Westbrook GL (1999) The incorporation of NMDA receptors with a distinct subunit composition at nascent hippocampal synapses *in vitro*. J Neurosci 19: 4180-4188.

Trachtenberg JT, Chen BE, Knott GW, Feng G, Sanes JR, Welker E, Svoboda K (2002) Long-term *in vivo* imaging of experience-dependent synaptic plasticity in adult cortex. Nature 420: 788-794.

Trachtenberg JT, Thompson WJ (1997) Nerve terminal withdrawal from rat neuromuscular junctions induced by neuregulin and Schwann cells. J Neurosci 17: 6243-6255.

Tweedle CD, Hatton GI (1984) Synapse formation and disappearance in adult rat supraoptic nucleus during different hydration states. Brain Res 309: 373-376.

Ullian EM, Sapperstein SK, Christopherson KS, Barres BA (2001b) Control of synapse number by glia. Science 291: 657-661.

van den Pol AN, Spencer DD (2000) Differential neurite growth on astrocyte substrates: interspecies facilitation in green fluorescent protein-transfected rat and human neurons. Neuroscience 95: 603-616.

VanSaun M, Werle MJ (2000) Matrix metalloproteinase-3 removes agrin from synaptic basal lamina. J Neurobiol 43: 140-149.

Vaughn JE (1989) Fine structure of synaptogenesis in the vertebrate central nervous system. Synapse 3: 255-285.

Verderio C, Bacci A, Coco S, Pravettoni E, Fumagalli G, Matteoli M (1999) Astrocytes are required for the oscillatory activity in cultured hippocampal neurons. Eur J Neurosci 11: 2793-2800.

Vicario-Abejon C, Collin C, McKay RD, Segal M (1998) Neurotrophins induce formation of functional excitatory and inhibitory synapses between cultured hippocampal neurons. J Neurosci 18: 7256-7271.

Vicario-Abejon C, Owens D, McKay R, Segal M (2002) Role of neurotrophins in central synapse formation and stabilization. Nat Rev Neurosci 3: 965-974.

Volterra A, Magistretti PJ, Haydon PG (2002) The Tripartite Synapse: Glia in Synaptic Transmission. Oxford: Oxford University Press.

Walsh MK, Lichtman JW (2003) *In vivo* time-lapse imaging of synaptic takeover associated with naturally occurring synapse elimination. Neuron 37: 67-73.

Wang CX, Shuaib A (2002) Involvement of inflammatory cytokines in central nervous system injury. Prog Neurobiol 67: 161-172.

Wang S, Barres BA (2000) Up a notch: instructing gliogenesis. Neuron 27: 197-200.

Weldon PR, Cohen MW (1979) Development of synaptic ultrastructure at neuromuscular contacts in an amphibian cell culture system. J Neurocytol 8: 239-259.

Yamada K, Fukaya M, Shibata T, Kurihara H, Tanaka K, Inoue Y, Watanabe M (2000) Dynamic transformation of Bergmann glial fibers proceeds in correlation with dendritic outgrowth and synapse formation of cerebellar Purkinje cells. J Comp Neurol 418: 106-120.

Yang JF, Cao G, Koirala S, Reddy LV, Ko CP (2001) Schwann cells express active agrin and enhance aggregation of acetylcholine receptors on muscle fibers. J Neurosci 21: 9572-9584.

Zhang W, Benson DL (2000) Development and molecular organization of dendritic spines and their synapses. Hippocampus 10: 512-526.

Zito K, Svoboda K (2002) Activity-dependent synaptogenesis in the adult mammalian cortex. Neuron 35: 1015-1017.

17.7. Abbreviations

AChR	Acetylcholine receptor
ADNF	Activity-dependent neurotrophic factor
AMPA	α-amino-3-hydroxy-5-methyl-4-isoxazole propionate
CNS	Central nervous system
ECM	Extracellular matrix
GCM	Glia conditioned medium
MARIA	Muscarinic acetylcholine receptor inducing activity
MMP	Matrix metalloproteinase
NMDA	N–methyl–D-aspartate
NMJ	Neuromuscular junction
NT	Neurotrophin
PNS	Peripheral nervous system
RGC	Retinal ganglion cell
SC	Schwann cell
TNF	Tumor necrosis factor
VIP	Vasoactive intestinal peptide

Index